SIXTH EDITION

Introduction to
Human
Disease

Pathophysiology for Health Professionals

Agnes G. Loeffler, MD, PhD

Director, Surgical Pathology
Associate Professor, School of Medicine and Public Health
University of Wisconsin-Madison

Michael N. Hart, MD

Professor and Chair, Department of Pathology
University of Wisconsin-Madison

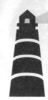

JONES & BARTLETT
LEARNING

World Headquarters
Jones & Bartlett Learning
5 Wall Street
Burlington, MA 01803
978-443-5000
info@jblearning.com
www.jblearning.com

Jones & Bartlett Learning books and products are available through most bookstores and online booksellers. To contact Jones & Bartlett Learning directly, call 800-832-0034, fax 978-443-8000, or visit our website, www.jblearning.com.

Substantial discounts on bulk quantities of Jones & Bartlett Learning publications are available to corporations, professional associations, and other qualified organizations. For details and specific discount information, contact the special sales department at Jones & Bartlett Learning via the above contact information or send an email to specialsales@jblearning.com.

Production Credits

Chief Executive Officer: Ty Field
President: James Homer
Chief Product Officer: Eduardo Moura
Executive Publisher: William Brottmiller
Executive Editor: Rhonda Dearborn
Editorial Assistant: Sean Fabery
Production Editor: Jessica Steele Newfell
Art Development Editor: Joanna Lundeen
Production Assistant: Eileen Worthley

Marketing Manager: Grace Richards
VP, Manufacturing and Inventory Control: Therese Connell
Composition: Cenveo Publisher Services
Cover Design: Kristin Parker
Photo Research and Permissions Coordinator: Amy Rathburn
Cover and Title Page Image: Courtesy of The National Library of Medicine
Printing and Binding: Courier Companies
Cover Printing: Courier Companies

To order this product, use ISBN: 978-1-284-03881-1

Library of Congress Cataloging-in-Publication Data
Hart, Michael Noel, 1938– author.
   Introduction to human disease : pathophysiology for health professionals / by Agnes G. Loeffler and Michael N. Hart. — Sixth edition.
      p. ; cm.
   Author's names reversed on the fifth edition.
   Includes bibliographical references and index.
   ISBN 978-1-284-03466-0 — ISBN 1-284-03466-6
   I. Loeffler, Agnes Gertrud, 1966– author.   II. Title.
   [DNLM: 1. Pathologic Processes—physiopathology.   QZ 140]
   RB111
   616.07—dc23
                                   2013027711
6048

Printed in the United States of America
18 17 16 15 14   10 9 8 7 6 5 4 3 2

This book is dedicated to students beginning their careers in the allied health sciences.

Brief Contents

SECTION IV   Multiple Organ System Diseases   393

Contents

Preface

The scope and purpose of this text has not changed since it was first published in 1979, and the intentions expressed in the preface to the *First Edition* are just as applicable to the *Sixth Edition. Introduction to Human Disease: Pathophysiology for Health Professionals* introduces the basic principles of disease to allied health professions students. Our intent is to provide comprehensive information on all aspects of human disease with minimal requirements for prerequisite knowledge. Over the course of the previous five editions, we have noticed that lay people and medical students—overwhelmed by the volumes of detailed and technical information delivered to them in print and, increasingly, on the Internet—turn to this text for a basic outline of how the health profession approaches particular diseases or where a specific disease fits into the medical nosological scheme. While we are happy they derive benefit from the discussions of diseases laid forth in this text, the intended readership is students wishing to pursue a career in nursing, pharmacy, dentistry, physical or occupational therapy, nutrition, or other allied health professions fields who require a broad understanding of disease epidemiology, cause, diagnosis and treatment, and a basic grounding in the specialized medical lexicon.

We have been pleased by the continued use of previous editions by instructors who teach pathology courses to a variety of allied health professions students. We believe all health professions students have a need for a common vocabulary and a broad-based understanding of human disease. Thus, we define terms as clearly and specifically as possible and attempt to describe the most common and important diseases of humans, including mental illnesses. In fact, a special effort is made in this text's format to make the reader aware of the most frequent and significant diseases in each organ category.

In this *Sixth Edition*, new illustrations have been added, and the content has been considerably updated to reflect the current state of medical knowledge and practice. Specifically, Chapter 24 (Mental Health) and Chapter 30 (Nutritional Disorders) received a major overhaul of content to reflect state-of-the-science advances in the fields, incorporate up-to-date epidemiologic information, and focus the discussion on diseases and disorders that are most relevant to medical practice today. The basic format of this text, which has made it so popular over the course of editions, has been retained, including the comprehensive list of learning objectives at the beginning of each chapter and a set of practice questions at the end of each chapter. Each chapter has been critiqued by pathophysiology instructors for content, accuracy, and presentation. Based on reviewers' and readers' suggestions for each successive edition, we have added more clinical information, including general and specific treatments for diseases. Consequently, although *Introduction to Human Disease* remains primarily a pathology text, the clinical information provides a more circumspect foundation for the reader.

This text is divided into four sections. Section I provides fundamental vocabulary and concepts, a broad analysis of the most common and significant diseases, and a discussion of the tools and processes of diagnosis. Section II provides a framework for the basic types of human disease: reactions to injury, neoplasia, genetically determined disease, and intrauterine injury. In Section III, each chapter discusses the diseases of a specific organ system. We review the anatomy and physiology of that organ, provide an overview of the most frequent and important diseases encountered, discuss diagnostic techniques (symptoms, signs, laboratory tests, and radiological and clinical procedures), profile the diseases, and discuss the consequences of failure of the organ to function. Section IV presents diseases that tend to affect multiple organs and share causative mechanisms within each group. Included topics are infections, immune reactions, external injury by physical and chemical agents, and disorders caused by nutritional deprivations and excesses. We believe these chapters are easier to learn after diseases of the organs have been studied; however, they can be inserted earlier in a course without any prerequisites other than Sections I and II.

We hope that this *Sixth Edition* continues to be of use to students embarking on a career in the allied health professions. The sheer volume of medical knowledge can appear overwhelming, and the technical vocabulary used can seem like a foreign language to students at the beginning of their studies. By reading and studying the content in *Introduction to Human Disease, Sixth Edition*, students should be well on their way to gaining the basic foundation they need for a rewarding and exciting career in medicine.

Features of This Text

Pedagogy

Introduction to Human Disease: Pathophysiology for Health Professionals, Sixth Edition incorporates a number of engaging pedagogical features to aid in the student's understanding and retention of the material.

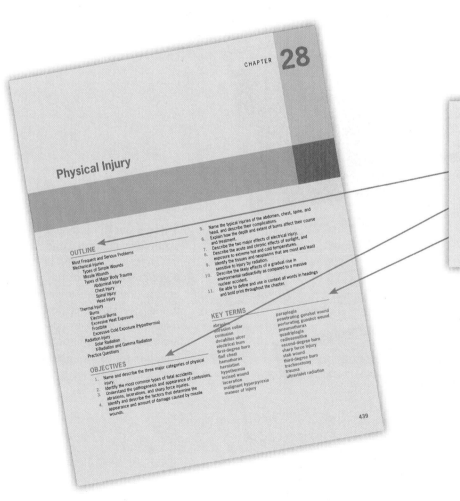

Each chapter begins with a framework for learning the most important topics covered, utilizing an Outline of material to be discussed, a list of learning Objectives, and an inventory of the Key Terms defined in the content.

Each chapter concludes with **Practice Questions** to assess comprehension of concepts.

154   CHAPTER 11   Bleeding and Clotting Disorders

Practice Questions

1. Which of the following accurately states the difference between hemostasis and coagulation?
   A. Hemostasis refers to the pathologic stagnation of blood in vessels, whereas coagulation refers to the solidification of plasma.
   B. Hemostasis primarily involves endothelial cells, whereas coagulation primarily involves platelets.
   C. Hemostasis refers to the formation of a thrombus, whereas coagulation refers to activation of the clotting cascade.
   D. Hemostasis refers to cessation of blood flow through an injured vessel, whereas coagulation refers to solidification of plasma.
   E. Hemostasis and coagulation are synonymous terms.

2. Proteins of the coagulation cascade, and their inhibitors, are primarily produced by
   A. enzymes in the liver.
   B. stem cells in the bone marrow.
   C. reticuloendothelial cells in the spleen.
   D. endothelial cells lining blood vessels.
   E. the coagulation cascade.

3. Factor IX is activated by
   A. tissue factor/factor VII complex.
   B. activated factor XI.
   C. activated factor X.
   D. thrombin.
   E. calcium.

4. A 64-year-old woman with hypersplenism runs the risk of spontaneously bleeding into her joints when the platelet count drops below which level?
   A. 100,000 per microliter
   B. 50,000 per microliter
   C. 25,000 per microliter
   D. 10,000 per microliter
   E. 5,000 per microliter

5. Of the following genetic conditions discussed in this chapter, which is the result of an inherited problem with platelet function?
   A. Hemophilia A
   B. Hemophilia B
   C. Von Willebrand disease
   D. Gaucher disease causing hypersplenism
   E. Factor V Leiden deficiency

---

and precipitating a brisk acute inflammatory reaction. Other, more virulent organisms may infect the lesions secondarily, producing tiny abscesses.

The severity of acne varies greatly among individuals, suggesting hereditary and hormonal influences on sebaceous glands. Acne may be aggravated by emotional stress and administration of corticosteroids. Severe cases lead to scarring, which may be disfiguring. Treatment is directed toward reduction of follicular plugging by gentle washing of the face, reduction of bacterial burden with topical or oral antibiotics, regulation of the development of the squamous lining of the hair follicle and sebum production with topical or oral retinoid drugs, and, in very severe cases, reduction of inflammation with steroids.

Specific Diseases   301

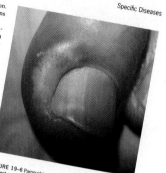

FIGURE 19–6 Paronychia, with swelling due to collection of purulent exudate around the nail. (Courtesy of Yale Residents' Slide Collection, Dermatology Department, Yale University School of Medicine.)

BOX 19–3   Acne

Causes

Plugs of keratin and sebum in hair follicles

Propionibacterium acnes

Chemical irritation

Secondary infection

Endocrine factors (androgen release during puberty)

Hereditary factors

Lesions

Comedone

Inflammatory papules and pustules

Manifestations

Open and closed comedones and pustules

Occurs in adolescents and young adults

Facial scarring (late)

Abscess

Skin abscesses are localized skin infections forming walled-off collections of pus. *S. aureus* is the most common infectious organism. Skin abscesses can occur at sites of skin trauma, around hair follicles, and around embedded foreign material, such as splinters. Paronychia is the occurrence of abscesses in the folds around the nails (**Figure 19–6**). A pilonidal cyst is an abscess occurring around ingrown hair in the skin just above the gluteal fold. Other common sites of abscess formation are around the anus and on the back of the neck. Small abscesses centered about a hair follicle are known as furuncles or boils. These begin as painful, elevated, red areas, and then develop a white, soft center that represents liquefaction necrosis of tissue with accumulation of purulent exudate. If uncomplicated, the furuncle is gradually walled-off, ruptures to release the exudate, and then collapses to heal with a small scar. Healing of an abscess is accelerated by incision and drainage. Recurrent abscesses, such as pilonidal cysts, may require excision of the sinus tract or marsupialization (incising the cyst

and suturing the exposed flap to adjacent tissue) so that the cyst is open and can drain to the surface. Splinters and other foreign materials should be removed, preferably before an abscess develops. A carbuncle is a group of furuncles with associated connecting sinus tracts and multiple openings on the skin. This uncommon lesion usually occurs on the back of the neck. Diabetics are especially prone to develop carbuncles because of their reduced resistance to infection.

BOX 19–4   Abscess

Causes

Trauma

Foreign bodies

Lesions

Abscess in dermis or subcutis

Furuncle carbuncle

Paronychia

Pilonidal cyst

Manifestations

Pain, swelling, heat, redness

Purulent discharge

Impetigo

Impetigo is a superficial bacterial skin infection that occurs predominantly in children and is characterized by flaccid bullae that easily rupture to form crusted erosions

Throughout the text, key points are illustrated and important information is highlighted in **Boxes** to ensure comprehension and to aid the study of critical materials. **Key Terms** also are bolded throughout the chapters for ease of discovery.

> A colorful and engaging layout enables easy reading and supports the retention of important concepts. Additionally, more than 400 full-color, medically accurate photographs, illustrations, and tables provide valuable insight into disease epidemiology and diagnosis.

---

of origin (Figure 5–5). Some benign neoplasms, such as smooth muscle tumors of the uterus, may become very large without causing any symptoms. Others, such as a meningioma in the brain, may cause symptoms or even death despite their small size, because they impinge on vital structures. Whether they are large or small, produce symptoms or not, benign neoplasms generally remain in the tissue in which they originated and do not spread to others. Malignant neoplasms, in contrast, are defined by their potential to invade and metastasize. Invasion refers to direct extension of neoplastic cells into surrounding tissue without regard to tissue boundaries (Figures 5–6).

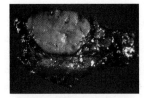

FIGURE 5–5 Benign neoplasm in the parotid gland.

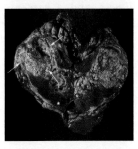

FIGURE 5–6 Invasion. This is an image of a carcinoma in the kidney. The kidney has been cut in half and opened, so the two sides are mirror images of one another. The benign renal parenchyma is the brown tissue at the bottom, marked with a white asterisk. The carcinoma is the yellow nodule between the white arrows. Note that the carcinoma has replaced the renal parenchyma and is invading out beyond the confines of the kidney into the perirenal adipose tissue (left-hand arrow). Compare to Figure 5–7.

For example, a malignancy arising from the epithelial cells of the colon does not remain localized to the colonic mucosa, as a benign polyp does, but rather develops the ability to invade the deeper tissues of the colonic wall—that is, the richly vascular connective tissue of the submucosa and the smooth muscle layer deep to it. In other words, invasion is continuous growth of the tumor into and through other tissue types adjacent to its site of origin. Metastasis means transplantation of cells to an entirely new site. For this to occur, the neoplastic cells must be transported through vascular channels or body spaces and must be able to grow at the new site. Cancers most often metastasize to the lymph nodes, lungs, liver, and bone (Figure 5–7). Usually, tumors that have metastasized are no longer curable. Some cancers can be lethal by invasion alone (e.g., if a lung cancer erodes into an artery, the patient may die of massive hemorrhage), but usually patients do not die until the tumor has metastasized.

The suffix -oma refers to a tumor. It does not necessarily distinguish between a neoplastic or non-neoplastic growth. For example, a hematoma is a localized collection of blood that often produces a swelling; a granuloma is an aggregate of inflammatory cells that forms a discrete, rounded lesion in tissues. The suffix is most commonly used in conjunction with neoplasms, however, and for all intents and purposes -oma signifies a neoplastic growth. Tables 5–1 and 5–2 list names given to benign and malignant neoplasms. Benign neoplasms usually are named by the suffix -oma appended to the name of the tissue of origin. Malignant neoplasms are usually called carcinoma or sarcoma. Carcinoma refers to a malignant neoplasm of epithelial tissue (e.g., squamous cell carcinoma of the skin). Sarcoma is used if the malignancy arises from mesenchymal tissue (e.g., osteosarcoma of bone). A few neoplasms of nonepithelial or ambiguous origin and unpredictable clinical behavior have names that do not follow this classification system (e.g., gastrointestinal stromal tumor, pancreatic neuroendocrine tumor). Other clearly malignant

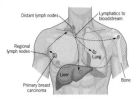

FIGURE 5–7 Typical pattern of metastasis from a breast cancer. For carcinomas, metastasis via lymphatics usually precedes metastasis via the blood.

TABLE 5–1 Names of Benign Neoplasms	
Cell or Tissue of Origin	**Name**
Squamous epithelium	Squamous papilloma
Glandular or surface columnar epithelium	Adenoma
Fibrous tissue	Fibroma
Adipose tissue	Lipoma
Cartilage	Chondroma
Bone	Osteoma
Blood vessels	Hemangioma
Smooth muscle	Leiomyoma
Nerve sheath	Neurilemmoma

TABLE 5–2 Names of Malignant Neoplasms	
Cell or Tissue of Origin	**Name**
Epithelium	
Site not specified	Carcinoma
Squamous epithelium	Squamous cell carcinoma
Basal cells of epithelium	Basal cell carcinoma (unique to skin)
Colonic mucosa	Adenocarcinoma of colon
Breast glands	Adenocarcinoma of breast
Bronchial epithelium of lung	Bronchogenic carcinoma
Prostatic glands	Adenocarcinoma of prostate
Bladder mucosa	Urothelial carcinoma
Endometrium	Adenocarcinoma of endometrium
Cervix	Squamous cell carcinoma of cervix
Stomach mucosa	Adenocarcinoma of stomach
Pancreatic ducts	Adenocarcinoma of pancreas
Connective tissue and muscle	
Site not specified	Sarcoma
Lymphoid tissue	Lymphoma
Bone marrow	Leukemia
Plasma cells in bone marrow	Multiple myeloma
Cartilage	Chondrosarcoma
Bone	Osteosarcoma
Fibrous tissue	Fibrosarcoma
Smooth muscle	Leiomyosarcoma
Other	
Site not specified	Malignant neoplasm
Glial cells	Glioma
Melanocytes	Malignant melanoma
Germ cells	Teratoma

neoplasms have been given names that make them sound benign, when in fact they are glaringly malignant. It is very important to recognize these as malignant neoplasms. A lymphoma is a malignancy of lymphoid cells; a melanoma is a malignant neoplasm of melanocytes; glioma is used to refer to all neoplasms, benign or malignant, of the supporting cells of the brain (glial cells); and hepatoma is an old name that has been replaced with the more accurate hepatocellular carcinoma.

Benign Neoplasms

Benign neoplasms are relatively easy to recognize grossly and microscopically because they produce a single mass that is discrete from surrounding tissue (Figure 5–5). When originating on a body surface, benign neoplasms extend outwardly, producing a polyp (Figure 5–8). A polyp is any abnormal protrusion from a mucosal surface. Polypoid growth is characteristic of benign neoplasms; however, polypoid growth sometimes occurs with other types of lesions, such as inflammation or hyperplasia, and polyps may harbor malignant neoplasms.

Benign neoplasms that originate within solid organs or connective tissue usually compress tissue around them to form a fibrous rim or capsule (see Figure 5–8). Because they are so circumscribed, benign tumors are easily separated from surrounding tissue during surgical removal. Histologically, benign neoplasms very closely resemble their cells of origin and demonstrate minimal degrees of cellular atypia (Figure 5–9). The most important morphologic criteria for benign neoplasms are the discreteness of the lesion and the uniform, relatively mature appearance of the cells.

Malignant Neoplasms

Two characteristics define a malignant neoplasm: cellular atypia, invasion, and metastasis. If a neoplasm has metastasized at the time of discovery, it is per definition

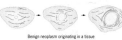

Benign neoplasm originating in a tissue

Benign neoplasm originating on a surface

FIGURE 5–8 Comparison of a benign neoplasm within solid tissue such as breast (above) with a benign neoplasm developing in an organ with a mucosal surface such as the colon (below). The breast neoplasm is encapsulated; the colon neoplasm is polypoid.

Student Resources

The Navigate Companion Website includes useful study activities to aid the learning process. To redeem the Access Code Card available with your new copy of the text, visit go.jblearning.com/humandisease6CWS. To purchase access to the website separately, call 800-832-0034 and request ISBN-13: 978-1-284-03570-4.

The Navigate Companion Website features the following tools:

- **Practice Quizzes:** Complete a quiz at the end of each chapter to assess your knowledge of key concepts. Results can be emailed to your course instructor.
- **Crossword Puzzles:** Enjoy an interactive overview of terms from each chapter with real crossword puzzles created with terms from the text.
- **Interactive Flashcards:** Enhance retention as these helpful tools guide you through the key terms vital to understanding important topics.
- **Interactive Glossary:** Search for key terms and their definitions alphabetically or by chapter.
- **Matching Exercises:** Engage in an enjoyable online activity to connect concepts and terms with their meanings.
- **Web Links:** Explore external sites that provide additional information about topics covered in this text.

Instructor Resources

Qualified instructors can receive the full suite of Instructor Resources, including:

- PowerPoint Presentations featuring more than 250 slides
- A Test Bank containing more than 200 questions
- Instructor's Manual including a sample syllabus and an answer key for the end-of-chapter practice questions.

To gain access to these valuable teaching materials, contact your Health Professions Account Specialist at go.jblearning.com/findarep.

New to the *Sixth Edition*

- New photos and illustrations.
- New and updated resources for instructors and students.
- Updated content reflects the current state of medical knowledge and practice.
- More clinical information, including general and specific treatments for diseases with an emphasis on common laboratory tests.
- *Chapter 26: Infectious Diseases* and *Chapter 27: Immunologic Diseases* are revised and now included in *Section 4: Multiple Organ System Diseases.*
- *Chapter 24: Mental Illness* and *Chapter 30: Nutritional Disorders* are significantly revised and up-to-date with current health problems, concepts, and terminology.

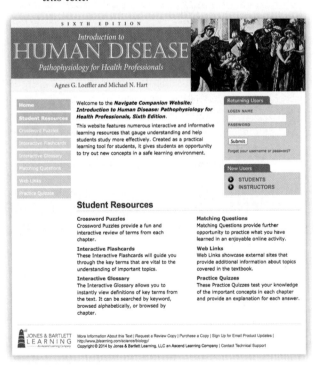

Acknowledgments

Foremost, we want to acknowledge the contributions of Thomas Kent, MD, who was the senior author of *Introduction to Human Disease* through the first four editions. Dr. Kent was a leading medical educator for many years and was cofounder of the Group for Research in Pathology Education (GRIPE), a consortium that shares pathology education materials amongst more than 75 medical schools. In 1975, Dr. Kent had students at the University of Iowa's College of Medicine take tests on the computer, a further example of his prescience in education. Dr. Kent is now retired from pathology teaching, but the success of the first four editions of this text is in no small measure the result of his vision in creating the style and format of the text, plus his insistence that the content be directed to an understanding of the most common and important diseases. We strive to carry forward his vision into the *Sixth Edition*.

In June of 2008, we received a letter from Jones & Bartlett Learning. The publisher had received a note from a person who "was extremely sad" to see *Introduction to Human Disease* "leave the shelves" after the fourth edition, and we were asked if we would consider revising the book. Thus began our relationship with Jones & Bartlett Learning, and we have been extremely pleased with the help we have received along the way from Kristine Johnson, Maro Gartside, Renée Sekerak, Jessica Elias, Teresa Reilly, Jess Newfell, Sean Fabery, Amy Rathburn, Joanna Lundeen, and other members of the editorial, marketing, and production teams.

Bringing this text up-to-date required the concerted effort of numerous colleagues. Not only did the text have to be revised, sometimes substantially, to reflect progress in medical knowledge, but we also wanted to enhance the text with high-quality, color photographs and illustrations. We would like to thank the following individuals who contributed significantly to the *Fifth Edition* and *Sixth Edition* of this text by reviewing chapters, contributing illustrations, or both: Rashmi Agni, Daniel Albert, Richard Antaya, Luis Brandi, Alan Bridges, Darya Buehler, Chiling Chai, Robert Corliss, Kirkland Davis, Charles Ford, John Frey, Andreas Friedl, Michael Fritsch, Molly Gurney, Josephine Harter, Michael Hartman, Eleanor Knopp, Catherine Leith, Bradley Maxfield, Patrick McBride, Fern Murdoch, Kenneth Noonan, Terry Oberley, Scott Perlman, Myron Pozniak, Gordana Raca, Shahriar Salamat, Lonie Salkowski, Suzanne Selvaggi, Donald Schalk, Lynette Scott, Carol Spiegel, Jose Torrealba, Patrick Turski, Art Walaszek, Stacy Walz, Eliot Williams, Donald Yandow, David Yang, and Weixiong Zhong.

Special thanks also are due to Taiya R. Bach, Elizabeth Way, Joan Miller, and Korise Rasmusson, who provided excellent secretarial, editorial, and administrative support during the revision process.

An Overview

The purpose of this section is to give you (1) the general vocabulary used to discuss and classify diseases, (2) a feeling for the general frequency and significance of particular diseases, and (3) an overview of the resources commonly used in diagnosis that bridge the gap between pathophysiology and the care of patients.

Introduction to Pathology

OBJECTIVES

1. Define disease and state the philosophic tenet of disease causation that forms the basis of allopathic medicine.
2. Define pathology and describe what pathologists do.
3. Define manifestation as used in the context of the workup of an ill patient, and describe the general categories of manifestations that healthcare practitioners use to identify diseases.
4. Compare and contrast functional and organic (structural) disease.
5. List, define, and give examples of the three major forms of organic disease.
6. Identify the three basic categories of exogenous causes of diseases.
7. Identify the three basic categories of endogenous causes of diseases.
8. Describe the steps involved in the workup, diagnosis, and treatment of a patient.
9. Describe some of the social, scientific, and economic obstacles to patient care.
10. Define and use in proper context all words and terms in this chapter that are in headings and in bold print.

KEY TERMS

allopathic medicine
anatomic pathology
cellular basis of disease
clinical pathologist
clinicopathologic
  observations
complications
cytopathology
developmental disease
diagnosis
differential diagnosis
disease
endogenous
etiology
evidence-based medicine
exogenous
experimental pathologist
external agents of injury
follow-up
functional disease
genetic disease
history
homeostasis
hyperplasia
iatrogenic

idiopathic
immunologic disease
infection
inflammation
internal mechanism of injury
laboratory finding
lesion
metabolic disease
neoplasia
nosocomial
organic disease
pathogenesis
pathology
pathophysiology
physical examination
prognosis
repair
sign
surgical pathology
symptom
syndrome
trauma
vascular disease
workup

Disease

Disease is a structural or functional change in the body that is harmful to the organism. Some changes in the body are perfectly normal, such as puberty, pregnancy, or increasing muscle mass in an athlete undergoing training. Also, the cells and tissues in the body can adapt to minor fluctuations in their environment, thereby maintaining a state of **homeostasis**. Disease occurs when the cellular environment changes to such a degree that tissues are no longer able to perform their function optimally. For example, with cataracts, the crystalline lens of the eye undergoes degenerative changes over the course of a person's lifetime and becomes cloudy, obstructing the passage of light and causing decreased visual acuity. In diabetes, the extracellular tissue of blood vessel walls undergoes changes that lead to narrowing of the blood vessels, which in turn leads to decreased blood flow, decreased oxygen delivery, and eventually irreversible damage to tissues such as the retina, skin, heart, and kidney. In cancer, mutations accumulating in the nucleic acids of cells result in distorted structure and function of proteins, which in turn affect the way the cells interact with or react to other cells, growth factors, hormones, and the extracellular matrix in their environment. In multiple sclerosis, destruction of the protective myelin sheath around axons in the brain results in decreased electrical conduction, which manifests in neurologic signs and symptoms such as weakness, double vision, and incoordination. In each of these conditions, the ability of cells or tissues to optimally perform their function is compromised, with deleterious consequences to the organism.

Every society identifies conditions that are abnormal and has devised means of treating illness, but there is great variation between cultures and even within subcultures in what constitutes "normal," "abnormal," "disease," or "feelings of ill health." Over time and over place, the explanations that have been given for ill health have varied from spirit possession, witchcraft, sorcery, the anger of ancestors, balance or imbalance of energy, elements or "humors," nutrition, and the will of God, to the bad influence of the climate, weather, or environment. Treatments have accordingly been as various as exorcism, prayer, shamanic rites, rituals that bring the ill person back into the social and universal order, herbs and foods that restore the balance of internal elements, physical manipulations that restore the flow of energy in the body, the "laying on of hands," and arming the ill person with amulets that provide protection against potentially harmful forces. Obviously, the diseases identified or named by all these various systems are not comparable to one another. Imagine the perplexity of a Western medical doctor if s/he were confronted with a patient who claimed to have been possessed by an ancestor's spirit, to be suffering a blockage in the flow of *chi* (the energy at the root of Chinese medicine, including acupuncture), or to be suffering an attack of "nerves" (Latin America: *susto*) brought on by witnessing the traumatic death of a close family member.

Although these conceptualizations of ill health are at variance with the definition of disease set forth in this textbook, it is necessary to recognize that they are millennia old, are based on a vast amount of experiential evidence, and are as real to the sufferers and the people who take care of them as are notions of cancer and infection to Western health practitioners. Though we may not

understand them, and may argue that they have no basis in science, we have no right to dismiss them or belittle them as "superstitious" or "uneducated" because this does no service to the patient who is suffering. Instead, we need to attempt to translate the patient's distress into something that does make sense in terms of our own notions of disease causation.

With the Enlightenment, people began to look at the workings of the body in a scientific manner—in other words, through repeated observations made under controlled circumstances. As knowledge about the way the body works accrued, scientifically oriented doctors began to formulate the idea that disease is not some external force that takes possession of the body, but rather arises from organs and tissues and leaves visible traces there. Physicians gained these insights by closely observing the course of disease on a patient's body, often over weeks or months, and then correlating the clinical findings with the appearance of the organs after death, as seen at autopsy. On the basis of these **clinicopathologic observations**, a philosophy developed that is called the **cellular basis of disease**. This states that diseases can be traced to deranged structures or functions of organs, tissues, and cells. Nowadays, we have expanded the definition to include changes at the molecular level, including proteins and, ultimately, genes. The medical tradition that has evolved from this philosophy is variously called **allopathic medicine**, biomedicine, or Western medicine.

Pathology

The term **pathology** has several meanings. In the broadest sense, pathology is the study of disease. All people working in a health-related field are lifelong students of pathology because, in one way or another, all are interested in altering the course of disease through scientific understanding of its nature. A course in pathology, such as the one you are taking, provides a concentrated study of the nature of disease and lays the foundation for its further study within specific disciplines. Pathology includes the study of basic structural and functional changes associated with a disease, as well as the sequence of events that leads from structural and functional abnormalities to clinical manifestations. This sequence is referred to as the **pathogenesis** of disease; its study is called **pathophysiology**. The term **etiology** means the study of causes, but it is also commonly used simply to connote the cause of disease.

Pathology is also the name of one of the specialties of medicine, one that deals with analysis of body fluids and tissues for diagnostic purposes and with teaching and research relating to fundamental aspects of disease (**Table 1–1**). Pathologists usually practice laboratory medicine or study basic aspects of disease within a department of pathology associated with a hospital and/or medical school. The field of pathology is

TABLE 1–1 Roles of a Pathologist	
Role	**Subject**
Experimental pathology	Research
Academic pathology	Teaching, research, anatomic, and/or clinical pathology
Anatomic pathology	Morphologic examinations
Autopsy pathology	Postmortem study of the body
Surgical pathology	Biopsies and resected tissues
Cytopathology	Individual cells removed by scraping or washing
Clinical pathology	Laboratory tests
Chemistry	Chemical analysis
Microbiology	Microorganisms
Hematology	Blood cells and bone marrow, blood clotting
Blood banking	Blood transfusion services
Immunopathology	Antigen and antibody detection
Molecular diagnosis	Nucleic acid (DNA and RNA) analysis

itself subspecialized. There are experimental pathologists, anatomic pathologists, and clinical pathologists. **Experimental pathologists** are basic scientists who spend the majority of their time in research, investigating the causes and mechanisms of disease. **Anatomic pathologists** perform autopsies, examine all tissues removed from live patients (**surgical pathology**), and examine cell preparations to look for cancer cells (**cytopathology**). **Clinical pathologists** analyze various specimens removed from patients, such as blood, urine, feces, spinal fluid, or sputum, for chemical substances, microorganisms, antigens and antibodies, nucleic acids, atypical blood cells, and coagulation factors. Anatomic and clinical pathologists are primarily concerned with diagnosing diseases, but, especially at hospitals associated with medical schools, they may also be engaged in research and teaching.

Manifestations of Disease

We use the term *manifestation* to refer to all the data gathered about a disease as it occurs in a patient. The manifestations that are of interest to the allopathic doctor are symptoms, signs, and laboratory abnormalities (**Table 1–2**). **Symptoms** are evidence of disease perceived by the patient, such as pain, a lump, or diarrhea. Health practitioners carefully elicit these during an interview with the patient and record them in the patient's chart as the *history*. **Signs** are physical observations made by the person who examines the patient. Examples include tenderness, a mass, or abnormal heart sounds. Signs are elicited and observed during the *physical examination*, the results of which are also recorded in the patient's chart. **Laboratory findings** are observations made by the application of tests or special procedures, such as x-rays, blood counts, or biopsies. **Diagnosis** is the process of assimilating the information from the history, physical examination, and laboratory findings to identify the condition causing the disease. Diagnosis also refers to the name given to that disease, such as "multiple sclerosis" or "diabetes." This name is a shorthand way of communicating and thinking. It sums up all the essential information from the history, physical examination, and laboratory findings so that a prognosis can be rendered and appropriate therapy can be initiated. Underlying diagnosis and treatment is, of course, the assumption that diseases of the same name run a predictable course that can be altered, to lesser or greater degree, by medical intervention.

Sometimes, a diagnosis cannot immediately be made. For example, Alzheimer disease cannot be definitively diagnosed until a patient's brain is examined after his or her death. Obviously, it is too late to do anything about it then, so, while the patient is alive, the patient is given a provisional diagnosis of "Alzheimer-type dementia." Other diseases, such as rheumatologic, neurologic, or gastrointestinal ones, may also be vaguely identified (for example, "paralysis of unknown cause") and treated symptomatically until the disease "declares itself," or develops some features that allow its unique identification. In such cases, the clinical problem—paralysis, dementia—is used as the focus of symptomatic treatment until the patient's disease can be definitively identified.

Clusters of findings commonly encountered with more than one disease are called **syndromes**. For example, leakage of protein into the urine, low serum

TABLE 1–2 Manifestations of Disease		
Type of Manifestation	**Nature of Data**	**Name for Collection of Results**
Symptoms	Patient's perceptions	History
Signs	Examiner's observations	Physical examination
Laboratory abnormalities	Results of tests and special procedures	Laboratory findings

protein, and edema are a common set of findings in the "nephrotic syndrome," which can be caused by a number of different diseases that affect the renal glomeruli. The syndrome is a description of a constellation of symptoms, and though treatments can be initiated to alleviate the symptoms and laboratory abnormalities, specific treatment of the disease causing the syndrome is still necessary.

Structural Diseases

Structural diseases, or **organic diseases**, are characterized by structural changes within the body. Structural changes are called **lesions**. Until recently, lesions were visually identified, either by changes visible to the naked eye or changes visible through the light or electron microscope. With the advent of molecular medicine, health professionals also recognize lesions that occur at the level of proteins and genes. Three broad categories suffice to classify most structural diseases (**Table 1–3**). As with all classification schemes, there are always some items that do not fall easily into just one category, and some items are simply difficult to classify. Nevertheless, the scheme does capture most structural diseases, so it is useful to start sorting the vast numbers of diseases you will learn about.

Genetic diseases are caused by abnormalities in the genetic makeup of the individual, either at the level of chromosomes, such as increased chromosome numbers or translocations, or at the genetic level, such as mutations. **Developmental diseases** are ones that developed during an individual's life *in utero*—in other words, during embryonic and fetal development. The range of genetic and developmental abnormalities is very broad, extending from deformities present at birth, to biochemical changes caused by genes but influenced by environment so that they appear later in life, such as diabetes mellitus.

Degenerative and inflammatory diseases are caused by forces or agents that destroy cells or intercellular substances, deposit abnormal substances in cells and tissues, or cause the body to injure itself by means of the inflammatory process. **External agents of injury** include physical and chemical substances and microbes. The major **internal mechanisms** of injury are vascular insufficiency, immunologic reactions, and metabolic disturbances. There are two general reactions to injury: inflammation and repair. **Inflammation** is a vascular and cellular reaction that attempts to localize the injury, destroy the offending agent, and remove damaged cells and other materials. **Repair** is the replacement of damaged tissue by new tissue of the same type and/or fibrous connective tissue. Inflammation is a stereotyped response with several important variations. Unlike necrosis and inflammation, repair is greatly influenced by the type of tissue or organ that has been injured.

Hyperplastic and neoplastic diseases include those in which the basic abnormality is an increase in cell populations. **Hyperplasia** is a proliferative reaction to a prolonged external stimulus and usually regresses when the stimulus is removed. **Neoplasia** results from genetic changes that favor the growth of a single population of cells. Neoplasms are divided into two groups, benign and malignant, based on whether the cells remain localized or develop the ability to grow into surrounding tissue or even migrate to other tissues. *Cancer* is the colloquial term for malignant neoplasm. Certain types of hyperplasias can slowly evolve, presumably through a series of genetic changes induced by external agents, into malignant neoplasms.

Functional Diseases

Functional diseases are those in which there are no visible lesions, at least at the onset of the disease. The basic change is a physiologic or functional one. Two of the most common functional disorders are tension headache and irritable bowel syndrome, disorders that may be the result of unconscious stimulation of the autonomic nervous system.

Other examples of common functional disorders are diabetes and hypertension. These diseases are diagnosed by laboratory evidence of increased circulating glucose in the blood and increased blood pressure readings, respectively. Only over time do structural changes become evident, first in blood vessels and then in the form of end-organ damage, such as necrosis of renal tissue and its replacement by fibrosis. By this time, the disease has progressed to such a degree that complications (stroke, heart disease, blindness, and kidney disease, among others) are inevitable. Many mental illnesses are considered functional disorders; however, there is increasing evidence that they may, indeed, have an organic basis. The same is true for many other functional disorders, including diabetes and hypertension. In fact, most diseases have a genetic basis. Even how people respond to external stimuli such as infectious agents, alcohol, or environmental toxins is genetically based. The classification of such diseases as "functional" may therefore be an oversimplification, but for the present purposes it is still of heuristic value.

Causes of Disease

Diseases are initiated by injury, which may be either external or internal in origin. Agents acting from without are termed **exogenous**; those acting from within are referred to as **endogenous**.

TABLE 1–3   Major Categories of Structural Diseases
• Genetic and developmental diseases
• Acquired injuries and inflammatory diseases
• Hyperplasias and neoplasms

Exogenous causes of disease are divided into physical, chemical, and microbiologic (**Table 1–4**). Direct physical injury is called **trauma**. Physical agents causing disease include extremes of heat and cold, electricity, atmospheric pressure changes, and radiation (electromagnetic and particulate). Chemical injuries are generally subdivided by the manner of injury into poisoning (accidental, homicidal, or suicidal) and drug reactions (toxic effects of prescription or proprietary drugs taken to treat disease). Microbiologic injuries are usually classified by the type of offending organism (bacteria, fungi, rickettsiae, viruses, protozoa, and helminths) and are called **infections**.

Endogenous causes of disease fall into three large categories (**Table 1–5**). **Vascular diseases** include obstruction of blood supply to an organ or tissue (e.g., myocardial ischemia secondary to atherosclerosis), hemorrhage (e.g., a ruptured abdominal aortic aneurysm), or altered blood flow (e.g., microvascular changes in diabetes or hypertension). **Immunologic diseases** are those caused by aberrations of the immune system. Failure of the immune system to work when it is needed results in immunodeficiency disease. Overreaction of the immune system causes allergic, or hypersensitivity, diseases. Abnormal reaction of the immune system to endogenous substances causes autoimmune diseases. The category of **metabolic diseases** encompasses a wide variety of biochemical disorders that may be genetically determined or secondary effects of acquired disease. Metabolic diseases are most commonly categorized as abnormalities primarily involving lipids, carbohydrates, proteins, minerals, vitamins, and fluids.

Some diseases cannot be classified according to internal or external causes because the cause is not known. Diseases of unknown cause are termed **idiopathic**. Adverse reactions resulting from treatment by a health specialist produce **iatrogenic** disease. **Nosocomial** diseases are those acquired from a hospital environment.

The Care of Patients

The typical approach to disease in allopathic medicine is to wait for the patient to seek help because of bothersome symptoms. The health practitioner, presented with a sick patient, proceeds in a systematic fashion to help the patient (**Table 1–6**). The **workup** of a patient encompasses three major steps: (1) taking the **history**, which involves listening to the patient or to the patient's relatives to ascertain the patient's symptoms, and reviewing any other past or present medical problems that might relate to them; (2) performing a **physical examination**, or systematically looking, feeling, listening, and sometimes even smelling accessible parts of the body for signs of illness; and (3) when needed, ordering laboratory tests, radiologic imaging tests, and specialized clinical procedures to detect chemical and physiologic abnormalities. After acquiring the history, performing the physical examination, and reviewing initial ancillary tests, the health practitioner makes a list of possible diagnoses. This is called a **differential diagnosis**. Additional tests are ordered to exclude specific diagnoses on the list so that in the end one diagnosis is made that is the best interpretation of the symptoms, signs, and laboratory data.

A diagnosis is simultaneously a summing up of a patient's problem, a prediction about the course the disease will take, or **prognosis**, and a guide for treatment.

TABLE 1–4	Exogenous Causes of Disease

Physical injury
- Trauma
- Heat/cold
- Electricity
- Pressure
- Ionizing radiations

Chemical injury
- Poisoning
- Drug reactions

Microbiologic injury
- Bacteria
- Fungi
- Rickettsiae
- Viruses
- Protozoa
- Helminths

TABLE 1–5	Endogenous Causes of Disease

Vascular
- Obstruction
- Bleeding
- Deranged flow

Immunologic
- Immune deficiency
- Allergy
- Autoimmunity

Metabolic
- Abnormal metabolism or deficiency of:
  - Lipids
  - Carbohydrates
  - Proteins
  - Minerals
  - Vitamins
  - Fluids

TABLE 1–6	Steps in the Care of a Patient's Illness

1. Gather facts:
   - History
   - Physical examination
   - Laboratory and radiology tests
2. Interpret the facts and render a diagnosis.
3. Treat the patient, if feasible.
4. Follow up on results of treatment.

Therapy is undertaken in an attempt to alter the natural course of the patient's disease. The goal of therapy depends on the disease. The goal of treating a middle ear infection in a child is to eradicate the infection. The goal of treating diabetes is to prevent complications. The goal of surgery after a patient has been in a motor vehicle accident and has a major internal hemorrhage is to stop the hemorrhage and thereby avert the patient's death. The goal of treatment of widely metastatic cancer is no longer to cure but to alleviate pain in the last days or weeks of a patient's life. Whatever the goal of treatment, **follow-up** of the patient is essential to monitor progress toward the goal; determine whether **complications**, or secondary problems that emerge as a consequence of treatment, have developed; and alter therapeutic efforts accordingly.

Diagnosis of specific diseases is useful not only for determining treatment and prognosis in any specific instance of disease but also to future patients. It is through collection of data by disease category that knowledge of prognosis, effectiveness of treatment, and frequency of complications is derived. Sometimes these data also further the health profession's understanding of the cause of a disease. This is particularly true when the distribution of the disease gives clues as to possible causative factors. For example, our knowledge about how the human immunodeficiency virus (HIV), the cause of AIDS, is spread began with the insight that the first patients to come down with this disease in the United States were (homosexual) men practicing unprotected sex with multiple sexual partners.

Obstacles to Patient Care

The process of patient care described here is limited by availability of resources, the nature of particular diseases, and clinicians' ability to understand disease processes. The greatest improvements in our health care have come from preventive measures, including sanitation, improved nutrition, immunization, control of infectious diseases, and avoidance of toxic substances. Whereas infections were once the major cause of death in Western nations, reducing life expectancy to the 40- to 50-year range, we now have the means to prevent, control, and eradicate these diseases. However, as the recent example of AIDS has shown, the amount of initiative, time, and money that it takes to spread knowledge about diseases and convince people to adopt protective measures is exorbitant. It also paints a very stark line between societies that have such resources and those that do not. Whereas in the United States we might claim that AIDS is more or less under control, the incidence of this disease having been pretty stable since the late 1990s (around 56,300 new cases per year), it is primarily under control among white men and women. Blacks, especially young African American women, are at seven times greater risk of contracting the disease than are whites.[1]

Worldwide, AIDS is one of the major killers: 2.0 million people died of AIDS in 2008, and more than three-quarters of these deaths occurred in poverty-stricken nations of sub-Saharan Africa.[2] There, as in Asia, the people most vulnerable to contracting the disease are poor women, and, by extension, their children. The reasons for this are multifactorial, but they can be summarized as lack of resources: poverty driving women to trade sex for food, no health education to learn how to prevent contracting the disease, and no access to therapies that slow progression of the disease.

Moreover, the application of new knowledge about a disease process or therapeutic intervention lags far behind discoveries. Smoking is an illustrative example. As early as the 1920s, autopsy series documented the strong link between smoking and lung cancer. By 1964, a special commission set up by President John F. Kennedy was able to review more than 7,000 scholarly articles, many of them meticulously researched and prepared by the American Cancer Society, on the effect of smoking cigarettes on health. The resultant Surgeon General's report stunned the nation by detailing the magnitude of the effect of smoking on health, attributing 70% increased mortality and a 9- to 10-fold increase in the incidence of lung cancer in smokers as compared to non-smokers. Despite the incontrovertible scientific evidence that smoking is harmful to health, cigarette consumption actually increased over the next decades. It was not until 1987 that the first anti-smoking law, banning smoking on airlines, was passed in the United States. It took another several years for cities and states to begin banning smoking in public places, such as the workplace, restaurants, and bars. Of course, there is a lot more to smoking, beginning to smoke, and quitting smoking than personal will and judgment based on scientific evidence: peer pressure, social expectations and values, and addiction are major influences, if not determinants, of smoking behaviors. But similar lag times are well known for other scientific insights, as well. It is estimated that it takes 15 to 20 years for a scientific discovery to be translated into a standard of practice.

Standards of allopathic practice, though based in scientific evidence, are not universally adhered to. It has been well documented now for several decades that hypertension is a major risk factor for stroke and heart disease, yet the percentage of Americans who are adequately treated for hypertension is only about 30–40%. It is senseless and possibly harmful and counterproductive to take antibiotics, which inhibit the growth of bacteria, for conditions not caused by bacteria, yet many doctors continue to prescribe antibiotics for diseases that are caused by a virus (for example, upper respiratory tract infections and middle ear infections in children). These are only two examples, yet variability in patient assessment and care is such a matter of fact that patients often visit more than one doctor—and may even be encouraged to do so by their first doctor—for the same condition to gather a second opinion that will help them make a more informed or confident decision about their therapeutic plan. While in some cases the second opinion is the same as the first, it may not be. This leads to frustration on the part of the patient, who is expecting a single "answer" based on scientific data. It also leads to frustration on the part of doctors who believe that, for the maximal benefit of patients, medicine should be practiced strictly along guidelines formulated on the basis of a thorough review of the scientific literature. These practice guidelines, issued by expert panels, form the core of **evidence-based medicine**.

Although evidence-based practice guidelines ensure that physicians know what the standard of care should be, there is still a great amount of variation in how patients are treated. Economic factors, including the resources available at a particular clinic or hospital, the patient's insurance status, the age of the patient, other illnesses the patient has, religious beliefs, personal experiences of the physician in treating similar patients, and personal wishes of the patient all influence the treatment plan.

Moreover, the focus of treatment varies widely by clinic type and demographic factors. In large hospitals affiliated with universities, so-called academic hospitals, patients are treated at the forefront of scientific advances: organ transplantations, experimental cancer treatments, and treatment of rare and complicated diseases are the main focus at such centers. Conversely, in inner-city clinics, the main focus is on preventive care, such as maternal and child health, and on management of diseases that are most common in that population, such as diabetes and heart disease.

Scientific and technical knowledge and progress are not the only factors affecting health and health care. The United States is one of the world leaders in scientific and technical advances in the healthcare field, and it spends more money than any other nation on health care, yet it ranks very low in general measures of health, such as infant mortality and life expectancy. There is no doubt that the largest challenge faced by healthcare workers in the United States is equitable distribution of resources. Health practitioners have the knowledge to prevent many diseases and delay if not entirely avoid complications of others, but a large percentage of the population is denied access to this knowledge, either because of lack of the ability to pay for it, lack of health education, or lack of clinics and healthcare workers willing to serve an underprivileged community. In addition, U.S. society must confront the issue of cost containment in terminally ill patients, for whom procedures are often performed with costs that are out of proportion to the benefit received. This will mean engaging in economic studies, ethical debates, and legal reforms that will hold the healthcare industry accountable for the money it consumes. Such debates need to be informed by a solid understanding of the pathophysiology of diseases. The information in this text will allow you to become an informed participant in the healthcare debate.

The Structure of This Text

This text presents a basic classification scheme for diseases and an introductory discussion of their causes. The first part of the text discusses disease processes that are applicable to all tissues in the body, such as genetics, inflammation, and neoplasia. The second part of the text discusses diseases by organ system. The third part presents diseases that affect many different organs simultaneously, such as infections and immunologic diseases.

Each chapter begins with a short review of the structure and function of the organ system under discussion. It should be stressed that this is a review: though you probably do not need to have a background in physiology to understand the diseases as they are presented here, it is certainly advisable for you to have had a course in physiology to better understand pathophysiology.

After the review of structure and function, we list the diseases of that organ system that are most common. This means there is a certain degree of redundancy in the text because we might explain some aspect of pathophysiology in this section and reiterate this or explain it in greater detail later in the chapter. This is intentional. Getting a sense of how common a disease is and what impact it has on a population enhances learning about the disease, and repetition is one of the key factors in retention of information.

Although the diseases included for discussion in this text are those that are most common, or classically illustrate a disease process, the list of diseases is long and the reading will unfortunately get tedious. In addition, the discussion for some diseases may not be as detailed as you would like. Several excellent resources are available that provide more information. Robbins and Cotran's *Pathologic Basis of Disease* (edited by Vinay Kumar, Abul Abbas, Nelson Fausto, and Jon Aster, Saunders, 2009) and *Rubin's Pathology* (edited by Raphael Rubin and David Strayer, Lippincott Williams and Wilkins, 2007) are pathology texts used in medical schools that have detailed explanations and many pictures and diagrams that aid in understanding disease processes. If you have access to a health library, the electronically published *UpToDate* (of which there is also a "patients" edition that is free to general readership) provides information on pathophysiology and gives much more detailed information on diagnostic and treatment strategies than we provide in this text. The Internet is also an invaluable resource. Numerous excellent web pages have been designed by disease interest groups. These are governmental, such as the National Institutes for Health (NIH) and the Centers for Disease Control and Prevention (CDC); private or nonprofit, such as the American Heart Association; and driven by physician (e.g., Mayo Clinic or Cleveland Clinic Web pages) or patient groups (e.g.,

Susan G. Komen "for the [breast cancer] Cure" organization). Although you do need to be careful about believing everything you read on the Internet, by carefully searching and questioning the sources, you can gather much information from these web pages, in a concise and readable format.

We hope that the information you find in this text helps you in your career. It is important to have a broad foundation of knowledge about basic pathophysiologic principles and causes of common diseases, such as is presented in this text, before becoming enmeshed in the details of an area of specialization. In addition, such knowledge should help you formulate your own informed opinions about how best to help patients and where to most effectively put our society's resources to prevent disease and alleviate patients' suffering.

Practice Questions

1. A 54-year-old woman has a breast biopsy. Which of the following pathologists will look at and diagnose the biopsy?
   A. Surgical pathologist
   B. Cytopathologist
   C. Clinical pathologist
   D. Research pathologist
   E. Microbiologist

2. The three categories of endogenous causes of disease are
   A. microbiologic, immunologic, metabolic.
   B. physical, vascular, metabolic.
   C. metabolic, immunologic, vascular.
   D. chemical, microbiologic, vascular.

3. An ulcerating sore on a person's skin is
   A. an infection.
   B. a lesion.
   C. a functional change.
   D. a complication.

4. A 55-year-old man complains to his physician of extreme tiredness. This is an example of
   A. a symptom.
   B. a sign.
   C. a manifestation.
   D. a complication.

5. Which of the following is the basic philosophical tenet of allopathic medicine?
   A. Disease is caused by external agents that leave visible traces on organs and tissues.
   B. Disease is caused by deranged structure and/ or function of tissues, cells, or molecules.
   C. Diseases cause visible changes in tissues and organs.
   D. Diseases are caused by structural changes in genes that result in functional changes in tissues.
   E. Diseases can be diagnosed by the scientific method.

6. Which of the following is not a manifestation of disease?
   A. Ultrasonographic evidence of abnormal heart chambers in a fetus
   B. Fever, leukocytosis, and abdominal pain in a child with appendicitis
   C. A history of breast cancer in a close family member
   D. A necrotizing skin ulcer
   E. A feeling of shortness of breath and abnormal lung sounds in a patient with pneumonia

7. Care of a symptomatic patient includes all of the following except which one?
   A. Taking a history
   B. Performing a physical exam
   C. Performing screening procedures
   D. Seeing the patient in follow-up
   E. Prescribing treatment plans

8. A differential diagnosis is
   A. a list of possible diseases a patient may have, generated during the workup of a patient.
   B. a constellation of symptoms that is not unique to a particular disease.
   C. a diagnosis that is made presumptively, without confirmatory laboratory tests.
   D. the opinion of a second physician, which is different from that of the first physician consulted.
   E. a diagnosis rendered by a practitioner of alternative medicine.

REFERENCES

1. Hall HI, Song R, Rhodes P, et al. Estimation of HIV incidence in The United States. *JAMA*. 2008;300:520–529.
2. UNAIDS. Epidemiology slides: 2009 AIDS epidemic update. Available at www.unaids.org/en/KnowledgeCenter/HIVData/Epidemiology/2009_epislides.asp. Accessed August 24, 2010.

Most Frequent and Significant Diseases

OUTLINE

OBJECTIVES

1. List the leading causes of death and what percentage of people dies from each.
2. Define incidence, prevalence, and mortality rates, as well as other measures of the impact of diseases on populations such as disability and healthcare costs. State what the statistics are useful for.
3. State the relative frequency of the leading causes of acute disease and how they relate to age.
4. List the most common chronic diseases and state whether they are age-related or age-dependent.
5. List the acute and chronic diseases that most frequently bring patients to the doctor's office.
6. State which factors determine the limits of life expectancy.
7. Be able to define and use in proper context all words and terms in bold print in this chapter.

KEY TERMS

acute diseases
age dependent
age related
aging
atherosclerosis
cancer
cerebral vascular
  accident (CVA)

heart disease
incidence
indirect cost
life expectancy
morbidity
mortality
mortality rate
prevalence

chronic diseases
chronic pulmonary disease
direct cost
disability

prognosis
stroke
survival rate
trauma

Causes of Death (Mortality)

Causes of death (mortality) are compiled by government agencies from death certificates, which must be filled out by trained personnel at the time of a person's death. Approximately 70% of all deaths in the United States are accounted for by the five most frequent causes (see Table 2–1). The causes of death vary considerably by age. The most common causes of death of children aged 1–14 years are given in Table 2–2. In children less than 1 year, the most common causes of death relate to congenital anomalies, low birth weight, and complications of premature birth.

Heart disease accounted for 25% of deaths in the United States in 2011. The vast majority of these deaths are caused by atherosclerosis, a degenerative disease of arteries. Over the course of many years, lipid-rich deposits develop in the arterial lining. These areas of thickening may induce the sudden development of a thrombus that completely occludes the vessel and obstructs the flow of blood to a portion of myocardium (heart muscle), which subsequently dies. This is a "heart attack," or myocardial infarct. Myocardial infarcts are more frequent and occur at an earlier age in men than in women under the age of 50, but after this the incidence of myocardial infarct equalizes between the two sexes. Myocardial infarcts can be lethal by causing sudden death (death within an hour of the onset of symptoms), or they can induce degenerative

TABLE 2–1 Overall Leading Causes of Death, United States, 2011

Cause of Death	Number of Deaths
1. Heart disease	596,339
2. Cancer	575,313
3. Chronic pulmonary disease	143,382
4. Cerebrovascular disease (stroke)	128,931
5. Accidents	122,777
6. Alzheimer dementia	84,691
7. Diabetes	73,282
8. Pneumonia and influenza	53,667
9. Kidney disease	45,731
10. Suicide	38,285
11. Septicemia	35,539
12. Chronic liver disease	33,539
13. Hypertension	27,477
14. Parkinson disease	23,107
15. Pneumonitis due to aspiration	18,090
— all other causes	512,723

Data from Hoyert DL, Xu J. Deaths: preliminary data for 2011. *National Vital Statistics Reports*. October 10, 2012;61(6). National Center for Health Statistics, CDC.

TABLE 2–2 Leading Causes of Death in Children Aged 1–14 Years, United States, 2006

Cause of Death	Number of Deaths
1. Accidental trauma	3,868
2. Cancer	1,284
3. Congenital anomalies	859
4. Homicide	756
5. Heart disease	314
6. Sepsis	172
7. Influenza and pneumonia	149
8. Cerebrovascular disease	165
9. Benign neoplasms	136
10. Chronic lower respiratory disease	119

Reproduced from Heron M. Deaths: leading causes for 2006. *National Vital Statistics Reports*. March 31, 2010;58(14). National Center for Health Statistics, CDC.

and compensatory changes in the heart that can be lethal from days to years after the infarct, such as sudden rupture of the myocardial wall or congestive heart failure.

Cancers are the second leading cause of death in the United States, accounting for 23% of deaths. The most lethal, in the sense of causing the largest number of deaths, is lung cancer. Cancer of the sex organs (breast, uterus, ovary, prostate) and gastrointestinal tract are the next most common cancers. The frequency of cancer overall increases dramatically between the ages of 50 and 80 years, but the median age of incidence varies considerably by cancer type. For example, prostate cancer is primarily a disease of old men, while testicular cancer is primarily a disease of young (20- to 40-year old) men. In addition, some cancers are much more rapidly lethal than are others. Pancreatic cancer has a median survival of only about 18 months, while thyroid cancer is typically cured with surgery. Overall, however, the burden caused by cancer in terms of lives lost and cost of care is staggering and is expected to increase. Within a decade, cancer is expected to take the place of heart disease as the number one cause of death in the United States.

Chronic pulmonary disease is the third leading cause of death (approximately 6% of the total), with most of these deaths the result of chronic obstructive pulmonary disease caused by cigarette smoking.

Stroke is the fourth leading cause of death in the United States, accounting for 5% of deaths. Stroke is the common name for **cerebral vascular accident (CVA)** and is caused by injury to an area of the brain due to vascular obstruction or bleeding into the brain. As in the heart, vascular obstruction results from atherosclerosis and overlying thrombus formation. Atherosclerosis of the arteries leading to the brain predisposes an individual to a cerebral infarct, or death of the brain tissue supplied by that artery. Strokes caused by bleeding usually result from high blood pressure or rupture of an aneurysm (a dilated outpouching of an artery). Strokes are most common in older adults and commonly present with weakness of one side of the body or difficulty with speech.

Trauma caused by accidents is the fifth leading cause of death in the United States, accounting for 5% of deaths. Automobile accidents are the most common cause of traumatic death. It is estimated that 50% of drivers responsible for automobile accidents are under the influence of alcohol. Young people and older adults are most commonly affected by accidents.

When comparing the overall causes of death by numbers in 2011 with those from 1990, only mortality resulting from heart disease, pneumonia, and influenza has decreased, while deaths due to cancer, stroke, accidents, chronic pulmonary disease, diabetes, and chronic liver disease have all increased. AIDS was the 10th leading cause of death in 1990, but, fortunately, is no longer within the top 15 in the United States.

From the list of the most common causes of death, it is apparent that common risk factors underlie many of these diseases: atherosclerosis, hypertension, smoking, and obesity. Atherosclerosis induces myocardial infarcts and cerebral infarcts; hypertension causes heart disease and intracerebral hemorrhages; smoking aggravates atherosclerosis, is the leading cause of chronic pulmonary disease, and induces the development of several cancers including lung cancer; and obesity favors the development of atherosclerosis, heart disease, and cancer. Reducing mortality from these diseases therefore requires not only better interventions, such as better drugs with which to treat cancer, but also encouraging healthier lifestyles among the American people.

Causes and Measures of Disability (Morbidity)

Mortality is a crude measure of the effect of a disease on a population. It documents the frequency of lethal diseases, but it does not capture the burden of ill health in a population. Health, and not death, is what workers in the medical field need to be most concerned about anyway. But measures of ill health are not as easy to standardize or use as those for mortality because there is no one clear definition of what constitutes "ill health" or which illness is "significant," and not everyone who has a disease will come to medical attention and so be counted or included in the statistic.

When people develop an illness they often go to see a doctor. One could therefore count the reasons why people go to see doctors and use these statistics as an estimate of which diseases are most troublesome (see **Table 2–3**). As you can see from the list, the top two reasons for office visits in the United States are not feelings

TABLE 2–3	Top 20 Reasons for Office Visits to a Physician in the United States

1. Routine infant or child health check
2. Hypertension
3. Acute upper respiratory infections
4. Arthritis and related conditions
5. Diabetes
6. Spinal disorders
7. Specific procedures
8. Malignant neoplasms
9. Normal pregnancy
10. Rheumatism
11. Gynecologic examination
12. Otitis media
13. Follow-up examination
14. General medical examination
15. Nonischemic heart disease
16. Sinusitis
17. Allergic rhinitis
18. Ischemic heart disease
19. Asthma
20. Cataracts

Reproduced from Cherry DK, et al. National Ambulatory Medical Care Survey: 2006 summary. *National Health Statistics Reports*. August 6, 2008;3.

of ill health at all: they are screening procedures. Most routine well-child checks are performed on well children, with the goal of detecting the earliest signs of disease, providing immunizations, and counseling new parents on safety and nutrition, while visits for essential hypertension are routinely scheduled to monitor the effectiveness of therapy at maintaining healthy blood pressure readings. These two reasons for office visits therefore do not reflect what makes Americans feel ill. The next most common reason for visits to doctors is acute upper respiratory tract infections: the common cold. The common cold is a self-limited illness with no long-term sequelae. As much as it is a nuisance, it hardly reflects the severity of Americans' ill health. Not until you move farther down the list do you begin to see the names of those diseases that have a significant impact on people's lives, consume a large portion of healthcare resources, and often result in death—namely, diabetes, cancer, and heart disease.

The statistics of reasons for doctor visits not only encompass a mixture of screening tests, acute and self-limited illnesses, and serious diseases that require long-term care, but they are also not universally valid, even for the American population. People who can go see a physician when they are ill are insured, and people who are insured generally have a level of health education, or shared understandings of what causes disease and what constitutes ill health, that will prompt them to see a physician for routine blood pressure readings, well-baby checks, arthritis, and monitoring of diabetes. This is not necessarily the case for the multitudes of poor and rural Americans, inner-city populations that may additionally be suffering mental health problems and drug addiction, or immigrants who come with cultural understandings of health at variance with the dominant American medical one. Many of these people rely on home health remedies, native healers, scarce public health clinics, and emergency departments for their health care, and their experience of ill health is not captured by the statistics that merely count visits to doctors' offices.

Another way of measuring ill health would be to identify people who are disabled and document the reason for their **disability**. Disabilities are health problems that interfere with a person's normal physical, mental, or emotional functions. For example, after a person has experienced a heart attack, s/he may feel depression, which may even be severe enough to induce suicidal intentions, and, if the damage to the heart is severe enough, may not be able to go about activities of daily living as before. This means the person may not be able to hold a job and may need help with routine activities such as bathing or going to the bathroom. The emotional and financial burden of disability is severe. Not only does care of people disabled by disease require money for doctor visits, therapies, special equipment (for example, wheelchairs), and pharmaceutical drugs but it also imposes a financial burden on society in terms of days lost from work. More important, the adverse psychological effects of dependency and lost productivity are severe and can themselves require additional health care and support.

It is not as easy to measure the degree of disability or its frequency as it is to measure mortality. The frequency of disability within a population is called morbidity. In the United States, the top three causes of disability, defined as conditions requiring the use of an assistive device such as a cane or wheelchair, or interfering with activities of daily living, a job, or business, are arthritis, back or spine problems, and heart disease (Table 2–4). Note that mental or emotional problems are number four: it behooves health practitioners to remember that mental ill health is a significant cause of morbidity. The problems with measuring morbidity in this way are that it relies on self-reporting or reporting done through doctors' offices, so again it does not capture the experience of people who are not in the healthcare loop. Moreover, the definition of disability is arbitrary. How would the statistics look if, for example, one defined disability as being confined to a wheelchair or bed or, at the other extreme, as a single day lost from work or school because of a health-related issue?

Most diseases incur a financial cost. Insights into where Americans as individuals and as a society spend money on health care are also informative about the burden of ill health. Direct cost refers to the amount of money spent on treatment and management of a specific disease; indirect cost is a measure of the money lost by an ill person not performing his or her usual job and requiring disability payments. The amounts incurred by

specific diseases are staggering. In 2007, for example, the cost of diabetes was $174 billion, including the cost of treatment of complications and indirect costs. The care of people with cancer was $104 billion in 2006. The costs of different diseases can be compared, as can the cost of the same disease in different years, so as to monitor trends in healthcare costs. But the financial cost of a disease is simply that: it does not take into consideration the degree of disability incurred by a disease or the psychological impact of the disease on the patient. Moreover, it obscures the fact that the treatment for some diseases is more costly than it is for others. For example, chemotherapy and radiotherapy for cancer are much more costly than are the drugs commonly used to keep diabetes in check. However, treatment of diabetes must continue over a lifetime, whereas treatment for cancer is limited to weeks, months, or a few years. These subtleties are not captured by measuring only the costs of health care.

The most commonly used measure of the impact of a disease on a population is its frequency, or the number of people affected by a disease in comparison to the number of people in the population. The frequency of disease can be measured at a given time or over a period of time. Incidence is a measure of the number of newly diagnosed patients in a given time period, usually a year. Persons who had the disease diagnosed before the year began are not counted. Prevalence refers to the number of persons with a disease at any one time, regardless of when they were diagnosed. For example, the incidence rate of breast cancer between 2003 and 2007 (SEER data) was 123 per 100,000 population, meaning that for every 100,000 women, 123 got breast cancer every year.[1] The prevalence of breast cancer in the United States on January 1, 2007, was 2,591,855 women: this included women with active disease, those undergoing treatment, and those who were diagnosed with breast cancer at any time in the past, including those who are considered to be cured. When discussing incidence and prevalence, it is important to specify both the time interval over which the observation is made and the specific population under study. For example, you can discuss incidence and prevalence of a disease in all of the people living in one state, or all of the men in one state, or all of the women in the state aged 50 to 59, or black women as compared to white or Hispanic women.

Incidence is a useful measure of the impact of acute diseases in a population. Acute diseases are those that come on abruptly and last a short amount of time, such as a few days or a few weeks. Acute conditions include such things as the common cold, urinary tract infection, appendicitis, or a broken leg or arm. Because the condition is of short duration, the prevalence of the disease is not very helpful in managing the disease; it is more important to identify who will get the disease and design methods of avoiding it. Thus, incidence is a measure of the risk of developing a disease. Prevalence is a more useful tool for measuring the impact of chronic diseases,

| TABLE 2–4 | Leading Causes of Disability Among Adults and Percentage of All Disabilities |

Condition	Percentage
Arthritis	19
Back and spine problems	17
Heart trouble	7
Mental or emotional problems	5
Lung, respiratory trouble	5
Diabetes	4.5
Deafness or hearing problems	4
Stiffness or deformity of limbs/ extremities	4
Blindness	3
Stroke	2

Reproduced from Centers for Disease Control and Prevention. Prevalence and most common causes of disability among adults—United States, 2005. *Morb Mortal Wkly Rep.* 2009;58(16): 421–426.

or diseases that last for a long time and that may not be cured. Examples of chronic diseases are diabetes, Alzheimer disease, rheumatoid arthritis, and cancer. Although it is important to know the incidence of these diseases so as to determine risk factors and design preventive strategies, the majority of patient care revolves around management of the disease for a long period of time. It is therefore essential to know how many people have the disease at any one time so as to adequately allocate healthcare resources.

Mortality rate is a measure of the number of people dying in a given time period. It is usually expressed as the number dying per 100,000 population per year. **Survival rate** is the percentage of people with a particular condition who live for a given period of time after diagnosis. For example, the 5-year survival rate of breast cancer is the percentage of all women with breast cancer who are alive 5 years after diagnosis, regardless of whether they still have cancer, are about to die of metastatic disease, or are considered cured of cancer. The age-adjusted or relative survival rate adjusts the rate for those who might have died from other causes based on their age. The term **prognosis** refers to the outcome of a disease. Prognosis includes both morbidity and mortality estimates.

Frequency of Acute Diseases

Almost half of acute diseases are respiratory illnesses, mostly acute viral diseases (**Figure 2–1**). Approximately one-sixth of acute diseases result from injuries of various types. Another one-third of acute diseases are divided among nonrespiratory infections and a variety of noninfectious-, noninjury-type diseases. The frequency of acute illnesses decreases with age. For example, children younger than 6 years of age have three acute illnesses per year compared to one per year for persons older than age 44.

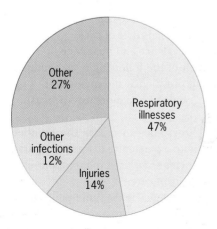

FIGURE 2–1 Approximate frequency of acute diseases.

Frequency of Chronic Diseases

Unlike acute disease, the frequency of chronic disease dramatically increases with age. One of the most prevalent chronic diseases is periodontal disease (inflammation of the gums), which affects about one-third of persons between 45 and 65 years of age and about one-half of persons older than age 65. Patients often do not report periodontal disease as a disabling condition, so it is not listed in comparative data. Mental diseases are also quite prevalent but are not necessarily accurately reported. Most of the leading causes of chronic disease reported in a national survey are associated with aging. Arthritis occurs predominantly in older adults. Diabetes mellitus, back ailments, hearing impairments, and visual impairments are other common chronic diseases that increase in frequency with age. Two chronic conditions that are about equally frequent in young and old persons are chronic bronchitis and asthma.

Certain physical conditions, although not diseases per se, contribute to the development of diseases. A good example is obesity, which is associated with enhanced development of hypertension, diabetes, and atherosclerosis—all three of which contribute to earlier onset and greater incidence of heart disease and strokes. Chronic disease accounts for 70% of all U.S. deaths and for more than 75% of all medical care costs.

Aging

Humans, like other species, have a finite life span. This life span is determined by the process of **aging**, a normal process affecting all individuals that is progressive and irreversible. Over the past century in the United States, a combination of sanitation, healthier lifestyles, better preventive care such as immunizations, and better medical care for previously fatal or potentially fatal conditions such as acute cholecystitis or traumatic accidents have markedly prolonged the life span. For example, in the 1920s, the **life expectancy**, or the amount of time an infant could expect to live, was around 55 years. In 2004, the life expectancy of an infant was around 80 years. It is estimated that by the middle of the 21st century, life expectancy will be close to 90 years. Although for many people this means they have a longer time to be active and enjoy life, it also means that many people will suffer chronic diseases for a longer period of time.

The aging process begins at physical maturity—in other words, at the end of adolescence, usually around age 17 through 20 years. It does not have a marked influence on death rate until much later in life. The mechanism of death from aging is increased susceptibility to disease. For example, aged individuals can die from respiratory infections, accidents, or exposure to cold that would not have killed them at a younger age.

There is no simple explanation for aging. Both genetic and acquired factors are involved. From a genetic standpoint, each species has a maximum life span that is attained by a few individuals. The maximum life span of about 110 years for humans has not changed during the time that the average life expectancy has risen so dramatically in developed nations. Some families or inbred groups of people tend to live longer than others, perhaps because of a lesser tendency to develop certain diseases. Conversely, individuals with the rare genetic disease called progeria show the changes of aging at a very young age.

From an experimental standpoint, cells in culture undergo a limited number of cell divisions before dying out. Apparently, cell metabolism and cell turnover rates decrease with age, possibly secondary to the accumulation of acquired injuries. Mutations, damage to DNA, and cell death resulting from radiation or the formation of oxygen-derived free radicals may account for decreased cell turnover and decreased cell function. Cross-linking of collagen and other long-lived connective tissue substances makes them more rigid and less functional, leading to changes such as degenerative arthritis, wrinkling of the skin, and cataracts.

Diseases that increase in frequency with age can be roughly divided into those that are age dependent and those that are age related. **Age-dependent** diseases occur to some extent in all individuals with time. Examples include degenerative arthritis, osteoporosis, presbyopia, endocrine changes associated with atrophy of ovaries and testes, and hyperplasia of the prostate. **Age-related** diseases are not part of the aging process itself because not all individuals are affected. Examples include many types of cancer, actinic and seborrheic keratoses of the skin, atherosclerosis, hypertension, Alzheimer disease, diverticulosis of the colon, and cataracts. Still another group of diseases accumulates in frequency with age, although their onset is not age related. Examples include chronic lung disease from smoking and gallstones.

There is considerable variation in the degree to which body systems are affected by aging. Decrease in immunity is not overtly obvious but is expressed by an increased susceptibility to and severity of infections in older adults and by an increased rate of development of cancer caused by a failure of the immune system to reject cancer cells as foreign. Manifestations of aging in the endocrine system include impaired glucose tolerance that predisposes individuals to diabetes mellitus, decreased thyroid function, and decreased gonadal function leading to osteoporosis and other changes. Neuronal loss is part of the aging process. The musculoskeletal system and skin are also affected by aging. It becomes more difficult for older adults to maintain muscle strength and the skin becomes thin and loses its elasticity. Decrease in function of the heart, lungs, liver, and kidneys can be demonstrated, but the direct changes of aging have relatively little effect on them. Most of the decreased function of these organs is the result of major diseases such as atherosclerosis, emphysema, and diabetes, which may be age related but not age dependent. The intestines show little

morphologic evidence of aging, but decreased motility is frequently manifested by constipation and diverticulosis in older persons.

As you have seen, most deaths in the United States result from heart disease, cancer, and stroke. Heart disease and stroke deaths are in part the result of aging itself, but there is also an environmental factor that causes accelerated atherosclerosis in the United States as compared to societies with a low-cholesterol diet such as in Japan. Japanese, like Americans, die from the effects of aging on the vascular system, but they rarely die at an early age from myocardial infarcts. This evidence suggests that some gain toward the ideal health curve could be made by a change in diet. The same could be said for many of the other factors that predispose to heart disease, cancer, and stroke, such as smoking, sedentary lifestyle, and obesity. It is clear that the major challenge in health care in the United States in the near future is to alter disease-promoting behaviors. Aging may not be reversible, but people can strive to live as long as their genes will let them.

Practice Questions

1. The leading causes of death
   A. are the same all over the world.
   B. are the same in children and adults.
   C. are compiled from death certificates.
   D. are stable over time.
   E. are unrelated to aging.
2. Which are currently the three leading causes of death in the United States?
   A. Stroke, lung disease, myocardial infarct
   B. Heart disease, lung cancer, breast cancer
   C. Heart disease, cancer, stroke
   D. Atherosclerosis, myocardial infarct, stroke
   E. Cancer, stroke, lung disease
3. Which of the following are not measures of ill health?
   A. Death certificate statistics
   B. Reasons for doctor office visits
   C. Measures of disability
   D. Financial costs of care
   E. Prevalence and incidence
4. Which of the following is an accurate statement about prevalence and incidence?
   A. Incidence is a more useful measure of chronic disease.
   B. Prevalence measures the number of people with a particular disease at a particular time.
   C. Incidence is used to assess direct and indirect costs of care.
   D. Prevalence is the same as prognosis.
   E. Prevalence measures the number of people who develop a disease in a particular time period.

5. The most common causes of disability (as defined in this chapter) are
   A. acute infections, pregnancy and the neonatal period, and chronic obstructive pulmonary disease.
   B. Alzheimer disease, mental illness, and aging.
   C. heart disease, cancer, and stroke.
   D. heart disease, arthritis, and mental illness.
   E. arthritis, back pain, and heart disease.

6. The most common cause of death in the pediatric population is
   A. accidents.
   B. leukemia.
   C. heart disease.
   D. solid-organ cancer.
   E. stroke.

7. A 76-year-old woman who is otherwise perfectly healthy, does not smoke, and does not have hypertension develops pneumonia. She is at greater risk of dying from this disease than a 42-year-old woman would be because of age-related changes in her
   A. heart.
   B. liver.
   C. brain.
   D. immune system.
   E. endocrine system.

8. Life expectancy is
   A. the same for everyone all over the world.
   B. influenced by genetic and environmental factors.
   C. lower now than it was 100 years ago.
   D. unrelated to aging.
   E. influenced most by access to medical care and pharmaceutical drugs.

REFERENCE

1. Surveillance Epidemiology and End Results (SEER). SEER Stat Fact Sheets: Breast. Available at http://seer.cancer.gov/statfacts/html/breast.html. Accessed August 24, 2010.

Diagnostic Resources

OUTLINE

OBJECTIVES

1. Define symptomatic disease, asymptomatic disease, and potential disease.
2. Name the strategies that healthcare practitioners use to detect and diagnose symptomatic disease, asymptomatic disease, and potential disease.
3. List some of the common diseases or conditions for which a screening test or procedure is available, and name that test procedure.
4. Explain the role of the primary care physician, medical specialist, radiologist, pathologist, and public health laboratory in diagnosing diseases.
5. Identify the tests or procedures performed by radiologists, anatomic pathologists, and clinical pathologists.
6. Describe the role of molecular procedures in the diagnosis and treatment of disease.
7. Define and be able to use in context all the words in headings and bold text throughout the chapter.

KEY TERMS

auscultation
autopsy

nuclear medicine
ophthalmoscope

bacterial culture
biopsy
blood bank
   (transfusion medicine)
chemistry
clinical pathology
complete blood count
   (CBC)
computed tomography
   (CT)
cytogenetics
cytology
family history
fine-needle aspiration
   (FNA)
fluoroscope
forensic pathology
frozen section
hematology
history
immunopathology
laboratory medicine
magnetic resonance
   imaging (MRI)
management of disease
microbiology

otoscope
palpation
Pap smear
percussion
pharmacogenomics
physical examination
polymerase chain
   reaction (PCR)
positron emission
   tomography (PET)
preventive medicine
procedure
proteomics
public health laboratory
radiation therapy
radiology
resection
screening
surgical pathology
T1 images
T2 images
targeted therapy
test
ultrasound
vaginal speculum
x-ray

Approach to Patient Care

Symptomatic Disease

The process of working up a patient who comes to a health practitioner for some perceived abnormality in health, or symptom may take minutes or weeks, depending on the complexity of the disease. Most diagnoses can be made from a detailed history and physical examination. In the history, the patient presents the circumstances surrounding the emergence of the problem and describes the severity, quality (e.g., sharp, dull, aching), and timing (e.g., morning or evening, before or after meals, better or worse during activity) of the symptoms. In the **physical examination**, the practitioner looks and listens for further manifestations of disease. This includes visual inspection of skin, nails, and oral mucous membranes, as well as the use of specialized instruments for inspection of structures hidden in recesses of the body, such as the **otoscope**, which allows the practitioner to look into the curved ear canal; the **ophthalmoscope**, which allows inspection of the retina in the back of the eye; and the **vaginal speculum**, which allows visual inspection of the upper vagina and outer cervix. Physical examination also includes **auscultation**, or listening for heart sounds and breath sounds with the stethoscope; **percussion**, or gentle tapping over body cavities to detect changes in the resonance of the chamber, as occurs, for example, with the accumulation of abnormal fluid; and **palpation**, or applying gentle pressure to feel for abnormal growths.

The history and physical examination are usually supplemented by special procedures, radiologic tests, and laboratory tests that explore hypotheses about the patient's condition and provide additional data that support or refute a diagnosis. These procedures can range from endoscopic visualization of the gastrointestinal tract, to radiologic assessment of the integrity of bones, to visualization of the patency of arteries, to tests that measure the amount of metabolic breakdown products in the blood or assess the functional status of an individual organ.

The symptomatic approach to patients is appropriate for acute diseases or conditions such as sinusitis, urinary tract infections, fractures of the bones, myocardial infarction, or middle ear infections in children. However, most of the diseases of industrialized countries are chronic diseases that have a very poor outcome if not treated in their initial stages. These include atherosclerosis, diabetes, hypertension, cancer, and autoimmune diseases. Once these manifest, or become symptomatic, there is usually little that can be done for the patient: the disease may be managed, but the patient will not be cured. For this reason, more and more emphasis in recent years has been put on detecting disease before the patient notices it.

Asymptomatic Disease

In general, the earlier a diagnosis of a chronic disease is made, the better it can be **managed**—in other words, the better its complications can be delayed, if not halted entirely. This approach requires frequent, regular examinations, or checkups, in the form of dental appointments, well-baby examinations, and periodic physical examinations. The attempt to discover disease before it manifests in a patient is called **screening**. The goal of screening is either to cure a disease by catching it early (e.g., cancer) or to begin treatment early to delay the progression of the disease (e.g., hypertension).

Although there are currently many different screening procedures available for many different diseases, it is not advisable to screen everyone for everything. Who and when to screen depend on the likelihood of a patient developing a particular disease, the availability of a treatment for the disease, and the cost of the screening test. For example, radiographic techniques can detect lung cancer when it is still small and limited to the lung and therefore potentially curable. However, radiographic techniques are expensive and confer potential harm to the patient in the form of exposure to ionizing radiation, so they are not ideal for a screening procedure. Instead of screening the entire population, health practitioners perform periodic radiographic exams of the lungs only in patients who have the highest risk of developing lung cancer: those with a smoking history. By comparison, hypertension, which has an onset at all ages and is a strong risk factor for many serious, chronic diseases, can easily be screened for and treated. All screening requires is a blood pressure cuff and stethoscope, and treatment involves some lifestyle modifications as well as relatively inexpensive pharmaceutical drugs. Therefore, it makes sense to screen all patients at each visit to a practitioner's office—and even in between—for hypertension.

There is no doubt that screening procedures are powerful in the sense that diseases can be managed, or even cured, by early detection. For example, the **Pap smear** for cervical cancer, by which cells are scraped from the surface of the cervix, smeared on a slide, and examined microscopically, has dramatically reduced mortality from cervical cancer. This is because precancerous cells can be seen microscopically and the patient treated by biopsy or limited excision of the cervix so that the lesion cannot progress to invasive cancer.

Screening procedures are reactive, not proactive: they allow health practitioners to effectively treat a disease in its early stages, but they do not prevent the occurrence of the disease in the first place. For most people, prevention of disease occurrence would be the most desirable approach to disease.

Potential Disease

The discipline that deals with prevention of disease is called **preventive medicine**. Most of the classic infectious diseases that formerly killed a significant proportion of the population, such as smallpox, bubonic plague, typhoid fever, typhus, measles, diphtheria, and whooping cough, now fall into the category of diseases that are preventable by immunization and good sanitation. Other outstanding examples of preventable diseases are dental caries and periodontal disease, which have been greatly reduced by addition of fluoride in drinking water and preventive dentistry. The link between lifestyle or behaviors and many other diseases is by now well documented: alcohol is linked to traumatic accidents and liver disease; smoking is linked to many different kinds of cancer, most strongly to lung cancer; unprotected sex puts a person at risk for sexually transmitted diseases including gonorrhea, syphilis, cervical cancer, and HIV infection, not to mention a potentially undesired pregnancy. A sedentary lifestyle and a diet high in fat have been linked to many of the chronic diseases plaguing developed nations, including diabetes, obesity, atherosclerosis, and various forms of cancer.

Statistics accrue almost daily on the harmful effects of eating the way we do and living the way we do. Reason does not beget change, however. In addition to vaccination and public health, a large part of the effort of preventive medicine revolves around disseminating information about healthful lifestyles and encouraging people to participate in smoking cessation programs, nutrition counseling, and exercise programs.

The other problem with prevention is reaching people who are most in need of preventive services. Going to see a doctor for screening or prevention is not part of the mind-set of people the world over, including certain populations of the United States, who still hold the idea that one goes to see a doctor only when one is sick or symptomatic. Inner cities, poor and rural areas, and Native American populations have some of the highest incidences of complications of preventable diseases, ranging from poor pregnancy outcomes to complications of diabetes, hypertension, hyperlipidemia, and atherosclerosis. To have a healthy nation, it is not enough to discover new screening tests and pharmaceutical drugs and risk factors: society must be able to make them available to those who need them. This requires establishment of public health departments and public health workers who are dedicated to improving the health of underserved and underprivileged populations.

Screening

The techniques of screening for asymptomatic disease are the same as those used to investigate symptomatic disease: gathering a patient history, conducting a physical examination, and performing targeted laboratory tests. The history allows for exploration of risk factors that predispose the patient to developing disease. For example, during a routine physical exam the health practitioner should ask the patient whether s/he uses a seat belt while riding in a car, has unprotected sex with multiple partners, or smokes. The practitioner must be prepared to provide counseling and education should the patient be engaging in risky behavior. Inquiring into the **family history** of diseases exposes ones the patient might also be prone to developing. For example, if multiple close relatives have developed breast or ovarian cancer at a young age, the patient is also at risk of developing one of these cancers and should be offered an evaluation by a geneticist, which could include genetic testing. Examples of screening by physical examination include dental examination for caries, palpation of breasts for lumps, and

TABLE 3–1 Screening Tests and Procedures	
Test or Procedure	**For Detection of**
Cervical (Pap) smear	Cervical cancer
Blood count	Anemia, leukemia
Urinalysis	Kidney disease
Fecal occult blood test	Colon cancer
Serum lipids (especially cholesterol)	Risk factor for atherosclerosis
Serology	Syphilis, prior to pregnancy
Dental x-rays	Caries
Chest x-ray	Lung cancer, tuberculosis
Mammography	Breast cancer
Visual acuity tests	Problems with vision
Audiograms	Problems with hearing
Tuberculin skin test	Tuberculosis
Sigmoidoscopy	Colon cancer
Serum PSA (prostate-specific antigen)	Prostate cancer
Sphygmomanometry	Hypertension

frequent well-baby checks to monitor growth and development. Laboratory tests and radiographic procedures are used to test for specific diseases, such as serum PSA for prostate cancer and mammography for breast cancer. Some of the more important and widely used screening tests and procedures are listed in **Table 3–1**.

Diagnostic Tests and Procedures

Test is used here to refer to an analysis performed on a specimen removed from a patient. A **procedure** involves doing some manipulation of the patient beyond that usually done during physical examination. Some procedures are done to obtain specimens for a test. Most tests are performed by or supervised by a pathologist. Procedures are performed by various types of physicians, including radiologists and primary care providers.

Clinical Procedures

Primary healthcare practitioners may perform some common or simple tests and procedures themselves. For example, urinalysis, vaginal smears to look for fungi, and throat cultures can be done in a physician's office. The primary care physician may also procure samples that are then sent to the laboratory for analysis. These might include skin biopsies, the Pap smear, and blood draws for serologic tests. Manipulative procedures such as sigmoidoscopy (examination of the distal colon by a scope inserted through the anus) and those that require specialized equipment (such as the slit lamp examination of the globe of the eye) are performed by specialists.

Radiologic Procedures

Radiology is the discipline of medicine that uses techniques such as x-rays, computed tomography (CT) scans, ultrasound, and nuclear medicine to diagnose disease. In addition, one of the fields of radiology is radiation therapy, where ionizing radiation is used to induce cancer cell death. Some of the more common radiologic procedures used for diagnosis are listed in **Table 3–2**.

X-ray procedures are dependent on differing absorption properties of tissues as x-rays pass through them. In conventional x-ray techniques, the net amount of x-radiation that passes through the body exposes film to produce a roentgenogram (commonly called an x-ray). Radiodense material, such as bone, absorbs the x-rays that pass through the tissue, leaving a white shadow on the film. In contrast, air-filled cavities, through which the x-rays pass without any impedance, appear dark (**Figure 3–1**). Alternatively, the x-rays that pass through the body can be viewed with a **fluoroscope**, an instrument that uses a fluorescent plate to detect x-rays. A roentgenogram is a static image; a fluoroscopic image is

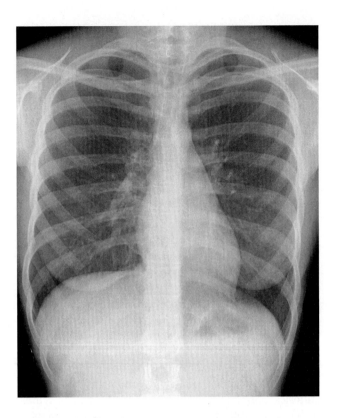

FIGURE 3–1 Chest x-ray. Normal chest x-ray in an 18-year-old woman, showing white bones and dark lung fields. The heart and subdiaphragmatic organs are also white because of the density of the soft tissue through which the x-rays pass. (Courtesy of Dr. Donald Yandow, Department of Radiology, University of Wisconsin School of Medicine and Public Health.)

TABLE 3–2	Radiologic Procedures
Test or Procedure	**Lesions Commonly Detected**
X-rays	Structures of bones and teeth (e.g., fractures, dental caries)
Sinus films (x-ray or CT)	Sinusitis
Chest x-ray	Any lesion that replaces normally air-filled lungs
Upper gastrointestinal series	Ulcers or tumors of the esophagus, stomach, and upper small intestine
Barium enema	Tumors, ulcers, and diverticula of the colon
Intravenous urogram	Decrease in kidney function, obstruction of the urinary tract
Myelogram	Obstruction of the space surrounding the spinal cord
Arteriogram	Obstruction or displacement of arteries
Computed tomography	Tumors, infarcts, blood clots, abscesses, and other lesions
Ultrasound	Gallstones, cysts, twin pregnancy
Magnetic resonance imaging	Tumors, infarcts, blood clots, abscesses, and other lesions
Nuclear isotope scans	Tumors, altered tissue uptake of specific substances

dynamic and allows the radiologist to watch movements such as the passage of barium down the esophagus.

Computed tomography (CT) is a sophisticated x-ray technique in which the x-ray absorption patterns through planes of tissue are recorded and analyzed by a computer. The x-ray generating tube and the x-ray detector (analogous to the x-ray film) rotate around a patient and take more or less continuous images. The computer integrates this information and creates cross-sectional images of the body. Various contrast agents can be used to further highlight internal structures. Lesions can be more sharply defined and precisely localized than with conventional plain films. CT is now the preferred diagnostic modality for detecting acute and potentially lethal processes such as intracerebral hemorrhages, pulmonary embolism, and aortic dissection, as well as delineating deep-seated lesions such as kidney and pancreatic cancer, liver abscesses, and gallstones (**Figure 3–2**).

Magnetic resonance imaging (MRI) also uses a computer to record tissue characteristics in tissue planes but differs in that it does not use x-rays. The image is produced by displacing protons in atomic nuclei with radiofrequency signals while the body is surrounded by a strong magnet. The affected protons release a radiofrequency signal that can be evaluated by a computer to produce images of a section through the body. Different

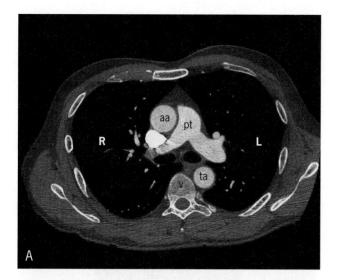

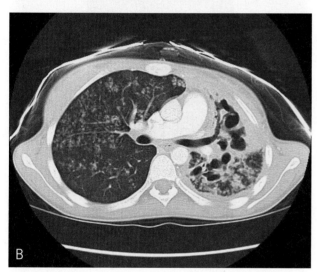

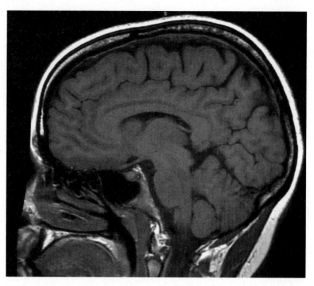

FIGURE 3–3 MRI. Normal brain in sagittal view. The nose is on the left of the image. Notice how clearly the fissures and folds (sulci and gyri) over the surface of the brain can be seen, as well as the distinction between gray and white matter. (Courtesy of Dr. Patrick Turski, Department of Radiology-MRI, University of Wisconsin School of Medicine and Public Health.)

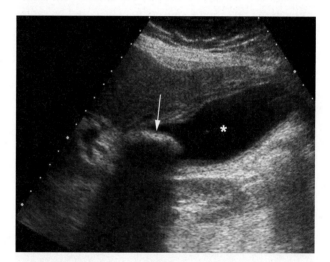

FIGURE 3–2 Computerized tomography. **A.** Normal cross-sectional image of the chest. v = vertebra, pt = pulmonary trunk (the left and right pulmonary arteries can be seen branching from it), aa = ascending aorta, ta = thoracic aorta, R = right lung, L = left lung. As in a regular radiograph, dense structures, such as bones and vessels containing blood, are white or gray, whereas the air-filled lungs are black. **B.** Cross-sectional image at approximately the same level of the chest as in A. This patient has tuberculosis. The left lung is scarred, cystic, and smaller than the right lung, which also contains numerous small white nodules of infection. The midline structures (aorta, pulmonary trunk) are shifted to the left as the left lung is scarred down. (Courtesy of Dr. Donald Yandow, Department of Radiology, University of Wisconsin School of Medicine and Public Health.)

FIGURE 3–4 Ultrasound. This gallbladder (dark, sharply demarcated longitudinal structure with white asterisk in the center) contains a stone (white crescent at the left edge of the gallbladder, white arrow) that is casting a shadow opposite the ultrasound probe because the sound waves are not passing through it. (Courtesy of Dr. Myron Pozniak, Department of Radiology, University of Wisconsin School of Medicine and Public Health.)

physical characteristics of protons among the elements allow production of two types of images. **T1 images** give a strong signal for lipids and **T2 images** give a strong signal for water. MRI does not expose the patient to radiation, but the patient must hold still for a very long time in a very noisy, enclosed space. The confinement and noise are often intolerable to patients, and the time and expense involved in obtaining MRI images are also prohibitive against its routine use. MRI is used especially in orthopedic (bone and joint) and neurologic (brain and

nerve) imaging. The anatomic detail provided by MRI is illustrated in **Figure 3–3**.

Ultrasound measures the reflection of high-frequency sound waves as they pass through body tissues. The greatest contrast is provided by interfaces of soft tissues and liquids; therefore, this technique has its greatest usefulness in studying cystic structures such as the gallbladder, urinary bladder, and the gravid (pregnant) uterus. It is the procedure of choice for detecting gallstones (**Figure 3–4**).

In pregnancy, it can be used without risk of radiation to the fetus. Twins and ectopic pregnancies are easily detected, and structural anomalies of the developing fetus and placenta, such as heart defects or disorders of placentation, can also be detected.

The subspecialty of **nuclear medicine** involves the injection of various radioactive materials into the bloodstream and subsequently determining their degree of localization within tissue. The body is scanned externally for radioactivity and the results recorded as a nuclear isotope scan. The functional activity of an organ can also be evaluated. For example, the amount of radioactive iodine taken up by the thyroid gland reflects thyroid function. **Positron emission tomography (PET)** involves injection of positron-emitting radionucleotides, such as carbon, nitrogen, or oxygen into the body (**Figure 3–5**). The positrons collide with electrons and matter is converted to energy. All nuclear medicine techniques have the ability to portray the functional status of tissues rather than merely their anatomy; however, they are quite expensive and do expose the patient to radiation, so their use in medicine is limited.

Radiation therapy is the branch of radiology involved in treatment of cancer and other conditions with x-rays and gamma rays. Some cancers may be cured by radiation. Others are irradiated to slow the progress of the disease and delay complications.

Anatomic Pathology Tests and Procedures

Surgical pathology involves the diagnosis of lesions in pieces of tissue removed from a patient. Diagnosis is based on gross (naked-eye) and microscopic examination by a pathologist (**Figure 3–6**). **Biopsy** is the procedure for obtaining small specimens. Partial (incisional) biopsy specimens include only part of the lesion and are done

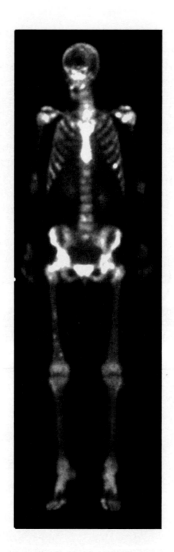

FIGURE 3–5 Nuclear isotope bone scan. Numerous small white dots, for example, in the right femur, represent the spread of cancer to bone. (Courtesy of Dr. Scott Perlman, Department of Radiology, University of Wisconsin School of Medicine and Public Health.)

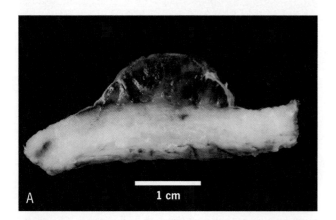

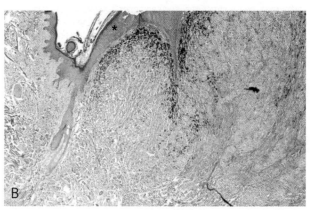

FIGURE 3–6 Pathologic examination of a resected specimen. This is a melanoma. **A.** Gross appearance. A brown nodule is sitting on the superficial aspect of a portion of excised skin. This is a wide and deep skin excision, extending to subcutaneous adipose tissue. The specimen has been cut down the middle, so you are looking at the cut surface of the lesion and skin. The gross description records the size, color, and texture of the lesion as well its relationship to surrounding structures. **B.** Microscopic appearance. The epidermis, or superficial part of the skin, is the dark pink layer marked by an asterisk. Notice how deeply the tumor cells (right side of the image) are infiltrating the dermis, or tissue underlying the epidermis. For prognostic purposes, the microscopic depth of infiltration needs to be precisely measured.

primarily for diagnosis. Needle biopsy, which involves the insertion of a needle into a solid organ and aspiration of a core of tissue, is widely used for the diagnosis of liver, kidney, and prostate disease. Excisional biopsy specimens include the entirety of a small lesion and are done for both diagnosis and treatment. The removal of large specimens in the operating room is called **resection**. Resected specimens are usually removed primarily for treatment purposes. Biopsy and resection specimens ordinarily require 1 to 2 days for preparation of microscopic slides and microscopic examination and diagnosis by a pathologist. When more rapid diagnosis is needed because a therapeutic decision needs to be made immediately, a **frozen section** can be prepared in a few minutes for interpretation by the pathologist.

Cytology specimens consist of cells sloughed or scraped from body surfaces. These are examined primarily to detect cancer cells (**Figure 3–7**). Ordinarily, a cytotechnologist examines the stained smears, and a pathologist interprets any abnormalities. Any body fluid, such as urine, sputum, cerebrospinal fluid, and pleural fluid, can be used for cytologic study. The majority of cytology specimens are from the uterine cervix (Pap smears). **Fine-needle aspiration (FNA)** is a technique that uses a small-caliber needle to obtain material for cytologic examination. The specimen can be collected directly across the skin if the lesion is superficial, such as a thyroid nodule, or it can be obtained under radiographic or endoscopic guidance, such as from masses in the lungs or pancreas. Fine-needle aspiration is faster and less expensive than open biopsy for the diagnosis of certain lesions but may not always provide a specimen that is adequate for diagnosis.

An **autopsy** is the postmortem examination of a body. Organs of the neck, chest, abdomen, and cranium are ordinarily examined to make a final evaluation of the nature and extent of disease and to determine the probable cause of death. Autopsies are important tools for observing and describing new diseases, such as AIDS or the recent "swine flu," but one of their most critical roles is to teach medical students, residents, and other healthcare workers about disease processes and to provide the treating physician with information about the extent of disease or confounding factors that may have interfered with his or her treatment plan. Biochemical, microbiologic, and immunologic tests can be performed if needed.

Forensic pathology is a subfield of pathology in which accidental and criminal deaths are investigated. Most forensic pathologists work in large metropolitan areas. In most communities, the investigation of accidental, sudden, or suspected criminal deaths is carried out by the county medical examiner or coroner, who is appointed or elected and who may not be a physician. When an autopsy is needed, the county medical examiner calls on a pathologist to perform the autopsy. Forensic pathology is technically a medical field, but it works very tightly with law enforcement, criminal investigation, and public health. Many of the laws or behaviors people take for granted, such as wearing seat belts while riding in a car and occupational safety regulations, came from lobbying for consumer and worker protection on the basis of evidence derived from forensic investigations.

Clinical Pathology Tests and Procedures

Clinical pathology or **laboratory medicine** is the branch of pathology that performs laboratory tests on tissues and fluids. The clinical pathology laboratory is subdivided into sections of **chemistry, hematology, blood bank (transfusion medicine), immunopathology, microbiology**, and **cytogenetics**. Biochemical tests on blood account for the largest number of tests done. Biochemical tests may be used to evaluate organ function or to detect relatively specific abnormalities. Some of the more common biochemical tests are for blood glucose, cholesterol and other lipids, and kidney and liver function tests. A **complete blood count (CBC)** is the most common hematologic test and consists of measurement of hemoglobin, counting of white and red blood cells, and microscopic evaluation for morphologic changes in the blood cells. Special hematologic tests are available for evaluation of various types of anemia and evaluation of blood coagulation. Transfusion medicine involves the procurement, typing, testing, processing, storage, and administering of blood components as well

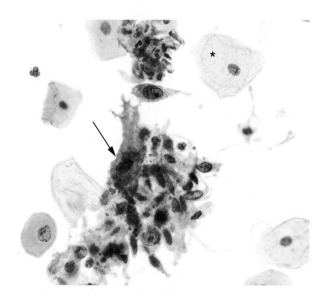

FIGURE 3–7 Pap smear. Compare the appearance of a normal cervical squamous cell (asterisk), which has abundant cytoplasm and a small, smoothly contoured nucleus, to that of a malignant squamous cell (arrow), which has irregular cell contours and two dark, abnormally shaped nuclei. (Courtesy of Dr. Josephine Harter, Department of Pathology and Laboratory Medicine, University of Wisconsin School of Medicine and Public Health.)

as evaluation of adverse reactions to transfusion therapy. Immunopathology involves the detection of antigens and antibodies in blood and tissue and the study of lymphocytes. Immunologic techniques are used to detect a wide variety of diseases including immunodeficiencies, allergic (hypersensitivity) diseases, and certain cancers. **Bacterial culture** is the most common test performed in the microbiology laboratory because bacteria are easily grown and can be tested for their sensitivity to antibiotics. The ease and means of detection of other types of microbes such as parasites and viruses are variable. Cytogenetics involves examining the chromosomal and genetic makeup of cells to diagnose and detect disorders such as trisomies, translocations, and deletions known to cause disease.

Molecular Diagnosis and Proteomics

Molecular methods have become extremely important adjunctive diagnostic tools. Conventionally, anatomic pathologists have used pattern recognition to diagnose tumors and other lesions on sections of tissue, and microbiologists have relied on cultures to identify pathogens. Molecular diagnosis goes beyond what can be seen by the eye to determine the "molecular signature" of neoplasms or microorganisms. Each microorganism and, presumably, tumor has a unique signature of genes that pathologists can use to identify it. This entails sequencing DNA or RNA that is known to be unique to that microorganism or neoplasm. Many microorganisms that require growth in culture for 24–48 hours or more for identification can now be identified in just a few hours with molecular techniques. Also, tumors that appear identical under the microscope, yet have vastly different prognoses, and thus require different treatments, can now be separated on the basis of their DNA profiles.

The sequencing of short stretches of a gene is done by **polymerase chain reaction (PCR)**. This involves amplifying or increasing the numbers of a particular gene or short sequence of nucleic acids to aid their detection. For example, if infection by a particular virus is suspected, PCR with a primer complementary to the viral nucleic acids can be performed on the patient's blood sample to increase their copy number, and then be detected by addition of fluorescent probes for that nucleic acid sequence. **Proteomics** refers to the mapping of the patterns of proteins involved in supporting cancerous growths. The uniqueness of these patterns forms the basis for identification of various tumors as well as their growth patterns. The proteins are identified by mass spectroscopy.

The ability to amplify and sequence large numbers of genes and then detect either gene sequences or particular genetic defects is leading to the discovery of new insights into pathophysiologic processes that can be harnessed for targeted care. **Pharmacogenomics** involves predicting a particular patient's response to particular drugs on the basis of the person's genetic makeup. The genes that encode for enzymes used in drug metabolism are determined so that the proper dose of the drug can be calculated according to predicted enzymatic activity before the drug is administered. This is particularly useful when treatment involves a drug that is notorious for eliciting an "idiosyncratic," or unpredictable, response yet is very dangerous if therapeutic levels are exceeded.

Targeted therapy refers to treatment with particular drugs if the substrate on which they act is known to be present. For example, breast cancer is routinely tested for the presence of estrogen and progesterone receptors and a particular growth factor receptor. If these are present, they can be blocked by pharmaceutical agents so that the tumor cells cannot respond to the growth-promoting effects of estrogenic hormones or the growth factor. This kind of therapy is becoming the model for treatment of neoplastic diseases. Other molecules, such as tyrosine kinase inhibitors, are increasingly being tested for in specific instances of disease to tailor therapy to the genetic makeup of the tumor.

In addition, pathologists apply molecular methods to diagnose inherited disorders, cardiovascular diseases, and immunoglobulin abnormalities. Identification of the perpetrator of a crime by DNA profiling using molecular methods has become a standard procedure in criminal investigations and law enforcement.

Public Health Laboratories

Public health laboratories are established by governments to help in the control of communicable diseases. For this reason, they perform many microbiologic tests, such as blood tests for syphilis and rabies and viral cultures and PCR to identify epidemics of virus infection. Water testing is another important aspect of community health. State health laboratories may serve as a reference laboratory and provide a link with the National Communicable Disease Laboratory in Atlanta, Georgia. Certain highly contagious diseases require reporting to state authorities.

Practice Questions

1. The attempt to discover disease in its earliest stage is referred to as
   A. preventive medicine.
   B. diagnostic testing.
   C. screening.
   D. public health.
   E. physical examination.

2. Which of the following is not a screening procedure?
   A. Mammography
   B. Liver biopsy
   C. Dental x-rays
   D. Visual acuity tests
   E. PSA test

3. A 34-year-old woman is found to have a lump in her breast by mammography. To make a diagnosis, the next procedure that should be performed is
   A. a PET scan.
   B. chemistry tests.
   C. magnetic resonance imaging (MRI).
   D. biopsy.

4. A 26-year-old man develops seizures. Which of the following procedures would best demonstrate that the seizures are caused by an abnormal mass in the brain?
   A. X-ray
   B. Ultrasound
   C. Magnetic resonance imaging (MRI)
   D. Fine-needle aspiration

5. A 67-year-old woman is diagnosed with breast cancer. Which of the following is a technique that could reasonably be used to detect whether the cancer has spread to other organs?
   A. Magnetic resonance imaging (MRI)
   B. Polymerase chain reaction (PCR)
   C. Positron emission tomography (PET)
   D. Ultrasound

Basic Disease Processes

The purpose of this section is to give you an overview of the fundamental mechanisms of disease processes. The principles we present here apply to almost every disease described throughout the rest of the book. We choose to present this material rather concisely so that we can spend more time on individual diseases later. We recommend that you study these chapters very thoroughly, review them as you progress through the book, and consult other texts to broaden your understanding of these topics.

Injury, Inflammation, and Repair

OUTLINE

OBJECTIVES

1. Understand how the duration of an injury affects the interrelationships between injury, inflammation, and repair.
2. Name the major causes, lesions, and manifestations of necrosis, inflammation, and repair.
3. List the functional and histologic changes that indicate cell death.
4. Distinguish cell necrosis from apoptosis.
5. Discuss the difference between metastatic and dystrophic calcification.
6. Compare acute inflammation, chronic inflammation, and granulomatous inflammation in terms of cause, histologic appearance, and manifestations.
7. List the sequence of events in a typical acute inflammatory reaction.
8. Describe how chemical mediators, including cytokines and chemokines, control the acute inflammatory response.
9. Explain how serous, fibrinous, and purulent exudates differ in composition and gross appearance.
10. Explain how abscesses, cellulitis, and ulcers differ in gross appearance and location within the body.
11. Describe abscesses in terms of cause, appearance, location, and resolution.
12. Understand what determines whether repair is by regeneration or fibrous connective tissue repair. Understand the sequence of each and how the outcomes differ.
13. Distinguish healing by primary union from healing by secondary union.
14. List the modifiers of inflammation and repair.
15. Be able to define and use in proper context all words and terms in bold print in this chapter.

KEY TERMS

abscess
accumulation
adhesion
adiposity
allergy
amyloid
anaphylaxis
anoxia
antibody
apoptosis
arachidonic acid
atrophy
autoimmune reaction

boil
bradykinin
brown atrophy
C3a
C5a
cardinal signs of
    inflammation
caseous necrosis
cell membrane
cellular immunity
cellulitis
chemokines
chemotaxis

coagulation (clotting)
  system
coagulation necrosis
collagen
comedone
complement proteins
complement system
cytokines
cytoplasmic organelles
debridement
degeneration
denervation atrophy
disuse atrophy
dystrophic calcification
edema
embolus
emigration
empyema
endocrine atrophy
endoplasmic reticulum
enzymatic fat necrosis
epithelial cells
epithelioid cells
exudate
factor XII
fatty change
fibrin
fibrinogen
fibrinous exudate
fibrous connective tissue
  repair
foreign body granuloma
free oxygen radical
furuncle
gangrenous necrosis
  (gangrene)
giant cells
glycogen storage
Golgi apparatus
granulation tissue
Hageman factor
heat
hemochromatosis
hemosiderosis
histamine
histiocyte
humoral immunity
hyaline
hyperemia
hypoxia
immunologic
infarct
infection
inflammation
inhibitors
ischemia

karyolysis
karyorrhexis
kinin system
kinins
leukocyte
leukotrienes
lipofuscin pigment
liquefaction necrosis
loss of function
lymphocyte
lysis
lysosome
macrophage
margination
mast cell
membrane attack complex
metastatic calcification
mitochondria
monocyte
necrosis
necrotizing fasciitis
neutrophil
opsonin
organ
organization
pain
parenchymal
paronychia
phagocyte
phagocytosis
pressure atrophy
prostaglandins
protein
purulent exudate
pus
pyknosis
pyogenic
regeneration
repair
resolution
ribosomes
sarcoidosis
scar
senile atrophy
serous exudate
sublethal (reversible) cell
  injury
suppurative inflammation
thrombus
tissue
toxic shock syndrome
transudate
trauma
ulcer
vasoactive amine

Review of Structure and Function

The body is made up of cells and intercellular substances that are capable of undergoing dynamic change to carry out body functions, including self-renewal. One or several of the more than 100 cell types, along with appropriate intercellular substances, make up a tissue. The term **tissue** is typically used to refer to a functional grouping of cells and intercellular substances. An **organ** is one or more tissues arranged into a structure that carries out a major body function. For example, liver tissue forms one massive organ called the liver, whereas loose connective tissue is a general type of tissue that may be a part of many organs. The cells that carry out the main function of an organ, and are usually most abundant and often unique to the organ, are called **parenchymal** cells. For example, hepatocytes, renal tubular epithelial cells, cardiac muscle cells, and osteocytes are the parenchymal cells of the liver, kidney, heart, and bone, respectively.

Typical components of a cell are illustrated in **Figure 4–1**. The nucleus is surrounded by a nuclear membrane and contains loosely arranged chromatin, which stains with basic dyes such as hematoxylin because of its high content of deoxyribonucleic acid (DNA). During cell division, the chromatin aggregates into discrete strands, or chromosomes, which replicate and separate to form two daughter cells. The nucleus is vital to the cell because the genetic code in its DNA is the ultimate regulator of cell function. Histologically, changes in the nucleus are reflective of abnormal processes, including malignant transformation, responses to inflammation and cell death.

The cytoplasm of a cell contains **cytoplasmic organelles**, with specialized functions, and a soluble component called the cytosol. The cytoplasm is enclosed by a highly specialized **cell membrane** that protects the cell from physical injury and selectively regulates the entrance and exit of various ions and nutrients, including amino acids, sugars, electrolytes such as sodium, potassium, and calcium, and fluid. Movement of water to and from the cell is largely dependent on the movement of ions across the cell membrane. A large amount of a cell's energy is spent on actively maintaining an electrical and osmotic gradient across the cell membrane and maintaining precise control over intracellular pH, osmolality, electrolyte concentration, and fluid balance. Cytoplasmic organelles include structures such as **mitochondria**,

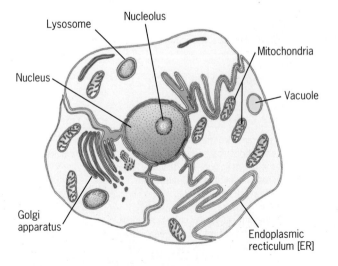

FIGURE 4–1 Components of a cell.

rough and smooth **endoplasmic reticulum**, **Golgi apparatus**, and **lysosomes**. Mitochondria are complex, membranous structures that generate energy for use by the cell. Injuries that interfere with energy production often cause the mitochondria to swell and later condense. The endoplasmic reticulum is a tortuous set of membranes. Rough endoplasmic reticulum is lined with small basophilic granules called **ribosomes** because of their high content of ribonucleic acid. Proteins produced under the enzymatic control of ribosomes are carried along the rough endoplasmic reticulum to the Golgi apparatus, where they are modified, sorted, and stored for secretion. The smooth endoplasmic reticulum also serves to transport materials through the cell and is the site of production of many biochemical substances other than proteins. Lysosomes are membrane-bound packets of digestive enzymes. Lysosomes may coalesce to surround and digest foreign substances that have been engulfed (phagocytosed) by the cell. Worn out or injured parts of the cytoplasm may also be digested by lysosomes, a process known as autophagocytosis.

A simple classification of tissue components is shown in **Table 4–1**. The two most varied classes of cells are epithelial cells and connective tissue cells. The distinction between these two classes of cells is very important in pathology because they react quite differently in disease situations. **Epithelial cells** work with each other as coherent units to carry out specialized functions, such as protection of body surfaces, secretion of specific products, and special metabolic functions. Injury interferes with their specialized function and causes them to revert to a more primitive stage for purposes of reproduction to replace cells that have been killed. Connective tissue cells are more loosely arranged and are involved in general support functions, such as providing physical support and facilitating the movement of fluids and nutrients. An example of the arrangement of the various cell types into a tissue is shown in **Figure 4–2**.

White blood cells (**leukocytes**) are mobile connective tissue–type cells that are specialized to attack foreign substances. Each type has a characteristic morphologic appearance (**Figure 4–3**). **Neutrophils**, also called polymorphonuclear leukocytes or "polys," and **monocytes** can engulf (phagocytose) and digest foreign materials such as bacteria. When monocytes leave the bloodstream

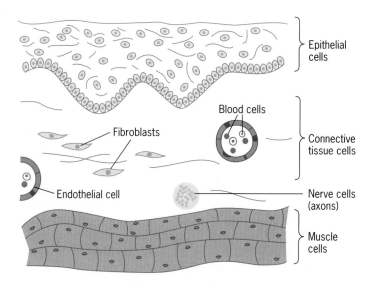

FIGURE 4–2 Major cell types in the wall of the oral cavity.

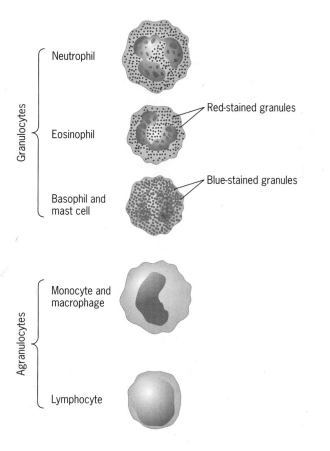

FIGURE 4–3 Types of white blood cells.

TABLE 4–1	Structural Elements of Tissues

Cells
- Epithelium (e.g., mucosal cells of the gastrointestinal tract, epidermis of skin)
- Connective tissue cells
  - Fixed: Fibrocytes, chondrocytes, osteocytes, endothelial cells
  - Mobile: Blood cells
- Muscle cells (e.g., skeletal muscle, cardiac muscle, smooth muscle of uterus, gastrointestinal tract, bladder)
- Nervous tissue cells

Intercellular substances
- Basement membranes
- Ground substance
- Collagen
- Elastin
- Cartilage
- Bone

they differentiate into another type of motile phagocyte called **macrophages** or **histiocytes**. **Lymphocytes** direct the attack against persistent foreign materials by remembering their chemical structure. Lymphocytes release substances (cytokines and chemokines) that kill cells in the area of the foreign material and other substances that attract macrophages to the area. The macrophages, in turn, can phagocytose both the foreign material and dead cells to prevent further spread of the injurious material. Some lymphocytes (B cells) also transform into plasma cells to produce **antibodies**. Antibodies attach to the unique chemical structure of the foreign substance (antigen) to aid in neutralizing or destroying it. The other two types of white blood cells, basophils and eosinophils, are much less abundant. Both are involved in allergic reactions.

The connective tissue structure of the body provides physical support and facilitates transportation. Tissues that give physical support include bone, cartilage, ligaments, tendons, fascia, and other fibrous tissues. At the microscopic level, connective tissues contain ground substance, which allows passage of fluid and nutrients. Basement membranes surround epithelial clusters and allow passage of fluid and nutrients to and from the epithelial cells. **Collagen** is the most abundant component of connective tissues. The amount of collagen relates to the strength and fibrous nature of the connective tissue. Thus, loose connective tissue, such as fascia, contains little collagen, and dense connective tissue, such as tendons, contains much collagen. Vessels course through the supporting connective tissue to allow fluids to be carried close to epithelial cells and other active tissues such as muscle.

Regulation of tissue fluids is a function of movement of water in and out of small blood vessels (capillaries and venules) and uptake of fluid by lymphatics. Fluid and nutrients pass out of the small blood vessels and diffuse through the ground substance and basement membranes so that exchange with cells can occur. Reverse movement can occur back into blood vessels or into lymphatic vessels. The most important factors in this regulatory process are the pressure in the vessels, the osmotic pressure difference between tissue and blood resulting from the relative amount of large protein molecules present, and the size of the pores between endothelial cells in the lining of small vessels. This regulatory process is important in situations of injury because larger amounts of fluid and nutrients are needed to react to the injury.

Physiologic replacement of cells is a normal process that closely relates to the repair of injuries to be discussed later in this chapter. Certain body cells wear out rapidly and are continually being replaced. These include blood cells and cells lining body surfaces such as skin and intestinal mucosa. Most glandular epithelial cells and cells that form the supportive connective tissue undergo very slow replacement but are capable of more rapid replacement if necessary. Other types of cells, such as cardiac muscle cells and neurons, are replaced only rarely, if at all.

Events Following Injury

The events following injury involve, in varying proportions, necrosis, inflammation, and repair. You can think of these processes as a temporal and morphologic continuum. **Necrosis** is the death of cells or tissue as a result of an endogenous or exogenous injury. Mild forms of injury may produce sublethal cell injury without necrosis, changes that are referred to as **degeneration**. Lethal and sublethal cellular changes occur together in varying proportions. **Inflammation** is the vascular and cellular response to necrosis or sublethal cell injury and is the body's mechanism of limiting the spread of injury and removing necrotic debris. **Repair** refers to the body's attempt to replace dead cells, whether by regeneration of the original tissue or replacement by connective tissue.

Another type of cell death is **apoptosis**, often referred to as programmed cell death. Apoptotic cell death is not necessarily an indication of injury. It occurs, for example, during embryogenesis when not all cells generated are needed. It is also the mechanism of ridding the body of excess lymphocytes following resolution of an inflammatory or immune event, of hormone-dependent cell death after the hormonal stimulus has been removed, and of tumor cell death. It may, however, also occur following injury from a variety of agents that might cause necrosis under other conditions. Apoptosis is referred to as *programmed* because it results from the activation of specific genes following appropriate stimuli. In tissue sections, it differs in appearance from necrosis (**Figure 4–4**) in that the cell shrinks, the nuclear chromatin condenses into dense masses, blebs form in the cytoplasm, and the apoptotic cells are phagocytosed by macrophages or adjacent parenchymal cells. Importantly, apoptosis does not elicit inflammation. Mainly for the latter reason, further discussion of cell death in this chapter concerns only necrosis.

The relative intensities of necrosis, inflammation, and repair depend on the magnitude of the injury, the duration of injury, and, to some extent, on the location within the body and the nature of the injury. Some examples of how necrosis, inflammation, and repair vary with intensity and duration of injury are shown in **Figure 4–5**. In general, inflammation begins immediately after cell injury. Repair is usually not well established until necrosis ceases, although in very chronic injuries, all three processes are likely to occur together. Inflammation itself, when intense, is a cause of necrosis. The body, in a sense, sacrifices some of its own tissue to isolate an injurious agent.

Injury

Acute injury most prominently affects cells because cells are more susceptible to injury than are the noncellular connective tissue elements. Cells may be injured by any of the exogenous and endogenous causes listed in **Table 4–2**.

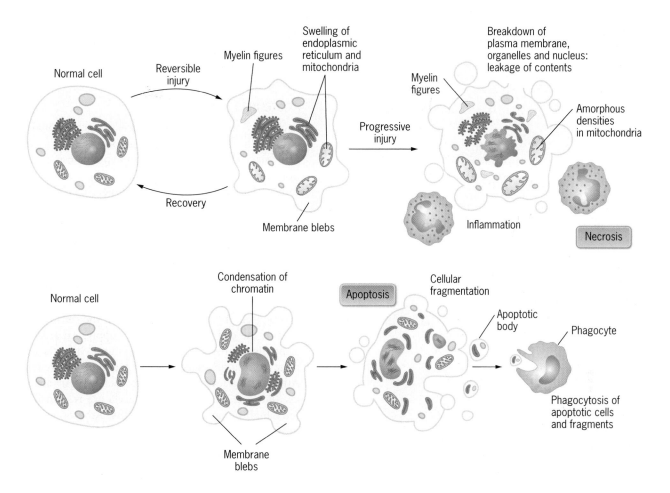

FIGURE 4–4 Differences between necrosis and apoptosis.

The critical difference between **sublethal (reversible) cell injury** and necrosis is whether the cell can recover or is dead. Certain changes in the nucleus, as seen in microscopic sections, indicate cell death. Nuclear changes may include condensation of the nucleus (**pyknosis**), fragmentation of the nucleus (**karyorrhexis**), and lysis or fading of the nucleus (**karyolysis**) (Figure 4–4 and **Figure 4–6**). These nuclear changes take a number of hours to develop, so cells may not show these changes histologically even though they are dead. For example, heart tissue in a person who dies within 12 hours of sustaining a myocardial infarct (heart attack) may not show the histologic changes of necrosis. If the patient had lived, some of the myocardial cells would have developed the histologic changes of necrosis, whereas others may have developed reversible changes and then recovered. Reversible cell injury is characterized by preservation of the nucleus and variable changes in the cytoplasm such as swelling or condensation of the cell, nucleus, and/or cytoplasmic organelles. These histologic changes reflect biochemical changes in the cell. There is no exact biochemical end point that determines cell death, but depletion in the cell's energy system (especially adenosine triphosphate [ATP]) and alteration of cell membrane permeability are critical events leading to cell death.

Many different types of cell injury result, at least in part, from the generation of **free oxygen radicals** that damage vital cell structures such as membranes. Free radicals are unstable oxygen molecules having only a single unpaired electron in their outer orbit and are generated by the reduction of molecular oxygen to water. They react with proteins, lipids, and carbohydrates, releasing energy that damages membranes and DNA.

TABLE 4–2 **Endogenous and Exogenous Causes of Tissue Injury**

Endogenous	Exogenous
• Tissue necrosis • Ischemia • Anoxia • Immune reactions • Allergies • Autoimmune diseases • Hypersensitivity reactions	• Infections (bacterial, viral, or parasitic) • Trauma (blunt or penetrating) • Physical agents • Burns • Frostbite • Irradiation • Chemical agents • Acids • Bases • Environmental toxins • Foreign bodies

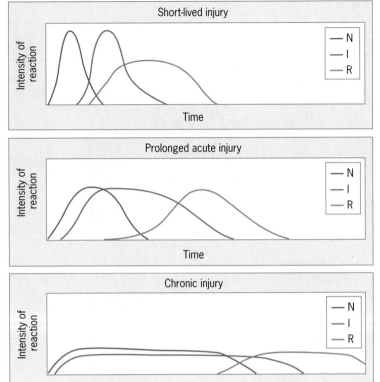

FIGURE 4–5 Time sequences of necrosis (N), inflammation (I), and repair (R).

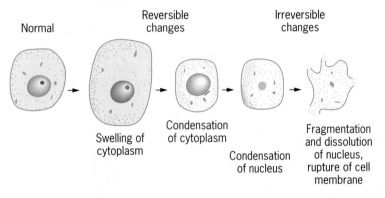

FIGURE 4–6 Cellular changes leading to cell death (necrosis).

Once the nucleus is destroyed or the cell membrane disrupted, the cell cannot recover. After cell death, enzymes released from the cell's own lysosomes begin to digest the remains of the cell. Other events associated with necrosis include influx of calcium, dissolution of ribosomes, clumping of DNA followed by its enzymatic digestion, and finally rupture of the cell membrane. These changes elicit an inflammatory response. In fact, necrotic tissue is a very potent stimulus of inflammation.

Acute changes resulting from sudden injury to a cell or tissue lead to cell death or recovery within a short time. Necrosis is often associated with acute injury. Chronic injury (mild continuous injury) leads to cumulative effects on the cells and the tissues. Necrosis is not usually prominent and may be of such a low degree as to be imperceptible in histologic sections.

Acute Injury and Necrosis

Lack of oxygen (**anoxia**) or reduced oxygen (**hypoxia**) is one of the most common causes of acute injury and necrosis. Cells are vulnerable to hypoxia in proportion to their oxygen requirements; thus, metabolically active cells are selectively vulnerable. Selective vulnerability is well illustrated by cases of systemic anoxia from such causes as carbon monoxide poisoning, blood loss, or suffocation. In these situations, neurons in the brain and the kidneys' tubular epithelial cells are more vulnerable to necrosis than are other types of cells. Localized hypoxia resulting from poor blood flow is called **ischemia**. When severe, ischemia leads to necrosis of the cells in the area of the compromised blood supply. An area of ischemic necrosis is called an **infarct**. Infarcts are most commonly caused by obstruction of arteries. Atherosclerotic plaques that obstruct coronary arteries and lead to myocardial infarcts are responsible for a high percentage of all deaths. Atherosclerotic obstruction also is important in producing infarcts of the brain, legs, kidneys, and other sites.

Thrombi and emboli are also important causes of ischemic necrosis. A **thrombus** is a blood clot that forms during life in a blood vessel as a result of activation of the coagulation mechanism. It is composed of layers of fibrin and entrapped blood cells. An **embolus** is any particulate object that travels in the bloodstream from one site to another. It most commonly arises from a thrombus but may be composed of other substances such as bone marrow, fat, air, or cancer tissue. Thrombotic emboli most commonly originate in the leg veins and travel through the vena cava and right heart to the pulmonary arteries or from the left side of the heart through the aorta to various organs such as brain, legs, kidneys, spleen, and intestines. Bone marrow and fat emboli occur from trauma to bones; when severe, the fat globules pass through the pulmonary vessels and gain access to the systemic circulation where they may cause obstruction of the small vessels of the brain.

Trauma, infection, and hypersensitivity are other common causes of acute injury and necrosis. **Trauma** disrupts cells by direct physical force; the effects are dependent on the site injured and nature of the force applied. Although there are many types of **infections** and the degree of injury varies widely, most of the damage is produced by the body's own inflammatory reaction to the invading microorganism. **Immunologic** mechanisms are an important part of the inflammatory reaction and also contribute to the damage produced by inflammation, but the immune damage is usually less than the potential damage that could be inflicted by the offending agent. When an immunologic or presumed immunologic reaction occurs in sensitized individuals only, the reaction is called a hypersensitivity reaction or **allergy**. Poison ivy, hay fever, hives, and contact dermatitis are common examples. Sometimes the body's immune system reacts to its own tissues (**autoimmune reaction**), producing destructive diseases such as rheumatoid arthritis, lupus erythematosus, and thyroiditis.

The morphologic changes of reversible cell injury and necrosis form a continuum. If the injury is mild and functional changes following the injury go away in a few hours, the cells involved undergo sublethal changes with an eventual return to their normal appearance. If functional changes persist, it is likely that at least some cells will undergo necrosis; recovery then depends on regeneration, a process discussed later in the chapter. Study of biopsy specimens or tissues removed at autopsy allows the pathologist the opportunity to evaluate the extent of injury. Changes in reversibly damaged cells are limited to the cytoplasm; necrotic cells have both cytoplasmic and nuclear changes. Typically, the early change is cytoplasmic swelling, producing enlarged cells with pale cytoplasm. Later, the cytoplasm may be shrunken and more densely eosinophilic than normal. The development of nuclear changes—pyknosis, karyorrhexis, or karyolysis—indicates progression to necrosis. Thus, when reversible changes predominate, a tissue is enlarged; when necrosis predominates, a tissue is of normal size or shrunken.

Necrotic tissue takes on different gross and microscopic appearances depending on circumstances; recognition of these differences suggests the cause of the necrosis. The following types of necrosis are descriptive.

Coagulation necrosis is most commonly caused by anoxia, whether it be generalized or ischemic. In many tissues, the coagulation process evolves slowly, over a number of days, producing the characteristic preservation of cell and tissue outlines until the later stages of the process. The pathologist can recognize the coagulation necrosis of an infarct by its pale yellow color and solid but soft texture. The location, size, and shape of the infarct depend on the area supplied by the blocked artery.

Liquefaction necrosis is most commonly caused by certain types of bacteria, known as pyogenic bacteria. Pyogenic bacteria attract neutrophils into the area and the enzymes released by the neutrophils liquefy the dead tissue. The resultant thick, creamy mixture of dead tissue and neutrophils is called **pus** or **purulent exudate**. When cut into, an area of liquefaction necrosis exudes pus and leaves a hole in the tissue.

Caseous necrosis is most commonly caused by *Mycobacterium tuberculosis*, the bacterium that causes tuberculosis, or by certain types of fungi. Caseous necrosis looks different because it is necrosis of diseased tissue. The causative organisms are attacked by large numbers of lipid-containing macrophages.

Necrosis of these macrophages produces a solid, amorphous, cheesy mass. Microscopically, a confluent mass of red cytoplasm with scattered nuclear dust remains. The alert pathologist, however, uses special staining techniques to demonstrate the causative organisms in the caseous material and sometimes the organisms can be cultured.

Enzymatic fat necrosis, which occurs following injury to the pancreas and surrounding adipose tissue as a result of leakage of that organ's digestive enzymes, produces chalky, yellow-white nodules somewhat resembling caseous necrosis. The location, however, is limited to the pancreas and surroundings.

Gangrenous necrosis (gangrene) is coagulation necrosis with superimposed decomposition by saprophytic bacteria. It is similar to postmortem decomposition except that only a portion of the body is dead. In gas gangrene, however, the organisms causing the gangrene include a strain of bacteria of the genus *Clostridium* that produces gas and a necrotizing toxin. The toxin of gas gangrene can spread to normal tissue and produce lethal effects.

Chronic Injury

Chronic injury may produce a decrease in tissue size (**atrophy**) or **accumulation** of material within cells or between cells. Atrophy may be the result of a decrease in the size of cells, a decrease in the number of cells, or both. A gradual loss of cells is the most common mechanism. Chronic injuries associated with accumulation of substances are quite different from atrophy. Many times, cells slowly accumulate their own metabolic products or exogenous materials, with a resultant decrease in cell function. The storage of these materials may even result in an enlarged cell, albeit one with decreased function. The types of chronic cell or tissue degeneration are classified according to the cause of the atrophy or type of material accumulated.

Atrophy

Senile atrophy is caused by aging. Tissues often become smaller and decrease in functional capacity, presumably as a natural part of the aging process. For example, the brains of older people become smaller, while decreased memory and slowed thought processes provide some evidence of decreased cellular function.

Disuse atrophy occurs when the cells are unable to carry out their normal function. For example, when an arm or leg is placed in a cast, the muscle cells gradually become smaller and show a decreased ability to contract. Disuse atrophy may be reversible. Once the cast is removed and the limb is exercised, the atrophic muscle cells can regain their prior function and structure. However, if muscle cells are immobilized because of permanent loss of nervous stimulation—for example, after the traumatic severance of a nerve—they will stay atrophied. This type of atrophy is called **denervation atrophy**.

Pressure atrophy results from steady pressure on tissue, such as might be produced by the mass of an expanding tumor. Bedsores are another common example. They occur in chronically bedridden patients because of continued external pressure on the skin.

Endocrine atrophy results from decreased hormonal stimulation. Certain organs are maintained in a functional state by the action of hormones on them. Insufficient hormonal stimulation results in atrophy in that organ. For example, the decrease in estrogen and progesterone at the time of menopause results in atrophy of the breasts and the uterus.

Accumulations

Various substances can accumulate within cells (**Figure 4–7**). Accumulation of lipid within cells is called **fatty change** or fatty metamorphosis. Fatty change should be distinguished from **adiposity**. In adiposity, there is an increased storage of fat in fat cells; in fatty change, fat droplets appear as an abnormality in parenchymal cells. Fatty change may be either acute or chronic and characteristically occurs in cells involved in fat metabolism, especially the liver. The liver takes in lipid in the form of triglycerides (from dietary absorption) and free fatty acids (from adipose tissue stores or absorption). The liver metabolizes triglycerides and free fatty acids to lipoprotein, a much more soluble form of lipid that can be exported for use by other tissues. Droplets of triglyceride may form in hepatocytes because of decreased production of lipoprotein or increased uptake of lipid from the blood (Figure 4–7C). Causes of fatty liver include conditions that induce mobilization of more fat than the liver can handle, such as diabetes mellitus; excess dietary intake as in obesity; chemical injury, as in alcoholism or carbon tetrachloride poisoning; and acute starvation, where there is depletion of the proteins needed to form lipoproteins. In chronic alcoholism, the liver may become more than twice its normal size as a

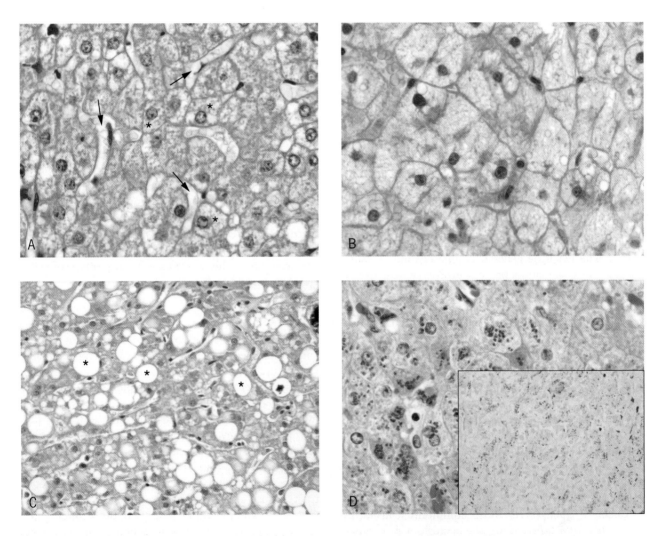

FIGURE 4–7 Examples of accumulations. **A.** Normal liver. Hepatocytes (*) have fluffy-appearing cytoplasm. Open spaces (arrows) are sinusoids. **B.** Liver in patient with glycogen storage disease. The hepatocyte cytoplasm is swollen and pale. The pallor comes from increased cytoplasmic glycogen. The sinusoids are inconspicuous because they are compressed by the swollen hepatocytes. **C.** Steatosis. Before tissue processing, the holes (*) were occupied by lipid droplets. **D.** Hemosiderosis. Brown granules have accumulated in hepatocytes. The Prussian blue reaction (inset) demonstrates that these brown granules are hemosiderin.

result of the accumulation of fat in hepatocytes. In diabetes mellitus, there is decreased uptake of fat in adipose tissue and increased accumulation in the liver. Alcoholism is the most common cause of clinically significant fatty liver in affluent societies.

Glycogen storage is an example of accumulation of carbohydrate. It occurs in rare genetic conditions where specific enzymes for glycogen breakdown are missing. The glycogen accumulates in various organs (Figure 4–7B) and eventually causes malfunction.

Excess **protein** can accumulate within cells and become compacted, producing a dense, homogeneous, eosinophilic deposit called **hyaline**. Excess collagen and compacted fibrin clots are the most common causes of hyalinization. **Amyloid** is a hyaline deposit that has a crystalline chemical structure, which polarizes light and stains with the dye Congo red. Certain small proteins can leak from the blood and crystallize to form extracellular deposits of amyloid. Examples of proteins that can form amyloid include immunoglobulin light chains derived from abnormal proliferations of plasma cells, serum amyloid-associated protein produced by the liver in prolonged chronic inflammation, and beta protein deposited in the brain in Alzheimer disease. Amyloid deposits develop very slowly, affect organ function late in the course of disease, and are not reversible.

Accumulations of minerals and pigments include calcification, hemosiderosis, and "brown atrophy." In some situations, the deposition of minerals or pigments is associated with obvious tissue injury, but in others it is difficult to prove that excessive accumulation of a given pigment or mineral is deleterious to that tissue. Calcification is of two types. Excessive blood calcium, which may result from certain metabolic disorders, leads to calcium accumulation in normal tissues, especially those that excrete acid from the body such as renal tubules, lung, and gastric mucosa. This is termed **metastatic calcification**. Dying cells take on calcium. When this calcium remains as a deposit in the area of necrosis, it is known as **dystrophic calcification**. Most dystrophic calcification causes no problem in itself, but because calcium is radiopaque, it allows the radiologist to spot areas of disease. For example, foci of caseous necrosis caused by tuberculosis undergo calcification and thereby remain visible on x-rays of the lungs for years after the primary infection has subsided, and calcifications on mammography alert radiologists to the presence of necrosis associated with breast cancer.

Hemosiderosis and **hemochromatosis** are terms applied to excessive iron accumulation in tissues; the former term implies iron accumulation in tissues, while the latter term implies a more serious condition associated with tissue damage. Typically, the absorption of iron from the intestines is carefully regulated so that the body has enough for production of red blood cells and other needs, but not too much. Excessive iron may be introduced into the body by blood transfusion or excessive absorption may occur as a result of genetic causes, dietary overload, or increased need because of destruction of red blood cells in hemolytic anemias. The excess iron in the form of ferritin combines with protein to form hemosiderin, a brown pigment that accumulates in cells, especially macrophages and hepatocytes (Figure 4–7D). Hemochromatosis is usually caused by a genetic defect in regulation of iron uptake, and its damaging effects are most felt in the liver and pancreatic islets with resultant cirrhosis of the liver and diabetes mellitus. Periodic withdrawal of blood lowers body iron stores and slows down the progression of this disease.

Brown atrophy is an old term applied to the brown color of the heart and the liver that develops with aging as a result of the accumulation of **lipofuscin pigment** in myocardial fibers and hepatocytes. This poorly defined pigment, composed of lipid, carbohydrate, and protein, is the residue of lysosomal digestion of cellular debris and has no clinical significance other than being a marker for aging or increased cellular damage.

BOX 4–1   Effects of Injury

Causes

Physical injury

Chemical injury

Infection

Anoxia/ischemia

Antigen–antibody reactions

Metabolic abnormalities

Radiation

Lesions

Reversible cell changes

Necrosis

Atrophy

Accumulations

Manifestations

Loss of cell function related to site involved

Inflammation

Inflammation is the protective response that the body mounts in response to injury. The term reflects the observation that an inflamed lesion is like fire: red, hot, and painful. As you have seen, necrosis reflects the destructive effects of injury to cells. Inflammation is a process by which fluid, chemicals, and cells are brought to an injured area to limit the extent of injury, remove necrotic debris, and prepare for the healing process. Inflammation involves very complex chemical and, to a lesser extent, neural mechanisms that serve to turn the "fire fighters" on quickly and mobilize more reserves, but also to turn the process off so that these cellular and chemical responses do not destroy any more normal tissue than is necessary to control the spread of injury.

The nature of the inflammatory response is stereotyped; the degree and duration vary depending on the cause and time course of the injury. The stereotyped response is described in the section titled "Acute Inflammation," and the variations produced by prolonged injury and certain agents are described in the section titled "Chronic Inflammation." Although inflammation is described as a protective response, it also has damaging effects. The potential for drugs to modify the inflammatory response has stimulated continued research to unravel its complex biochemical control mechanisms.

Acute Inflammation

Overview

Acute inflammation consists of tightly coordinated vascular and cellular responses to injury. The vascular response results in increased blood flow to the injured area and increased vascular permeability so that water, electrolytes, and serum proteins leak into the tissue spaces. The cellular response refers to the movement of leukocytes, predominantly neutrophils and monocytes, from the blood into the tissue.

These events produce the **cardinal signs of inflammation**: redness, swelling, heat, pain, and loss of function. The increased blood flow in dilated vessels is called **hyperemia** and causes redness. The leakage of fluid into the tissue is called **edema** and causes swelling. The increased blood in the area causes **heat**. **Pain** results from the pressure of the swelling and the action of kinins on nerve endings. **Loss of function** results from the attempt to protect the painful, swollen lesion from further injury.

The effects of inflammation are to destroy or limit the spread of the causative agent and to clean up the debris in preparation for repair. In simple injuries, such as a burn, a cut, or a chemical injury where the chemical has been diluted away, the causative agent is no longer a threat and the inflammatory reaction is proportional to the amount of tissue damage. Tissue damage itself incites a mild inflammatory reaction, enough to bring leukocytes to digest and remove the debris from the dead cells and increase lymph flow to carry away fluid from the lesion. Both neutrophils and macrophages engulf particulate matter, a process called **phagocytosis**. Microscopically, acute inflammation is characterized by the presence of abundant neutrophils, usually intermixed with a few macrophages (**Figure 4–8**).

Vascular and Cellular Events

Phagocytes (neutrophils and macrophages) play a key role in the inflammatory process. They move from their normal central location in the bloodstream to the periphery as the venule dilates and the flow of blood slows (**Figure 4–9**). This is called **margination**. The marginated leukocytes then stick to the endothelial cells

---

BOX 4–2 Acute Inflammation

Causes

All types of acute injuries (necrosis)

Pyogenic infections

Hypersensitivities

Lesions

Hyperemia

Exudate

Neutrophils and macrophages

Manifestations

Redness

Heat

Swelling

Pain

Loss of function

Fever

Leukocytosis

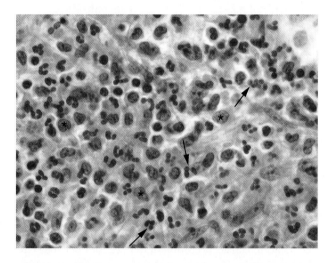

FIGURE 4–8 Acute inflammation is characterized by the presence of numerous neutrophils (polymorphonuclear leukocytes) (arrows). Notice that macrophages (*) are also numerous.

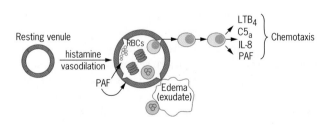

FIGURE 4–9 Vascular phase of acute inflammation.

(adhesion) because of complementary molecules on the leukocytes and endothelial cells that are activated by various chemical mediators of the inflammatory process. Once chemically stuck to the endothelial cell, leukocytes crawl between endothelial cells into the tissue (emigration). Neutrophils migrate fastest from the vessel to the injured site, arriving within minutes and accumulating over hours. Macrophages are slower moving and peak later than neutrophils. Neutrophils may die soon after arrival at the injured site to liberate their powerful digestive enzymes, or they may phagocytose and digest cellular debris and foreign material before dying.

Neutrophils are particularly important in certain types of bacterial infections such as those caused by *Staphylococcus aureus*, various streptococci (including *S. pneumoniae*), gonococci, meningococci, coliform bacteria, anaerobic bacteria from the intestines, and others. These organisms are responsible for a large number of infections because many are part of the normal flora of the skin, mouth, respiratory tract, and intestines, and they are ever ready to cause infection whenever host defense mechanisms break down. Neutrophils recognize and move toward certain chemicals contained in bacteria by the process of chemotaxis. Chemotaxis is the movement of white blood cells in response to a chemical gradient. The chemical gradient may be established by chemicals released from bacteria or by chemokines, small proteins produced endogenously (by the body itself) during the inflammatory response—for example, upon activation of the complement or coagulation cascades (discussed later).

Once at the site of an infection, neutrophils rapidly phagocytose the offending agent, including bacteria (Figure 4–10). Bacteria have evolved mechanisms of resisting phagocytosis, such as a thick polysaccharide capsule (*S. pneumoniae*) that evades host detection mechanisms. The host can counter by producing antibodies that attach to this capsule and are easily recognized by phagocytes. Such phagocytosis-promoting antibodies are called opsonins. Opsonins are important in the response to organisms that have been previously encountered or when antibodies have been artificially induced by immunization. The brisk neutrophil reaction to these bacteria often results in the death of many neutrophils and much tissue breakdown to produce pus; for this reason the organisms are referred to as pyogenic (pus forming).

Macrophages arrive later and are hardier than neutrophils; they carry the major load in cleaning up the inflammatory debris, including the dead neutrophils. The relative numbers of neutrophils and macrophages depend on the amount and nature of the dead tissue and whether highly chemotactic foreign substances, such as pyogenic bacteria, are present. A staphylococcal infection has lots of neutrophils; injured adipose tissue from trauma has mostly macrophages removing the spilled lipid. Macrophages also predominate in reactions to large inert foreign particles such as talc or suture material. They surround the foreign material and often form multinucleated giant cells, which remain for a long time in the tissue.

Phagocytosis by neutrophils and macrophages entails sequestration of the engulfed particle, whether bacterium or foreign material, into a cytoplasmic compartment where killing occurs mainly by the action of free oxygen radicals, such as hydrogen peroxide (H_2O_2), hydroxyl halide ($HOCl^-$), nitric oxide (NO), or hydroxyl ions (HO). Digestion of the particles follows release of hydrolases and other enzymes.

The role of noncellular elements in inflammation is very important as well. The increased fluidity of the lesion facilitates movement of cells and chemicals and promotes increased lymph flow to carry fluid debris away from the area. It may also serve to dilute offending agents such as toxins and antigens. Fibrinogen is a soluble blood protein that may leak into the inflamed site and be converted to a stringy polymer, fibrin. This process involves several enzymes and is activated by exposure to damaged tissue. The formation of fibrin serves as a barrier to prevent the spread of injury; for example, the scab formed over a scrape of the skin is composed largely of fibrin and serves to keep bacteria out and fluid in. Because fibrinogen is a very large protein, it leaks into tissue only when the increase in vascular permeability is severe; even then, some of the fibrin that is formed is lysed by the enzyme fibrinolysin. These control mechanisms prevent the formation of fibrin in mild injuries when it is not needed.

Patients who lack the ability to mount an acute inflammatory reaction succumb to infections that are easily warded off by people with an intact inflammatory response mechanism, so the reaction is obviously very important. The acute inflammatory reaction can also be very damaging, so its control is important. It must be activated quickly and turned off when no longer needed. The control mechanisms are complex and primarily involve chemical mediators of inflammation. The following discussion is intended only to introduce the most important classes of chemical mediators of inflammation. The interested reader is referred to standard pathology textbooks for more detailed discussion.

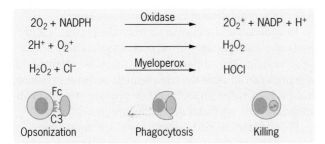

$$2O_2 + NADPH \xrightarrow{\text{Oxidase}} 2O_2^+ + NADP + H^+$$
$$2H^+ + O_2^+ \longrightarrow H_2O_2$$
$$H_2O_2 + Cl^- \xrightarrow{\text{Myeloperox}} HOCl$$

Opsonization Phagocytosis Killing

FIGURE 4–10 Phagocytosis.

Chemical Mediators

The inflammatory reaction is initiated by local factors in the injured tissue. Stimulation of small nerve endings causes arteriolar dilation, but this reaction is not an essential or prominent event. The release of **histamine** or other **vasoactive amines** from mast cells is an important initial event. **Mast cells** are scattered throughout the connective tissue of the body and contain large amounts of histamine in their dense granules. Histamine can be released from mast cells by two types of inflammatory reactions: immune complex reactions and atopic allergy. Histamine diffuses from the injured site to cause vasodilation and increased permeability of adjacent small venules. The venules leak plasma proteins, particularly albumin, which draw water into the tissue by osmotic pressure. Mast cells rapidly become depleted of histamine and the released histamine is diluted and inactivated by the influx of water into the tissue, so the inflammatory reaction cannot be sustained by this reaction alone.

Once initiated, the inflammatory reaction is rapidly and greatly amplified by chemicals circulating in the blood. Three chemical systems are involved: the **kinin system**, the **complement system**, and the coagulation system. In each case, an inactive protein precursor is activated by a series of enzymatic steps, with products of the reaction itself acting as catalysts to further speed up the reaction. To counter the dangers of accidental triggering or endless activation of these reactions, **inhibitors**—enzymes that destroy products of the reactions—are formed at the same time as the pro-inflammatory molecules, and the dilutional effect of the bloodstream decreases the concentration and therefore the cumulative effects of the activated inflammatory mediators.

When **kinins** leak through the venule made permeable by histamine, they are activated to become **bradykinin** (**Figure 4–11**). Bradykinin itself causes increased vascular permeability and is a major factor in sustaining the flow of fluid and chemicals to the inflammatory site by a self-perpetuating reaction. Bradykinin also acts on nerve endings to cause pain. At some point, bradykinin is deactivated faster than it forms and the vascular response gradually subsides.

When fibrinogen leaks through the permeable vessels along with other blood coagulation factors, the **coagulation (clotting) system** is activated (**Figure 4–12**). The end effect of this system is polymerization of fibrinogen to fibrin. As already mentioned, fibrin serves as a barrier to the spread of the injurious agent. Both the kinin and coagulation systems are initiated by a tissue factor known as the **Hageman factor** or **factor XII**.

The splitting of **complement proteins** into several active factors is initiated by complexes of antigen and antibody (**Figure 4–13**) or by an alternate pathway induced by bacterial endotoxins and some normal tissue proteins. Complement fragment **C5a** is an important mediator of chemotaxis and, along with fragment **C3a**, causes increased vascular permeability by stimulating release

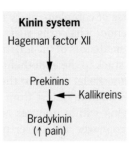

FIGURE 4–11 Kinin system.

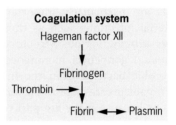

FIGURE 4–12 Coagulation system.

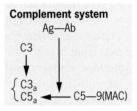

FIGURE 4–13 Complement system.

of histamine from mast cells. This vasoactive effect is called **anaphylaxis**. The final product of the complement pathway is the **membrane attack complex**, a polymer of various complement proteins that punches holes in bacterial cell walls, effectively causing their **lysis** or death.

The exact role of each of these various chemicals or chemical systems in a particular inflammatory reaction is difficult to evaluate, and we have not mentioned here the multitudes of other chemical intermediates known to have varying degrees of inflammatory and catalytic activity. Rather than memorize these in detail, it is more important for you to appreciate that the blood plays a sophisticated role in the regulation of the inflammatory reaction.

In addition to the chemicals from the plasma, neutrophils and macrophages bring products that help amplify and sustain the inflammatory reaction. Neutrophil enzymes can activate the complement and kinin systems, but perhaps more important they provide essential substrates for the synthesis of prostaglandins.

Prostaglandins and **leukotrienes** are metabolites of **arachidonic acid** that are produced locally by cells and act as short-range hormones (**Figure 4–14**). The chemistry of these compounds is complex, the number of compounds

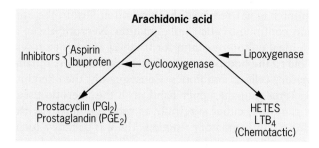

FIGURE 4–14 Arachidonic acid system.

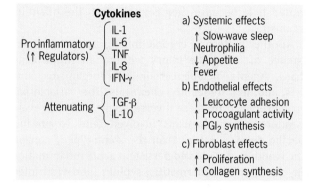

FIGURE 4–15 Cytokines.

produced large, and their effects are confusing because they are often contradictory. Suffice it to say that prostaglandins and leukotrienes are produced in response to inflammation and act locally to sustain the reaction. They are involved in vasoconstriction, vasodilation increased vascular permeability, chemotaxis, and fever. The anti-inflammatory action of aspirin and ibuprofen, at least in part, is the result of inhibition of prostaglandin synthesis.

The complement, arachidonic acid, and kinin systems all produce proteins that enhance the vascular phase of inflammation by dilating venules and increasing their permeability to fluids. Other proteins produced by these systems serve as chemotactic agents and opsonins.

In addition to the chemical systems just discussed, a variety of polypeptide **cytokines** and **chemokines** serve to up- and down-regulate inflammation (**Figure 4–15**). Tumor necrosis factor (TNF), interleukin-1 (IL-1), IL-8, and IL-6 are cytokines produced by leukocytes and endothelial cells; they enhance the acute inflammatory process locally by increasing leukocyte adhesion to endothelium, increasing blood coagulation properties, and stimulating the further production of prostaglandins. Systemically, these cytokines elicit fever and neutrophilia, increase sleep, and decrease appetite. Other cytokines, such as IL-10 and transforming growth factor (TGF), have a down-regulating effect and consequently aid in the resolution of acute inflammation.

We have already mentioned, in passing, some important variations in the inflammatory process. Reactions

with lots of neutrophils cause tissue destruction but are important in containing pyogenic bacteria. Macrophages are prominent when there is dead tissue to remove or foreign substances to surround or engulf. Edema predominates when lots of histamine is released, as in atopic allergy and immune complex reactions. Fibrin is a prominent part of the inflammatory process if a protective barrier is needed on injured surfaces. Chronicity, or prolonged duration, of inflammation introduces even more variations.

Chronic Inflammation

Overview

Chronic means persistent for a long time. In that sense, chronic inflammation may result from acute inflammation that persists because the cause is not completely eliminated, or it may be associated with a cause that never was acute but is continuing at a low level for a long time.

The term *chronic inflammation* is also used as a label for the histologic picture typically associated with prolonged inflammation. As will be discussed later, some chronic inflammations have a more specific appearance (e.g., granulomatous inflammation) and some clinically acute inflammations mimic chronic inflammation histologically. Let us first describe the typical appearance of chronic inflammation and then deal with the variations and their pathogenesis.

Because the injury in chronic inflammation is usually low grade, edema and hyperemia are less pronounced than in acute inflammation and few or no neutrophils are present. The area is infiltrated predominantly with lymphocytes, plasma cells, and, less conspicuously, macrophages (**Figure 4–16**). Plasma cells are often prominent

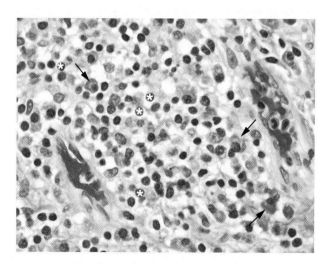

FIGURE 4–16 Chronic inflammation is characterized by an infiltrate composed of lymphocytes (white *), plasma cells (black arrows), and macrophages. Eosinophils are also present in this focus of chronic inflammation. Notice also the vascular congestion (bright red areas represent red blood cells in capillaries).

and easily recognized. They are derived from B lymphocytes in the tissue and their primary function is to produce antibodies. Antibodies produced by the plasma cells attach to foreign material in the area as opsonins, priming neutrophils, and macrophages to phagocytose this material. The lymphocytes, which are mostly nucleus with a small rim of cytoplasm, play a much larger role than their innocuous appearance suggests. Different types of lymphocytes can perform various functions. They can recognize foreign materials, kill host cells in the area of foreign antigens to isolate the foreign substance, transform into plasma cells to produce antibodies, and direct the traffic of other inflammatory cells, especially macrophages. However, histologically, it is not possible to tell which lymphocytes are doing what and why. Macrophages may play the same role as they do in acute inflammation (phagocytosis and digestion of debris), but they may also become directly cytotoxic to host cells under certain conditions. Lymphocytes produce cytokines and chemokines that attract macrophages to the area of inflammation, and macrophages in turn secrete cytokines and chemokines that attract and activate lymphocytes.

Another hallmark of chronic inflammation, regardless of type, is the laying down of new fibrous tissue. Whenever there is tissue injury in the presence of chronic inflammation, there is a fibrous tissue proliferation that tends to wall off the injured area and provide strength to the defective tissue. The chronicity of the inflammation can be estimated by judging the extent and the age of the new fibrous tissue. The process of fibrosis in repair is discussed later.

Clinically, chronic inflammation has the same features as acute inflammation—edema, redness, heat, pain, and loss of function—but these features are much less pronounced and more variable in their intensity. Contraction of the developing fibrous tissue may distort the lesion and surrounding tissue and give it a variegated, firm, glistening, gray appearance.

The pathogenesis of chronic inflammation involves persistence of the causative agent and a host reaction that is predominantly immunologic in nature. The immune response, which may be of one or several types, produces a more varied picture than the acute inflammatory response does. Chronic inflammation resulting from persistent acute inflammation is usually caused by pyogenic bacteria. Foreign bodies and necrotic tissue provide a haven for these organisms to proliferate and cause continuing foci of acute inflammation. The superimposed chronic inflammation is characterized by many plasma cells, which are producing antibodies to help fight the festering bacterial infection, and by fibrous tissue, which is attempting to wall off the area. The reaction to a splinter is typical of this situation.

If a splinter (foreign body) is removed, the acute inflammatory reaction will eliminate the bacteria and digest the small amount of necrotic tissue. But if the splinter is not removed, bacteria often lurk in the area and continue to elicit inflammation. Necrotic tissue is an ideal culture medium for bacteria and is not accessible to the body's vascular system that delivers inflammatory cells or antibiotics. Consequently, the offending bacteria gain the upper hand until the necrotic tissue is removed, either surgically or more gradually by the chronic inflammatory reaction. There is usually a focus of acute inflammation near the splinter, surrounded by a zone of chronic inflammation. Such lesions are sometimes called subacute inflammation or combined acute and chronic inflammation. Therapy should be directed at the removal of the cause; antibiotics are often of limited help because they cannot reach the offending organisms.

Another pattern of chronic inflammation is the persistence of low-grade injury without an initial acute phase. Agents include certain microorganisms, antigens, and, less frequently, chemicals. The variable patterns produced by these diverse agents and the several immunologic mechanisms involved tend to produce specific diseases rather than the stereotyped, nonspecific reaction of acute and persistent acute inflammation. Hay fever, contact dermatitis, syphilis, and viral infections are examples of the diversity of manifestations of chronic inflammation. The common denominator of these chronic inflammatory reactions is that they employ T lymphocytes to attack the offending agent (**cellular immunity**) and/or B lymphocytes to produce antibody to it (**humoral immunity**). Consequently, lymphocytes and plasma cells predominate in the lesions.

BOX 4–3   Chronic Inflammation

Causes

Prolonged injury

Prolonged infection

Certain types of infection

Antigens (immune reactions)

Lesions

Less exudate than acute

Lymphocytes and plasma cells

Occurs with fibrous repair

Manifestations

Same as acute, but less severe and more variable

Scar tissue

Granulomatous Inflammation

Granulomatous inflammation is a specific type of chronic inflammation characterized by focal collections of closely packed, plump macrophages (**Figure 4–17**). Granulomatous inflammation occurs in response to certain indigestible organisms and other foreign materials

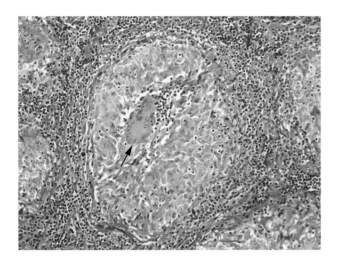

FIGURE 4–17 A granuloma consists of a collection of plump histiocytes (macrophages) surrounded by a rim of lymphocytes. In the center of this granuloma are a few dead cells and a giant cell (arrow). The edges of other granulomata can be seen at the periphery of the picture.

and involves an element of cell-mediated immunity to the foreign material. In granulomatous inflammation, T lymphocytes become sensitized to the offending agent and recruit large numbers of macrophages that engulf the antigenic agent. These macrophages are called **epithelioid cells** because their abundant cytoplasm and close approximation to each other in aggregates make them resemble epithelial cells.

The macrophages in a granuloma can form **giant cells**, or very large cells with numerous nuclei. Granulomas often become large enough to produce grossly visible, pale yellow nodules. Central, caseous necrosis can also occur, especially in larger granulomas. Small granulomas heal by fibrosis. Large caseous granulomas are walled off by a fibrous rim and eventually calcify.

The classic cause of granulomatous inflammation is tuberculosis. Other microorganisms, particularly the fungi causing histoplasmosis, coccidioidomycosis, blastomycosis, and cryptococcosis, produce granulomatous disease that is very similar in appearance to tuberculosis.

Another relatively common granulomatous disease is **sarcoidosis**, a disease of unknown cause characterized by widespread noncaseous granulomas. It produces a mild to moderately debilitating illness usually involving lungs and lymph nodes, though it can affect many other organs as well. It is more common in young adult women, in black people, and in the southern United States. Most patients are asymptomatic or have a mild illness that disappears in a few years. A few die from progressive granulomatous involvement of the lungs or complications of the lesions.

Foreign body granulomas are less stereotyped than the tuberculoid or sarcoid granulomas described earlier. They result from indigestible foreign material being surrounded by epithelioid cells and giant cells. Common causes are suture material, splinters, talc, mineral oil inhaled into the lung, crystalline cholesterol deposits derived from blood or bile, and large organisms such as helminths. The foreign body is usually quite evident within the granuloma.

BOX 4–4   Granulomatous Inflammation
Causes
Tuberculosis
Fungal infections
Foreign bodies
Sarcoidosis
Lesions
Focal collections of plump macrophages and giant cells
Often multiple foci
May have central, caseous necrosis
Manifestations
Nonspecific, may be none
Positive tests for causative organisms
Tissue destruction that may affect organ function

Transudates and Exudates

A **transudate** is a collection of fluid in tissue or in a body space that accumulates because of increased hydrostatic or decreased osmotic pressure in the vascular system. Transudates are watery and have a low protein content. **Exudates** are the result of increased osmotic pressure in the tissue because of high protein content and are caused by inflammation or obstruction of lymphatic flow. Thus, a swelling with cloudy or protein-rich fluid is caused by inflammation or lymphatic obstruction, whereas a swelling with thin, watery fluid might be caused by heart failure with its increased venous pressure or by depleted serum proteins. Exudates tend to be more localized than are transudates because most inflammations are localized, whereas the effects of increased hydrostatic pressure or depleted serum proteins are usually generalized.

A **serous exudate** contains fluid as well as small amounts of protein and often implies a lesser degree of damage. For example, the fluid content of blisters that follow skin burns is serous exudate.

A **fibrinous exudate** is an exudate composed of large amounts of fibrinogen from the blood that is polymerized to form fibrin. For example, in bacterial pneumonia fibrinous exudate forms a mesh that helps trap the bacteria; on a skin wound, dried fibrinous exudate forms a scab. The coagulation system plays a large role in the formation of a fibrinous exudate.

Purulent exudate (also called pus) is an exudate that is loaded with live and dead leukocytes, mostly neutrophils.

An inflammatory reaction with much purulent exudate is called **suppurative inflammation**. A localized collection of pus is an **abscess**. When pus fills a body cavity such as the pleural cavity, the term **empyema** is used.

Gross Appearance of Inflammatory Lesions

Lesions with a relatively specific gross appearance include abscess, cellulitis, and ulcer. An abscess is a localized, usually spherical lesion containing liquefied dead tissue and neutrophils (purulent exudate) (**Figure 4–18**). Pyogenic bacteria are the most typical cause of abscesses because they liberate chemotactic factors and proliferate to produce an exuberant acute inflammatory reaction. The host is induced to destroy and liquefy its own tissue to limit the spread of the offending agent. Abscesses are typically caused by bacteria of the skin (staphylococci), oral cavity (streptococci including pneumococci, anaerobic bacteria), and lower intestinal tract (coliform bacteria and anaerobic bacteria). Examples of abscesses include the **boil** or **furuncle** caused by an obstructed skin appendage or foreign body, a **paronychia** caused by purulent infection around a fingernail, and the pimples or **comedones** of acne that form when greasy secretions obstruct sebaceous glands and become the culture medium for bacteria. Abscesses also occur in areas where there is change from one tissue type to another such as around the nostrils, teeth, and anus. The combination of foreign material, necrotic tissue, and bacteria trapped in wounds or in operative incisions is particularly likely

to produce an abscess. In more serious breakdowns of the body's defense mechanisms, such as perforation of the intestines or necrosis of tissue in organs open to the bacterial environment (lung, intestine, skin), anaerobic organisms of intestinal, oral, or soil origin often cause abscesses.

The typical small abscess is red, hot, swollen, and quite painful. When the abscess reaches a head, the center is liquefied and fluctuant and the edge is beginning to wall off. Puncture of the abscess causes an outpouring of pus, relief of pain, and more rapid healing. If punctured before this stage, the abscess may be spread. Larger abscesses are more irregular and may spread in tissue spaces and cause extensive damage. An abscess is walled off and replaced by fibrous tissue after drainage or resolution (resorption) of the purulent exudate. If uncontained, an abscess may enlarge, spread, and kill the host. For example, acute appendicitis with abscess formation can lead to death; early appendectomy prevents such an outcome.

Cellulitis refers to a spreading acute inflammatory process. This type of inflammation is commonly seen with streptococcal bacterial infections and is caused by the body's inability to confine the organism. Cellulitis is seen in the skin and subcutaneous tissue and is characterized by nonlocalized edema and redness. A related condition is **necrotizing fasciitis**, caused by similar organisms and usually located in deep tissues, such as the fascia around muscles or subcutaneous tissues. Cellulitis and necrotizing fasciitis caused by streptococcal bacteria can lead to **toxic shock syndrome**, a life-threatening condition manifested by severe respiratory distress and renal failure.

An **ulcer** is a local excavation of an epithelium, such as skin or mucous membranes. The epithelium is usually damaged by a combination of an injurious agent and the acute inflammatory response that attempts to contain it. Ulcers are commonly seen in the stomach and duodenum secondary to local injury by acid from the stomach. Bedsores, resulting from pressure atrophy, are another example of ulcers.

Repair
Regeneration

The body's two basic methods of repair following tissue destruction are **regeneration** and **fibrous connective tissue repair** (scarring or fibrosis). Regeneration is replacement of the destroyed tissue by cells similar to those previously present—that is, the parenchymal cells of the organ are reconstituted. For example, the epidermal surface of a cut is replaced by epidermis, fractured bone is united by bone, and scattered dead liver cells are replaced by new liver cells (**Figure 4–19**). In fibrous connective tissue repair, tissue previously present is replaced by fibrous tissue (scar). For example, the dermal edges of a cut are united by scar, a bone fracture that is not properly united is healed by scar tissue, and extensively damaged liver

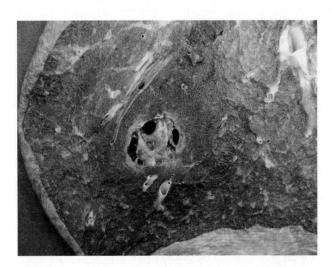

FIGURE 4–18 Abscess. There is a hole filled with necrotic debris in this section through lung tissue. The brown tissue is the pulmonary parenchyma; tan vessels are coursing through the parenchyma (the lumena of some of them are seen in cross section); and the smooth, gray border at the bottom and left of the image is the pleural surface. The brown and green color of the parenchyma is an artifact of fixation. Note that the abscess is sharply circumscribed, has a tan rim, which is the result of an increased density of cells that are attempting to wall off the inflammatory process, and is surrounded by a red border. The redness is imparted by congested vessels.

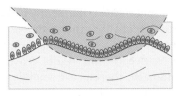

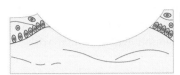 Superficial scrape

Epithelium removed

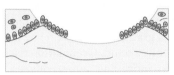 Regenerating basal cells from margin

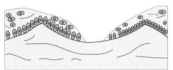 Regenerating cells mature

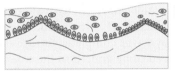 Normal structure restored

FIGURE 4–19 Complete regeneration of lost surface epithelium.

may be replaced by fibrous tissue. Many tissue injuries heal in part by regeneration and in part by fibrosis.

Regeneration is the most desirable form of repair because normal function is restored. Regeneration of functional tissue is particularly important when there has been widespread damage to a vital organ. As a prerequisite to regeneration, cells next to those that have died must be able to multiply. Some cells, such as neurons and cardiac muscle fibers, do not undergo cell division in adults; therefore, these cells cannot regenerate after injuries. In contrast, tissues that are continuously replacing their cells under normal circumstances, such as the cells of the epidermis, gastrointestinal tract, or bone, have a great capacity for regeneration. When a patient sustains generalized hypoxia (for example, from septic shock, prolonged cardiac arrest followed by successful resuscitation, or carbon monoxide poisoning), renal tubular cells, hepatocytes, and neurons are most susceptible to necrosis because of their high metabolic requirements. Renal and hepatic function is likely to be restored because the few surviving cells can regenerate. Brain function, however, cannot be restored because neurons cannot effectively regenerate.

The epidermis and intestinal mucosa can repair defects up to several centimeters in diameter through the process of regeneration. Bone marrow can replace itself even when only a few cells survive an injury. Its tremendous capacity to regenerate from only a few cells is exploited therapeutically in bone marrow transplants. The diseased bone marrow is first ablated by toxic drugs, and then a few cells from a donor are introduced and completely reconstitute functional bone marrow. Most of the tissues of the body normally undergo cell replacement at a slow rate and are intermediate in their ability to regenerate. Regeneration can usually occur in parenchymal organs if the architectural framework is not destroyed. Complex structures composed of interrelating tissue types, such as the gas-exchanging membranes of the lung and renal glomeruli, do not regenerate.

Fibrous Connective Tissue Repair (Scarring or Fibrosis)

Fibrosis can occur in any tissue and produces the same result regardless of site—namely, the formation of a dense, tough mass of collagen called a **scar**. Unlike regeneration, replacement by fibrous tissue does not restore the original function. The purpose of fibrosis is to provide a strong bridge across the damaged area.

The process of fibrous repair is also called **organization** and consists of a granulation tissue stage and a scar formation stage. **Granulation tissue** consists of capillaries and fibroblasts. Repair is initiated by the ingrowth of new capillaries and fibroblasts into the injured area. The capillaries bring blood to provide the nutrition for the repair process. Capillaries also carry away liquid remains of dead tissue and particulate material removed by macrophages. The removal process is called **resolution**. The fibroblasts proliferate rapidly and then initiate the stage of scar formation by laying down collagen. Initially, there are small amounts of loose collagen within the mass of capillaries and fibroblasts. With time, more collagen is formed and the number of capillaries and fibroblasts decreases. The final stage, which takes weeks to months, involves shrinking and condensation of the fibrous scar (**Figure 4–20**).

Wound Repair

The process of repairing wounds is artificially separated into repair by primary union and secondary union, depending on whether the wound edges are placed together or left separated. The best example of repair by primary union is that which follows a clean surgical incision of the skin in which there is minimal tissue damage and the edges of the wound are closely approximated by tape or sutures. In this example, the narrow space between the two wound edges fills with a small amount of serum, which quickly dries and clots, forming a scab. Within 1 to 2 days, the narrow zone of acute inflammation at the wound edges has lessened and new capillaries begin to bridge the gap across the defect. By this time, the

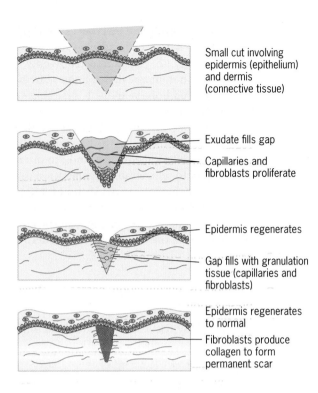

Small cut involving epidermis (epithelium) and dermis (connective tissue)

Exudate fills gap

Capillaries and fibroblasts proliferate

Epidermis regenerates

Gap fills with granulation tissue (capillaries and fibroblasts)

Epidermis regenerates to normal

Fibroblasts produce collagen to form permanent scar

FIGURE 4–20 Fibrous connective tissue repair and epithelial regeneration in a skin cut.

epithelium has already grown across the surface of the gap. Within a few more days, fibroblasts grow across the subepithelial portions of the wound and begin to deposit collagen, which eventually contracts, pulling the wound edges together and giving them strength. Although this incision may appear well healed by about 2 weeks, it may take a month or more for the strength of the scar tissue to approximate that of the original tissue.

Repair by secondary union uses the same basic process as primary union, except that there is greater injury with consequent greater tissue damage and more inflammation to resolve (**Figure 4–21**). To fill the void left by tissue damage, there is a tremendous proliferation of capillaries and fibroblasts, which actually start growing after the injury is just a few days old and acute inflammation may still be intense. After a week or more, the wound will be filled with this granulation tissue, composed largely of capillaries, fibroblasts, variable numbers of residual acute inflammatory cells, and some chronic inflammatory cells. This tissue is friable and red and oozes blood. You are familiar with the appearance of granulation tissue if you have ever picked a scab off a skin wound. Granulation tissue eventually is replaced as more and more collagen is deposited by fibroblasts. Fibroblasts and collagen have inherent contractile properties, which aid in shrinking a wound and drawing the edges together. Fibroblast proliferation and collagen synthesis by fibroblasts are both stimulated by pro-inflammatory cytokines such as TNF and IL-1. It may take a long time for a wound that heals by secondary union to achieve strength approximating that of the normal tissue. If a skin wound is very large, the epithelium may never completely bridge the wound, and skin may need to be grafted to the wound site from another area of the body. Transplanted skin usually grows quite readily in such a situation because the underlying granulation tissue is so rich in capillaries. One of the greatest impediments to healing and repair of a wound is the amount of dead tissue and foreign material (e.g., dirt, bacteria, shrapnel) present. It might take the body's inflammatory cells many months to phagocytose a large amount of dead tissue and foreign material, and the presence of bacteria in a wound may produce necrotic tissue and inflammatory cells as

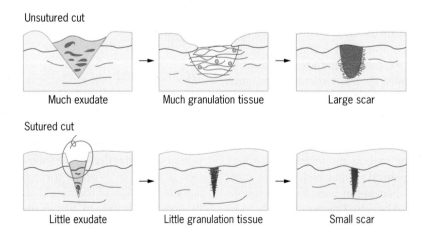

Unsutured cut

Much exudate → Much granulation tissue → Large scar

Sutured cut

Little exudate → Little granulation tissue → Small scar

FIGURE 4–21 Repair of an unsutured and sutured skin cut leading to secondary and primary union, respectively.

fast as they are removed. For this reason, the medical care of a large wound should always include thorough cleaning and **debridement** (removal of foreign material and necrotic tissue).

Inflammation and subsequent repair of tissue are very dynamic processes that are influenced by numerous modifying factors. The following factors may detract from the body's ability to deal effectively with an injury:

1. *Virulence of the infective organisms*: For example, staphylococcal bacteria are more capable of destroying tissue than are alpha-streptococci.
2. *Advancing age*: Elderly people heal more slowly than do younger people, for various reasons.
3. *Poor nutrition*: Protein and vitamin C are needed to produce collagen.
4. *Diabetes*: Small blood vessels are abnormal in diabetics and consequently they do not deliver materials to the tissues optimally.
5. *Steroid therapy*: Steroids inhibit the inflammatory response by preventing vascular permeability, hindering cellular digestion of debris, and blocking antigen–antibody reactions. Steroids can be very useful in those situations where inhibition of inflammation is desired, for example, to slow the destructive inflammation of rheumatoid arthritis.

BOX 4–5   Repair

Causes

Necrosis from injury

Lesions

Parenchymal cell proliferation

Fibrosis

Manifestations

Return of partial function

Stabilization of tissue

Practice Questions

1. Mitochondria, Golgi apparatus, and lysosomes are examples of
   A. endoplasmic reticulum.
   B. organelles.
   C. ribosomes.
   D. cytoplasm.
2. Proteins that attach to invasive organisms and aid in phagocytosis are called
   A. opsonins.
   B. cytokines.
   C. chemokines.
   D. peptides.

3. Necrosis and apoptosis are both manners of cell death. They differ in which of the following ways?
   A. Necrosis occurs with infection and apoptosis occurs with ischemia.
   B. Necrosis is associated with inflammation and apoptosis is not.
   C. Necrosis involves activation of genes that regulate cell death while apoptosis results from an external injurious stimulus.
   D. Necrosis may occur as part of normal physiologic or developmental processes while apoptosis is always pathologic.
4. Which sequence best describes the cellular events in acute inflammation?
   A. Margination, exocytosis, chemotaxis, phagocytosis
   B. Chemotaxis, opsonization, necrosis, antigen presentation
   C. Exocytosis, phagocytosis, oxidative burst, apoptosis
   D. Margination, opsonization, arachidonic acid metabolism
   E. Vasodilation, margination, exocytosis, oxidative burst
5. An older woman has a history of leg fracture when she was a teenager, peptic ulcer disease, numerous strokes, and a recent urinary tract infection. Of these conditions, which will not have healed by regeneration?
   A. The ulcer in the stomach
   B. The infection in the bladder
   C. The infarcts in the brain
   D. The bone fractures
   E. None will have healed by regeneration.
6. Hepatitis C virus infects the liver and causes chronic inflammation. A biopsy of a liver with chronic hepatitis C virus infection may show all of the following except which one?
   A. Fibrosis
   B. Lymphocytes
   C. Necrosis of hepatocytes ✓
   D. Suppurative inflammation
   E. Destruction of liver parenchyma
7. A middle-aged man sustains a myocardial infarction. He survives the infarct but dies 4 years later in a motor vehicle accident. At autopsy, the heart muscle
   A. will look normal because myocardial cells have regenerated in the area of injury.
   B. will have a soft and yellow patch because of coagulative necrosis of the infarcted area.
   C. will have a scar in the area of the prior infarct.
   D. will have granulation tissue in the area of the prior infarct.
   E. will have evidence of numerous other myocardial infarcts.

8. A woman slips on ice while getting out of her car and twists her ankle. It becomes red, swollen, and painful, and she hesitates to put any weight on it. Her physician recommends she take some ibuprofen, and within half an hour her discomfort has improved considerably. This is because
   A. ibuprofen inhibits chemotaxis by neutrophils.
   B. ibuprofen inhibits the release of histamine.
   C. ibuprofen inhibits chemokine production by lymphocytes.
   D. ibuprofen inhibits the production of arachidonic acid–derived inflammatory mediators.
   E. ibuprofen inhibits the mediation of pain by injured nerve endings.

5

Hyperplasias and Neoplasms

OUTLINE

Review of Structure and Function
Significance of Hyperplasias and Neoplasms
Classification of Neoplasms
    Benign Neoplasms
    Malignant Neoplasms
Natural History of Hyperplasia and Cancer
Practice Questions

9. Describe how carcinomas and sarcomas differ in tissue of origin and spread.
10. Understand the concept of staging a malignancy, and demonstrate how stage relates to prognosis and therapy.
11. Define, describe, and use in context all the words in bold print in this chapter.

OBJECTIVES

1. Review the names of different cell types, and understand on what basis they are classified as labile, stable, or permanent.
2. Understand the pathogenesis and clinical implications of hyperplasias and neoplasms.
3. Understand the difference between hypertrophy and hyperplasia, understand the difference between physiologic and pathologic hypertrophy or hyperplasia, and learn which cell types undergo hypertrophy and which undergo hyperplasia.
4. Understand the difference(s) between hyperplasia/hypertrophy, atrophy, metaplasia, and dysplasia.
5. Compare inflammatory lesions, hyperplasias, benign neoplasms, and malignant neoplasms in terms of behavior, morphology, and treatment.
6. Describe the conventions used in naming benign and malignant neoplasms.
7. Understand histomorphologic criteria that are used to diagnose and describe cancer.
8. Understand the relationship between mutation, transformation, premalignant lesions (dysplasia), *in situ* cancer, local invasion, and metastasis.

KEY TERMS

atrophy
benign
cancer
carcinoma
cellular atypia
columnar epithelium
connective tissue cells
curative therapy
differentiation
dysplasia
epithelial cells
germ cells
hyperplasia
hypertrophy
in situ
invasion
labile cells
malignant
metaplasia
metastasis

muscle cells
neoplasia
nervous tissue cells
palliative therapy
pathologic hypertrophy
permanent cells
physiologic hypertrophy
pluripotent
polyp
premalignant lesion
sarcoma
somatic cells
stable cells
stem cell
stratified squamous
    epithelium
transitional epithelium
tumor
tumor stage

Review of Structure and Function

All the cells of the body are derived from one cell, the fertilized ovum. During embryonic development, successive cell divisions lead to more and more specialized (differentiated) cell types and the less differentiated embryonic cells disappear. Even in the mature organism, differentiation, or the maturation from a nonspecific cell type, or stem cell, to a specialized cell, occurs in many tissues of the body. Stem cells are pluripotent, meaning they can differentiate into many different types of adult cells. Their main function is to divide and produce daughter cells. The daughter cells pass through several intermediate stages of differentiation until they become mature, differentiated cells. For example, in the bone marrow, undifferentiated stem cells give rise to white blood cells, red blood cells, and platelets through progenitor cells that mature through well-recognized stages. Similarly, in the glandular epithelium of the gastrointestinal tract (GI), a stem cell at the base of the gland divides, and the daughter cells, as they migrate up to the surface of the epithelium, gradually specialize and acquire mucus-secreting or absorptive functions. In general, the more differentiated a cell type becomes, the more its capacity to proliferate decreases. In the blood, the functional red blood cells do not replicate; all new red blood cells must come from the stem cells in the bone marrow. The same is true in the gastrointestinal tract. The mature surface epithelial cells do not replicate; replication occurs at the base of the gland.

To some degree, the propensity of cells to proliferate beyond what is needed for normal homeostasis reflects their ability to replicate in normal, mature tissue. As already discussed in the context of injury and repair, certain cells (e.g., skin, bone) are able to replicate and reconstitute an injured tissue, while others (e.g., nerve, muscle) cannot. The ability of cells to divide is the basis for categorizing cells as labile, stable, or permanent. **Labile cells** (e.g., skin, GI tract, bone) are continuously dividing and thus can regenerate or, in the context of this chapter, undergo excessive growth (hyperplasia) or new growth (neoplasia). **Stable cells** (e.g., liver, kidney) normally divide only in response to injury, and **permanent cells** (e.g., cardiac muscle, neurons) do not normally undergo division once they are mature. Most abnormal growths thus occur in tissues composed of labile cells.

The cells of the developed organism can be divided into **germ cells** (normally confined to the gonads) and **somatic cells**. Somatic cells are classified into four major categories: epithelial cells, connective tissue cells, muscle cells, and nervous tissue cells.

Epithelial cells arise from the embryonic ectoderm and endoderm to form the skin, lining of body spaces, and the various glands. Surface lining cells are of squamous, transitional, or columnar types. **Stratified squamous epithelium** forms a tough protective barrier and can be keratinized or nonkeratinized. Keratinized squamous epithelium makes up the outer layer of the skin, and nonkeratinized epithelium lines the mouth, pharynx, larynx, esophagus, vagina, and anus. **Transitional epithelium** is also multilayered but lacks the surface layer of keratin and the intercellular bridges of squamous epithelium. Transitional epithelium is confined to the urinary tract, including the renal pelvis, ureter, bladder, and urethra. **Columnar epithelium** is usually composed of one layer of tall cells, which often are mucus secreting. Columnar epithelium forms the mucous membranes lining the nose, trachea, bronchi, stomach, small intestine, colon, cervix, uterus, and many of the ducts leading from glands, such as the bile ducts.

Epithelial cells can be arranged as glands (acini) or in tubules or cords. Glandular organs include breast, salivary glands, thyroid, and pancreas. The kidney is an example of an organ composed predominantly of tubules. The liver, adrenal glands, and pituitary are arranged in cords or sheets, with blood sinusoids (cavities) between the sheets of cells. In general, epithelial cells are labile: stem cells in the various epithelial tissues are continuously replacing mature cells that have outlived their usefulness and are induced to die.

Connective tissue cells, which are mostly derived from mesoderm, are recognized by their lack of close approximation with other cells and by the substances they produce. Fibroblasts produce and are associated with collagen, chondrocytes with cartilage, osteocytes with bone, and endothelial cells with blood vessels. Connective tissue cells have a great capacity to proliferate and blood cells are replaced continuously from the bone marrow. These are labile cells. Fixed connective tissue cells (fibroblasts, osteocytes) are replaced more slowly but can be stimulated to divide more rapidly by injury (stable cells).

Muscle cells are also derived from mesoderm but resemble epithelial cells in their close approximation to each other. They differ from epithelium by their elongated fiber-like structure and abundant contractile cytoplasm. Heart muscle cells cannot be replaced, and skeletal muscle cells have very limited replacement capacity. Smooth muscle cells, especially those in small blood vessels, can proliferate.

Nervous tissue cells are derived from ectoderm and include neurons and their supporting cells. Neurons have very long processes (axons), which carry electrical impulses. The supporting cells in the brain and spinal cord are glial cells (astrocytes and oligodendroglia). Supporting cells in peripheral nerves are Schwann cells. Supporting cells can proliferate and do so more rapidly in response to injury, but neurons have limited capacity for replacing themselves following injury.

Definitions

- **Tumor** refers to any mass or swelling. It is one of the cardinal signs of inflammation, but in daily usage this word most commonly refers to a growth.
- **Hyperplasia** and **hypertrophy** are exaggerated responses to a growth stimulus, resulting in an increase in volume in the tissue.

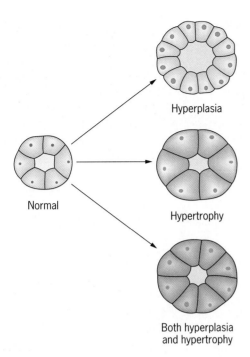

Hyperplasia

Normal

Hypertrophy

Both hyperplasia
and hypertrophy

FIGURE 5–1 Hyperplasia and hypertrophy of a gland.

- ■ **Neoplasia** literally means "new growth." More specifically, a neoplasm is a proliferation of cells that are independent of normal growth control mechanisms.
- ■ **Malignant** or malignancy refers to a neoplasm that has the potential to spread widely throughout the body and cause death of the organism.
- ■ **Cancer** is a synonym for a malignant neoplasm.

Hyperplasia and hypertrophy are responses of tissues to increased demand. The demand may be functional, such as when the skeletal muscle has to do increased work when a person undergoes athletic training; it may be hormonal, as when the endometrium proliferates in response to estrogen; it may be in response to an inflammatory stimulus, as when the lymph nodes enlarge while a person is fighting an infection; or it may be in response to chronic irritation, as when pressure is consistently applied to the skin of the toes by a poorly fitting shoe. Whether tissues respond to increased demand by hyperplasia or hypertrophy depends on the ability of their constituent cells to divide. **Figure 5–1** demonstrates the differences between hyperplasia and hypertrophy. Labile cells, such as epithelial cells, respond by increasing in number; this is called hyperplasia (**Figure 5–2**). Stable cells increase in size; this is called hypertrophy (**Figure 5–3**). Some tissues respond to increased demand by demonstrating both hyperplasia and hypertrophy. This is true, for example, of the uterus, which adapts to accommodate a growing fetus by increasing both the number and the size of the smooth muscle cells in its wall.

Hyperplasia and hypertrophy often occur in response to physiologic demands. The increase in the size of the uterus during pregnancy, the increase in the size of skeletal muscle in response to weight training, and the increase in size of breast lobules in girls during puberty are examples of **physiologic hypertrophy**. When an increase in the size of a tissue occurs because of an abnormal condition it is called **pathologic hypertrophy**. Thus, the increase in size of breast lobules in men because of a prolactin-producing pituitary adenoma is pathologic. The increase in size of the thyroid because of abnormal stimulation by thyroid-stimulating hormone (TSH) is pathologic. The increase in size of the heart muscle because it has to generate more force to pump against increased peripheral resistance (hypertension) is pathologic.

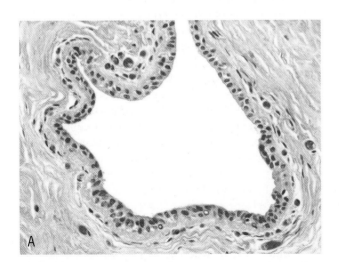
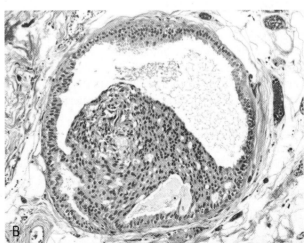

FIGURE 5–2 Hyperplasia. Breast ducts are normally lined by an epithelium that is only two cell layers thick (**A**). In benign ductal hyperplasia (**B**), the epithelial cells proliferate and grow into the duct lumen.

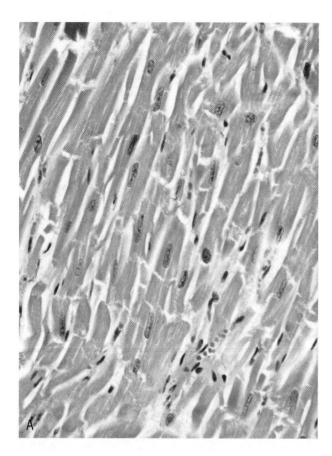 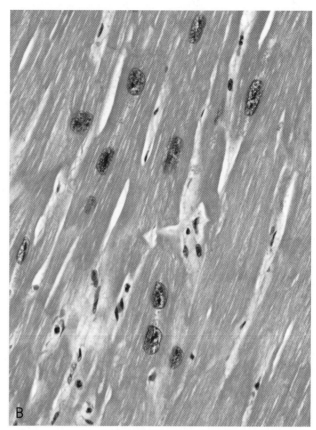

FIGURE 5–3 Hypertrophy. Heart muscle is photographed in both images at the same magnification. The muscle cells in **A** are of normal size. In **B**, they have undergone hypertrophy, or increase in size, in response to systemic hypertension. Note that both the nuclei and the cytoplasm have undergone hypertrophy.

Whether the stimulus to increase in size is physiologic or pathologic, hyperplastic and hypertrophic cells and tissues may return to normal if the stimulus is removed, provided permanent structural changes have not occurred. Again, think of the hypertrophied uterus and how it rapidly reduces in size after the fetus is delivered. Or, sadly, think how rapidly you lose muscle mass if you interrupt your exercise schedule.

Although not necessarily harmful, hyperplasia can be a premalignant process. A **premalignant lesion** is one that has an increased likelihood of developing into cancer compared to adjacent tissues. Hyperplasias of epithelial surface cells are particularly important as sites of cancer development in some organs. Surface hyperplasias produce slightly raised lesions resulting from piling up of cells. Where they can be visualized grossly (for example, in the skin, oral cavity, respiratory tract, or cervix), these lesions appear more opaque than the surrounding surface. Microscopically, their hyperplastic nature is evident, but the pathologist must judge whether it is a simple innocuous hyperplasia or whether it is premalignant hyperplasia.

Cells, tissues, and organs can also undergo a decrease in size. This is called **atrophy**. A terminological distinction is not made between decreased number of cells and decreased size of cells; both processes are called atrophy.

Atrophy can also be physiologic or pathologic, and the causes of atrophy are numerous. Decreased stimulation by hormones, pressure from an adjacent growing mass, decreased work of muscle cells because of a loss of innervation, or age can all result in atrophy of organs. Atrophy itself is usually not a premalignant condition.

Another change in tissues is metaplasia. **Metaplasia** is replacement of one tissue type by another. Most commonly this involves a change from columnar epithelium to stratified squamous epithelium (squamous metaplasia), such as occurs at the junction of the esophagus and the stomach or in the cervix, where the columnar epithelium lining the inner portion of the cervix turns into squamous epithelium lining the outer portion of the cervix (**Figure 5–4**). Again, metaplasia can be physiologic or reflect a pathologic process. The columnar epithelium of the bronchus may change to squamous epithelium in response to chronic irritation by cigarette smoking, for example. Such pathologic metaplastic epithelium is at increased risk for developing neoplasia.

Hyperplasia and neoplasia both refer to increased cell proliferation resulting in increased tissue mass. They differ in that, whereas hyperplasia is a response to a physiologic or pathologic stimulus, neoplasia is an autonomous growth, meaning that the cells grow in

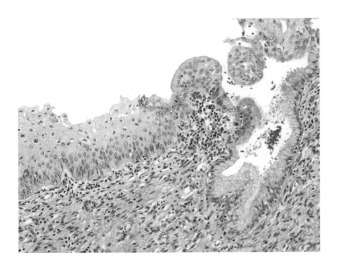

FIGURE 5–4 Squamous metaplasia in the cervix. The glandular epithelium of the endocervix (right side) abruptly changes to squamous epithelium that covers the ectocervix (left side).

the absence of a growth-promoting stimulus. They do so because of genetic changes that confer on the cells a growth advantage so that they proliferate independently of normal growth control mechanisms. They therefore behave as if they were an independent parasitic organism.

Significance of Hyperplasias and Neoplasms

Hyperplasias and neoplasms commonly produce masses that are discovered by direct vision, palpation, radiographic imaging, or presumption from the effects of the mass on organ function. Once discovered, their nature (whether caused by inflammation, hyperplasia, or neoplasia) must be histologically determined because the treatments for these processes are radically different. Subclassification within each category allows for even more rational treatment based on past experience with similar lesions.

With inflammation and hyperplasia, therapy focuses on removing the causative stimulus. With some forms of hyperplasia, the potential development of cancer is also a concern, and it may be necessary to remove the hyperplastic tissue surgically. With a benign neoplasm, therapeutic concern is limited to accurate diagnosis and removal (if necessary) of the lesion. With a malignant neoplasm, therapy is based on an estimate of the possibility for complete destruction of the neoplasm. **Curative therapy** is the attempt to remove all of the cancer, whether by surgical operation, radiation, or administration of drugs. **Palliative therapy** focuses on attempting to control the effects of the cancer, such as pain, when there is no possibility of cure. Palliative therapy may also be surgical, radiologic, or chemotherapeutic.

To illustrate these varying approaches to a mass, consider the case of a woman who discovers a lump in her breast. The mass is first biopsied using a thin, hollow needle that extracts a core of tissue. The pathologist examining the biopsy tissue must determine whether the mass is benign or malignant. If it is benign, nothing further need be done, unless the patient is discomfited by excretions produced by the lesion and expressed through the nipple. In this case, the surgeon may completely excise the lesion. If the pathologist determines that the lesion is a malignant neoplasm, further studies must be done to determine whether the cancer has spread to other tissues in the body, such as the axillary lymph nodes, lungs, or liver. This is called the **tumor stage**. It is on the basis of the stage of the tumor that decisions are made as to what kind of therapy to offer the patient: the wider the cancer has spread, the more aggressive the treatment necessary to eliminate it. A small cancer confined to the breast can be cured with an excisional biopsy or "lumpectomy" that removes the tumor with a rim of normal tissue; a larger cancer or one that has spread to lymph nodes requires more extensive surgery and additional radiotherapy and/or chemotherapy; and a cancer that has spread widely throughout the body may not be curable at all. Ductal hyperplasia of the breast usually does not come to attention by producing an observable mass lesion, but it may be seen in biopsies procured for other reasons. The exact stimulus for ductal hyperplasia in the breast is not known. Sometimes, the appearance of the hyperplasia suggests that it is precancerous or may indicate the potential for cancer to develop anywhere in the breast, not just at the site of the hyperplasia. In this case, the patient should probably be seen at more frequent intervals so that cancer, if it does develop, is picked up while it is still at a curable stage.

Although hyperplasia is not usually life-threatening, it may cause significant discomfort to the patient when the tissue itself swells and impinges on neighboring tissues or organs. The classic example for this is the age-related enlargement of the prostate in men. Prostatic hypertrophy refers to the increase in size of the prostate gland secondary to hyperplasia of its glandular and stromal cells. The enlarged prostate can impinge on the urethra and bladder neck, causing difficulties with urination, including frequent nighttime voiding, incomplete voiding, urinary retention, and urinary tract infection. Hypertrophic prostates are not at increased risk of developing carcinoma in comparison to normally sized prostate glands, but surgery may still be necessary to reduce the size of the prostate and improve urine flow.

Classification of Neoplasms

Most neoplasms can be classified as benign or malignant; a few are not clearly either but exhibit "uncertain malignant potential." **Benign** neoplasms are generally localized, discrete masses of cells that remain confined to their site of origin (**Figure 5–5**). Some benign neoplasms, such as smooth muscle tumors of the uterus, may become very large without causing any symptoms. Others, such as a meningioma in the brain, may cause symptoms or even death despite their small size, because they impinge on vital structures. Whether they are large or small, produce symptoms or not, benign neoplasms generally remain in the tissue in which they originated and do not spread to others. Malignant neoplasms, in contrast, are defined by their potential to invade and metastasize. **Invasion** refers to direct extension of neoplastic cells into surrounding tissue without regard to tissue boundaries (**Figures 5–6**).

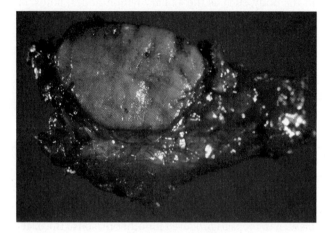

FIGURE 5–5 Benign neoplasm in the parotid gland.

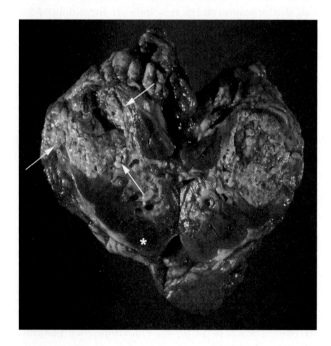

FIGURE 5–6 Invasion. This is an image of a carcinoma in the kidney. The kidney has been cut in half and opened, so the two sides are mirror images of one another. The benign renal parenchyma is the brown tissue at the bottom, marked with a white asterisk. The carcinoma is the yellow nodule between the white arrows. Note that the carcinoma has replaced the renal parenchyma and is invading out beyond the confines of the kidney into the perirenal adipose tissue (left-hand arrow). Compare to Figure 5–7.

For example, a malignancy arising from the epithelial cells of the colon does not remain localized to the colonic mucosa, as a benign polyp does, but rather develops the ability to invade the deeper tissues of the colonic wall—that is, the richly vascular connective tissue of the submucosa and the smooth muscle layer deep to it. In other words, invasion is continuous growth of the tumor into and through other tissue types adjacent to its site of origin. **Metastasis** means transplantation of cells to an entirely new site. For this to occur, the neoplastic cells must be transported through vascular channels or body spaces and must be able to grow at the new site. Cancers most often metastasize to the lymph nodes, lungs, liver, and bone (**Figure 5–7**). Usually, tumors that have metastasized are no longer curable. Some cancers can be lethal by invasion alone (e.g., if a lung cancer erodes into an artery, the patient may die of massive hemorrhage), but usually patients do not die until the tumor has metastasized.

The suffix *-oma* refers to a tumor. It does not necessarily distinguish between a neoplastic or non-neoplastic growth. For example, a hematoma is a localized collection of blood that often produces a swelling; a granuloma is an aggregate of inflammatory cells that forms a discrete, rounded lesion in tissues. The suffix is most commonly used in conjunction with neoplasms, however, and for all intents and purposes *-oma* signifies a neoplastic growth. **Tables 5–1** and **5–2** list names given to benign and malignant neoplasms. Benign neoplasms usually are named by the suffix *-oma* appended to the name of the tissue of origin. Malignant neoplasms are usually called carcinoma or sarcoma. **Carcinoma** refers to a malignant neoplasm of epithelial tissues (e.g., squamous cell carcinoma of the skin). **Sarcoma** is used if the malignancy arises from mesenchymal tissue (e.g., osteosarcoma of bone). A few neoplasms of nonepithelial or ambiguous origin and unpredictable clinical behavior have names that do not follow this classification system (e.g., gastrointestinal stromal tumor, pancreatic neuroendocrine tumor). Other clearly malignant

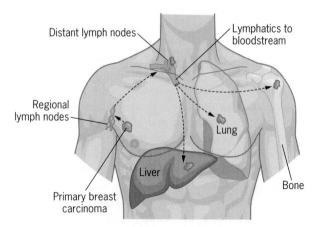

FIGURE 5–7 Typical pattern of metastasis from a breast cancer. For carcinomas, metastasis via lymphatics usually precedes metastasis via the blood.

TABLE 5–1	Names of Benign Neoplasms
Cell or Tissue of Origin	**Name**
Squamous epithelium	Squamous papilloma
Glandular or surface columnar epithelium	Adenoma
Fibrous tissue	Fibroma
Adipose tissue	Lipoma
Cartilage	Chondroma
Bone	Osteoma
Blood vessels	Hemangioma
Smooth muscle	Leiomyoma
Nerve sheath	Neurilemmoma

TABLE 5–2	Names of Malignant Neoplasms
Cell or Tissue of Origin	**Name**
Epithelium	
Site not specified	Carcinoma
Squamous epithelium	Squamous cell carcinoma
Basal cells of epithelium	Basal cell carcinoma (unique to skin)
Colonic mucosa	Adenocarcinoma of colon
Breast glands	Adenocarcinoma of breast
Bronchial epithelium of lung	Bronchogenic carcinoma
Prostatic glands	Adenocarcinoma of prostate
Bladder mucosa	Urothelial carcinoma
Endometrium	Adenocarcinoma of endometrium
Cervix	Squamous cell carcinoma of cervix
Stomach mucosa	Adenocarcinoma of stomach
Pancreatic ducts	Adenocarcinoma of pancreas
Connective tissue and muscle	
Site not specified	Sarcoma
Lymphoid tissue	Lymphoma
Bone marrow	Leukemia
Plasma cells in bone marrow	Multiple myeloma
Cartilage	Chondrosarcoma
Bone	Osteosarcoma
Fibrous tissue	Fibrosarcoma
Smooth muscle	Leiomyosarcoma
Other	
Site not specified	Malignant neoplasm
Glial cells	Glioma
Melanocytes	Malignant melanoma
Germ cells	Teratoma

neoplasms have been given names that make them sound benign, when in fact they are glaringly malignant. It is very important to recognize these as malignant neoplasms. A lymphoma is a malignancy of lymphoid cells; a melanoma is a malignant neoplasm of melanocytes; glioma is used to refer to all neoplasms, benign or malignant, of the supporting cells of the brain (glial cells); and hepatoma is an old name that has been replaced with the more accurate hepatocellular carcinoma.

Benign Neoplasms

Benign neoplasms are relatively easy to recognize grossly and microscopically because they produce a single mass that is discrete from surrounding tissue (Figure 5–5). When originating on a body surface, benign neoplasms extend outwardly, producing a polyp (**Figure 5–8**). A **polyp** is any abnormal protrusion from a mucosal surface. Polypoid growth is characteristic of benign neoplasms; however, polypoid growth sometimes occurs with other types of lesions, such as inflammation or hyperplasia, and polyps may harbor malignant neoplasms.

Benign neoplasms that originate within solid organs or connective tissue usually compress tissue around them to form a fibrous rim or capsule (see Figure 5–8). Because they are so circumscribed, benign tumors are easily separated from surrounding tissue during surgical removal. Histologically, benign neoplasms very closely resemble their cells of origin and demonstrate minimal degrees of cellular atypia (**Figure 5–9**). The most important morphologic criteria for benign neoplasms are the discreteness of the lesion and the uniform, relatively mature appearance of the cells.

Malignant Neoplasms

Two characteristics define a malignant neoplasm: cellular atypia, invasion, and **metastasis**. If a neoplasm has metastasized at the time of discovery, it is per definition

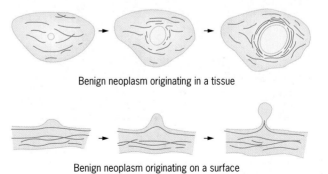

Benign neoplasm originating in a tissue

Benign neoplasm originating on a surface

FIGURE 5–8 Comparison of a benign neoplasm within solid tissue such as breast (above) with a benign neoplasm developing in an organ with a mucosal surface such as the colon (below). The breast neoplasm is encapsulated; the colon neoplasm is polypoid.

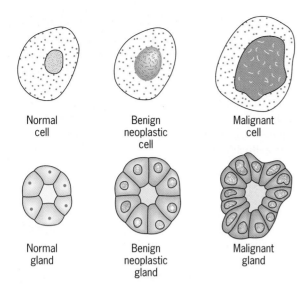

FIGURE 5–9 Comparison of cells and glands from normal tissue, benign neoplasm, and malignant neoplasm.

microscope. Microscopic or morphologic criteria for identification of malignant cells include **cellular atypia**, or the degree to which the cells resemble mature, non-malignant cells (**Figure 5–10**), and the presence of invasion. Features of atypia include enlarged nuclei, decreased amounts of cytoplasm, irregular nuclear placement in a cell, multiple nucleoli, large nucleoli, and frequent mitotic figures.

A growth may be atypical in appearance but still localized to its tissue of origin. This type of abnormality is a **dysplasia**. Dysplastic cells have acquired some of the genetic alterations necessary for the development of overt malignancy, but they do not necessarily become malignant. Dysplasias are recognized precursor lesions for carcinomas, but the precursors of sarcomas are unfortunately not morphologically recognizable. Examples of dysplastic epithelial lesions include the common tubular adenoma of the colon, a type of polyp that, if left in place, has a high likelihood of developing into colon cancer over the next 10 years, and dysplasia of the cervix, or cellular atypia and disregulated growth of the squamous lining of the outer portion of the cervix induced by the human papillomavirus (HPV). Dysplasias can range from low grade, or exhibiting minimal atypia, to high grade, or exhibiting the amount of atypia one

malignant, but fortunately most cases of malignancy are detected before they have metastasized. The nature of the cells has to be determined simply on the basis of their morphology, or how they appear under the

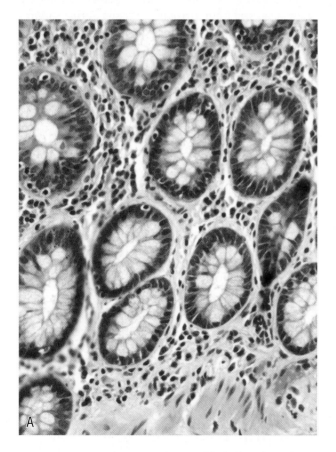

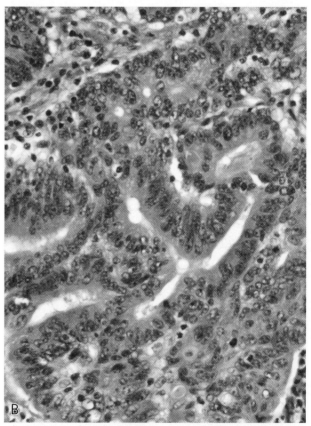

FIGURE 5–10 Atypia. In comparison to the cells in **A**, those in **B** are atypical. A shows normal colonic glands. The nuclei of the cells are arranged at the periphery of the glands, and a droplet of mucin distends the cytoplasm toward the lumenal surface. The cells and their nuclei are uniform in size. In the colonic carcinoma in B, the cells are no longer arranged in a regular pattern, the nuclei are overlapping one another and have irregular shapes and sizes, and the cells do not contain mucin droplets.

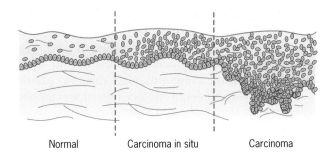

FIGURE 5–11 Invasion of the basement membrane differentiates invasive carcinoma from carcinoma *in situ*.

would expect to see in an invasive lesion. High-grade dysplasias are considered to be *in situ* lesions, or cancers that are still "in place."

What differentiates an *in situ* from an invasive carcinoma is whether the cells have broken through the basement membrane to which epithelial cells are normally anchored (**Figure 5–11**). To invade, malignant cells must be able to elaborate enzymes that destroy the basement membrane and the underlying connective tissue. Once they can do this, malignant cells can infiltrate the tissue, and in doing so they form a poorly circumscribed mass whose exact margins are difficult to delineate (**Figure 5–12**). The secondary effects of invasion often bring the tumor to clinical attention. For example, a colon cancer that has invaded through the bowel wall could present with colonic perforation; cervical cancer that has widely infiltrated the pelvis can cause ureteral obstruction; a carcinoma arising in the head of the pancreas can cause jaundice by obstructing the common bile duct.

Additional morphologic features that are helpful but not entirely specific for separating malignant from benign neoplasms include firmness (many malignant neoplasms provoke proliferation of fibrous tissue, or scar), necrosis (areas of cell death resulting from the cancer outgrowing its blood supply), ulceration (necrotic tissue of surface cancers sloughs, leaving an ulcer defect), and hemorrhage (cancer cells can erode through vessels, or new vessels that are forming may be leaky). Malignant neoplasms are usually larger than benign neoplasms, but this is a very unreliable generalization. Both benign and malignant neoplasms are usually solitary in their origin; however, a few benign neoplasms are characteristically multiple (nevi, leiomyomas of the uterus, neurofibromas, and sometimes adenomas of the colon).

The terminology used to describe malignant and premalignant lesions is admittedly confusing, and various terms may describe the same process but in different organs. For example, in the breast, carcinoma *in situ* describes a preinvasive malignancy of breast epithelium, but it could as well be described as high-grade dysplasia. Also, the differentiation between ductal epithelial atypia and carcinoma *in situ* is somewhat arbitrary by microscopic examination.

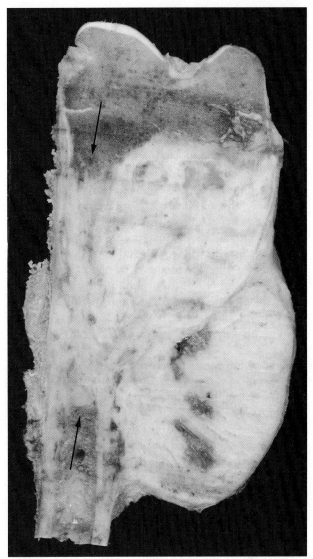

FIGURE 5–12 This is an image of a sarcoma that has invaded the tibia. The tumor is the dense white tissue. The granular red and yellow tissue at either end of the specimen is the marrow cavity of the bone. Note the irregular margins of the sarcoma where it is growing diffusely through the marrow space. Compare to Figure 5–6.

Natural History of Hyperplasia and Cancer

Cancers have a long life history, most of which occurs before there is any lesion that can be called a cancer, or even dysplasia. Early events in the development of cancer are known through experimentation and inference rather than through direct observation because most cancers develop in areas of the body that are not conducive to direct visualization and experimentation.

Genetic alterations are the basis for the development of a cancer. As already mentioned, malignant cells have acquired some advantage in growth potential; this advantage is genetically programmed and transmitted to daughter cells, which accumulate more genetic alterations. The mutations and epigenetic events that lead to the development of cancer are just beginning to be unraveled for most cancers, but a few generalizations can be made.

Most cancers do not develop from a mutation in a single gene. Instead, numerous genes have to be altered for a cell to develop a growth advantage and the ability to invade and metastasize. Cancer development therefore occurs through "multiple hits" on the genome, each of which contributes to the malignant phenotype eventually seen in the clinics and through the microscope.

It is tempting to think of hyperplasia, dysplasia, and neoplasia as occurring on a continuum of cancer development, with additional mutations slowly and steadily nudging the vulnerable population of cells toward malignancy. Whereas this may be the case for some cancers, several observations indicate that this continuum model is too simplistic to be realistic. Dysplasias and hyperplasias do not precede all cancers, and not all hyperplastic or even dysplastic lesions develop into cancer.

Hyperplasia and hypertrophy are responses to increased demand, or chronic irritation, and they recede once the stimulus for their development is withdrawn. They may cause organ dysfunction or symptoms, but in and of themselves they are not necessarily harmful to the organism. Metaplasia and atrophy can also be reversed if the underlying etiology can be addressed. Occasionally, if a stimulus persists and cells are chronically proliferating at a higher rate than normal, genetic alterations that confer a growth advantage can become fixed in the cells and transmitted to daughter cells, setting the stage for eventual malignant transformation.

There are some lesions from which cancers arise with noticeable frequency and which are therefore recognized as predisposing lesions. Examples are hyperplasia of the gums resulting from ill-fitting dentures and squamous metaplasia of bronchi in a chronic smoker. But predisposing or premalignant lesions for all cancers are not known. Adenocarcinoma of the esophagus serves as an illustration of the complex interrelationships between physiologic responses to demand and the development of cancer.

The normal squamous epithelium of the esophagus changes abruptly to columnar gastric epithelium at the squamocolumnar junction, which is normally at the same place as the anatomic esophageal–gastric junction. In patients with chronic gastric reflux, or backflow of the acidic gastric contents into the esophagus, the squamous mucosal lining of the esophagus can undergo metaplasia to a columnar gastric-type epithelium. This is thought to occur as a protective response against the acidic fluid from the stomach: the columnar, mucin-producing cells afford the esophageal wall greater protection from the acidic fluid than the squamous lining

does. The squamocolumnar junction thereby moves higher up into the esophagus. This change can be seen endoscopically in the form of tongues of pink gastric mucosa extending up into the normally white squamous mucosa of the esophagus. Over time, the gastric mucosa can itself undergo another type of metaplasia, called intestinal metaplasia. The mucosa is still columnar but has the phenotype (observable characteristics) of intestinal mucosa rather than gastric mucosa. In the esophagus, intestinal metaplasia, also called Barrett's esophagus, is a precursor lesion for the development of carcinoma. Adenocarcinoma arises from intestinal metaplasia through low-grade and then high-grade dysplasia. Because these dysplastic lesions can be identified by tissue biopsies, patients with Barrett's esophagus should undergo frequent screening via endoscopy and biopsy to monitor for this development. Various treatment modalities, ranging from phototherapy to mucosal (endoscopic) resection to surgical resection of the distal esophagus, are available for these lesions. Again, the goal of treatment is to catch the malignancy before it has invaded or metastasized to the lymph nodes or distant organs.

Many people experience gastric reflux. About 30–60 million people in the United States experience reflux more than twice a week. About 10% of these will develop Barrett's esophagus; of these, 5–20% will develop dysplasia, and of those with high-grade dysplasia, about 50–60% develop carcinoma within 3–5 years (overall, about 10% of patients with Barrett's esophagus progress to develop adenocarcinoma). If you do the calculations, you will see that by far the majority of patients with reflux do not develop intestinal metaplasia, and by far the majority of patients with intestinal metaplasia do not develop dysplasia, and most dysplasias do not progress to cancer. All the other metaplastic and dysplastic lesions stabilize, spontaneously regress, or the patient dies of some other disease before malignant transformation occurs. Currently, it is not possible to identify which of these premalignant lesions will progress to adenocarcinoma and which can be safely followed with longer screening intervals. Obviously, the lesions identified as premalignant and dysplastic are heterogeneous in their molecular biology and behavior.

Practice Questions

1. A 36-year-old woman has an enlarged thyroid on physical exam. A subsequent biopsy shows an increased number of enlarged thyroid cells. This is an example of
   A. hyperplasia.
   B. hypertrophy.
   C. atrophy.
   D. Both A and B.
   E. Both A and C.

2. A cancer of epithelial cells is called a (n)
   A. sarcoma.
   B. carcinoma.
   C. melanoma.
   D. lymphoma.
   E. adenoma.
3. A 67-year-old man who has used chewing tobacco for 40 years is found to have a small protruding growth in his mouth. The pathologist reading the subsequent biopsy notes dysplastic cells that are confined to the epithelial (mucosal) layer. This is an example of
   A. carcinoma *in situ*.
   B. sarcoma.
   C. hyperplasia.
   D. papilloma.
   E. metaplasia.
4. Which of the following pairings is correct?
   A. Neuron–labile cell
   B. Squamous mucosa at gastroesophageal junction–stable tissue
   C. Squamous cells of skin–labile cells
   D. Muscle cells of uterus–permanent cells
   E. Bone cells–permanent cells

5. A 28-year-old woman is told she has evidence of dysplasia in her cervix. This means that
   A. the squamous epithelial cells are piling up, creating a thickened, white patch, but microscopically they are normal in appearance.
   B. the glandular epithelium of the inner part of the cervix is turning into squamous epithelium.
   C. there is a premalignant lesion in the cervix.
   D. there is invasive carcinoma in the cervix.
   E. the squamous cells of the cervix are larger than normal.
6. A young adult long-distance runner who has competed in marathons for years has an x-ray done of the chest. It demonstrates an enlarged heart. The heart is most likely enlarged because of
   A. physiologic hyperplasia.
   B. physiologic hypertrophy.
   C. pathologic hyperplasia.
   D. pathologic hypertrophy.
   E. neoplasia.

Cancer

OUTLINE

OBJECTIVES

1. List the most common carcinomas and indicate how they differ in frequency, sex ratios, and survival rate.
2. List the cancers that occur predominantly in each of the first three decades of life, in middle-aged persons, and in older adults.
3. Describe how a cell becomes neoplastic—that is, the relationship of initiation and progression to transformation.
4. Describe the role of oncogenes and tumor suppressor genes in cancer development.
5. Describe what is meant by the multistep model of carcinogenesis.
6. Describe the types of agents that have been implicated in the development of cancers (chemical carcinogens, radiation, oncogenic viruses, and inherited mutations).
7. List the manifestations of cancer and describe how cancer causes them.
8. Describe and compare the major forms of cancer therapy.
9. Define stage, describe how it is determined for different cancers, and describe how it correlates with prognosis and survival.
10. Define, describe, and use in context all the words in bold print in this chapter.

KEY TERMS

anorexia
cancer
carcinogen
carcinoma
chemical carcinogen
chemotherapy
differentiated
etiology
5- or 10-year survival
grade
hormonal therapy
inherited genetic mutation
initiation
leukemia
lymphoma
occult blood
oncogene

oncogenic virus
paraneoplastic syndrome
Pap smear
progression
promotion
prostate-specific antigen (PSA)
radiation
radiation therapy
sarcoma
screening procedure
stage
surgical removal
tissue diagnosis
TNM system
transformation
tumor suppressor gene

The previous content covered the basic concepts of cell proliferative disorders, differentiating hyperplasias from neoplasms and benign from malignant neoplasms. The emphasis in this chapter is on malignant neoplasms, or **cancers**: their frequency and significance, etiology, manifestations, natural history, and treatment.

Frequency and Significance

Cancer ranks as the second leading cause of death in the United States. The term *cancer* encompasses a large number of specific types of malignant neoplasms whose behavior, treatment, and causes vary considerably. The prognosis of a cancer depends on the natural history of that type of cancer, the extent of spread at the time of discovery, and the efficacy of existing therapy for that particular type of cancer. In general, the incidence of malignant tumors is about twice the mortality rate. Stated differently, the overall survival rate of cancer is approximately 50%. However, there is great variability in the behavior of different cancers. Some types, such as carcinoma of the pancreas, almost always kill the patient, whereas others, such as basal cell carcinoma of the skin, are more of a nuisance than a threat to life if adequately treated.

Three important variables relating to cancer frequency and significance are site of development, gender, and age. Cancers developing from epithelium (**carcinomas**) outnumber cancers from nonepithelial cells (**sarcomas**, **leukemias**, and **lymphomas**) by 6 to 1. The most common cancers of humans are actually basal and squamous cell carcinomas of the skin, accounting for about 40% of all cancers and 99% of all skin cancers. Despite their frequency, they are very seldom fatal because they are readily detected, grow slowly, metastasize only rarely, and can be completely excised. In contrast, malignant melanoma represents only 1% of all skin malignancies but is fatal in about 20% of patients. Thus, the least common type accounts for a large proportion of the mortality associated with cancers of the skin. In addition to being the most common cancers, basal and squamous cell carcinomas are the only common cancers that are frequently treated in a physician's office and thus escape hospital statistics. Consequently, these two common skin cancers are often omitted from overall collections of cancer statistics.

Aside from skin cancers, carcinomas of the lung, colon, breast, prostate, and uterus are the most common types of cancer. The most common types of cancer in men and women are given in **Table 6–1**.

Lung cancer is responsible for about one-third of cancer deaths in males and one-fourth of cancer deaths in females. Treatment is relatively ineffective (approximately 13% 5-year survival), but prevention by avoidance of cigarette smoke could dramatically reduce its incidence. Surgical removal of colon cancer cures more than 50% of patients, and screening colonoscopy can identify precancerous lesions of the colon before they progress to cancer. It appears that dietary factors contribute to the development of colon cancer, but precisely what these factors are is not known and, therefore, its development cannot entirely be prevented. Breast and uterine cancers are often detected early and are quite accessible to surgical and radiation therapy, but their high frequency still accounts for a large number of cancer deaths. Prostate cancer is a disease of older men, so its impact on mortality statistics is lessened by the fact that these patients are likely to die of other diseases that afflict older adults. Leukemias and lymphomas have variable survival rates, depending on the specific type. Aggressive radiation and chemotherapy of leukemias and lymphomas consume a disproportionate share of medical resources and are associated with more complications than surgical therapy, which is the first-line treatment for most solid cancers.

In general, cancer is much more common in older persons; this is particularly true for carcinomas. Of the 10 most common carcinomas, most have a peak frequency in the 70s (see **Table 6–2**). Cancers of the breast and female genital tract tend to occur in midlife. Cancer of the lung also presents somewhat earlier than carcinomas

---

TABLE 6–1 **Frequency of and Deaths from Common Cancers in Men and Women**

Males/Females	Relative Incidence (%)	Cancer Deaths (%)	Relative 5-Year Survival (%)
Prostate/breast	33/31	9/15	~100/88
Lung	13/12	31/26	15
Colon	10/11	10/10	64
Bladder	6/2	3/<2	82
Uterus (not including cervix)	6	3	84
Leukemias/lymphomas	7/4	7/7	Highly variable

Data from Jemal A, et al. Cancer statistics. *CA Cancer J Clin.* 2006;56:106–130. (Published by the American Cancer Society.)

TABLE 6–2 Peak Age of Occurrence of Particular Kinds of Malignancies

0–10 Years	10–20 Years	20–30 Years	30–40 Years	40–50 Years	50–60 Years	60–70 Years
• Acute lymphocytic leukemia • Neuroblastoma • Wilms' tumor of kidney • Retinoblastoma • Medulloblastoma of cerebellum	• Osteogenic sarcoma • Leukemias	• Hodgkin lymphoma • Thyroid cancer • Testicular cancer	• Cervical cancer • Melanoma	• Breast cancer	• Endometrial carcinoma • Ovarian carcinoma • Non-Hodgkin lymphoma • Lung cancer	• Prostate cancer • Colon cancer • Pancreatic cancer • Bladder cancer • Stomach cancer

in general, with the peak number of new cases occurring in the 60s. Melanoma, however, is a cancer that typically arises in a younger age group: 20–40 years. Of the many other less common types of cancer, most have a characteristic age incidence. Although cancer is much less frequent in younger people, some types occur predominantly in the young. All of the common cancers of young people listed in Table 6–2 are non-epithelial, except for adenocarcinoma of the thyroid, a carcinoma most common in young adult women.

Etiology

Etiology literally means the "study of the cause," but it is taken to mean simply "cause." The etiology of cancers is varied (**Table 6–3**). Cancers arise in a variety of circumstances, which suggests that more than one factor is involved in the development of any neoplasm. Experimental studies indicate that cancers go through progressive changes before becoming clinically evident. Recall that a neoplasm is a proliferation of cells that is relatively independent of normal growth control mechanisms, and that this independence is achieved through genetic alterations that are passed to daughter cells. Genetic alteration is therefore the basis for the development of cancer. However, of all the mutations that occur in cells, very few lead to cancer, and most cells with the potential to develop overt malignancy do not do so. A cell must undergo an alteration or series of alterations called **initiation** to acquire autonomous growth potential. Agents that trigger cells to develop cancer are called **carcinogens**. Carcinogens may be physical (e.g., trauma, radiation), chemical (e.g., cigarette smoke, methylcholanthrene), or biologic agents (e.g., microorganisms—especially viruses). An initiated cell, in turn, divides to form a discrete population of altered cells (a clone). At this point the process is reversible. Selective growth of the initiated cells is called **promotion** and does not involve new mutations. Promoter agents can affect only cells that have already been initiated. Some carcinogens act as both initiators and promoters, but many others serve only one function or the other. **Progression** is the acquisition of additional DNA mutations resulting in multiple

clones that constitute the neoplasm (**Figure 6–1**). If a new clone has a higher rate of cell division than the old clones, the new will outgrow the old. As a general rule, the more a cell deviates in character from analogous normal cells (i.e., the more poorly differentiated it becomes), the more rapidly it grows. The more poorly

TABLE 6–3 Examples of Known Causes of Cancers

Cause of Cancer	Cancer Type
Chemical carcinogens	
Coal tar	Scrotal cancer
Aflatoxin	Liver cancer
Vinyl chloride	Liver cancer
Industrial dyes	Bladder cancer
Cigarette smoke	Lung cancer, bladder cancer, kidney cancer
Hormones (e.g., excessive estrogen)	Uterine cancer
Radiation	
Ultraviolet	Skin cancers
X-radiation	Thyroid cancer, skin cancer, leukemia/lymphoma
Oncogenic viruses	
Human papillomavirus (HPV)	Cervical cancer
Epstein-Barr virus (EBV)	Burkitt lymphoma
Hepatitis C virus	Liver carcinoma
Inherited genetic mutations	
Retinoblastoma gene (*Rb*)	Retinoblastoma
Adenomatous polyposis coli gene (*APC*)	Familial adenomatous polyposis/colon cancer
BRCA1 and *BRCA2* genes	Breast cancer
p53 gene	Diverse cancers

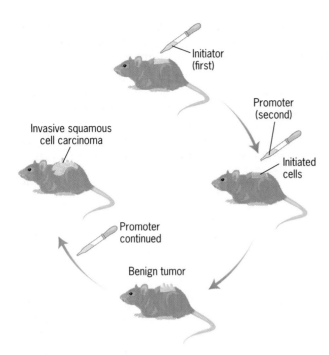

Initiator
(first)

Promoter
(second)

Invasive squamous
cell carcinoma

Initiated
cells

Promoter
continued

Benign tumor

FIGURE 6–1 Initiation, promotion, and progression of cancer.

differentiated cells are usually more invasive and more likely to metastasize.

The mechanism of action of the initiating carcinogen is direct or indirect alteration of **oncogenes** or tumor suppressor genes. Oncogenes code for growth-enhancing products, such as growth factors, that can contribute to increased proliferation of the cell. Initiators mutate the oncogenes so that they are permanently "turned on" and drive the cell to increased proliferation. Cells also contain **tumor suppressor genes** (e.g., *p53*) that typically keep the oncogenes in check. When there is a mutation in a tumor suppressor gene, it no longer functions as a control on an oncogene. The net result is replication of DNA and consequent cell division outside of the normal control mechanisms. Thus, the development of cancer is an extremely complex process that entails changes in multiple genes. The challenge in attempting to find a "cure for cancer" becomes apparent when you appreciate the complexities of the developmental events.

Transformation is the process by which normal cells first lose important checks on their growth. The cancer cells proliferate rapidly, thereby expanding the size of their population. In addition, they acquire new mutations, some of which allow them to become even more autonomous: to evade external checks on their growth, for example, or to elaborate enzymes that allow them to invade and metastasize.

These colonies of aberrant cells are not necessarily neoplasms. Most populations of aberrant cells are hyperplasias, metaplasias, or dysplasias—in other words, non-malignant or pre-malignant lesions. These are

amenable to surgical removal if they can be clinically discovered. Unfortunately, it is not possible to detect pre-neoplastic phases for most types of neoplasms.

Ultimate prevention and cure of cancer will depend on discovery and targeted manipulation of oncogenes and tumor suppressor genes. It is particularly important to understand what initiating agents cause the original genetic change and the circumstances that cause malignant transformation of mutated cells. At the present time, three general initiating factors have been identified—**chemical carcinogens**, **radiation**, and **oncogenic viruses**.

The recognition of a high incidence of scrotal skin cancer in London chimney sweeps led to the discovery that repeated occupational exposure to coal tar was carcinogenic. Later, through experimentation, methylcholanthrene, a chemical coal tar, was identified as a specific polycyclic hydrocarbon that could cause cancer. Since then, a large number of natural and synthetic compounds have been discovered that are potentially carcinogenic.

The mechanism of chemical carcinogenesis is complex. Generally, carcinogens must be metabolized by cells to an active metabolite, which in turn interacts with deoxyribonucleic acid (DNA), ribonucleic acid (RNA), or cell proteins. The interaction with DNA is potentially mutagenic. The cell has an enzyme system that normally repairs DNA defects, such as those caused by carcinogens. It appears that the establishment of a carcinogenic effect depends on failure of these enzymes to repair DNA. The appearance of tumors takes months to years after exposure to a carcinogen (latent period). What happens in this intervening time is not well known. The latent period can be reduced by increasing the frequency of exposure and size of the dose of the carcinogen. Other factors modifying the effects of chemical carcinogens include age, sex, diet, genetic factors, and immune deficiencies.

Many types of human cancer are known to be associated with exposure to carcinogenic chemicals in the workplace. Carcinogenic compounds implicated in various industries include certain dyes, vinyl chloride, alkylating agents, and asbestos. Hormones can also be considered to be chemicals that can initiate certain types of cancer. For example, administration of estrogen for the treatment of symptoms of menopause in women has been shown to increase the incidence of uterine cancer. Based on present knowledge, the cancer-inducing chemical agent(s) affecting the largest number of people is/are contained in cigarette smoke. Smokers have a 10- to 50-fold greater chance of developing bronchogenic carcinoma than do nonsmokers, and the risk can be significantly correlated with the number of packs smoked per day and duration of smoking. Squamous cell carcinomas of the oral region, larynx, and esophagus and carcinomas of the urinary bladder are also significantly associated with cigarette smoking.

Ultraviolet radiation, x-radiation, and gamma radiation are all carcinogenic, with the effect dependent on dose, duration, and the portion of the body exposed. As with chemical carcinogens, a latent period of years to decades intervenes between exposure and the appearance of neoplasms. Just how radiation initiates cancer is not known, although it is known that radiation produces localized breaks in DNA strands that cannot always be repaired, thereby introducing errors in transcription and translation.

Examples of radiation-induced cancer include skin cancers developing in sun-exposed areas of the body and thyroid carcinoma and leukemia developing in victims of the Hiroshima and Nagasaki atomic blasts and victims of the Chernobyl nuclear power plant accident. Before the adverse effects of ionizing radiation were discovered, up to 75% of thyroid carcinomas in children were preceded by "therapeutic" radiation to the head and neck, often for benign conditions such as acne or acute tonsillitis, and radiologists not uncommonly developed skin cancers before protective shielding was utilized. The strongest risk factor for the development of melanoma of the skin is a history of blistering sunburns, and the incidence of melanoma is highest in fair-skinned individuals living in sunny locations (Florida, Australia) or engaged in occupations where they are exposed to ionizing radiation from the sun (fishing, farming).

Both RNA- and DNA-containing viruses have oncogenic (tumor-producing) potential. In the DNA groups, members of the papova, herpes, pox, and adenovirus groups have been found to produce tumors in animals. Tumor-producing RNA viruses are called oncornaviruses (onco + RNA) or retroviruses. In cells infected by DNA oncogenic viruses, the viral genome is incorporated into the host cell genome and is expressed with it. This insertion of viral genome occurs in only a few cells of an infected population. In cells infected by RNA oncogenic viruses, the virus carries an enzyme, reverse transcriptase, that makes a copy of DNA complementary to the virus's RNA, and this DNA becomes inserted into the host genome.

Specific strains of human papillomavirus (HPV) play an important role in the etiology of carcinoma of the uterine cervix. Papovaviruses cause squamous papillomas in humans including the common wart (verruca vulgaris), venereal warts (condyloma acuminata), and laryngeal papillomas. Epstein-Barr virus (EBV), the cause of infectious mononucleosis, has been associated with Burkitt lymphoma, a neoplasm most prevalent in Africa, and with undifferentiated nasopharyngeal carcinoma. Hepatitis B and C viruses have been associated with carcinoma of the liver. Though it is known that these viruses are important in the development of the respective cancers, their exact role in initiation and progression has not been established, and in fact, most people with these viruses do not get cancer.

Another important predisposing factor for the development of cancer is an **inherited genetic mutation** that accelerates the development of cancer in affected individuals. The classic example is the development of retinoblastoma in children who inherit a defective tumor suppressor gene called *retinoblastoma (Rb)*. The familial occurrence of many different types of cancer is increasingly being linked to specific tumor suppressor genes. Inheritance of the defective tumor suppressor genes *BRCA1* and *BRCA2* is responsible for most familial breast and ovarian carcinomas, the defective tumor suppressor gene *APC* is implicated in familial (colonic) adenomatous polyposis, and a germline mutation of the oncogene *p53* can be responsible for neoplasms developing in a wide variety of organs, including the thyroid, stomach, breast, and soft tissues. Generally, cancers occur about 10 years earlier in patients with an inherited mutation than in the general population.

Local and Systemic Manifestations

Local manifestations of malignant neoplasms include a mass, pain, obstruction, hemorrhage, pathologic fracture, and infection. Systemic manifestations include infection, anemia, cachexia, and hormone production. Most cancers are asymptomatic until late in their course, so manifestation of local or systemic signs is associated with cancers that have already invaded widely, locally, or metastasized to different parts of the body.

Mass

Neoplasms are autonomous proliferations of cells, so it stands to reason that they form abnormal growths, or masses (**Figure 6–2**). If a cancer becomes very large or

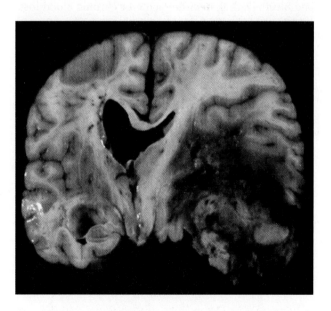

FIGURE 6–2 Mass effect of cancer. A neoplasm is invading and destroying the right side of the brain. It is such a large space-occupying lesion that it has pushed the remaining white matter against the ventricle, essentially causing it to collapse, and has pushed the midline structures to the left. (Courtesy of Dr. M. Shahriar Salamat, Department of Pathology and Laboratory Medicine, University of Wisconsin School of Medicine and Public Health.)

is situated in a location that is readily visible or palpable, the mass may be easily noted. With the increasing use of imaging techniques such as mammography, computed tomography (CT) scan, and magnetic resonance imaging (MRI), cancers are more likely to be detected as a mass lesion. Often, however, one or more of the complications discussed subsequently may become evident before a mass is noted.

Pain

Cancer produces pain by local destruction of tissue, by invasion of nerves, by obstructing hollow organs such as the intestine, and by causing inflammation. In advanced cases, surgical interruption of nerve tracts is sometimes needed to relieve otherwise uncontrollable pain.

Obstruction

Body passageways may be obstructed by tumors growing within their lumens or by external compression. Symptoms depend on the site involved. Examples of internal obstruction include the obstruction of a bronchus by lung cancer or bowel obstruction by colonic carcinoma (**Figure 6–3**). An example of external obstruction is compression of the common bile duct by a carcinoma of the pancreas. Infection is often a complication of obstruction because blockage of any lumen leads to accumulation of secretions that serve as good culture media for bacteria.

Hemorrhage

Cancers on mucosal surfaces or the skin may ulcerate and bleed, leading to either acute or chronic blood loss. Inapparent blood in feces (**occult blood**) can be detected by a simple chemical test. Initial signs of cancers of the gastrointestinal tract and bladder are likely to be blood in the stool and urine, respectively.

Pathologic Fracture

Primary bone cancer or metastatic cancers may invade and locally destroy bone, weakening it so that it fractures with minimal injury. Cancers of the lung, breast, and prostate are especially likely to metastasize to bone. Multiple myeloma, a neoplastic proliferation of plasma cells, is a primary cancer of bone marrow that commonly destroys adjacent bone. A third mechanism by which a neoplasm can cause pathologic fracture is by induction of osteoporosis. Osteoporosis may be caused by inactivity due to general malaise caused by cancer or by rare tumors secreting high levels of corticosteroids or adrenocorticotropic hormone (ACTH).

Infection

Infection is a common and often disastrous complication of neoplasia. A variety of overlapping mechanisms produce infections in patients with cancer. At the local level, erosion or ulceration of epithelial surfaces by a tumor allows entry of microorganisms through impaired defenses. Obstruction results in pooling of secretions and their subsequent colonization by organisms. Impaired host responses can arise from a number of causes. Leukopenia may result from extensive replacement of bone marrow in leukemias and lymphomas or in other metastatic cancers. In leukemias and lymphomas, the circulating neoplastic leukocytes are deficient in phagocytic ability. Inadequate nutrition and other factors in the terminally debilitated cancer patient may be associated with a decline in the general capacities of the immune system. Chemotherapy for cancer treatment has a side effect of suppressing the bone marrow's production of leukocytes. Because lymphocyte quantity and quality are often deficient in neoplastic disease, cell-mediated immunity may be particularly impaired. Immune deficiency is manifested by the occurrence of unusual infections caused by fungi, protozoa, viruses, and bacteria that are ordinarily not pathogens.

Anemia

Anemia is one of the most frequent manifestations of malignant neoplasms. Major mechanisms include decreased erythropoiesis (production of red blood cells) resulting from the effects of chemotherapeutic drugs or radiation on bone marrow, bone marrow replacement by neoplastic cells, and blood loss caused by ulceration of the cancer.

Cachexia

Cachexia is the generalized wasting that occurs in the terminal cancer patient. It is probably caused by a combination of **anorexia** (loss of appetite), the nutritional

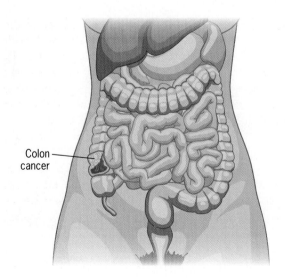

Colon cancer

FIGURE 6–3 Bowel obstruction. The portion of bowel proximal to the colon cancer becomes dilated, resulting in excruciating abdominal pain.

demands of the rapidly growing neoplasm, and cytokines produced by the body's inflammatory response to the tumor that suppress the appetite.

Hormone Production

A few neoplasms secrete hormones that lead to specific manifestations. Benign neoplasms of the endocrine glands most commonly cause overproduction of hormones. Occasionally, malignant endocrine gland neoplasms or other neoplasms such as small cell carcinoma of the lung produce hormones in sufficient quantity to cause clinical effects. Manifestations of aberrant and uncontrolled hormone production by a malignant neoplasm are called **paraneoplastic syndromes**.

Death

Infection is the most common cause of death in cancer patients. Commonly, as the terminally ill patient with a malignant neoplasm becomes more and more immobilized and bedridden, the lungs fail to remove secretions, allowing bacteria to proliferate and cause pneumonia. Infections of the genitourinary tract are also common in terminally ill patients. Whatever the initial site of the infection, many patients eventually develop bacteremia, with spread of the infectious organisms to other organs. The predisposing factors for terminal infections are the previously mentioned immune and white cell deficiencies, immobilization, obstruction of body passageways, and general debilitation. Cachexia, metabolic and endocrine effects, and hemorrhage are occasional causes of death in cancer patients. Often, a single immediate cause of death in a patient with terminal cancer is not identifiable: the various adverse results of the tumor burden collectively lead to death.

Diagnosis

The diagnosis of cancer is based on investigation of the cause of a patient's symptoms or on screening. The diagnosis is confirmed by biopsy or sometimes by blood smear or cytology. The astute physician who recognizes that a patient's symptoms may be caused by cancer performs the appropriate physical examination and orders appropriate laboratory tests, radiologic procedures, endoscopic examinations, and other diagnostic procedures. Before carrying out irreversible treatments that always entail some risk, a **tissue diagnosis** based on microscopic examination of a biopsy sample should be made. Otherwise, treatment protocols could be based on an erroneous assumption of cancer or on less than optimal knowledge of the type of cancer present.

Discovery of cancer, especially in older adults, often occurs when a physician sees the patient for some other disease. Physicians may detect asymptomatic cancer of the breast, prostate, or testis by palpation, and they can inspect the skin for malignant melanoma and carcinoma.

However, many cancers are hidden from the physicians' gaze and do not present with symptoms. In addition, cancers are ideally diagnosed when they are still small, or when they are still in a premalignant stage, because the larger they have grown and the more widely they have spread through the body, the more difficult it becomes to achieve a cure. Routine **screening procedures** are therefore recommended for the most common cancers.

Effective screening procedures that are simple and not very expensive have greatly reduced the incidence of two previously very prevalent diseases: cervical cancer and late-stage cancer of the prostate. The **Pap smear** identifies precancerous lesions of the uterine cervix so that these can be eliminated before they have a chance to develop into invasive carcinoma, and a blood test for **prostate-specific antigen (PSA)** allows for detection of most prostate cancers when they are still small and localized to the prostate gland. Mammography detects *in situ* and invasive breast cancers, and colonoscopy can detect dysplastic lesions of the colon that are at high risk of developing into cancer if left in place. Unfortunately, cost-effective screening tests are not available for most cancers, including those of the lung, ovary, and pancreas. These cancers have poor survival statistics because they are usually not detected until they are advanced. Abnormalities detected on screening procedures require follow-up with more specific tests and tissue samples for microscopic examination before a definitive diagnosis of cancer or a premalignant lesion can be made. The biggest problem with screening tests, however, is that they are underused or unavailable to the large numbers of uninsured who do not have primary healthcare coverage.

Prognosis

In general, the more widely a cancer has spread in the body at the time it is detected, the more likely it will result in death. However, the characteristics of a malignancy that correlate with survival and its pattern of spread vary from one type of tumor to the next. To prognosticate and design therapy that is most likely to be effective, the **stage** of the tumor must be determined. Stage describes the extent of spread of a cancer in the body. Universally, it is designated by the **TNM system**, whereby *T* describes the tumor itself, *N* describes the extent of lymph node metastasis, and *M* describes whether distant metastasis has occurred. Usually, the N and M designations simply reflect whether metastases to the lymph nodes or distant organs, respectively, are present, although for some cancers (e.g., breast cancer) further separation of N according to the number of involved lymph nodes and the size of the metastatic deposit within them is also necessary for accurate stage designation. T is the most variable factor. The characteristics defining T vary from one organ to the next but generally consist of a combination of the size of the tumor and the extent to which it has invaded surrounding

TABLE 6-4 TNM Grouping Criteria for Colon Carcinoma

Tumor characteristics	
T1	Tumor invades through basement membrane into submucosa of bowel wall
T2	Tumor invades through the submucosa and into the smooth muscle layer of the bowel wall
T3	Tumor invades through the smooth muscle of the bowel and into the pericolic fat
T4	Tumor invades all the way through the bowel wall; malignant cells are present on the peritoneal surface of the bowel or the tumor has invaded adjacent organs or structures
Lymph node characteristics	
N0	No regional lymph node metastasis
N1	Metastasis to 1–3 regional lymph nodes
N2	Metastasis to 4 or more regional lymph nodes
Distant metastasis	
M0	No distant metastasis
M1	Presence of distant metastasis

tissues. **Table 6-4** lists the TNM grouping criteria for colon carcinoma.

The possible combinations of T, N, and M correspond to different stages of cancer spread. For all cancers, there are four stages, with stage I representing the most localized manifestation and stage IV connoting metastatic spread. How the various T, N, and M classifications are combined in stages again varies from one organ to the next. These classifications are based on numerous studies and observations and are continuously being revised as more data about the natural history of the tumors and their responses to therapies are collected. **Table 6–5** shows the stage grouping for colon carcinoma.

TABLE 6-5 Stage Grouping by TNM Classification for Colon Carcinoma

Stage	T	N	M
Stage I	T1	N0	M0
	T2	N0	M0
Stage IIA	T3	N0	M0
Stage IIB	T4	N0	M0
Stage IIIA	T1 or T2	N1	M0
Stage IIIB	T3 or T4	N1	M0
Stage IIIC	Any T	N2	M0
Stage IV	Any T	Any N	M1

TABLE 6-6 5-Year Survival of Breast and Colon Cancer Patients by Stage

Stage	5-Year Survival	
	Breast Cancer (%)	Colon Cancer (%)
Stage I	100	93
Stage IIA	92	85
Stage IIB	81	72
Stage IIIA	67	83
Stage IIIB	54	64
Stage IIIC	N/A	44
Stage IV	20	8

Note. N/A = not applicable.

When predicting the behavior of cancers, the measurement of **5- or 10-year survival**, or what percentage of patients with that particular neoplasm will still be alive (with or without disease) 5 or 10 years after the initial diagnosis, is used. This prognostication of tumor behavior is far from exact. One person with a malignant metastatic neoplasm may die within months of diagnosis, whereas another patient with the same type of neoplasm may live for several years. In general, though, as you can see from **Table 6–6**, stage groupings do correlate with survival: most patients with stage I cancer who receive appropriate treatment are alive after 5 years, while survival rates for patients with metastatic disease (stage IV) are dismal.

Cancers of different organ systems spread in predictable ways. Carcinomas tend to metastasize first to regional lymph nodes and then to the liver, lung, and bone (**Figure 6–4**), while sarcomas are rarely carried

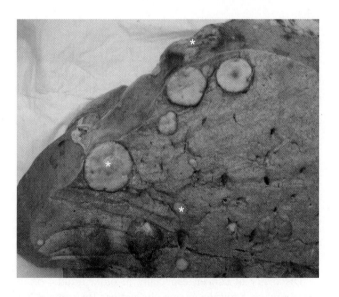

FIGURE 6–4 Metastasis. This is a cross section of a liver. There are numerous nodules in the liver, some even apparent on the capsular surface (top). These are metastases from a pancreatic adenocarcinoma.

through lymphatics but disseminate via the blood vessels, primarily to the lung. Some patterns of spread are idiosyncratic: prostate carcinoma does not metastasize to the brain, while breast and colon cancer commonly do; the spleen and kidney rarely harbor metastases; lobular carcinoma of the breast often causes insidiously infiltrative metastases that do not form a mass lesion and thus evade detection by imaging modalities; and melanoma breaks all rules by metastasizing to unusual sites such as the mucosa of the gastrointestinal tract and adrenal gland. Cancers may come to clinical detection because of the secondary effects of metastatic lesions. Metastases can cause pleural effusions, bone fractures, compression of bile ducts, neurologic manifestations, or lumps in the skin.

Another factor taken into consideration in prognostication is the **grade** of the tumor. This is the assessment of how aggressive the growth looks under the microscope, or how **differentiated** it appears. Malignant cells that resemble the tissue of origin are called "well differentiated," while those that have an atypical appearance with great variation in size and shape of cells, high nuclear to cytoplasmic ratios, and frequent mitotic figures are "poorly differentiated" (**Figure 6–5**). Differentiation correlates with grade, or degree of cellular atypia. Thus, the degree of differentiation and grade are a rough estimate of a tumor's malignant potential: poorly differentiated, high-grade cancers tend to behave more aggressively than do well-differentiated, low-grade ones. In general, high-grade lesions grow to a larger size, invade tissues extensively, and metastasize early. As with all other factors, these are only general observations: some high-grade lesions may remain completely localized and be cured with limited surgery, while some low-grade malignancies may already have metastasized widely at the time of detection.

Treatment

The basic modality of cancer treatment is **surgical removal**. Surgical removal of most cancers is necessary for accurate staging: both tumor characteristics and the presence of lymph node metastases require gross and microscopic examination by the pathologist. However, whether the cancer can be removed operatively depends on its accessibility to surgical removal and its amenability to other modes of therapy. For example, a surgeon may remove very little of a cerebellar medulloblastoma because surgical exposure of the tumor is difficult and there is a risk of destroying

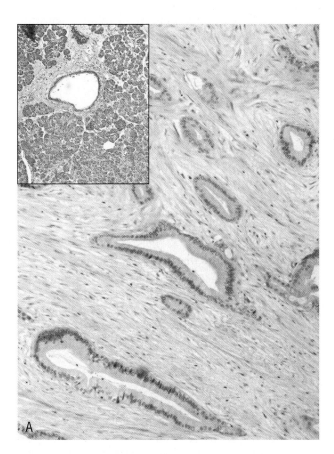
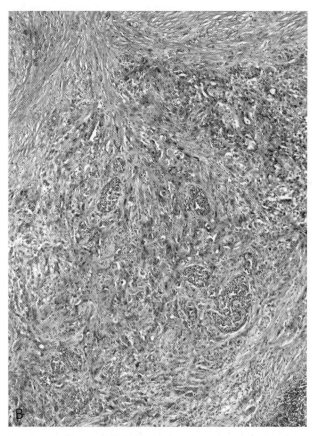

FIGURE 6–5 Differentiation. The inset shows a normal pancreatic duct surrounded by pancreatic acinar cells. The duct has a rounded contour, and the cells are small and inconspicuous. **A** shows a well-differentiated pancreatic ductal adenocarcinoma. The cells do not look much different from those in the normal duct, but the duct outlines are irregular and angulated. **B** shows a poorly differentiated pancreatic ductal adenocarcinoma. There is no gland formation. The cells are not clearly discernible because they are growing in irregular clusters.

adjacent brain structures. In addition, this type of cancer responds readily to radiation therapy; thus, removal of a very small amount of tissue to establish a tissue diagnosis is sufficient. If a tumor has spread very widely, such as ovarian carcinoma, which can fill the entire abdomen and pelvis, surgery may not be feasible; the patient is given chemotherapy to reduce the volume of the carcinoma before surgery is attempted. Conversely, when a cancer is discovered in the large bowel, total removal is anticipated because the tumor is usually accessible to the surgeon in its entirety. In the latter example, even if metastasis has already occurred, removal of the primary tumor may prevent bowel obstruction.

Radiation therapy is generally most effective with tumors composed of rapidly dividing cells. It is employed in the treatment of localized neoplastic masses that are not surgically accessible (inoperable) or in situations where surgery would be impractical or deleterious to the patient. Radiation therapy is also used to treat residual neoplasm following surgery. Another use of radiation therapy is in the treatment of lymph nodes in the expected metastatic pathway of a particular type of neoplasm. For example, carcinoma of the medial aspect of the breast would be expected to metastasize via the internal mammary lymphatic channels; consequently, these lymph node channels are often irradiated prophylactically following mastectomy. Only a limited number of cancer types can be cured by radiation. For many types of cancers, radiation therapy is palliative—that is, it temporarily abates the progress of a cancer without curing it.

Chemotherapy employs a wide variety of powerful metabolic inhibitors and other cell-killing chemicals that are used alone or in various combinations. The rationale behind the use of all chemotherapeutic agents is that they will kill or inhibit the growth of neoplastic cells to a greater degree than that of the body's normal cells. However, in some instances not enough differential response exists, and consequently, serious side effects from chemotherapy can occur. Side effects result from the harmful effects on rapidly metabolizing and rapidly regenerating normal body tissues such as bone marrow and gastrointestinal mucosa. Chemotherapy has been most successful for certain types of cancers that have a very high prolifertive rate, such as some aggressive leukemias and lymphomas. There are no effective chemotherapeutic treatment modalities for slowly growing cancers such as indolent lymphomas or prostate cancer.

Hormonal therapy may cause significant regression of some cancers of the breast and prostate gland and prolong life. The response may be induced by administering hormones or by removing hormone-producing organs such as testes, ovaries, adrenal glands, or pituitary gland. The growth-promoting effect of estrogen on breast cancers can be blocked by administration of the anti-estrogenic agent tamoxifen. Similarly, some prostate cancers regress when testosterone levels are lowered by castration or by administration of the opposing hormone estrogen.

This chapter provides an overview of cancer: how malignancies arise, how they are diagnosed, which factors clinicians consider in determining prognosis and therapy, and which types of therapeutic modalities are available.

Practice Questions

1. Which of the following statements about the epidemiology of cancer is correct?
   A. The incidence of cancers in the population is the same regardless of age, race, and sex.
   B. The types of cancers that affect children are different from those that affect adults.
   C. All cancers have the same survival statistics.
   D. Carcinomas are less frequent than sarcomas.
   E. Cancers are most common in the pediatric population.

2. A 63-year-old woman develops breast cancer. Which of the following tests would not provide information regarding the stage of her disease?
   A. A CT scan demonstrating nodules in the lung
   B. A biopsy of a suspicious nodule in the liver
   C. Removal and microscopic examination of the axillary lymph nodes on the same side as the breast cancer
   D. Counting the number of mitotic figures in the breast cancer

3. Which of the following is the most common cause of death from cancer?
   A. Obstruction
   B. Hemorrhage
   C. Cachexia
   D. Anemia
   E. Infection

4. Which of the following statements about carcinogenesis is correct?
   A. It usually takes only one mutation to cause transformation of a cell.
   B. Viruses, chemicals, and radiation are types of promoters.
   C. Mutations that cause transformation of a cell must be transmitted to the cell's progeny for progression to occur.
   D. Mutations in oncogenes result in slowing down of the cell cycle, so more mutations can accumulate.

5. Tumor suppressor genes are
   A. rarely mutated in cancers.
   B. more commonly mutated in carcinomas than in sarcomas.
   C. genes that are involved in accelerating or enhancing growth.
   D. genes that encode proteins that control oncogenes.
   E. rarely implicated in genetic forms of cancer.

6. So that appropriate therapy can be given for any cancer, which of the following is necessary?
   A. The presence of a mass
   B. X-ray diagnosis
   C. The presence of systemic manifestations
   D. The presence of metastases
   E. A tissue diagnosis

7. An old adage in medicine is "iron-deficiency anemia in an adult man is colon cancer until proven otherwise." Why do you think colon cancer would cause anemia?
   A. Colon cancer metastasizes to bone, replacing the blood-forming elements in the marrow.
   B. The cells of the colon carcinoma require iron, so they "steal" it from the blood.
   C. Red blood cells are lysed (killed) as they pass through the malignancy.
   D. Blood is lost across the ulcerated surface of the cancer into the gut lumen.
   E. Metastatic colon cancer destroys the kidneys, so they cannot put out the hormone that stimulates red blood cell formation.

8. Which of the following statements about therapy for cancer is correct?
   A. Surgery is usually not necessary for staging purposes.
   B. Radiation is useful for tumors that are rapidly dividing.
   C. Chemotherapy does not affect normal cells in the body.
   D. Hormonal therapy can be used to induce regression of certain types of cancers.
   E. Surgery is more effective for late-stage disease than for localized cancers.

Genetic and Developmental Diseases

OUTLINE

OBJECTIVES

1. Review human development from gametogenesis through fertilization, the embryonic and fetal periods, infancy, childhood, and adolescence, and describe how the etiology and incidence of diseases differ in each of these stages.
2. Define genetic and chromosomal diseases, congenital anomalies, and teratogenic effects, and describe at what stage of development these diseases originate and at what stage they become manifest.
3. Differentiate congenital, familial, and genetic diseases and give examples of each.

4. Differentiate monogenetic from polygenetic diseases and give examples of each.
5. Describe the inheritance patterns of genetic diseases.
6. Describe what is meant with "non-Mendelian inheritance" and give examples.
7. Define teratogen, describe how teratogens interfere with normal embryonic and fetal development, and give examples of well-known teratogenic agents, including infectious agents and pharmaceutical drugs.
8. Illustrate how fetal and perinatal diseases relate to the intrauterine environment, including the effects of maternal health and placental abnormalities.
9. Describe tests that are available for the detection of genetic and chromosomal diseases, such as karyotyping, DNA analysis, amniocentesis, and newborn screening.
10. List and describe the most common diseases occurring in the embryonic, fetal, and neonatal periods and in infancy.
11. Describe the common monogenetic diseases discussed in this chapter, including the approach to their treatment and management.
12. Define and use in context all terms in bold print throughout the chapter.

KEY TERMS

allele (dominant, recessive)
amniocentesis
autosomal chromosome
childhood
chromosomal disease
congenital
cyanotic heart defect
cystic fibrosis
developmental abnormality
Down syndrome (trisomy 21)
Duchenne muscular dystrophy
embryonic development
erythroblastosis fetalis

familial disease
fertilization
fetal period
fragile X syndrome
gamete
gene
genetic disease
genotype
gestational age
hemophilia
hemosiderosis
homologous chromosomes
imprinting

inborn error of metabolism
infancy
karyotyping
Klinefelter syndrome
meiosis
mitochondrial disease
mitosis
monogenetic
monosomy
mosaicism
mutation
neonatal period
non-Mendelian inheritance
perinatal period
phenotype

phenylketonuria
polygenetic
prematurity
quad test
sex-linked
sickle cell anemia
somatic cells
teratogen
tetralogy of Fallot
TORCH
translocation
triple screen test
trisomy
Turner syndrome
zygote

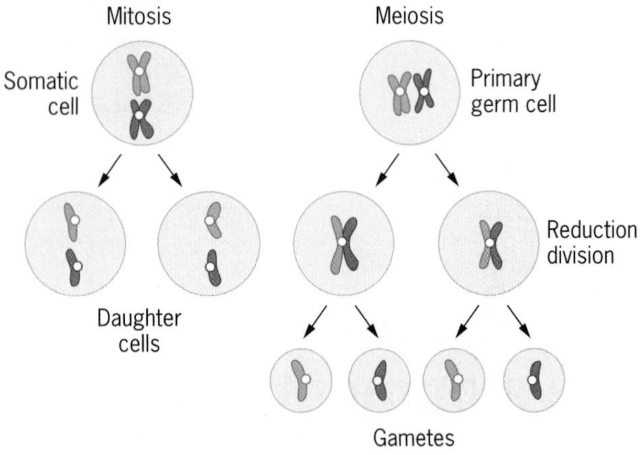

FIGURE 7–1 Comparison of mitosis in somatic cells with meiosis in germ cells. A homologous pair of chromosomes that have already duplicated but are still connected by a centromere are illustrated at the top. In mitosis, each daughter cell receives one of each of the duplicated chromosomes from each pair. In meiosis, the paired chromosomes align opposite each other and are separated at the first (reduction) division. The second division sends only one chromosome duplicate from the original pair to each gamete.

Review of Structure and Function

The development of a mature individual takes approximately 18 years. It can be divided into seven stages or periods: fertilization, embryonal period, fetal period, perinatal period, infancy, childhood, and adolescence. The organism's development and interaction with the environment are different in each of these stages. Consequently, the diseases that arise at each stage are different.

Fertilization involves the uniting of a sperm and ovum, with each contributing 23 chromosomes to the **zygote**. These chromosomes contain all of the genetic information needed to control the succeeding stages of development. Many human diseases result from abnormalities in genetic makeup as a result of events going awry before and during fertilization.

All of the cells of a normal person have 23 pairs of chromosomes (46 total) including 22 pairs of autosomes and 1 pair of sex chromosomes. One of each of these pairs comes from one of the parents. These chromosomes may duplicate and divide to form two daughter cells, each with 46 chromosomes. This process is called **mitosis** and occurs in most of the cells in the body (**Figure 7–1**). The germ cells that develop into sperm and ova undergo a different type of cell division, called **meiosis**. In meiosis, only one chromosome from each pair is passed on to each **gamete** (sperm or ovum) (Figure 7–1). Thus, each gamete has only 23 chromosomes.

Because of the vast amount of genetic information carried on each chromosome, a zygote may be severely affected by abnormalities of cell division. Chromosomes may not separate normally during meiosis, or they may break. Abnormalities in chromosome number result from *nondisjunction*, which results in two **homologous** (belonging to the same pair) chromosomes going to one gamete and none to another (**Figure 7–2**). If fertilization occurs with such a gamete, the zygote formed has three homologous chromosomes (**trisomy**) or only one (**monosomy**). Abnormalities in chromosome structure result from breakage of chromosomes during the process of cell division. Resulting fragments may pass to the wrong daughter cells, resulting in *duplication* or *deletion* of parts

of a chromosome, or fragments may exchange places with sequences on nonhomologous chromosomes, resulting in **translocations** (**Figure 7–3**). Occasionally, nondisjunction, duplication, deletion, or translocation occurs in the first or second cell division after fertilization, resulting in an individual with cells of differing chromosomal makeup. This is called **mosaicism**.

Chromosomes are made of deoxyribonucleic acid (DNA) molecules wrapped around and interacting with numerous proteins. The DNA represents the critical

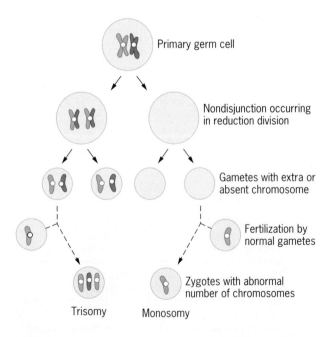

FIGURE 7–2 The results of nondisjunction at reduction division of meiosis.

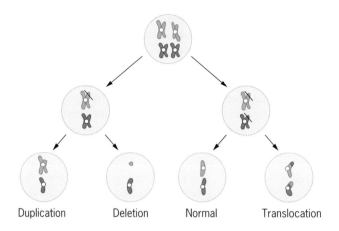

Duplication   Deletion   Normal   Translocation

FIGURE 7–3 Illustration of how breaks in chromosomes can result in duplication, deletion, and translocation.

genetic material that encodes the information necessary for cellular function. DNA is arranged into specific sequences, or **genes**, which define the subunits of a chromosome. One or more genes are responsible for determining a genetic trait. An abnormality in a gene may result in the genetic trait being expressed in an abnormal way. Genes can be altered in various ways, one of which is **mutation**, or chemical alteration in a sequence of DNA. When a mutation occurs during meiosis, the resulting sperm or ovum can pass the abnormal gene to the zygote. This abnormal gene will be present in all the cells of the new individual and will be passed to subsequent generations by the germ cells. Thus, abnormal genes can pass from one generation to the next or can arise by new mutations in germ cells. Mutations can also occur in nongerm cells (**somatic cells**), but the effects are limited to the individual and not transmitted to the next generation. As noted earlier in this text, neoplasms result from mutations in somatic cells.

Not all abnormal genes result in expression of abnormal genetic traits. Each genetic trait is influenced by two genes, one on each of the paired chromosomes. The two genes are called **alleles**. One of the alleles of a pair may be **dominant** over the other—that is, it determines how the genetic trait is expressed. A **recessive** gene results in an abnormal trait only when both alleles are defective or if the gene is located on the X chromosome of a male. Some of the genes on the female, or X, chromosome are not present on the Y chromosome, so a gene on the X chromosome is expressed in a dominant fashion in a male, whereas it is recessive in a female. Genes that are located on the X or Y chromosomes are called **sex-linked**, while those occurring on any of the other 44 chromosomes are called **autosomal**.

The genetic makeup of individuals is called the **genotype**. Although it is the genes that carry the blueprints for cellular structure and function, the genetic makeup alone does not determine how genes are expressed. Sometimes an abnormal dominant gene or pairs of abnormal recessive genes fail to result in an abnormal trait. This is called *nonpenetrance*. An abnormal trait may be expressed differently in individuals with an identical genotype for the alleles responsible for the trait. This is called *variable expressivity*. The expression of some genetic traits is dependent on multiple factors, such as how they interact with other genes and with the environment. In addition, one of the intracellular organelles, the mitochondrion, contains its own DNA that is derived only from the mother. *Paternal imprinting* silences certain genes that are derived from the father so that only the maternal allele is expressed. *Epigenetic phenomena*—modification of the DNA by methylation or addition of protein groups to certain portions of genes, for example—modify the manner in which a gene is expressed without altering the actual sequence of nucleic acids. For all these reasons, the **phenotype**—the physical and functional manifestation of genetic traits—is not simply a reflection of the genotype. Moreover, most of the abnormal genes in the population are not manifest. They are discovered only by inference, by establishing which family members have the disease and deducing which ones carry the abnormal genes.

Embryonic development occurs in the first 8 weeks after fertilization. The cells undergo rapid mitotic division during this stage, and are therefore very sensitive to cytotoxic and mutagenic insults, such as poor nutrition, infection, various chemicals, including pharmaceutical agents, toxins such as alcohol, and radiation exposure. During the embryonic period, the fertilized egg is transformed into a fetus with a body structure and organs. Obviously, abnormalities in chromosome number and structure may have an adverse effect on this tightly controlled developmental sequence. Most spontaneous abortions occurring during this period involve embryos with severe chromosomal abnormalities.

The **fetal period** spans the time from the eighth week after fertilization to birth. This period is primarily one of growth and maturation of organs and tissues and results in an individual who can survive and grow without the direct support of a maternal blood supply. The lungs, kidneys, liver, and brain require the longest time to reach maturation. Fetal growth depends not just on a sound chromosomal makeup but also on a healthy uterine environment. Maternal diseases that interfere with blood supply to the placenta can result in stunted growth or intrauterine fetal demise; intrauterine infections can cause severe damage to developing fetal tissues; abnormal implantation of the placenta and true knots in the umbilical cord can jeopardize blood flow to the fetus; and amniotic bands can wrap around fetal body parts and cause asymmetric development or even infarction. These abnormalities are called **congenital**: they are present at birth, but not necessarily genetic in origin.

Pregnancy in humans takes about 38 weeks, counting from fertilization. The first eight weeks is the embryonic period, and the rest of the time is the fetal period.

Because it is difficult, in most pregnancies, to ascertain when fertilization occurred, pregnancies are practically dated in reference to the last menstrual period, or roughly fertilization plus two weeks. This is termed the **gestational age**. Gestational age makes the embryo/fetus roughly two weeks older than it actually is and makes pregnancy 40 weeks long rather than 38.

The **perinatal period** is defined as the period from two weeks before birth to four weeks after birth. The **neonatal period** is the time from birth to four weeks after birth. The major event of the perinatal/neonatal period is adjustment to life outside the womb. The newborn's lungs and vascular system must take on the work of respiration formerly performed by the placenta. Kidney and liver function increases at this time, also to meet the demands formerly met by the placenta and the flow of blood from the mother. Functional derangements of the heart, lungs, kidney, and liver that had not interfered with fetal development may manifest at this stage of life.

The period of **infancy** is defined as one month to one year of age. Major events during this period include growth, development of motor and intellectual functions, and development of immunologic defenses against foreign substances. The period of **childhood** covers the period from infancy to puberty and is primarily one of growth and refinement of motor and intellectual

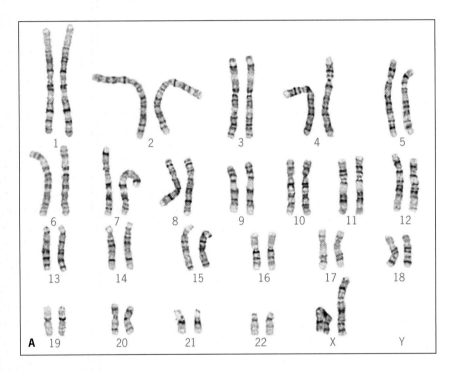

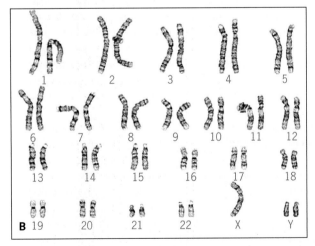

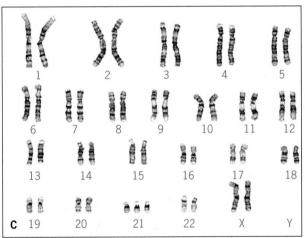

FIGURE 7–4 Karyotypes. Paired chromosomes are of the same size and have identical banding patterns. **A** shows a normal 46,XX karyotype. In **B**, there are two Y chromosomes and an X chromosome, so this individual has a sex chromosome trisomy (47,XYY). In **C**, there are three copies of chromosome 21, so this individual has the autosomal trisomy 47,XX+21, or Down syndrome. (Courtesy of Dr. Gordana Raca, Department of Pathology and Laboratory Medicine, University of Wisconsin School of Medicine and Public Health.)

functions. *Adolescence* is the final developmental period before the process of aging begins. Sexual maturation is the major physical event occurring in this period. Genetic derangements may first become manifest in any of these periods.

Definitions

Abnormalities of development may be the result of altered genetic structure or environmental effects or a combination of the two. The interaction of genetic and environmental factors is complex, and for any particular disease may not be well understood. We use the term **developmental abnormality** in a broad sense to refer to diseases that affect normal maturation.

A **genetic disease** is a disease caused by an abnormal gene. Simply having an abnormal gene is not a disease. Most abnormal genes are acquired at the time of fertilization, but most genetic diseases do not manifest until some time after birth. **Monogenetic** (single-gene) defects encompass the classic genetic diseases in which a single abnormal gene is responsible for the disease and can be traced through family trees. Examples of single-gene defects are phenylketonuria and sickle cell anemia. **Polygenetic** (multiple-gene) or complex gene defects involve more than one abnormal gene and sometimes interaction with environmental factors for their expression. Inheritance patterns of multiple- or complex gene defects are not clear-cut, but there is some tendency for these diseases to occur in families. Diabetes mellitus is an example of a complex genetic disease.

Chromosomal diseases are defined by microscopically visible structural changes in chromosomes. This can include changes in chromosome number (e.g., trisomy 21 or Down syndrome) or visually detectable translocations. Chromosomal diseases often result in genetic abnormalities so severe as to preclude reproduction and transmission of the abnormality. Chromosomes can be visualized by a process called **karyotyping**. This involves inducing cells to grow in cell culture, arresting the dividing cells during mitosis, and squashing and staining the cells so that the chromosomes can be seen under a microscope (**Figure 7-4**).

Abnormalities developing between the time of fertilization and birth can be classified according to whether they are initiated during the embryonic period (first eight weeks) or the fetal period (the final 32 weeks to birth); in reality, it is often difficult to tell when an insult occurred. Both can result in congenital diseases. Sometimes, embryonic and fetal anomalies may go undetected until adult life (e.g., two ureters on one side). Genetic and chromosomal diseases may also not manifest until sometime after birth.

Familial diseases are diseases in which several family members have the same genetically or chromosomally based disease. Genetic diseases are not necessarily familial. Many individuals with genetic diseases do not have a family history of the disease either because it is recessive (e.g., cystic fibrosis) or because the disease is caused by a new germ cell mutation. Some embryonic anomalies are caused by abnormal genes and may be familial (e.g., polycystic kidneys, cleft lip and palate). In the latter situation, the disease can be classified as both congenital and familial.

Frequency and Significance of Developmental Abnormalities

Approximately 2% of newborns have congenital anomalies. The causes of these anomalies can roughly be estimated as follows: 65% unknown, 20% genetic, 5% chromosomal, and 10% environmental. The overall frequency of genetic diseases is difficult to establish because of the delayed onset of some types and the variable effects of environmental factors on their expression. An estimate of the frequency of genetic diseases in children is given in **Table 7-1**.

Monogenetic Diseases

Monogenetic diseases are classified according to whether the abnormal gene is located on an autosome or sex chromosome, and whether it is dominant or recessive. Thus, there are four possible modes of inheritance: autosomal recessive, autosomal dominant, sex-linked recessive, sex-linked dominant. Autosomal diseases are much more common than sex-linked diseases, and recessive diseases are much more common than dominant diseases. Many of the thousands of types of genetic diseases are incompletely penetrant (not all persons with the affected genes will have the disease) and many are variably expressed (not all persons will have the disease to the same severity). Most genetic diseases are uncommon or rare; yet, when taken in aggregate, most families are influenced by some type of multifactorial genetic disease and may have members with single-gene diseases.

Dominant genes are easily recognized when completely penetrant because the presence of the disease identifies those individuals with the gene and the line of inheritance can be followed through each generation (**Figure 7-5**). Huntington disease, a devastating disease causing destruction of neurons in the brain, is an example

TABLE 7-1 Incidence of Genetic Diseases as Percentage of Live Births

Genetic Disease	Incidence (%)
Chromosomal abnormalities	0.4
Single-gene defects	2.0
Multigene disorders	2.6
Total	**5.0**

Data from National Health Education Committee. *The killers and cripplers: facts on major diseases in the U.S. today.* New York: D. McKay; 1976:127.

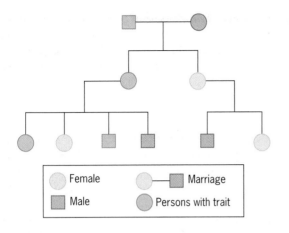

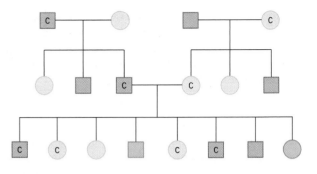

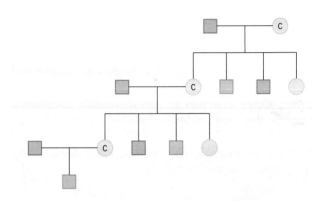

FIGURE 7–5 Family tree for a dominantly inherited trait. The abnormality appears in a parent of each involved individual.

FIGURE 7–6 Family tree for a recessively inherited trait. The trait appears in one-fourth of offspring when both parents carry the recessive gene. The trait is often absent in previous generations: carriers (represented by the letter c) do not manifest the trait.

FIGURE 7–7 Family tree for a sex-linked recessive trait. The trait appears only in males. Uncles or grandfathers are likely to be affected. The abnormal gene may be passed through carrier females for generations.

of an autosomal dominant disease with complete penetrance. Because it is a dominant trait, the offspring of an affected individual have a 50% chance of inheriting the defective gene, and because it is completely penetrant, if they inherit the gene, they will develop manifestations. Unfortunately, manifestations do not develop until the individual has reached middle age and has most likely already had children, so the gene has already been transmitted to the next generation.

Recessive disorders usually appear sporadically. When they occur, about one-fourth of siblings are affected because both parents must be carriers (the chance of a child getting both abnormal genes is $\frac{1}{2} \times \frac{1}{2}$). The family history will usually be negative unless the recessive gene has a very high frequency in the population or there was marriage among related individuals (**Figure 7–6**). Cystic fibrosis and sickle cell anemia are examples of autosomal recessive diseases. Carriers are not usually affected by the disease because both copies of the gene must be mutated to result in the abnormal phenotype.

Sex-linked recessive disorders appear in every other generation. Females with the abnormal gene on an X chromosome will not have the disease because they have a normal allele on the other X chromosome; males with the gene will have the disease because the Y chromosome has no allele to oppose the abnormal one on the X chromosome (**Figure 7–7**). If women inherit two defective copies of the gene, they usually have the disease in a more severe form. Duchenne muscular dystrophy and hemophilia are examples of sex-linked diseases.

The abnormal genes causing recessive diseases can be transmitted through many generations before two carriers mate and the genes' presence in families becomes manifest. Many dominant diseases arise as the result of sporadic mutations and, if severe, will disappear as involved individuals fail to reproduce. However, sometimes carrier status is not detected until later in life, after the gene has already been transmitted to the next generation. This is the case with Huntington disease or some forms of inherited breast cancer. Factors favoring the perpetuation of dominant diseases include late onset, mild disease, nonpenetrance, and variable expressivity.

Biochemical defects caused by abnormalities affecting a single gene can be subdivided into defects affecting structural proteins and defects affecting enzymes. An example of a structural protein defect is sickle cell anemia, in which the hemoglobin carried by red blood cells is defective, resulting in an abnormal red blood cell shape. Enzyme defects, or **inborn errors of metabolism**, are subdivided on the basis of the type of substrate affected into disorders of carbohydrate, protein, lipid, or mineral metabolism. An example of an inborn error of carbohydrate metabolism is glycogen storage disease, in which glucose can be converted into glycogen for storage, but one of the enzymes needed to convert the glycogen back to glucose is missing. This results in excessive storage of glycogen and enlargement of organs in which glycogen is stored.

The disorders discussed so far have all been examples of diseases caused by Mendelian inheritance, named after the scientist who first described how traits are passed to subsequent generations. Many genetic diseases are not expressed in families in manners predictable by Mendelian laws, however, and are the result of non-Mendelian inheritance. Mitochondrial genes are inherited only from the mother: the ovum contains the cellular machinery necessary for respiration, whereas sperm do not. The maternal mitochondria give rise to the mitochondria in the developing zygote. **Mitochondrial diseases** primarily affect the energy-producing apparatus and may manifest simply with exercise intolerance or with severe deficiencies in the function of "energy-hungry" tissues such as muscles, brain, and nerves. Some genes in humans are **imprinted**, or modified by alteration of molecules other than nucleic acids, such as proteins or methyl groups, that get attached to the gene during gametogenesis. Imprinting usually silences the gene, so only the allele inherited from the other parent is expressed. Imprinting occurs in a sex-specific manner: in some cases, the allele derived from the mother is silenced; in others, it is the paternal gene that is silenced. Prader-Willi syndrome is the result of failure of imprinting of a sequence of genes on the paternally derived chromosome 15. It manifests as obesity, excessive eating, flaccid muscles, small hands and feet, and mental retardation. Other examples of non-Mendelian inheritance patterns that may underlie diseases are trinucleotide repeat expansion (resulting in increasingly severe manifestations, for example, of mental retardation, in successive generations) and mosaicism.

Polygenetic Disorders

The exact genetic basis of polygenetic disorders is difficult to determine because inheritance patterns are not clear-cut and because similar disorders may be caused by nongenetic mechanisms. Diabetes mellitus is a good example. Diabetes tends to occur in families but not in a predictable manner, and some cases of diabetes are clearly the result of environmental factors or other diseases, such as an autoimmune process that destroys the pancreas. Some congenital anomalies, such as cleft lip and congenital heart disease, are presumed to be genetic because they have a definite tendency to occur in families, but their exact genetic basis remains elusive. In addition to the multigene disorders that are reasonably well established as genetic, there is a much broader category of multifactorial diseases that appear to be caused by the association of abnormal genes and environmental influences. Such multifactorial diseases include atherosclerotic heart disease, hypertension, obesity, and some forms of cancer.

Chromosomal Diseases

Most disorders of autosomal chromosomes are so severe as to be incompatible with embryonic development. These account for one-third of spontaneous abortions that occur during the first third of pregnancy. Of the types of chromosomal diseases compatible with survival beyond birth, Down syndrome (trisomy 21) is most common. Other autosomal chromosomal disorders usually produce severely deformed infants who die soon after birth. Abnormalities of sex chromosome number can produce relatively mild abnormalities that often are not detected until puberty, when secondary sex characteristics do not develop normally.

Environmental Factors

Environmental factors can interfere with development at any stage. Those that interfere with the development of an embryo or fetus are called **teratogens**. Teratogens can be infectious agents, drugs (pharmaceutical or recreational), maternal health factors such as diabetes mellitus, physical factors (e.g., radiation, hyperthermia), or environmental chemicals. In the embryo and fetus, organs are growing very rapidly, so toxins or infectious agents that interfere with cell growth and cell signaling can severely disrupt normal development.

Various infectious agents that cause only mild disease in the mother can cross the placenta and cause serious problems in the fetus, especially during the first 16 weeks of pregnancy. These are known by the acronym **TORCH**: toxoplasma, "other" (e.g., syphilis), rubella, cytomegalovirus, and herpes simplex virus. Toxoplasmosis is a parasitic infection carried by domestic cats and excreted in their stool. It is transmitted to humans via the oral route. If the mother contracts toxoplasma during pregnancy (e.g., by emptying litterboxes), the parasite can cross the placenta and cause serious impairment of the fetal neurologic system, resulting in blindness, mental retardation, and/or death. Rubella (German measles) is a self-limited viral infection in the mother, but can disrupt the development of the auditory apparatus, heart, and neurologic system and cause glaucoma and cataracts in the fetus. The other members of the TORCH group have equally potentially devastating consequences. For this reason, the mother is routinely tested for exposure to these agents and vaccinated against rubella early in pregnancy.

Maternal metabolic disorders, such as iodine deficiency or diabetes, can cause anomalies of embryonic and fetal development. The thyroid of the developing fetus is dependent on maternal iodine to be able to make thyroid hormone, so insufficient iodine in the maternal blood can result in hypothyroidism of the fetus and newborn. Excessive glucose in the blood of diabetic mothers can result in multiple severe congenital anomalies of various organ systems and/or excessive growth of the fetus and placenta, potentially resulting in obstetric problems and hypoglycemia in the neonatal period.

Drugs, environmental chemicals, and alcohol account for about half of the known nongenetic causes of developmental defects. Historically, the most notorious of these agents is thalidomide. This drug was given to pregnant women in the 1950s and 1960s to treat the nausea of pregnancy. Many babies were born to these mothers with short limbs, heart defects, and malformations of the eyes, ears, genitals, kidneys, digestive tract, and/or nervous system. The drug was taken off the market once its teratogenic effects were discovered. The devastating experience with thalidomide resulted in strict guidelines for drug testing and marketing. Nowadays, pharmaceutical drugs are classified as to their teratogenic potential. Nonteratogenic substitutes for these drugs are recommended, but if there is no substitute, women must be warned and counseled about the drug's potential harmful effects during pregnancy. Highly teratogenic drugs include retinoic acid (prescribed for intractable acne), warfarin (prevents blood clot formation), phenytoin and valproic acid (for epilepsy), and ACE inhibitors (antihypertensive drugs). Mothers developing cancer during pregnancy often face the agonizing decision whether to terminate the pregnancy or wait until the fetus has passed through the most vulnerable period before undergoing chemotherapy.

Unfortunately, alcohol is not covered by the safety measures in place for prescription drugs. Alcohol is a potent teratogen. Women who drink alcohol during pregnancy can give birth to babies with the fetal alcohol spectrum disorder. This is characterized by abnormal facial features, impaired growth during infancy and childhood, and neurologic problems, including mental retardation and impaired socialization. The teratogenic effect of other "recreational" drugs is not as clearly demonstrated, but cocaine is associated with an increased risk of stillbirth, and smoking cigarettes can result in impaired growth of the fetus.

Embryonic Anomalies

Among the various types of anomalies presumed to result from abnormal development in the embryonic period, congenital heart defects are the most common. They may not be manifest at birth but rather come to light as the infant grows, becomes more active, and requires a greater cardiac output. Most congenital heart defects can successfully be repaired surgically. Abnormalities of the kidney and urinary tract are also quite common. They are often not manifest at birth but are discovered later in life through complications such as repeated urinary tract infections. The gastrointestinal tract may manifest embryonic anomalies, such as fistulas (abnormal connections between parts of the gastrointestinal tract or between the gastrointestinal tract and other structures), most of which are surgically treatable. Anomalies of the central nervous system, in contrast, often are serious and nonrepairable. Approximately 15% of embryonic anomalies are multiple, involving several organs.

Fetal Diseases

It is often difficult to determine whether a disease is embryonic or fetal because development of organs occurs throughout both periods and the timing of an insult is not always known. Environmental insults can affect development during either stage.

A serious fetal disease is erythroblastosis fetalis, which is caused by the mother producing antibodies to the fetus's red blood cells. Red blood cells are coated with numerous antigens, including those of the ABO blood group system and Rh factor. If the mother's red blood cells do not carry Rh factor, she will produce antibodies to it when she is exposed to it—for example, when she receives a minute "transfusion" of fetal blood during delivery of an Rh factor–positive infant. In subsequent pregnancies, the mother's antibodies can leak into the fetal circulation and cause massive destruction of the baby's red blood cells, resulting in severe fetal anemia and, occasionally, death.

Infectious agents other than those resulting in congenital anomalies can cause significant problems in the fetal and neonatal periods. The placental membranes can become infected, usually by bacteria. This is called chorioamnionitis. If severe, chorioamnionitis can lead to premature delivery of the infant, neonatal sepsis, convulsions, and death.

The fetus is dependent on the mother for all its nutrients, so nutritional deficiencies in the mother, such as in iron, iodine, or folate, may affect the growth and development of the fetus. Likewise, anything resulting in impaired blood flow to the placenta, such as vasoconstriction caused by toxins in cigarette smoke, can result in impaired growth resulting from hypoxia.

Brain damage in the late fetal or perinatal period can result in cerebral palsy, a condition characterized by nonprogressive abnormal muscular coordination with or without mental retardation or seizure disorders. Cerebral palsy has variable clinical features and time of onset, and its cause is not clearly understood. Its development does seem to correlate with low birth weight, intrauterine infection, disorders of the placenta, and multiple gestation. The role of birth trauma in the development of cerebral palsy is contested.

Perinatal Diseases

Prematurity is the most important cause of disease during the perinatal period. **Prematurity** refers to births that occur 3 weeks or more prior to term (37 weeks gestational age or less). Approximately 10% of babies are born prematurely. Gestational age correlates directly with survival: infants born at 25 weeks gestational age have only about 50% survival, while those born at 37 weeks have almost 100% survival. Premature infants run the risk of developing pneumonia and hyaline membrane disease because of immaturity of the lungs, neurologic damage resulting from intracranial hemorrhages, necrotizing enterocolitis (severe infection of the intestinal tract), sepsis, and abnormal retinal development. Prematurity also correlates with low birth weight, which in itself is a risk factor for significant complications after birth. Prematurity is only one cause of low birth weight. Others include maternal nutritional deficiencies and conditions that cause insufficient blood flow through the placenta. Large infarcts of the placenta, or premature detachment of the placenta from the uterus, can lead to hypoxia and stunted growth of the fetus.

Many genetic and chromosomal diseases manifest during the perinatal or neonatal period. In the United States, neonates are routinely tested for some of the more common genetic diseases, such as phenylketonuria, galactosemia, and sickle cell anemia. Treatment, which may be as simple as dietary restriction, can prevent the development of serious disorders and even death, if the genetic anomaly is detected early. A thorough neonatal physical examination can also detect congenital anomalies such as undescended testicles, heart murmurs, and defects in neurologic development.

Diseases of Infancy

The five major causes of death in infants born in the United States are, in descending order, congenital and chromosomal abnormalities, prematurity and low birth weight, sudden infant death syndrome, complications of maternal diseases, and diseases of the placenta, cord, and membranes. As you can see from this list, genetic and chromosomal conditions and the intrauterine environment exert their effects beyond birth.

Infants are also at risk for developing infections because they have not had previous experience with infectious agents. Antibodies acquired from the mother tend to protect the infant for about six months. After this point, the infant must experience the infection or be immunized to develop antibodies against infectious agents.

A common nutritional problem in infants is failure to get enough iron. Babies fed on milk and fruit, without sources of iron such as cereals, will develop iron-deficiency anemia beginning around six months of age, when iron stores acquired from the mother are used up. Infectious and nutritional diseases are the most common causes of infant death worldwide.

Accidents and injuries also occur during this time. These may be inadvertent or the result of neglect (e.g., when babies put small objects in their mouths and suffocate, or fall from a bed or table), but they may also be inflicted. The shaken baby syndrome, which has gained much notoriety in the press, is thought to result from child abuse. Intracranial and retinal hemorrhages occur more easily in infants than in older children. Infants do not have the muscular strength to control their heads, so if they are shaken, their head is exposed to rapidly alternating mechanical forces that repeatedly throw the brain against the inside of the cranium and cause shearing of blood vessels. Babies can die from the neurologic injuries and intracranial hemorrhages that result.

Diseases of Childhood and Adolescence

Diseases of childhood and adolescence rarely relate to developmental problems, and they differ from diseases of older age groups only in relative frequency.

Accidents and infections are more common, whereas degenerative diseases and neoplasms are uncommon. Genetic and chromosomal diseases as well as the conditions resulting from the effect of teratogens are lifelong. Some genetic diseases, such as inborn errors of metabolism, may increase in severity during childhood or may not manifest until childhood as by-products of metabolism that cannot be cleared gradually and inexorably accumulate.

Symptoms, Signs, and Tests
Genetic Diseases

The Human Genome Project was completed in 2003. This was a massive and expensive undertaking with the—for its time—extraordinary and ambitious goal of sequencing all 3 billion base pairs and identifying all 20,000 to 25,000 genes of the human genome. The project also necessarily entailed developing computing strategies to manage the information, mine the data, and make the data available to the private sector. Ten years later, individual people can have their entire genome sequenced for about $40,000, and with a $0.99 app can not only explore their own genome down to individual variant base pairs but also determine the known implications of that variant for their health. The magnitude of knowledge literally available at one's fingertips is mind staggering, but it is not yet clear how it helps in medical management of diseases.

The problems with utilizing whole-genome sequencing routinely in medical care are manifold. Technologies are still in their infancy, so with 3 billion base pairs sequenced it is only to be expected that there would be errors in the detection or recording of the data. The technologies are expensive, and insurance companies are loath to pay for it if there is no dire medical necessity. Most of the genetic variations are of dubious significance: they may not result in any change in structure or function of the protein they code for. Most diseases are the result of gene–gene or gene–environment interactions, which have not been worked out. (Gene sequencing and information technologies will likely give a significant boost to our ability to discover the interplay between genes and the environment.) And the ethical issues surrounding the disclosure of genetic testing are still being debated in heated arguments: Should parents have the right to know their children's genetic makeup? What would you do if you knew you had a gene defect that might or might not predispose you to disease later in life? What is the purpose of knowing that there is a gene defect if nothing can be done about it?

Whole-genome sequencing has been helpful in the medical care of some children with very rare and baffling disease manifestations.[1] In these cases, mapping the entire genome can uncover genetic abnormalities that may be linked to the patient's life-threatening symptoms. While a cure is not always possible, such knowledge can help with symptomatic management of the disease manifestations.

For most genetic diseases, however, extensive genome sequencing is not necessary. Signs and symptoms are often quite suggestive of specific diseases. For example, cystic fibrosis presents with pneumonia and failure to thrive (slow or no weight gain), Friedreich ataxia presents with increasing clumsiness and gait disturbances, and retinoblastoma presents as a neoplasm in the eye in children. Inborn errors of metabolism present with manifestations specific to the metabolic product that is accumulating. Abnormal facial features, an unusual body odor, jaundice, or an enlarged liver and spleen may be indications of an underlying genetic error of metabolism. These specific manifestations can be followed up with tests targeted at common mutations in specific genes. For example, if a patient is suspected of having hemochromatosis or cystic fibrosis, tests are performed that specifically look at individual nucleic acid pairs or sequences in the genes known to cause these monogenetic diseases. Likewise, testing of family members of patients with a known genetic or familial disease, such as Marfan syndrome or breast cancer, is designed to detect the most common mutations associated with these diseases (and consequently, some cases of familial diseases caused by mutations at very rare locations are missed).

Genetic tests are used in several different areas of medicine. In microbiology, testing for specific RNA sequences allows for more rapid and specific identification of bacteria than traditional bacterial cultures. In pharmacology, identifying the genetic makeup of enzymes that are involved in drug metabolism allows fine-tuning of the dosage of drugs that have a notoriously variable clearance in different patients (e.g., warfarin). Increasingly, extensive panels of genes known to be associated with malignancies are tested in individual cancers, with the hope that therapy can be tailored to specific genes or combinations of genes that are known to be mutated in that individual cancer. Tests also can be performed for mutations in mitochondrial DNA. For the time being, however, most genetic testing is performed to look at variations in specific genes in the context of specific clinical manifestations.

Chromosomal Diseases

Chromosomal diseases are suspected and often diagnosed by physical examination. Karyotyping can be used to substantiate the diagnosis. Karyotyping is performed only at large referral centers but is essential for accurate diagnosis and counseling. The **triple screen test** and the **quad test** are performed on the serum of pregnant women to measure substances that are present in abnormal concentrations if the fetus has a neural tube defect (an embryonic anomaly resulting in malformation of the central nervous system) or trisomy 21. The difference between the two is that the triple screen test measures three substances (alpha fetoprotein, human chorionic gonadotropin, and estriol) whereas the quad test adds another (inhibin-A), and thereby increases the likelihood that babies with neural tube defects or Down syndrome will be identified. Both the triple and quad tests are only screening tests: they are not diagnostic. Abnormal test results have to be followed up by more sensitive, diagnostic procedures such as ultrasound or **amniocentesis** (testing of the amniotic fluid during pregnancy; **Figure 7–8**).

Embryonic Anomalies and Fetal Diseases

Anomalies of embryonic and fetal growth and development can be detected by physical examination, radiologic procedures, ultrasonography, or exploratory surgery.

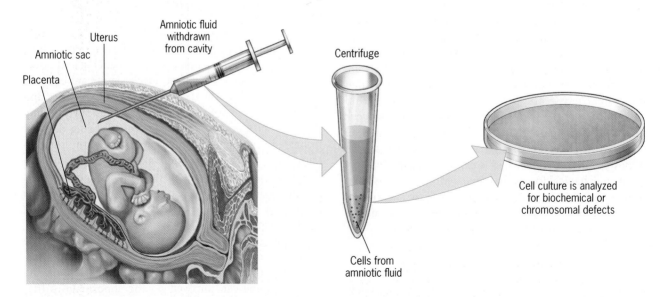

FIGURE 7–8 Amniocentesis to obtain fluid and cells for the detection of some genetic chromosomal diseases.

The method of diagnosis depends on the nature of the disease. Infections are diagnosed by culture or measurement of antibodies (e.g., serology for syphilis). Immunologic diseases are diagnosed by measuring antigen and antibodies (e.g., Rh factor in fetal and maternal red blood cells). Hydrocephalus, polycystic kidneys and congenital heart defects can be detected by ultrasound. Bone diseases are initially evaluated by radiographic techniques. Pathologic examination of the placenta should be performed on all neonates who are premature, of low birth weight, or suspected of having experienced some complication during pregnancy or delivery, such as infection. Several biochemical diseases, including sickle cell anemia, phenylketonuria, galactosemia, and hypothyroidism, are routinely tested for at birth, and early treatment can prevent long-term disability.

Specific Diseases
Genetic Diseases

There are numerous genetic diseases and new ones are added to the list every day as the molecular basis of diseases is uncovered. Here, we discuss only common or classic ones that illustrate how mutations in a single gene can result in disease and how these diseases can be treated.

The gene for **sickle cell anemia** causes a structural defect in the hemoglobin molecule that carries oxygen on red blood cells. The defect results from the substitution of a single nucleic acid in the DNA of the hemoglobin gene. The protein that is translated from this gene has a single amino acid substitution. This is sufficient for the hemoglobin to have an altered shape. The disease is transmitted in an autosomal recessive manner, so people may carry the defective allele for the hemoglobin molecule but not experience any symptoms. When an individual is born with two such genes, however, the blood cells become rigid and assume an abnormal, sickle rather than discoid, shape under stressful conditions. These cells are eliminated from the circulation in the spleen, causing anemia. The patient may become symptomatic from severe anemia. The abnormally shaped red blood cells can also get stuck in small capillaries, causing microinfarcts and severe, often crippling pain. Recurrent episodes of pain are called sickle cell crises. Eventually, the spleen, which plays a major role in preventing infection from certain pathogens, may be entirely replaced by fibrous tissue because of numerous, repeated microinfarcts, and the patient becomes susceptible to repeated infections, which themselves precipitate further sickling of red blood cells. Adequate care includes periodic transfusions to replace red blood cells, adequate oxygenation to prevent further sickling, and prompt pain management at the onset of a crisis. Currently, the median age at death of patients with sickle cell anemia is in the fifth decade.

Many monogenetic diseases result in deficiencies of function of enzymes and the resultant accumulation of abnormal amounts of substances. Ideally, gene therapy would replace or repair the defective DNA so that the patient's cells would be capable of producing the normal protein; however, despite significant advances in this field, gene therapy is still an elusive goal. Treatment for these diseases, therefore, is geared toward replacing necessary enzymes or their products, or eliminating the accumulating substance before it can cause damage. Both of these treatment strategies have inherent problems because the deficient product needs to be replaced repeatedly or the harmful accumulating substance cannot be entirely cleared from the system. Two diseases that illustrate these problems are hemophilia and hemosiderosis.

There are two types of **hemophilia**. Both are sex-linked disorders, so they affect primarily men. A specific enzyme in the blood-clotting cascade is deficient, leading to spontaneous bleeding into joints or uncontrollable bleeding even after minor trauma. Women who are born homozygous for the abnormal allele have more serious symptoms than do men: the onset of menstruation can be fatal. Hemophilia is a rare genetic disease, affecting about 2 per 100,000 persons, but it commands a large amount of medical resources. Patients are treated with a combination of prevention (avoiding anything that might precipitate bleeding, including schoolyard rough-and-tumble play) and prophylaxis. Prophylaxis involves replacement of the missing clotting factor. This is currently the mainstay of treatment. In the past, the clotting factor was concentrated from the blood of many blood donors, and replacement was therefore very expensive. Also, patients were at risk for contracting blood-borne, primarily viral, diseases, such as HIV. Better screening of donated blood has decreased this risk, and clotting factors produced in laboratories by recombinant methods are increasingly becoming available. Still, patients are frequent visitors in transfusion clinics and doctors' offices in their pursuit of normal blood clotting.

Hemosiderosis is also a monogenetic disease. This disease affects iron storage: the intestine absorbs greater than normal amounts of iron, which accumulates in various tissues including the liver and heart. The organs in which the iron accumulates gradually fail. The liver becomes severely scarred and is predisposed to the development of carcinoma, while the heart becomes stiff and cannot pump effectively. The treatment of hemosiderosis is theoretically and practically simple: bloodletting (phlebotomy) reduces the iron load in the body. Chelation therapy, whereby the iron is coated by substances that make it more easily cleared from the body, can also be performed, but phlebotomy is easier and less costly. Unfortunately, many patients live until adulthood without knowing that they have this disease, and it manifests with organ damage. At this time, there is no effective way of completely ridding the tissues of the accumulated iron.

Phenylketonuria is an autosomal recessive disease caused by an absence of the enzyme phenylalanine hydroxylase, which metabolizes phenylalanine to tyrosine. As a result of the absence of this enzyme, phenylalanine accumulates. Through unknown mechanisms, excessive amounts of phenylalanine result in mental retardation, apparently by inhibiting brain growth and myelination of nerve cell processes. The neonate is usually normal, but signs of impaired neurologic development begin to appear during infancy. Breast milk and infant formula contain high concentrations of phenylalanine. Avoidance of this amino acid in the diet is sufficient to prevent neurologic impairment. Diagnosis can be made by testing newborns for phenylketones in the blood and is mandatory in all 50 states.

Unfortunately, not all diseases are detectable at birth. It is not practical or cost-effective to screen for all known genetic diseases. Some of these cannot be detected by simple blood tests but require more elaborate tests, such as molecular analysis or karyotyping, for diagnosis. Others have no known treatment, so knowledge of the presence of the genetic defect would not help prevent or delay the development of the disease. This is the case with the most common type of muscular dystrophy, **Duchenne muscular dystrophy**. Duchenne muscular dystrophy is a sex-linked disorder, so it occurs primarily in males. The disease usually does not manifest until the second or third year of life, or possibly even later. It is caused by an abnormality in a muscle protein called dystrophin. As a result of this defect, skeletal muscles degenerate, and the patients develop muscle weakness, heart failure, and orthopedic and pulmonary problems. Patients are often wheelchair-bound by their early teens and do not survive beyond the early 20s. Diagnosis of Duchenne muscular dystrophy requires expertise in differentiating various genetic and acquired musculoskeletal disorders. There is no effective therapy for the disease: treatment involves managing its complications.

Another common genetic disease is **cystic fibrosis**. This is an autosomal recessive disorder caused by mutations in a gene that encodes the cystic fibrosis transmembrane regulator conductor (CFTR). CFTR regulates the movement of chloride across cell membranes. As a result of a defect in this protein, the concentration of ions in secretions, such as sweat and mucus in the respiratory tract, is abnormal. In the respiratory tract, the mucus becomes thick and tenacious, plugs airways, and becomes infected. Patients experience repeated episodes of pneumonia and inflammatory destruction of the lungs, which eventually become severely scarred and unable to function properly. The pancreas can also be affected. Blockage of ducts by thick pancreatic secretions leads to decreased delivery of pancreatic enzymes to the intestine and thus to poor digestion of food and failure to thrive. Until a few decades ago, children succumbed to bacterial infections of the lungs. With improved management of cystic fibrosis, which includes pancreatic enzyme replacement and prophylactic antibiotic administration, among others, patients with this disease are surviving longer into adulthood.

The diseases discussed here are examples of monogenetic diseases. As the understanding of the role of genes in other diseases increases, it is becoming clear that some of the most common diseases affecting the population in the United States have an inherited genetic basis. Diabetes mellitus, atherosclerosis, hypertension, obesity, and the predisposition to the development of certain neoplasms are examples. Although these are at least partially genetic, the effect of environment on their expression and management cannot be stressed enough. As you saw from the discussion of diseases such as phenylketonuria, sickle cell anemia, and cystic fibrosis, the course and outcome of even monogenetic diseases are modifiable. Close, effective management and prevention of complications, which can include diverse measures such as dietary avoidance of precipitating agents, dietary replacement therapy, physical therapy, preemptive administration of antibiotics, blood transfusions, nutritional support, and even psychosocial counseling, can significantly improve and prolong lives.

Chromosomal Diseases

The most common types of chromosomal disorders include increases (polysomy) or decreases (monosomy) in the normal complement of autosomal or sex chromosomes, translocations of parts of chromosomes, or damage to, deletion, inversion, or duplication of parts of one or more arms of chromosomes. Examples of chromosomal diseases include Down syndrome, Klinefelter syndrome, Turner syndrome, and fragile X syndrome.

Down syndrome (trisomy 21) occurs in 1 of every 1,000 newborns and is the most common genetic cause of mental retardation. It is a chromosomal disorder in which cells have three copies of chromosome 21. It is associated with mental deficiency and common dysmorphic characteristics, such as a round face with narrow palpebral fissures (the space between the eyelids), as well as cardiac defects, a predisposition to developing leukemia, and a predisposition to developing Alzheimer dementia at a very early age. It should be noted that the range of IQ in Down syndrome patients is very large, approaching normal in some cases, and with appropriate educational, vocational, and social opportunities, these patients can hold jobs and contribute to their communities. They often require surgical and medical treatment of anatomic, physiologic, and neoplastic disorders. In general, with medical and social interventions, the life expectancy and quality of life for persons with Down syndrome have markedly improved over the past few decades.

Klinefelter syndrome occurs in males who are born with one Y and two X chromosomes, so it is technically a sex chromosome trisomy. It is usually not diagnosed until puberty, when it comes to attention because of lack of male sexual development and breast enlargement. As with genetic diseases and Down syndrome, treatment of this condition requires management of its manifestations. Testosterone therapy can help these boys develop secondary sex characteristics and eventually father children. They may have a delay in language development, so appropriate intervention may be needed to help them with socialization. These individuals are also at risk for the development of breast cancer.

Turner syndrome is another anomaly of sex chromosomes: it is a sex chromosome monosomy. Affected individuals are females with a single X chromosome. At puberty, they fail to undergo normal female secondary sex development. They are short in stature and have a broad neck, but normal mentation. This condition is less common than Klinefelter syndrome.

Fragile X syndrome produces mild to moderate mental retardation and is the most common genetic cause of mental retardation in males. It is an example of a non-Mendelian trait. The "fragility" on the X chromosome is caused by trinucleotide repeats, which increase in length in successive generations. Males have a characteristic phenotype of long faces and enlarged ears, and affected individuals have variable degrees of mental retardation. The diagnosis is confirmed by DNA analysis of the fragile site.

Embryonic Anomalies

Congenital heart diseases are the most common kinds of embryonic anomalies. The heart develops from a muscular tube that twists, loops, and folds; establishes and remodels connections with the superior and inferior venae cavae, aorta, pulmonary veins, and pulmonary arteries; and develops various partitions to efficiently direct the flow of blood. After birth, the heart and its vessels have to rapidly respond to the need of respiration and reroute the flow of blood so that it can become oxygenated in the lungs. Structural abnormalities of the heart and the great vessels often come to attention around the time of birth. Decreased oxygenation of the blood gives the baby a blue hue, called cyanosis, but this occurs only with certain kinds of anomalies. Many structural heart defects are detected during newborn and infant well-baby checks because they result in a heart murmur.

The most common congenital malformation is a bicuspid aortic valve. The next most common malformation, and more likely to present in infancy, is a "hole in the heart," or a defect in the atrial or ventricular septa (**Figure 7–9**). Because the pressure of blood on the left side of the heart is higher than on the right side, oxygenated blood in the left side of the heart will pass through the defect and mix with blood in the right side of the

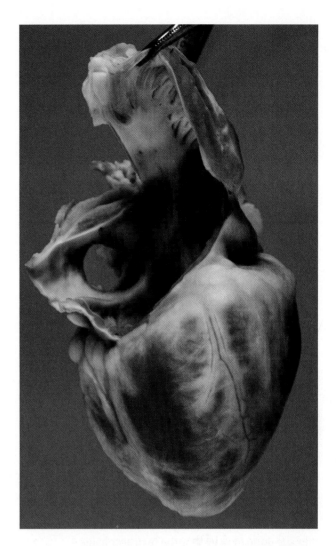

FIGURE 7–9 Atrial septal defect. This is the heart of a 1-year-old who died of acute leukemia and also had a large atrial septal defect. The left and right atria have been opened and you can see the blue background through the hole in the interatrial septum.

heart. The right side of the heart therefore has to pump more blood than normal, and the lungs have to process more blood than normal. This eventually leads to pulmonary hypertension and right heart failure. Depending on how large the defect is, the patient may develop heart failure shortly after birth or, if smaller, anytime during childhood or adulthood.

A right-to-left shunt occurs when there is an anomalous connection siphoning blood away from the lungs, so the blood in the systemic circulation is not as well oxygenated as it should be. This is the kind of shunt that makes a baby blue, or cyanotic. Congenital cardiac anomalies resulting in cyanosis are called **cyanotic heart defects**. These are less common than left-to-right shunts, but require surgical intervention early in life. The classic right-to-left shunt is the **tetralogy of Fallot**. This is a very complicated structural abnormality. If you would like to test your understanding of the anatomy of the heart, see if you can figure out why the baby with tetralogy of Fallot will be blue. The four features of the tetralogy are a defect between the two ventricles of the heart, misplacement of the aorta so that both ventricles empty into it (called an overriding aorta), obstruction of the normal outflow tract of the right ventricle, and hypertrophy of the right ventricle.

Other congenital diseases are much more rare but can affect any organ. One kidney may be small (hypoplastic) or missing (agenesis). This presents a problem only if the other kidney becomes diseased and needs to be removed. Otherwise, this anomaly may go undetected. Meckel's diverticulum is an outpouching of the distal small intestine. It is a remnant of an embryonic connection between the intestine and yolk sac. It occurs in 2% of the population and is usually harmless. Sometimes the diverticulum contains gastric epithelium that is capable of producing acidic secretions. A Meckel's diverticulum may, therefore, become symptomatic when the patients develop ulcers or perforations in the diverticulum. Meningomyelocele is an outpouching of the spinal cord and its covering, the meninges, through a defect in the bony structure of lumbar vertebrae. The brain stem often has an associated defect, with the brain being pushed into the foramen magnum, the hole at the base of the skull. Compression of the brain stem may block the flow of cerebrospinal fluid, resulting in hydrocephalus (enlargement of the brain and head resulting from increased fluid in the ventricles of the brain). Surgical repair of the meningomyelocele can prevent secondary infection of the protruding mass but cannot correct the damage done to nerves or the hydrocephalus.

Fetal Diseases

Examples of fetal diseases include erythroblastosis fetalis and congenital infections. These have to some extent already been discussed. **Erythroblastosis fetalis** occurs when maternal antibodies destroy fetal red blood cells. The timing and severity of the subsequent anemia vary greatly. The fetus may go into heart failure and die *in utero*, or the problem may not develop until after birth. Destruction of blood cells after birth results in jaundice. The bilirubin pigment responsible for the jaundice is a breakdown product of red blood cells. Bilirubin in high concentration can cause brain damage and mental retardation. It is now possible to limit maternal antibody production caused by leakage of fetal red blood cells into the maternal circulation at the time of delivery. Gamma globulin containing Rh-positive antibodies is given to the mother just after delivery. These antibodies tie up the Rh-positive antigen on the fetal cells that have leaked into the maternal circulation, thus preventing the mother's immune system from recognizing them as foreign and producing antibodies to them.

If this procedure is followed for each pregnancy involving an Rh-negative mother and an Rh-positive fetus, the incidence of erythroblastosis is reduced. Screening for maternal Rh status and administration of the gamma globulin when indicated have significantly decreased the incidence of erythroblastosis fetalis caused by Rh incompatibility. Other red blood cell antigens can also cause erythroblastosis fetalis, though this occurrence is quite rare.

Syphilis is an infection that may go unrecognized, especially in females, where the primary lesion is hidden in the vagina. The causative organisms of syphilis are spirochetes (a type of bacteria). These may circulate in the blood for months without being noticed. During the second half of pregnancy, the spirochetes are capable of crossing the placenta and infecting the fetus. The severity of the disease in the fetus varies greatly. It may cause death of the fetus and stillbirth or may be discovered only after birth when the infant shows signs of mental retardation or skeletal deformities. Congenital syphilis has become very rare in the United States because mothers are routinely screened for the disease during the first prenatal visit. If a pregnant woman tests positive, penicillin eradicates the infection without harming the fetus. Other infections, such as toxoplasmosis and rubella, can also be transmitted transplacentally and can cause acute illnesses, destructive neurologic lesions, or death.

A variety of maternal diseases and teratogenic agents can result in fetal growth restriction, neurologic defects including mental retardation, dysmorphic features, congenital heart defects, and various other structural and functional problems. Maternal hypertension, for example, can cause constriction of uterine arterioles supplying the placenta so that blood delivery to the fetus is impaired. Hypoxia impairs the growth of the fetus, resulting in low birth weight. Often, maternal diseases and exposure to teratogens result in more than one organ system being damaged, as for example in the fetal alcohol spectrum disorder.

Practice Questions

1. Trisomy 21 (Down syndrome) classically occurs through
   A. nondisjunction during mitosis.
   B. nondisjunction during meiosis.
   C. duplication of an autosomal chromosome.
   D. translocation between chromosomes.
   E. fertilization of one egg by two sperm.
2. The fetal period is defined as
   A. the time from fertilization to birth.
   B. the last month of intrauterine development.
   C. the eighth week of fertilization to birth.
   D. the first four weeks after fertilization.

3. A woman with epilepsy would like to become pregnant but is worried about the potentially teratogenic effects of the anti-epileptic drugs she is taking. Which of the following is true regarding her medications?

    A. The risk of harmful effects is greatest in the first 16 weeks of pregnancy.

    B. Pharmaceutical drugs for epilepsy currently on the market are safe to use during pregnancy.

    C. An epileptic seizure will be more harmful to the fetus than taking phenytoin.

    D. The drugs are more likely to cause chromosomal abnormalities than to interfere with the development of the embryo or the fetus.

    E. Pharmaceutical drugs do not cross the placenta and therefore will not harm the embryo or fetus.

4. Chorioamnionitis most commonly results in

    A. congenital birth defects such as cleft lip and palate.

    B. premature delivery.

    C. cataracts, auditory deficiency, and mental retardation.

    D. genetic diseases.

    E. erythroblastosis fetalis.

5. Many patients with monogenetic diseases, such as sickle cell anemia and cystic fibrosis, survive for much longer today than they did a few decades ago. What is the reason for this?

    A. The exact genetic abnormality is known and can be repaired.

    B. The product of the defective gene can be artificially synthesized and administered to patients.

    C. The diseases are becoming less virulent.

    D. There are better techniques for prevention and management of complications.

REFERENCE

1. Johnson M, Gallagher K. One in a billion: a boy's life, a medical mystery. *Journal Sentinel* (Milwaukee, Wisconsin), December 2010. Available at www.jsonline.com/features/health/111641209.html.

Major Organ-Related Diseases

The purpose of this section is to survey the diseases of humans as they manifest in organs and tissues. Most diseases present with a problem that can be associated with an organ, and often patients can tell you the organ that is causing their problem. For accurate diagnosis and treatment, it is necessary to know which diseases are most likely in each organ system, which kinds of symptoms they produce, how they can be detected by physical exam and laboratory tests, specific features of the possible diseases, and finally, what the systemic effects are when the organ "gives out" entirely.

With the exception of Chapter 11, "Bleeding and Clotting Disorders," and Chapter 24, "Mental Illness," each chapter is organized according to the following format:

- Review of structure and function
- Most frequent and serious problems
- Symptoms, signs, and tests
- Specific diseases
  Genetic/developmental diseases
  Inflammatory/degenerative diseases
  Hyperplastic/neoplastic diseases
- Organ failure

As you saw from their description in Chapter 7, genetic diseases cannot always be distinguished from developmental ones, so these are discussed together. Likewise, hyperplasia and neoplasia often exist on a continuum, so they are discussed under the same header. We use the term *degenerative diseases* as a nonspecific classification to include all acquired non-neoplastic conditions that are presumably the result of exogenous or endogenous injuries. In the section on organ failure, we discuss what happens when the organ that is the topic of the chapter ceases to function altogether.

Each chapter begins with a list of learning objectives that are intended to help you organize and comprehend the material, and at the end of each chapter are a few questions that help you to review the topic.

Vascular System

OUTLINE

OBJECTIVES

1. Review the structure and function of the vascular system, including the architecture of arteries, veins, capillaries, and lymphatics; how blood is returned to the heart; and the way in which blood pressure, volume, and extracellular fluid composition are regulated.
2. Name the most frequent and serious diseases involving blood vessels.
3. Describe diagnostic instruments and tests used to screen for and detect diseases of the vascular system.
4. Describe the most common congenital anomalies of the vascular system, and differentiate between hemangioma and lymphangioma.
5. Compare and contrast the terms arteriosclerosis, atherosclerosis, and arteriolosclerosis.
6. Discuss the pathophysiologic development of atherosclerotic plaques, and name the vessels most commonly involved with atherosclerosis.
7. Discuss four ways in which atherosclerotic lesions can cause complications.
8. Discuss the risk factors for the development of atherosclerosis, and discuss how the development of atherosclerotic lesions can be prevented.
9. Define hypertension, review the systolic and diastolic components of a blood pressure reading, differentiate between essential and secondary hypertension in terms of cause and treatment, and describe the symptoms and clinical manifestations of hypertension.
10. Recognize the critical role of screening, lifestyle modifications, and pharmaceutical therapy in decreasing morbidity and mortality associated with hypertension.
11. Define vasculitis, describe how it compromises organ function, and provide examples of vasculitic diseases.
12. Differentiate thrombophlebitis and varicose veins in terms of the vessels affected, etiology, complications, diagnosis, and treatment.
13. Define shock and compare and contrast the four types of shock in terms of cause, manifestation, treatment, and outcome.
14. Define and use in context the words and terms in bold print in the text.

KEY TERMS

acute respiratory distress syndrome (ARDS)
aldosterone
anasarca
aneurysm
angiography
angioplasty
angiotensin II
angiotensin-converting enzyme (ACE)
aortic dissection
artery
arteriole
arteriolosclerosis
arteriosclerosis
atherosclerosis
ascites
blood vascular system

capillary
congestion
dialysis
diastolic pressure
disseminated intravascular
    coagulation (DIC)
edema
elephantiasis
embolus
endarterectomy
endothelium
esophageal varices
essential hypertension
fatty streak
filariasis
funduscopic examination
HDL
hemangioma
hemorrhoids
hydrothorax
hyperlipidemia
hypertension
hypotension
infarct
intermittent claudication
ischemia
LDL
lipoprotein
lumen
lymphangioma
lymphatic vascular system
lymphedema
malignant hypertension

medial sclerosis
multiple organ system
    failure
ophthalmoscope
plaque (atheromatous)
polyarteritis nodosa
portal vein
pulmonary embolism
Raynaud's phenomenon
renin
secondary hypertension
shock (cardiogenic, septic,
    neurogenic)
sinusoid
sphygmomanometer
syncope
systemic lupus
    erythematosus (SLE)
systolic pressure
temporal arteritis
thrombophlebitis
thrombus
transudate
triglycerides
tunica adventitia
tunica intima
tunica media
varicose vein
vasoconstriction
vasodilation
vein
venule
VLDL

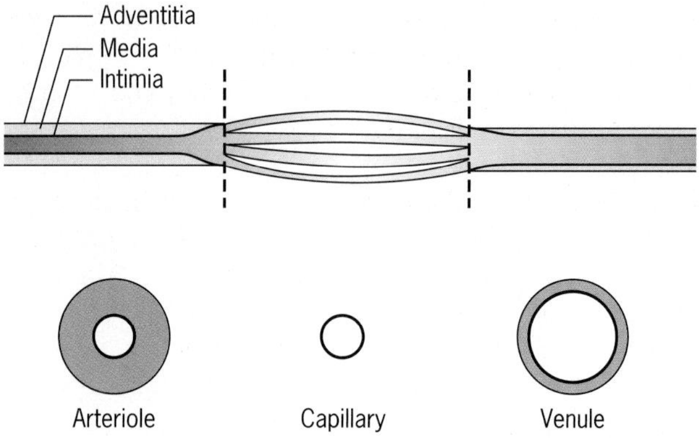

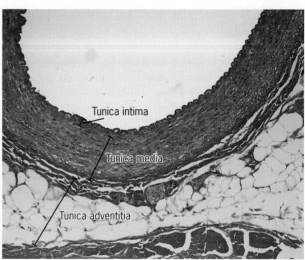

FIGURE 8–1 Comparison of arterioles, capillaries, and venules.

FIGURE 8–2 The wall of an artery, stained with hematoxylin and eosin. The tunica intima consists of a very thin layer of endothelial cells lining the lumen of the vessel. The tunica media is the thickest portion of the artery, consisting of smooth muscles cells aligned in concentric layers around the vessel. The tunica adventitia is the outer sheath of the vessel, consisting of fat and loose connective tissue. (© Donna Beer Stolz, Ph.D., Center for Biologic Imaging, University of Pittsburgh Medical School.)

Review of Structure and Function

The vascular system actually comprises two systems—the **blood vascular system** and the **lymphatic vascular system**. The blood vascular system is a continuous-flow system transporting blood to and from the heart via **arteries**, **capillaries**, and **veins**. Because the blood does not directly surround tissue cells, the vascular system must allow for exchange of gases, nutrients, and metabolic wastes across its walls. This exchange takes place primarily in the smallest component of the blood vascular system, the capillaries and **venules** (small veins) (**Figure 8–1**), where blood flow is slowest and the walls are thinnest.

The walls of arteries and veins have three concentric layers, or *tunicas*: the tunica intima, tunica media, and tunica adventitia (**Figure 8–2**). The **tunica intima** (usually just called *intima*) is lined by broad, flat endothelial cells anchored to a basement membrane and a few connective tissue cells for support. The continuous lining of endothelial cells is also called **endothelium**. The endothelial cells in smaller vessels control the exchange of nutrients, gases, and wastes between blood and tissue. The **tunica media** (or *media*) is composed of elastic tissue and smooth muscle. Either sympathetic (autonomic nervous system) stimulation or circulating adrenergic hormones (e.g., adrenalin) can produce contraction of the

muscle cells, which decreases the caliber of vessels. This is called **vasoconstriction**. Cholinergic hormones (e.g., acetylcholine) and, in some vessels, parasympathetic (autonomic nervous system) stimulation cause **vasodilation**. The **tunica adventitia** (or *adventitia*) is composed of supporting connective tissue cells. The space through which blood flows is called the **lumen**.

The maximum pressure as the heart muscle contracts, or **systolic pressure**, is approximately 120 mm Hg in most normal individuals, and the lowest pressure between heart contractions, or **diastolic pressure**, is approximately 80 mm Hg. Thus, the arterial side of the vascular system has intraluminal pressures of about 100 mm Hg throughout most of its length. Vessels are not merely conduits of blood: they actively control how much blood flows through tissues, and in so doing determine the systolic pressure. The major determinants of blood pressure are the amount of blood flowing through the vessels and the resistance of the vessels to this flow. Therefore, either an increased amount of blood or decreased vessel caliber will elevate the blood pressure. Normally, pressure is controlled mainly by the degree of dilation or constriction of arteries and **arterioles** (very small arteries).

The venous side of the vascular system has a mean pressure of less than 30 mm Hg. Veins have thinner muscular walls than do arteries and larger lumens to carry blood at a slower rate and under less pressure. The function of veins is to return blood to the heart from the tissue capillary beds. The force that pushes blood in the veins back to the heart is the pressure that remains after the passage of blood through arteries, arterioles, and capillaries. This force is only adequate to return blood to the heart when the body is in a horizontal position. Unless compensated for, blood in the head and upper parts of the body would gravitate to the abdomen and lower extremities in a person standing upright. Among the compensatory mechanisms to prevent this are reflexes that constrict the lower body veins, the massaging action of skeletal muscles on veins, and the action of respiratory movements on the great veins in the chest. In addition, veins contain valves, which aid in the flow of blood against gravity by preventing backflow. Obstruction of blood flow in veins by such mechanisms as compression, thrombosis (blood clots), or heart failure elevates venous and capillary blood pressures, causing accumulation of blood in these highly distensible structures. Distention of veins and capillaries caused by increased venous pressure is called **congestion**. Continued congestion results in leakage of fluids through capillary endothelium into tissues. This accumulation of fluid is called **edema**, and it results in a disturbance of tissue–capillary exchange of oxygen, nutrients, and metabolites.

The **portal vein** is an exceptional vein that collects blood from most of the intestinal tract and spleen and carries it to the liver, where nutrients and metabolic products are removed before it is returned to the heart via the hepatic vein.

Capillaries are small vessels lying between arteries and veins. They consist essentially of only an intimal layer. In aggregate, capillaries contain by far the largest volume of the vascular system, although most are in a state of collapse at any given time. Capillaries are extremely adaptable in being able to open in response to the needs of the tissue for increased blood flow and in being able to proliferate to help repair an injured area. Capillary flow is controlled by contraction or relaxation of arterioles and venules.

Capillaries regulate fluid, electrolyte, and nutrient exchange between the blood and the extracellular space. Three factors mediate this exchange: (1) the hydrostatic pressure transmitted from the venules, (2) the osmotic pressure determined by the amount of solutes (particularly protein) in blood and tissue fluid, and (3) the integrity of endothelial cells. Alteration in any of these factors can result in edema. If the hydrostatic pressure in veins is increased, as happens in heart failure, the pressure in capillaries will potentiate net movement of fluid out of them. If the osmotic pressure decreases, as happens with liver failure (albumin, produced by the liver, is the serum protein that contributes the most to osmotic pressure), there will also be a net movement of fluid out of capillaries. Disruption of capillary endothelial cell integrity or function leading to edema is usually a localized accompaniment of the inflammatory reaction caused in part by the release of vasodilating substances such as histamine.

In some organs, such as the liver, spleen, adrenal gland, and pituitary gland, the capillaries take the form of sinusoids. **Sinusoids** are dilated capillaries that are more continuously open to blood flow than are ordinary capillaries. Sinusoids are associated with specialized functions, such as filtering out particulate matter, including damaged blood cells in the liver and spleen, and hormone regulation in the adrenal and pituitary glands. The most structurally complex capillaries are found in the renal glomeruli, where they function to filter waste products into the urine.

The lymph vascular system (lymphatic system) is unique in that it has no vessels flowing into the system. Lymphatic vessels originate as blind-ended, thin-walled channels that drain local tissues and extend to lymph nodes. The lymph nodes in turn drain into larger lymphatic channels, which eventually empty into the thoracic duct. The thoracic duct flows into the superior vena cava, thus returning lymphatic fluid to the systemic circulation. To a lesser extent, lymphatic vessels also empty into other veins. Lymph is composed predominantly of water, proteins, and white blood cells, but not red blood cells. Lymphatic vessels function as a low-pressure drainage system as they return excess tissue fluid back into the venous system. Also, lymphocytes may reenter the circulation from tissue via this route.

Most Frequent and Serious Problems

Atherosclerosis is a disease characterized by lipid, calcium, and fibrous deposits in the intima of large and medium-sized arteries and is by far the most significant disease in the United States in terms of death and morbidity. The arteries to the brain are the second most important site of atherosclerosis. Cerebral infarcts (strokes) resulting from atherosclerosis of cerebral vessels are the fourth most common cause of death in the United States. Atherosclerosis of the arteries of the legs and of the main artery to the intestines (superior mesenteric artery) less commonly leads to arterial obstruction and infarction, but when it occurs, the effects are quite serious.

The formation of thrombi, or blood clots anchored to vessel walls, in the deep veins of the legs is a relatively common and sometimes serious problem that occurs particularly in bedridden patients. The most important complication of thrombi occurs when they break away from the vessel wall. Pieces of thrombi that are free-floating in vessels are called emboli. Emboli breaking away from thrombi in deep leg veins are carried through the veins to the right side of the heart, where they are pumped into the branches of the pulmonary arteries, causing obstruction of blood flow to portions of the lungs. This is called pulmonary embolism (PE). Depending on the size of the emboli and their number, they can have a range of effects, from pulmonary infarction to the gradual development of pulmonary hypertension to sudden death, if large pulmonary arteries are suddenly obstructed.

Varicosities are permanently dilated venous channels. They most commonly occur in the legs (varicose veins) and about the anus (hemorrhoids). Varicose veins may cause discomfort, disfigurement, edema, ulceration of the lower extremities, and predispose individuals to the formation of thrombi. Hemorrhoids may be asymptomatic or may cause itching, pain on defecation, bright red bleeding, or sudden, severe pain if thrombosis occurs.

High blood pressure, or hypertension, is one of the most important conditions for healthcare providers to understand because its recognition and treatment can prevent or delay serious complications, such as heart failure, kidney disease, or myocardial or cerebral infarcts. Most cases of hypertension are idiopathic, meaning they do not have a clear cause. Effective pharmacological treatments that reduce blood pressure are available, however. It takes many years for the effects of hypertension to become evident, so it is possible to detect and treat this disease early in its course, before it has become symptomatic.

Symptoms, Signs, and Tests

Occlusive conditions of the arteries (thrombi, emboli, atheromas, or inflammatory occlusions) manifest as infarcts or more gradual loss of tissue resulting from insufficient blood supply (ischemic atrophy). Either infarcts or ischemic atrophy results in loss of function in the organs supplied by the affected vessel. Pain may also occur.

The integrity of arteries can be directly evaluated by angiography, a procedure in which radiopaque dye is injected into arteries and successive x-ray films are taken to show the caliber of the vessels and distribution of blood flow. For example, a cerebral angiogram may demonstrate an aneurysm of a cerebral vessel or displacement of cerebral vessels by a tumor. Commonly, a carotid angiogram demonstrates atherosclerotic narrowing or occlusion of the carotid artery, a significant predisposing factor to strokes (**Figure 8–3**).

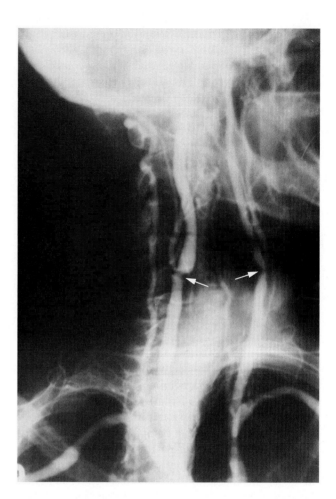

FIGURE 8–3 An angiogram of carotid arteries with areas of narrowing (arrows).

Functional diseases of arteries, causing high or low blood pressure, have entirely different symptoms than does arterial occlusion. Hypertension is usually asymptomatic, but it may manifest as headaches and dizziness. Low blood pressure (hypotension), if severe, manifests as symptoms of shock, which include faintness, cold skin resulting from vasoconstriction, and reduced blood flow to the brain and the kidneys. The functional status of the arterial system is usually evaluated by measuring the arterial blood pressure with a sphygmomanometer (pronounced "sfig-mo-ma-NA-meter") and by determining the fullness of the pulse by placing a finger over a pulsating artery.

The status of the venous system can be estimated by inspection or it can be measured using specialized instruments. Distention of neck veins when the patient is in an upright position is an obvious sign of increased pressure in the venous system. More subtle increases can be measured by inserting a pressure gauge into an arm vein. Rarely, when a patient is critically ill, the pressure gauge can be threaded through the veins into the heart to measure the pressures generated in the heart chambers during systole and diastole. Thrombosis of deep leg veins causes cyanotic congestion, edema, and sometimes pain. Ultrasound techniques measuring the Doppler effect provide a sophisticated method of evaluating venous flow (or the absence thereof) at deep sites, such as the deep veins of the legs. Incompetent valves in superficial leg veins lead to distended, tortuous, protruding, rope-like varicosities that are obvious on inspection. Likewise, hemorrhoidal and esophageal varicosities are evaluated by inspection of the anus and by endoscopy, respectively.

Some diseases, such as hypertension and diabetes mellitus, preferentially affect small vessels. They may cause skin ulcers, which heal poorly and become secondarily infected. They may also cause decreased visual acuity and even blindness. The only area in the body where the small vessels are readily visible is in the back of the eye, where they lie immediately beneath the highly translucent retina. Examination of the back of the eye with an **ophthalmoscope** is called **funduscopic examination**. Early evidence of hypertension and diabetic retinopathy can be detected by examining these vessels.

Specific Diseases
Genetic/Developmental Diseases

Congenital variations in the vascular system, such as angiomas, are common but rarely cause problems. Congenital heart diseases and anomalies of the great vessels can be life-threatening, however.

Angiomas

Hemangiomas are local proliferations of capillaries that may be present at birth. They are common in the skin, where they vary from small red dots to large cosmetically distracting "port wine stains" (**Figure 8–4**). Because the dilated vessels fill with blood, they are red to blue and blanch under the pressure of a finger as the blood is pushed out of them. Hemangiomas of the skin rarely cause any problem, but they are occasionally removed for cosmetic reasons. **Lymphangiomas**, dilated masses of lymphatics, are much less common. When they occur in the neck of an infant (*cystic hygroma*), they may be frightening in appearance, but they usually regress with age.

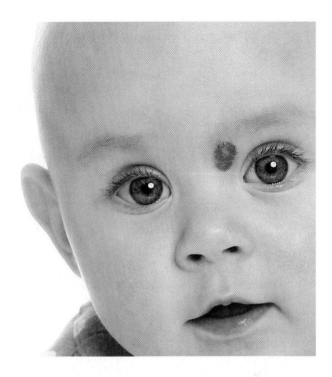

FIGURE 8–4 Hemangioma on the side of the face of an infant. (© Julie DeGuia/Shutterstock, Inc.)

Inflammatory/Degenerative Diseases

The terms used to describe thickening and hardening of arteries can be confusing. **Arteriosclerosis** means "hardening of the arteries" and is the generic term used to refer to three different processes (**Figure 8–5**): thickening of the intima and media of small arterioles (**arteriolosclerosis** or arteriolar sclerosis; **Figure 8–6**), calcification of the media of large arteries (**medial sclerosis** or medial calcification), and plaque formation in the intima of large arteries (atherosclerosis). Arteriolosclerosis occurs in response to prolonged hypertension. It is seen most commonly in the renal arterioles and may contribute to decreased renal function. Medial calcification occurs in the medium-sized to large arteries of the thyroid, brain,

---

BOX 8–1   Hemangiomas

Causes

Congenital anomalies

Lesions

Excessive capillary proliferation, often on the skin

Manifestations

Localized redness of the skin, which blanches with pressure

Rarely bleed

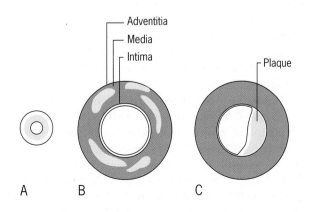

FIGURE 8–5 Types of arteriosclerosis: **A.** Arteriolosclerosis. **B.** Medial calcification. **C.** Atherosclerosis.

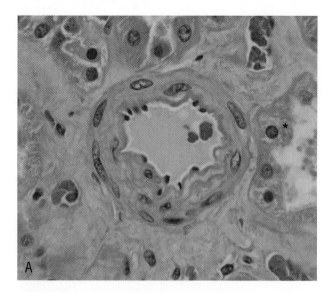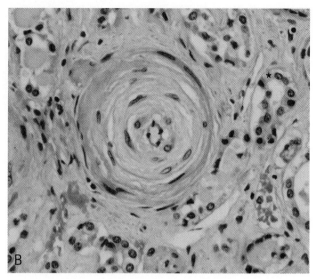

FIGURE 8–6 Changes in arteriole (on cross section) associated with severe hypertension. The renal arteriole in **A** is of normal size. Its wall is composed of a few concentric layers of smooth muscle cells with elongated nuclei. Notice that the wall of the arteriole is about as thick as the single layer of epithelial cells in the renal tubule next to it. (An asterisk appears on a renal tubular epithelial cell in this and the next picture.) The wall of the arteriole in **B**, which is from the kidney of a patient with severe and long-standing hypertension, is greatly thickened. Notice the numerous layers of cells in the wall and the reduction of the lumen to a pinpoint opening. The epithelial cells in the tubules surrounding the arteriole appear much smaller in relation to the thickness of the arteriole wall.

genital tract, and extremities with aging and is not considered to be a cause of significant disease. Because atherosclerosis and hypertension directly or indirectly cause so much morbidity in the population, we will discuss them here at greater length.

Atherosclerosis

Atherosclerosis is a degenerative condition: its prevalence and severity increase with advancing age. The basic lesion of atherosclerosis is a fibrofatty (i.e., composed of fibrous tissue and lipids) deposit in the intima of blood vessels, particularly in the major muscular arteries (**Figure 8–7**). This deposit is called an **atheromatous plaque**. Atheromas occur in large and medium-sized arteries, particularly the aorta and its major branches (the carotid, coronary, mesenteric, renal, iliac, and femoral arteries). The earliest visible lesions, called **fatty streaks** because they are composed almost entirely of lipid, can be found even in children dying of unrelated diseases, and most people older than the age of 30 years have grossly visible atherosclerotic lesions in their larger arteries. Complications of atherosclerosis—namely, decreased blood flow, thrombosis, or embolism—can begin to occur in persons in their 30s but usually do not manifest as signs or symptoms until much later. The increase in frequency of complications in women is usually delayed until after menopause, presumably because of a protective effect of estrogen and progesterone. The low-pressure pulmonary arteries are not usually involved.

It is not known exactly what stimulates atheromatous plaque formation, but most theories about the

pathogenesis of atherosclerosis implicate damage to the endothelium as the initiating event. A variety of agents, including toxins in cigarette smoke, diabetes, hypertension, turbulent flow at sites of bifurcation of arteries, and immune injury, could be responsible for the initial endothelial damage. Once the endothelial cells are damaged, they become leaky, and lipid droplets that are normally circulating in the blood diffuse across the endothelium and become deposited in the intima. In response, the endothelial cells recruit monocytes and lymphocytes. The monocytes scavenge the free lipid, and then remain in the tissue as lipid-laden macrophages. At the same time, smooth muscle cells migrate into the intima from the media, presumably also to limit the damage and restore function to the intima. The activity of the macrophages and smooth muscle cells is regulated by cytokines secreted by the lymphocytes. Accumulation of lipids within the macrophages and smooth muscle cells gives the intima the yellow color that is grossly appreciated as a "fatty streak."

As the atheromatous plaque matures, smooth muscle cells and macrophages become incontinent and release the lipids into the extracellular space again, thereby aggravating and accelerating the inflammatory process. The lipids are deposited extracellularly in the form of cholesterol crystals. As with any other chronic inflammatory lesion, fibrosis also occurs, and over time the plaques become scarred, or sclerotic. Also, cells within the lesion die, and their remains undergo dystrophic calcification. The atheromatous lesions therefore gradually enlarge over years and become progressively more fibrous and calcified (**Figure 8–8**). The white-yellow, shaggy, crusted

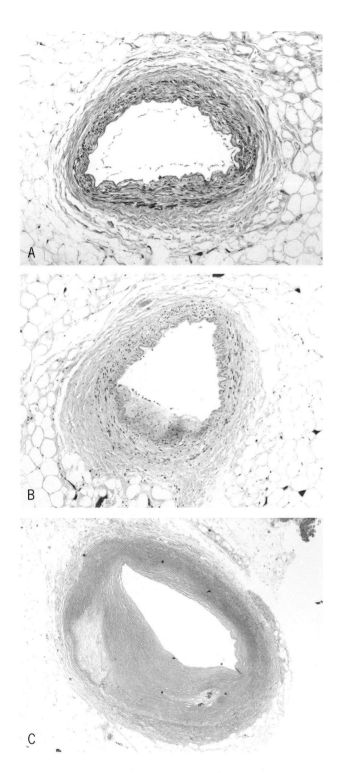

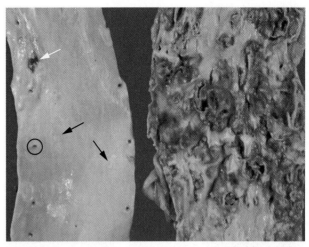

FIGURE 8–8 Atherosclerosis. The two aortas in this image have been opened posteriorly to expose the intimal surface. The regularly spaced holes on either side of the aorta on the left (black circle) are the openings to the vertebral arteries. The aorta on the left has a shiny, white intimal surface. Closer inspection reveals irregularly shaped patches of yellow discoloration (black arrows), or fatty plaques. The white arrow is pointing to a more advanced atherosclerotic lesion. The aorta on the right is severely affected with atherosclerosis. The white intimal surface is only apparent as small, ragged patches amid ulcerated, necrotic, and calcified atheromatous lesions.

FIGURE 8–7 Atherosclerosis. **A** shows a cross section of a coronary artery stained with trichrome, which colors collagen blue and muscle fibers red. A dense layer of collagen lines the lumen of the artery. This marks the boundary between the tunica media and the tunica intima. The tunica intima is inconspicuous, and the tunica media is composed of bright red muscle cells. The artery in **B** has been stained with hematoxylin and eosin. You can see the demarcation between intima and media as a corrugated, wavy, dark pink line around the lumen. In the lower left of the lumen, a heap of cells is layered on top of the intima. This represents focal intimal hyperplasia, an early stage in plaque formation. In **C**, the darker blue area is the approximate transition between the tunica media and the tunica intima. The lumen is more than 50% occluded by plaque. Atherosclerosis involves the entire circumference of the lumen.

appearance of advanced atherosclerosis is caused by crystallization of the cholesterol and calcification.

Atherosclerotic plaques can cause harm in several ways. The lumen of the blood vessel may become significantly narrowed, or occluded, by the plaque. This causes **ischemia** of the tissue normally supplied by that artery. The surface of a plaque can become ulcerated. Exposed collagen is very thrombogenic, and a thrombus can rapidly form over an ulcerated plaque. This can lead to acute occlusion and infarction of the tissue supplied by the artery. Or, bits of the thrombus can break off and travel distally before occluding a smaller-caliber vessel. The plaque may also damage the structural integrity of the vessel wall so that it balloons under pressure to form an **aneurysm** (**Figure 8–9**). If the wall becomes thin enough, the aneurysm can rupture, leading to life-threatening hemorrhage.

Different vessels tend to suffer different complications. Atherosclerosis in the coronary arteries, which are relatively small caliber, tends to produce narrowing of the lumen. Rupture of the plaque with thrombosis or hemorrhage into the plaque causes myocardial infarction. Plaques in the carotid arteries tend to cause occlusion. Atherosclerosis of the abdominal aorta, the most common site for atherosclerosis, may be asymptomatic even when extensive. Complications can occur if an atherosclerotic plaque overgrows the orifice (origin) of an aortic branch artery, if a thrombus forms and bits of it embolize to different tissues, or if an aneurysm forms. Atherosclerosis in the arteries of the lower limbs may cause an infarct of the foot resulting in an ulcer (**Figure 8–10**) or produce

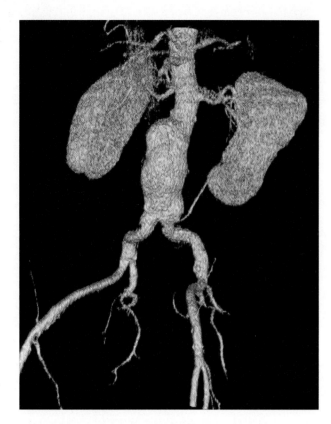

FIGURE 8–9 CT angiogram of an atherosclerotic aneurysm of the aorta. The two orange masses on either side of the aorta are the kidneys. The aortic aneurysm is the irregular dilatation of the aorta between the renal arteries and the bifurcation of the aorta. (Courtesy of Dr. Myron Pozniak, Department of Radiology, University of Wisconsin School of Medicine and Public Health.)

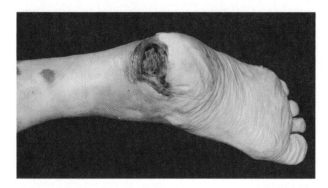

FIGURE 8–10 A deep, nonhealing ulcer due to tissue infarction on the heel of this foot necessitated amputation.

more gradual ischemic changes in the leg. Gradual ischemic changes are associated with atrophy of muscle and pain that is aggravated by walking and relieved by rest (**intermittent claudication**).

Although it is not fully understood what initiates and perpetuates the atherosclerotic process, it is generally agreed that atherosclerosis is a chronic inflammatory process, that endothelial injury plays a critical role in initiating the process, and that circulating lipids are key to perpetuation and evolution of the lesion. The

relationship between endothelial injury and lipid deposition is complex. Clearly, serum lipid abnormalities promote the development of atherosclerosis, but local factors are necessary for plaque development.

All people have some degree of atherosclerosis, yet one individual may die of a myocardial infarct from an occluded coronary artery at the age of 35, whereas another individual may die of cancer at the age of 90 with only mild atherosclerosis. In addition, some populations in the world have very little atherosclerosis, but when individuals from these populations move to areas where atherosclerosis is more prevalent, their risk for developing atherosclerosis and its complications increases. The recognition of such environmental and individual variations has led to the elucidation of risk factors, or conditions that, when present, render an individual more susceptible to development of the disease. The major risk factors for atherosclerosis are the following (**Table 8–1**):

1. *Hyperlipidemia:* Increased dietary intake and familial (genetically influenced) elevations of serum lipids are predisposing factors to atherosclerosis. Serum cholesterol values higher than 200 mg/dL are generally considered to confer an increased risk. Serum cholesterol levels represent the total of several forms of cholesterol in the serum, some of which are more strongly associated with the development of atherosclerosis than are others. **Lipoproteins**, the major carriers of cholesterol in the serum, have been classified on the basis of their density and electrophoretic migration. Elevated serum levels of low-density lipoproteins (**LDLs**) and very low-density lipoproteins (**VLDLs**) are associated with more severe atherosclerosis, whereas high-density lipoproteins (**HDLs**) are somewhat protective. Hyperlipoproteinemic states have been classified on the basis of serum levels of lipoproteins, cholesterol, and **triglycerides**. **Figure 8–11** illustrates the percent content of cholesterol and triglyceride in each of the three lipoprotein classes. Familial forms of **hyperlipidemia** confer a high risk for development of complications of atherosclerosis beginning at a relatively young age (30s and 40s, compared to 50s and 60s in the general population).

2. *Hypertension:* The higher the blood pressure, the greater the risk for development of atherosclerosis. The reason is not known, but it may be related to

TABLE 8–1 Atherosclerosis Risk Factors	
Major	**Minor**
• Hyperlipidemia	• Age*
• Hypertension	• Family history*
• Smoking	• Gender*
• Diabetes	• Stress
• Obesity	• Activity level
• Hyperhomocysteinemia	

* Indicates nonmodifiable risk factors.

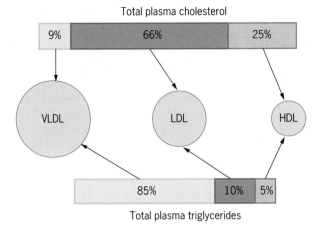

Total plasma cholesterol

| 9% | 66% | 25% |

VLDL   LDL   HDL

| 85% | 10% | 5% |

Total plasma triglycerides

FIGURE 8–11 Distribution of plasma lipids among the major lipoprotein classes.

trauma to the arterial intima, particularly at sites of turbulent blood flow, such as at bifurcations of arteries. In support of this hypothesis is the observation that when veins, which normally do not develop atherosclerosis, are transplanted to a position where they carry arterial blood—for example, when used as a coronary artery bypass graft—they can develop atherosclerotic lesions very rapidly.

3. *Cigarette smoking:* The death rate from coronary atherosclerosis in smokers is more than double that of nonsmokers.

4. *Diabetes:* Diabetics have more, and more significant, atherosclerosis on average than nondiabetics.

5. *Obesity:* People with obesity and/or high intake of calories, carbohydrates, and saturated lipids have a greater incidence of atherosclerosis.

6. *Hyperhomocysteinemia:* Homocysteine is an amino acid involved in the conversion of methionine to cysteine. When it is found in elevated levels in blood, it is associated with accelerated atherosclerosis and venous thrombosis. Again, the pathophysiologic links between elevated homocysteine levels and atherosclerosis are not understood. Hyperhomocysteinemia can be treated by a diet high in folic acid and vitamins B_6 and B_{12}.

7. *Age:* In general, the older a person, the more atherosclerosis is present.

8. *Gender:* Men have a higher incidence of atherosclerosis. In women, the severity of atherosclerosis and the frequency of its complications rapidly increase after menopause, to approach that of older men.

9. *Family history:* Some families have a much higher incidence of atherosclerosis and resulting diseases than do other families. In some instances, this may be related to a common diet, but in other cases, there is a clear genetic influence such as familial hyperlipidemia, risk of diabetes, or obesity.

10. *Activity level:* Reasonable and regular exercise reduces lipid levels, blood pressure, and weight, and thus the amount of atherosclerosis.

11. *Psychological factors:* Emotional stress and depression seem to be associated with an increased incidence of atherosclerotic coronary artery disease.

Of all these risk factors, the first six (hyperlipidemia, hypertension, smoking, diabetes, obesity, and hyperhomocysteinemia) are considered major, and the others, minor, meaning that the former have more of an impact on the development and severity of atherosclerosis than the others do. In addition, some of these risk factors are not treatable: age, gender, and family history are what they are. Modification of the other risk factors is possible by diet, exercise, smoking cessation, stress therapy, and pharmaceutical agents. Several pharmaceutical agents are now available that can very effectively reduce serum lipid levels. Finally, the effect of these risk factors on the development of atherosclerosis and its complications is exponential. The presence of one risk factor doubles the death rate; the death rate when there are two risk factors is double that when there is one; and so forth.

Once established, treatment of atherosclerotic lesions involves (1) preventing further lesions from developing and preventing growth of existing lesions, and (2) taking care of complications as they arise. It is important to remember that atherosclerosis is a dynamic lesion—that is, plaques change over time, and they can even, to some degree, be reversed or at least stabilized so that they do not grow further. The same measures that are known to reduce the risk of developing atherosclerosis can stabilize or decrease atherosclerotic lesions once they have formed. Early diagnosis and treatment of hypertension clearly have a beneficial effect. Cessation of smoking, even by those who have smoked for many years, reduces the frequency of atherosclerotic complications. Dietary preventive measures that reduce serum cholesterol have been proven to be effective at reducing the development of atherosclerosis. The use of statin pharmaceutical agents is a powerful means of reducing serum lipid levels, including cholesterol, and thereby reducing the development of atherosclerosis and its complications.

Surgical therapy for established atherosclerotic lesions and its complications has become very effective over the last several decades. Ultrasound techniques allow diagnosis and measurement of asymptomatic aneurysms so that they can be treated before they reach a critical size at which they are more likely to rupture. Treatment of abdominal aortic aneurysms entails bypassing the aneurysmal portion of the aorta with a tube of biologically inert material. Operations to remove atherosclerotic plaques from the lumens of carotid and coronary arteries are reserved for symptomatic patients, and then only after careful evaluation of potential risks and benefits. Carotid artery plaques, which occur at the bifurcation of the internal and external carotid arteries and reduce cerebral blood flow, are removed by opening the artery and "shelling out" the plaque, a process called **endarterectomy**. Treatment of atherosclerotic lesions in coronary arteries can be done by bypass surgery or **angioplasty**, whereby a deflated balloon is passed into the coronary artery and then inflated at the site of the plaque, effectively crushing it against the wall of the artery, and/or by placing a metal stent over the occluded area to keep the lumen propped open. Occluded leg or mesenteric vessels can be bypassed by insertion of grafts before the tissue distal to the occlusion becomes terminally damaged. Gangrenous legs or ischemic bowel can be removed by surgery.

Some complications are not amenable to surgical or medical treatment, however. Strokes can have devastating consequences, the first myocardial infarction is also often the fatal one, and removal of the intestines or legs is irreversible. Taking care of complications as they arise is therefore not an ideal option. In addition, an enormous portion of healthcare resources is used in managing the complications of atherosclerosis.

In recent years, attention to preventing or delaying the development of atherosclerosis by promoting preventive measures has produced some promising results. For example, although atherosclerotic cardiovascular disease has for decades been the number one cause of death of adults in the United States, mortality from cardiovascular disease has been declining steadily, and it is estimated that it will soon fall below mortality resulting from neoplastic diseases. This is in part secondary to better detection and treatment modalities so that more people with atherosclerotic cardiovascular disease survive for longer periods (and thereby die of other causes), but it is also in part the result of increasing awareness in the population of the importance of adopting healthy lifestyles. What impact the "obesity epidemic" will have on cardiovascular morbidity and mortality remains to be seen.

BOX 8–2   Atherosclerosis

Causes

Multifactorial

Known risk factors (e.g., hyperlipidemia, hypertension, smoking, diabetes)

Lesions

Atheroma

Superimposed thrombosis or hemorrhage

Infarcts

Ischemic atrophy

Aneurysms

Emboli

Manifestations

Related to site involved

Loss of function

Pain

Hemorrhage

Hypertension

Hypertension means high blood pressure. The upper limits of normal blood pressure are generally considered to be 80–90 mm Hg diastolic and 120–140 mm Hg systolic. As thus defined, more than 50 million persons in the United States have hypertension. Transient hypertension, such as is caused by anxiety or physical activity, needs to be distinguished from hypertensive disease in which there is sustained hypertension leading to gradual development of arteriolosclerosis and atherosclerotic lesions.

Systolic blood pressure is reflective of the force of the heart's contraction as it expels blood into the aorta. Large arteries expand to dampen the force of the pulse. Loss of the ability to expand, as occurs in the aorta with atherosclerosis, produces systolic hypertension. Systolic hypertension also may be produced by increased cardiac output, such as occurs with exercise, hyperthyroidism, or fever. Diastolic pressure represents the minimum pressure within arteries between heart contractions and is reflective of muscle tone in small arteries. Mean arterial pressure, which very roughly can be thought of as the average of the systolic and diastolic pressures, is the product of cardiac output and systemic peripheral resistance. In other words, blood pressure is a measure of both the amount of blood the heart is pumping per minute and the state of constriction of the small arteries and arterioles supplying capillary beds. The state of relaxation and the patency of these arteries are therefore crucial in regulating blood pressure.

Essential hypertension refers to primary or idiopathic hypertensive disease. *Idiopathic* means the cause is unknown. Essential hypertension is the most common form of the disease, accounting for more than 90% of cases. **Secondary hypertension** refers to hypertensive disease in which a cause, such as a tumor that is producing adrenalin, is evident (**Table 8–2**). Even though an identifiable cause is present in only 10% of patients with hypertension, it is important to look for one because treatment would focus on eliminating it rather than simply on treating the sign, which is the only option with essential hypertension.

Essential hypertension appears to be a multifactorial disease involving both genetic and environmental factors. That it is at least partially genetic is suggested by the tendency for it to be familial and by its high prevalence among American blacks. The genetic factor probably involves multiple genes and does not manifest in clear lines of inheritance. Among the many possible environmental factors, a high-salt diet, smoking, obesity, diabetes, a sedentary lifestyle, and high alcohol consumption are modifiable risk factors. Psychological stimuli, such as stress, also appear to aggravate hypertension in some individuals. It is possible that many cases of essential hypertension are perpetuated by hypertensive effects on the renal vessels, thereby resulting in a vicious cycle.

The kidney plays a critical role in the regulation of blood pressure (**Figure 8–12**). When specialized cells

TABLE 8–2 Causes of Hypertension

Essential (idiopathic)

Secondary

Renal
- Destruction of renal parenchyma (pyelonephritis, cystic disorders)
- Acute renal diseases (acute glomerulonephritis)
- Diseases of renal artery (atherosclerosis)

Endocrine
- Increased secretion of adrenal hormones (adrenalin, corticosteroids)
- Exogenous hormones (steroids)
- Hyperthyroidism or hypothyroidism

Neoplastic
- Pheochromocytoma
- Tumors producing hormones

Neurologic
- Increased intracranial pressure
- Sleep apnea
- Acute stress (e.g., surgery)

Cardiovascular
- Rigidity of aorta
- Coarctation of aorta
- Arteriovenous fistula
- Increased intravascular volume
- Increased cardiac output (e.g., pregnancy, anemia)
- Toxemia of pregnancy

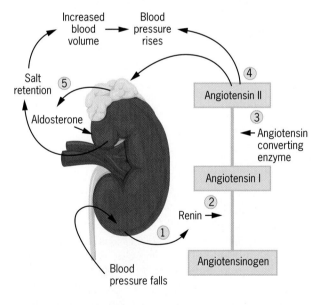

FIGURE 8–12 Role of kidney in hypertension: relationship of a fall in blood delivery to the kidneys to the renin–angiotensin–aldosterone axis.

in the kidneys sense decreased blood flow because of decreased blood volume, they secrete an enzyme, **renin**, which converts inactive serum angiotensinogen to angiotensin I, which is in turn converted to **angiotensin II** by **angiotensin-converting enzyme (ACE)** in the lung. Angiotensin II causes constriction of the smooth muscle

in the media of arteries and arterioles, thereby increasing the total peripheral resistance. It also stimulates the secretion of the hormone **aldosterone** from the adrenal gland. Aldosterone causes resorption of sodium and water in the tubules of the kidney, which translates into increased blood volume. In addition, when blood volume decreases, the glomerular filtration rate decreases, and this also causes the renal tubules to reabsorb sodium, thereby again contributing to the blood volume. Pharmaceutical agents used for the treatment of essential hypertension in part interfere with these processes: reducing total circulating blood volume by reducing sodium and water reabsorption in the renal tubules (diuretic agents, for example) or reducing the conversion of angiotensin I to angiotensin II (angiotensin-converting enzyme [ACE] inhibitors).

Given the central role of the kidney in regulating blood pressure, it is not surprising that the most common causes of secondary hypertension are renal diseases. Three types of renal disorders that produce hypertension are (1) chronic destructive renal diseases, such as chronic glomerulonephritis, chronic pyelonephritis, and polycystic kidneys; (2) acute renal disease, such as glomerulonephritis; and (3) narrowing of the renal artery because of atherosclerosis or smooth muscle hypertrophy. Chronic destructive renal disease is the most common cause of secondary hypertension. Partial occlusion of the renal artery results in decreased blood delivery to the kidney and subsequent release of renin. Renal arterial narrowing can be diagnosed by angiograms and treated with placement of a wire stent into the renal artery, but the benefit of such intervention on blood pressure control is modest at best.

Other causes of secondary hypertension (Table 8–2) include endocrine disorders, brain disorders, cardiovascular problems, and toxemia of pregnancy. There is not enough room to discuss all of these here, so we profile only a few to illustrate how diseases in various tissues can result in hypertension. Endocrine causes of hypertension usually can be related to increased secretion of adrenal hormones. Corticosteroids and aldosterone from the adrenal cortex cause salt retention and lead to hypertension if secreted in excess. Epinephrine and norepinephrine are produced by a rare neoplasm of the adrenal medulla called pheochromocytoma and cause hypertension by constricting blood vessels. Endocrine causes of hypertension are often treatable by removal of the tissue responsible for the production of the aberrant hormone.

Increased intracranial pressure is often associated with hypertension. Causes of increased intracranial pressure are numerous, from acute intracranial bleeding to generalized swelling secondary to trauma or neoplasms that take up scarce space in the cranium. Treatment of this kind of hypertension again involves addressing the underlying cause. Coarctation of the aorta is usually a congenital condition in which the aorta is focally constricted, or stenotic. This produces hypertension proximal to the coarctation by obstruction of the aorta. It is treatable by

TABLE 8–3	The Major Clinical Complications of Hypertension

Cardiovascular
- Heart failure
- Accelerated atherosclerosis
- Myocardial infarction
- Aneurysm
- Aortic dissection

Neurologic
- Cerebrovascular accident (stroke)
- Intraparenchymal bleeding
- Blindness
- Memory impairment

Renal
- Chronic renal failure leading to
- End-stage kidneys
- Dialysis dependence

surgical release of the coarcted segment. Arteriovenous fistulas are abnormal connections between arteries and veins that cause rapid drainage of blood from arteries directly into veins. This produces a low diastolic pressure, which the heart attempts to compensate for by increasing cardiac output and thereby increasing systolic pressure. Toxemia of pregnancy is a poorly understood condition causing hypertension in pregnant women.

Hypertension takes years to produce its damaging effects, but in the end, it can affect virtually any tissue or organ (**Table 8–3**). Hypertrophy of the left ventricle resulting from the increased pumping force required of the heart is an almost invariable finding. Acceleration of the development of atherosclerosis also occurs commonly in hypertensive patients. Many hypertensive patients die from heart failure. This results from increased work imposed on the left ventricle as well as from damage to the myocardium from the concomitant coronary artery atherosclerosis. Another common cause of death in hypertensive patients is a cerebrovascular accident, or stroke, that results from bleeding of damaged small arteries in the brain.

A catastrophic complication of hypertension, affecting the vasculature directly, is **aortic dissection** (**Figure 8–13**). Dissection means "breaking into," and aortic dissection refers to blood breaking into the media of the aorta through a tear in the intima. The intimal tear most commonly occurs at the very beginning of the aorta, before it bends to form the aortic arch. It is thought that the jet of blood ejected from the heart under high pressures in hypertensive patients injures the intima where it impacts the aortic wall just above the aortic valve. This is where an intimal tear is likely to occur. Aortic dissections are frequently rapidly fatal, because a large amount of blood escapes from the vascular system in a short amount of time. The blood can flow backward into the pericardium and fill the pericardial sac so that the heart can no longer expand during diastole; travel along the media for variable distances and extend into branch arteries, causing their occlusion; or break through the adventitia and escape into the thoracic or abdominal cavities. To add insult to injury, the clinical manifestations of aortic dissection are manifold. It might present with the classically described ripping, tearing,

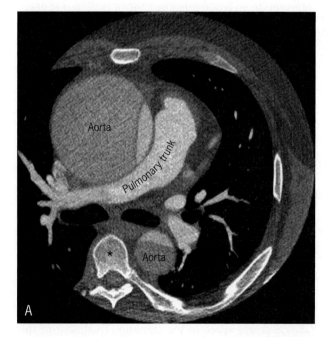

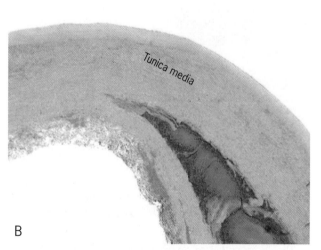

FIGURE 8–13 Aortic dissection. **A.** CT scan. Contrast material indicative of normally flowing blood is present in the pulmonary trunk, but only a small arc of contrast material is present in the ascending and descending aorta. Instead of flowing within the "true lumen," blood is tearing down the tunica media in the wall of the aorta, creating a "false lumen" and compressing the true, functional lumen to a narrow space. (Asterisk is on a vertebral body.) **B.** Photomicrograph illustrating blood (bright red) dissecting down the tunica media of the aorta. (Courtesy of Dr. Donald Yandow, Department of Radiology, University of Wisconsin School of Medicine and Public Health.)

crushing sensation in the chest, but it may also mimic the symptoms of heart attack or cause symptoms referable to major branches of the aorta that secondarily become involved with the dissection, such as mental confusion or dizziness (carotid artery) or pain or paralysis of the arms or legs (brachial arteries, iliac arteries). The diagnosis is unfortunately frequently missed because there is nothing specific about the presentation to remind doctors to think of it and ask for the appropriate tests (a computed tomography [CT] scan can demonstrate the dissection).

Chronic hypertension also often leads to kidney failure, manifested clinically as increasingly poor filtration of the blood and loss of protein in the urine. Patients with end-stage kidney disease, in which the kidneys are essentially not filtering the blood at all, require **dialysis**, in which the blood is passed through a machine that filters waste products from the blood before it is passed back into the body.

Small arteries are best visualized clinically in the retina, by funduscopic (ophthalmoscopic) examination. In patients with hypertension, these small vessels show thickening and focal narrowing. The degree of arteriolar involvement in the retina is an indication of the degree of arteriolosclerosis in other tissues, such as the kidney, which cannot so readily be examined. The sclerotic vessels in the retina may hemorrhage, or they may become so narrowed that they result in ischemia of the tissue. Either of these processes can result in blindness.

Rarely, the course of hypertensive disease may become accelerated, with severe renal and retinal vascular disease and very high blood pressure, even in the range of 250/130 mm Hg or more. Although hypertension is usually not symptomatic, accelerated, or **malignant hypertension** can manifest in the form of severe headaches and convulsions and lead to rapid death within months if not controlled.

Because most hypertensive disease is asymptomatic, it must be diagnosed by screening. This is performed by measurement of the blood pressure with a sphygmomanometer. Blood pressure measurement is a simple, noninvasive test that should be performed routinely on adult patients every time they come to the clinic. Three elevated blood pressure readings must be documented before a patient is diagnosed with hypertension. Symptoms, when they do develop, are usually complications of organ damage. Myocardial infarcts, heart failure, strokes, headaches, sometimes dizziness or light-headedness, blind spots in the field of vision, and renal failure are some of the more common complications of hypertension. Severe epistaxis (nosebleeds), hemoptysis (coughing up blood), and metrorrhagia (uterine bleeding at an abnormal time) may also occur. Obviously, the point of screening is to detect and treat hypertension before symptomatic complications can develop.

The prognosis for people with hypertension depends on many factors, such as how high the blood pressure is, occurrence with other potentiating diseases such as atherosclerosis, presence of a treatable cause, stage at time of diagnosis, ability to alter environmental factors such as stress and diet, and effectiveness of drug therapy in reducing the blood pressure. Untreated hypertensive disease might be expected to run a course of 20 years or so, with the first 15 years being asymptomatic. Although it is difficult to measure the effects of treatment in a predominantly older group of patients, there is no doubt that treatment adds years to the life of an average hypertensive patient and delays the development of complications.

The strategy of approach to hypertensive disease is threefold: (1) make the diagnosis early through screening, (2) perform a thorough medical investigation to discover the 10% of patients who have secondary hypertension that may be curable, and (3) reduce the blood pressure through environmental manipulation and drug therapy. *Environmental manipulation* refers to dietary modification, exercise, and attention to psychologic well-being. Note that the most important steps people can take to naturally reduce high blood pressure are also the ones that reduce the risk of progression of atherosclerosis. In addition, hypertension is a risk factor for the development of atherosclerosis, and atherosclerosis can potentiate high blood pressure (e.g., by causing obstruction of the renal artery), so paying attention to lifestyle issues actually allows patients to circumvent two potentially fatal vascular conditions at once.

Numerous drugs are available to treat hypertension. Among the more common are diuretics, which decrease the vascular volume; beta-adrenergic blocking agents, which decrease the heart rate and cardiac output by down-regulating the heart's response to stimulation by the sympathetic nervous system; calcium-channel blockers, which act directly on vascular smooth muscle to dilate peripheral blood vessels; and angiotensin-converting enzyme inhibitors and angiotensin II receptor blockers, which interfere with renal blood-pressure-elevating mechanisms. Drug therapy requires that the patient be under continuous medical surveillance. It is no wonder that hypertension is the most common chronic disease requiring visits to primary care physicians.

BOX 8-3 Hypertension

Causes

Unknown (most)

Secondary (see Table 8-2)

Lesions

Arteriolosclerosis

Left ventricular hypertrophy

Accelerated atherosclerosis

Aneurysm

Manifestations

Elevated blood pressure

Damage to brain, heart, eyes, vessels, and kidneys (see Table 8-3)

Vasculitis

Several uncommon, relatively low-grade, and sporadic noninfectious inflammatory diseases affect arteries and sometimes veins. Their exact causes are usually not known, but in most instances they appear to be autoimmune in nature. Histologically, they are characterized by accumulations of acute and/or chronic inflammatory cells in the walls of and scattered around vessels. Vasculitis poses significant diagnostic challenges because its variable distribution produces unpredictable and often myriad effects, depending on the organ system(s) involved. In general, vasculitides result in obstruction of vessels by inflammatory lesions. Patients therefore present with pain and symptoms related to ischemia or infarction of the tissue supplied by the involved artery. Occasionally, vasculitis might result in weakening and subsequent aneurysm formation or tearing of the artery. A small percentage of vasculitis cases are associated with hepatitis B virus (HBV) or with antineutrophil cytoplasmic antibodies (ANCA). Finding evidence of HBV or ANCA in the serum can aid in diagnosis. Some types of vasculitis manifest strictly as inflammation limited to blood vessels, whereas other cases are associated with systemic autoimmune diseases.

The most common type of vasculitis occurs with **systemic lupus erythematosus (SLE)**, an autoimmune disease that is quite variable in presentation because it affects numerous organs and organ systems. Patients can present with anything from a "butterfly rash" over the bridge of the nose to renal disease, pleuritic chest pain, arthritis, myalgias, fevers, hematologic abnormalities, or mental conditions such as psychosis or convulsions. A necrotizing (destructive) vasculitis appears to underlie many of the symptoms and can be seen in virtually any tissue. Serum antibodies to cell nuclei are the basis of the antinuclear antibody test (ANA), which is a sensitive test for this disorder.

Polyarteritis nodosa is another type of vasculitis. This results in nodular inflammatory thickening of medium-sized arteries, particularly those of the kidneys, intestines, and skeletal muscles. Inflammation of these arteries may lead to luminal occlusion, resulting in small to medium-sized infarcts in many organs.

The most common form of vasculitis in adults is **temporal arteritis**, which affects medium-sized muscular arteries of the temples. The symptoms are nonspecific, such as fever, fatigue, and weight loss accompanied by headache and pain over the course of the temporal artery, which lies rather superficially across the temporal bone and forehead. More ominous is the sudden loss of part or all of vision, if the inflammation extends into the ophthalmic branch of the temporal artery. Temporal arteritis responds very rapidly to steroid therapy. If a biopsy is performed before steroid therapy is initiated, it will demonstrate destruction of the arterial wall by giant cells and chronic inflammatory cells (**Figure 8–14**).

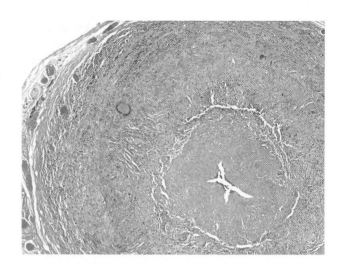

FIGURE 8–14 Temporal arteritis. The wall of the artery is greatly thickened and the lumen reduced to a slitlike opening. The muscular layer of the wall is heavily infiltrated by lymphocytes (tiny blue dots), and a multinucleated giant cell is present at the 10:00 position.

BOX 8–4   Vasculitis

Causes

Usually immunologically mediated

Lesions

Inflammatory cells in the walls
  of small and medium-sized vessels

Manifestations

Infarcts in the areas supplied by affected vessel,
  leading to, for example, renal failure, muscle
  weakness, and pain

Functional Vascular Disease

In various disease states, arterioles and venules constrict secondary to local influences such as precipitation of intraluminal proteins, chemicals applied to the adventitia, or disturbance of autonomic function. One of these states is **Raynaud's phenomenon**. In this condition, the small vessels of the hands and feet constrict excessively in an exaggerated response to cold, leaving the fingers or toes cold and blue. Psychological stress might also trigger this response. Raynaud's phenomenon also occurs with some collagen-vascular diseases, such as lupus erythematosus, but usually it is an isolated—and idiopathic—phenomenon.

Thrombophlebitis

Literally, **thrombophlebitis** means "thrombosis in an inflamed vein." The term *phlebothrombosis* may be more appropriate because the veins are not usually inflamed. Thrombophlebitis occurs most frequently in the deep veins of the legs or pelvis. It may also occur in arm veins as a complication of intravenous catheters that are left in place for several days. Sluggish and turbulent blood flow is probably more important in causing thrombosis than is inflammation. If the thrombi are dislodged from a vein wall, they can be carried to the lung (**Figures 8–15** and **8–16**), where they produce varying pulmonary symptoms and sometimes death.

Pulmonary emboli (PEs) from venous thromboses are common in hospitalized patients, particularly following surgical operations and childbirth, presumably because lack of exercise causes stasis of blood in leg veins and because blood platelet concentration is increased under these conditions. The prevention of thrombi in leg veins is the reason for insisting that patients ambulate early following an operation or childbirth. Most venous thrombi and even pulmonary emboli are undiagnosed. This is known because they are found frequently at autopsy when they were clinically unsuspected. Indeed, it is difficult to detect them clinically because they are often asymptomatic and no thoroughly sensitive test is available. To have a clinical suspicion (or think of the condition in patients at risk for the development of PEs) and act presumptively is often the most important thing a doctor can do. Local symptoms of thrombophlebitis may include leg pain and tenderness, but these symptoms are unreliable. Diagnosis depends on use of ultrasound to detect venous occlusions in the deep veins of the legs,

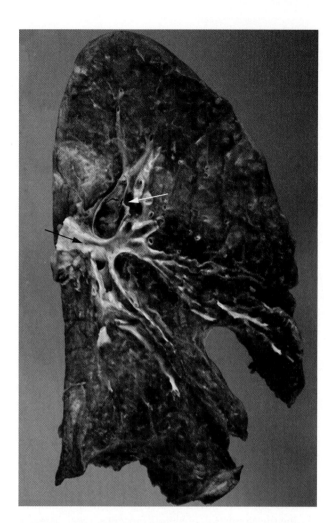

FIGURE 8–16 Pulmonary embolus. This is a cross section of the left lung of a patient who died of pulmonary emboli. The embolus plugs and distends a large-caliber artery (white arrow). The black arrow is pointing to the bronchus.

and sensitive computer tomography (CT) scans that can demonstrate clots in pulmonary vessels. Treatment consists of anticoagulant drugs and may involve surgical ligation of leg veins to prevent clots from moving to the lungs or placement of a filter in the inferior vena cava. With time, the thrombi are either dissolved or replaced by scar.

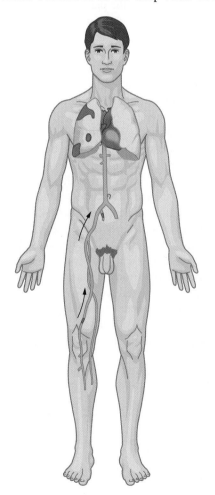

FIGURE 8–15 Thrombi in leg and pelvic veins leading to pulmonary embolism and infarcts. Arrows indicate direction of blood flow.

BOX 8–5   Thrombophlebitis

Causes

Stasis of venous blood

Increased platelet concentration

Venous injury

Lesions

Veins distended by blood clot

Manifestations

Possible pulmonary emboli

(rare) Swelling of affected area

(rare) Pain

Varicose Veins

Varicose veins are dilated, tortuous veins. Three important sites of development are the legs, anus, and lower esophagus. **Esophageal varices** are caused by increased pressure in the portal vein, usually resulting from cirrhosis of the liver, and may readily bleed, sometimes catastrophically, with a fatal outcome. Hemorrhoids are enlarged veins of the lower rectum and anus that are presumed to result from prolonged congestion of pelvic veins secondary to constipation or pregnancy.

Varicose veins of the lower extremities commonly involve the greater saphenous vein, a superficial vein just beneath the skin on the medial side of the leg. Normally, valves in the leg veins aid in the return of blood to the heart by preventing backflow once the blood has been forced upward by muscular activity. Varicose veins have incompetent valves, so hydrostatic pressure is transmitted through the entire course of the vein. The increased internal pressure leads to dilated, tortuous, and visible veins. Standing for long periods of time may further lead to edema and, eventually, ulceration of the skin from the pressure of the edema fluid. Venous valves often become incompetent with age. They are also more likely to become incompetent in overweight and inactive persons because the leg muscles that pump the blood upward also structurally support the veins, and the soft adipose tissue that replaces muscle does not offer sufficient support. Because there are many alternative venous routes for blood to return to the heart, these superficial varicosities can be removed by a surgeon without compromising the circulation of blood. Short of surgery, external compression by elastic stockings can help alleviate the symptoms.

BOX 8–6   Varicose Veins

Causes

Chronically increased venous pressure

Incompetent valves in legs

Lesions

Dilated tortuous veins including

    Esophageal varices

    Hemorrhoids

    Varicose leg veins

Manifestations

Edema

Visibility of veins

Hemorrhage

Hyperplastic/Neoplastic Diseases

Except for hemangiomas, discussed earlier, benign and malignant tumors of vessels are rare.

Organ Failure

Failure of the cardiovascular system to maintain adequate blood pressure is called **shock**, and it is clinically manifested by decreased blood pressure, increased heart rate, decreased urine output, and altered states of consciousness. Shock is a critical condition: patients who suffer it are usually very ill and require specialized care to bring their blood pressure to adequate perfusion pressures. **Table 8–4** lists the causes of the various types of shock. *Cardiogenic* shock results when the heart cannot pump enough blood under sufficient arterial pressure to maintain oxygenation of tissues. The best example of this is the cardiovascular collapse that occurs after a myocardial infarct, when the heart cannot effectively pump blood at adequate systolic pressures because some of the heart muscle is dead. *Hemorrhagic* shock results when massive bleeding leads to an insufficient amount of blood in the vascular system to maintain arterial pressure. In *septic* shock, overwhelming infections and toxins produced by Gram-negative bacteria cause vasodilation of peripheral vessels. Blood pools in the periphery, so an inadequate amount of blood returns to the heart to maintain adequate perfusion pressures. *Neurogenic* shock also results from dilation of small vessels, pooling of blood in the periphery, inadequate return of blood to the heart, and insufficient blood flow to the remainder of the vascular system. **Syncope** (fainting) is most often the result of neurogenic shock and may occur in response to emotional situations. Pooling of blood in the lower body results in brain ischemia. After approximately 10 seconds of ischemia, neurons cease to function properly and the person loses consciousness. Syncope is relieved by lowering the position of the head so that less pressure is needed to get blood to the brain.

Prolonged shock causes tissue injury secondary to prolonged ischemia: patients rapidly become obtunded or unconscious if their brain is not adequately supplied with oxygen, the liver can fail acutely, the gut may undergo ischemic necrosis with secondary leakage of gastrointestinal flora into the peritoneal cavity, and the epithelial cells of the tubules of the kidney undergo necrosis. In fact, any tissue of the body can undergo ischemic damage, but the ones listed here, particularly the brain and kidney, are the ones most likely to suffer damage. Very often, patients in shock develop more than one of these complications, a condition called **multiple organ**

TABLE 8–4   Types and Causes of Shock

Type	Cause
Cardiogenic	Inadequate pumping by the heart
Hemorrhagic	Loss of blood
Septic	Inappropriate dilation of small vessels, resulting in pooling of blood
Neurogenic	Inappropriate dilation of small vessels, resulting in pooling of blood

system failure. Prolonged and severe shock can lead to two rapidly progressive and fatal conditions. In **acute respiratory distress syndrome (ARDS)**, the epithelial cells lining pulmonary alveoli become damaged, and the lungs fill with edema fluid and blood, thereby severely hampering respiration. In **disseminated intravascular coagulation (DIC)**, damage to endothelial cells causes widespread activation of the clotting cascade with subsequent formation of microthrombi in small vessels and the subsequent paradoxical occurrence of microthrombi and hemorrhages through all tissues of the body.

As you can well imagine from this description, shock is an often fatal condition. It needs to be treated in intensive care units. The first goal of treatment is to remove the inciting agent, if possible. Antibiotics need to be administered in the case of septic shock, and blood loss from hemorrhage needs to be stopped with surgical repair of bleeding arteries. Supportive measures include increasing vascular volume by administering intravenous fluids, plasma, and/or blood products; improving myocardial contractility; increasing vascular tone in the periphery; providing supplemental oxygen if ARDS develops; and attempting to control coagulation if DIC develops.

Failure of the veins, capillaries, and the lymphatic system is usually not as precipitous as shock, though it may result in significant morbidity. When veins fail to return blood to the heart, they become engorged and dilated, or congested. If present close to visible surfaces, such as the skin or mucosal membranes that are amenable to endoscopic examination, they appear as blue, dilated, sometimes pulsating vessels. They may ulcerate or rupture, causing hemorrhage. This occurs, for example, when the portal venous system becomes obstructed. Obstruction of portal venous blood flow occurs in *cirrhosis* or fibrosis of the liver. Blood returning to the heart from the intestines bypasses the obstructed portal vein through systemic or anastomotic channels that occur at different sites in the abdomen. One of these sites is the distal portion of the esophagus. The veins here dilate to accommodate increased blood flow through them and are subsequently prone to rupture, causing massive and often fatal bleeding into the gastrointestinal tract.

When capillaries are not able to contain intravascular fluid, edema results. Edema can be a manifestation of any number of diseases. It can involve just the chest cavity (**hydrothorax**), just the abdominal cavity (**ascites**), or be generalized throughout the body (**anasarca**). Anasarca is particularly likely to occur when serum proteins are very low. The edema fluid produced by increased hydrostatic pressure or decreased osmotic pressure in the blood has a low protein content and is called a **transudate**.

Failure of the lymphatic system may result from permanent and extensive obstruction of the lymphatic channels. This is usually not a systemic disease but affects a particular region of the body. The result is chronic edema because excess fluid is not adequately drained from the tissue. This type of edema is called **lymphedema**.

It causes marked enlargement of the affected tissues, which acquire a firm, doughy consistency. It is on the basis of this characteristic appearance that it is also called **elephantiasis**. The most common cause of lymphedema is surgical removal of lymph nodes for cancer. Women who require radical mastectomy and removal of axillary lymph nodes for breast cancer are at risk for developing lymphedema of the arm on the side of the axillary lymph node dissection. In the tropics, chronic lymphedema is caused by a helminthic worm infection called **filariasis**. The worms cause fibrosis and blockage of lymphatic vessels.

Practice Questions

1. A 63-year-old woman has a myocardial infarct from which she recovers, followed eight months later by a stroke. Which of the following is the most likely underlying disease predisposing her to both of these conditions?
   A. Vasculitis
   B. Atherosclerosis
   C. Shock
   D. Thrombophlebitis

2. A 55-year-old man has had blood pressures in the range of 140–160/100–110 mm Hg for many years. After an episode of severe chest pain, he is hospitalized with a suspected myocardial infarct. An angiogram shows moderately severe atherosclerosis of the coronary arteries. His hypertension most likely contributed to the development of his atherosclerosis by which means?
   A. Damaging endothelium
   B. Elevating serum cholesterol
   C. Causing secretion of aldosterone
   D. Causing deposition of fibrous tissue
   E. Activating macrophages

3. Which of the following diseases or conditions occurring in veins is most serious in terms of potential mortality?
   A. Hemorrhoids
   B. Varicose veins
   C. Thrombophlebitis
   D. Vasculitis
   E. Congestion

4. Which of the following statements about essential hypertension is true?
   A. It is less serious than secondary hypertension.
   B. It has an unknown cause.
   C. It selectively affects the kidneys.
   D. It does not lead to malignant hypertension.

5. How are the effects of hypertension most easily observed?
   A. By taking a blood pressure reading
   B. By getting a kidney biopsy to demonstrate arteriolosclerosis
   C. By ophthalmoscopic examination
   D. By angiogram of cerebral vessels
   E. None of the above

Heart

OUTLINE

OBJECTIVES

1. Review the anatomy of the heart, the pathway of blood flow through the great vessels and cardiac chambers, and the origin of electrical impulses that coordinate myocardial contraction.

2. Define "cardiac death" and "sudden cardiac death," and name some of the major causes of each.

3. Describe common physical signs and symptoms that indicate heart disease, including angina pectoris, shortness of breath, pleural fluid, ascites, peripheral edema, neck vein distention, and murmurs.

4. Describe how each of the following tests or procedures is helpful in evaluation of a patient with heart disease: blood pressure, electrocardiogram, serum enzyme levels, echocardiogram, stress test, and cardiac catheterization.

5. Describe the most common congenital anomalies of the heart, what functional disturbance they cause, how they manifest, and how they lead to heart failure.

6. Describe the mechanisms by which coronary artery atherosclerosis can lead to myocardial infarction.

7. Describe the pathogenesis, complications, and manifestations of myocardial infarction.

8. Describe the pathogenesis of rheumatic heart disease and list its complications.

9. Discuss predisposing factors and consequences of infective endocarditis and myocarditis.

10. Compare and contrast the pathogenesis and effects of systemic and pulmonary hypertension on the heart.

11. Compare and contrast cardiogenic shock and congestive heart failure in terms of acuteness, severity, causes, and manifestations.

12. Be able to define and use in context all words and terms in bold print in this chapter.

KEY TERMS

angina pectoris
angiograms
angioplasty
aorta
aortic stenosis
arrhythmia
ascites
atherosclerosis
atrial and ventricular septal
   defects
atrial fibrillation
atrioventricular node
atrium
bicuspid aortic valve
brain natriuretic
   peptide (BNP)
cardiac catheterization
cardiac death
cardiogenic shock
cardiomyopathy
coarctation of aorta
congenital heart disease
congestive heart failure
cor pulmonale
coronary arteries
coronary artery bypass
   graft (CABG)
creatinine phosphokinase
   (CK)
cyanosis
diastole
dyspnea
echocardiography
electrocardiography
foramen ovale
heart transplantation
hepatosplenomegaly

hypertensive heart disease
hypertrophic
   cardiomyopathy
incompetent valve
infective endocarditis
interventricular septum
left heart failure
left ventricular assist
   device
mural thrombosis
murmurs
myocardial infarct
myocardial rupture
myocarditis
peripheral edema
pulmonary arteries
pulmonary edema
pulmonary veins
regurgitation
rheumatic heart disease
right heart failure
sinoatrial node
stent
stress test
sudden cardiac death
systole
tetralogy of Fallot
troponins
valves (tricuspid,
   pulmonary, bicuspid
   [mitral], aortic)
valvular stenosis
vegetation
venae cavae
ventricle
ventricular aneurysm
ventricular fibrillation

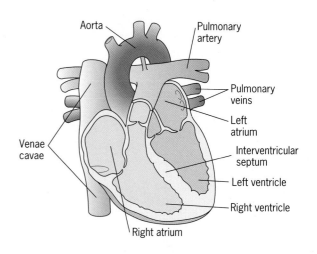

FIGURE 9–1 Great vessels and chambers of the heart.

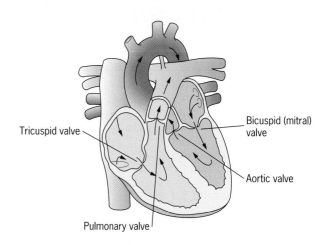

FIGURE 9–2 Blood flow and valves of the heart.

Review of Structure and Function

The heart functions as two pumps working synchronously to move blood throughout the body (**Figures 9–1** and **9–2**). The right side of the heart receives poorly oxygenated blood from the **venae cavae** and pumps it under relatively low pressure through the **pulmonary arteries** to the lungs, where it is oxygenated. The left side of the heart receives the oxygenated blood from the **pulmonary veins** and pumps it at high pressure into the **aorta**, from where it is delivered to all areas of the body. The right heart is less muscular than the left heart because the pulmonary vascular resistance against which it must pump is much less than the systemic vascular resistance. On each side of the heart, there is a receiving chamber (**atrium**) and a pumping chamber (**ventricle**). Delicate fibrous **valves** between the atria and ventricles and between the ventricles and large arteries open and close efficiently in response to pressure changes. These one-way valves control the inflow of blood into the ventricles and prevent backflow. If the valves fail to close completely, the ventricle pumps some blood back into the atrium during contraction (**systole**), or blood flows back into the ventricle from the major artery during relaxation (**diastole**). In either

case, the ventricle has to pump the blood more than once, with resultant loss of efficiency of the heart. If the valves fail to open completely, more pressure is needed to force the blood through the narrowed valve apertures. To some extent, the heart can gain this needed increased force by hypertrophy of its muscle fibers. Atrial muscle enlarges when the atrioventricular valves (**tricuspid** or **bicuspid** [**mitral**]) are narrowed and fail to open completely, and ventricular muscle enlarges when the **pulmonary** or **aortic** valves are narrowed and fail to open completely.

Cardiac muscle must have a generous supply of oxygenated blood to provide the fuel for its high energy needs. Blood is supplied to the muscle via two medium-sized arteries, the right and left **coronary arteries**, which originate from the aorta immediately above the aortic valve (**Figure 9–3**). In addition to the rich blood supply, an electrical pulse is needed to initiate each rhythmic contraction of the heart. This pulse is generated spontaneously within a pacemaker focus called the **sinoatrial node** and is conducted to the ventricles via the **atrioventricular**

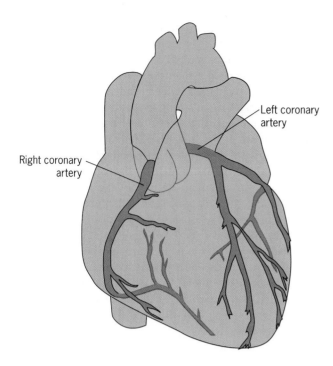

FIGURE 9–3 Coronary arteries.

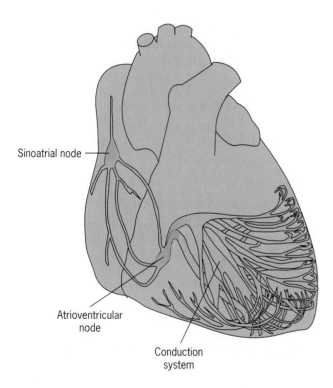

FIGURE 9–4 Conduction system.

node and by specialized bundles of muscle in the **interventricular septum** (the wall between the left and right ventricles) (**Figure 9–4**). The pulse may be disturbed by disease in the area of the nodes, by metabolic changes in the blood, such as changes in serum potassium level, and by a number of drugs.

Most Frequent and Serious Problems

Compromise of blood supply to the heart caused by obstruction of the coronary arteries from **atherosclerosis** is by far the most common cause of death in the United States and also the most common cause of death resulting from heart disease, or **cardiac death** (**Figure 9–5**). As you can see from Figure 9–5, of the top 10 causes of death in the United States, heart disease accounts for the largest fraction of mortality. For several decades, cardiac disease has been the number one cause of mortality in the United States. With advances in prevention, recognition, and treatment of heart disease, particularly atherosclerotic heart disease, the mortality figures have been slowly but steadily declining. It is projected that in the near future, neoplasia will become the leading cause of death in the United States.

Atherosclerosis leads to cardiac muscle dysfunction by interrupting the delivery of oxygen to myocardial tissue, which subsequently suffers ischemic injury. This can cause **myocardial infarct** and/or abnormal heart rhythms (**arrhythmias**). Coronary atherosclerosis not only is common as a cause of death, but is also common as a cause of disability, which may last for weeks to years prior to death. The major forms of disability are **angina pectoris** (cardiac chest pain) and **congestive heart failure**.

Atherosclerosis of the coronary arteries usually becomes manifest in adults. Until approximately the age of 65 years, men are more commonly affected than are women, but after this the incidence is about the same.

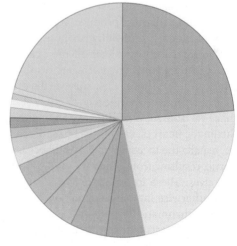

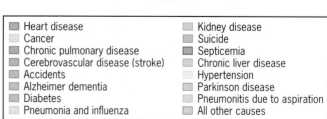

FIGURE 9–5 Top 10 leading causes of death. (Data from Hoyert DL, Xu J. Deaths: preliminary data for 2011. *National Vital Statistics Reports.* October 10, 2012;61(6). U.S. Department of Health and Human Services.)

Black people are more severely affected than are white people. The reason for these disparities is not entirely understood. About one-quarter to one-third of patients die suddenly (within 2 hours) of a myocardial infarct. Those who survive have an increased rate of death compared to the rest of the population because they are susceptible to the development of subsequent myocardial infarcts, and the permanent damage to the heart muscle incurred by an infarct may induce congestive heart failure.

Cardiac death also can be caused by damaged heart valves and by increased ventricular workload because of altered blood flow or high blood pressure in the pulmonary or systemic vascular circuits. **Hypertensive heart disease**, the second most common heart problem, is underestimated in the mortality figures because it often occurs in conjunction with coronary atherosclerotic heart disease. Hypertension is not a primary disease of the heart but is deleterious to the heart because high blood pressure in the systemic arteries increases the workload of the heart. The heart responds the same way as it does to **valvular stenosis**—namely, by undergoing hypertrophy. Over time, however, its ability to adapt to the increased pressure is overcome, and it fails to pump blood adequately. Patients then develop the signs and symptoms of heart failure. In addition, enlarged hearts are prone to spontaneously develop conduction disturbances, which can be lethal. Hypertensive heart disease is not rapidly fatal. Most deaths occur in older individuals who have had hypertension for several decades.

Congenital heart disease and rheumatic heart disease are less common causes of cardiac death but are particularly important causes of valve deformity. Many types of congenital heart disease produce abnormalities in the pathway of blood flow, leading to poor oxygenation of blood and increased workload on the heart. Most persons succumbing to congenital heart disease die in the first year of life. Those who survive have less severe anomalies or undergo surgical correction of their defect and have variable survival times extending to old age.

Rheumatic heart disease is the result of scarring of the valves, usually the bicuspid (mitral) and occasionally also the aortic, resulting from repeated bouts of inflammation of the valves. These inflammatory episodes are precipitated by otherwise innocuous infection by streptococcal organisms. Rheumatic heart disease is no longer as common a cause of heart failure as it has been even in recent history because eradication of the infection by early antibiotic administration has decreased its incidence, and the scarred valves can be surgically replaced when the damage is severe. Rheumatic heart disease also has a prolonged course, with most deaths occurring in older individuals.

Chronic lung disease can cause hypertension in the pulmonary arteries. Heart failure secondary to pulmonary hypertension is called **cor pulmonale**. The frequency of cor pulmonale as a cause of death is not known because lung disease is recorded as the cause of death, not right heart failure.

Sudden cardiac death, or cardiac death occurring within an hour of the onset of symptoms, is caused by dysfunction of the heart resulting in rapid cessation of circulation. It is most often associated with one of several complications of coronary atherosclerosis. Sudden death caused by a "heart attack" generally is the result of **ventricular fibrillation**, which is an uncoordinated, ineffective, weak contraction of ventricular muscle resulting from spontaneous generation of impulses within the muscle cells themselves rather than coordinated electrical stimulation through the conduction system. Overdosage with certain cardiac drugs may also produce ventricular fibrillation. Rupture of the heart is not common but does cause sudden death because the pericardial sac fills with blood and prevents adequate ventricular filling and pumping. Rupture may be the result of the softening of heart muscle in the region of a large myocardial infarct or to trauma (car accident, stabbing, gunshot wound). Marked narrowing of the aortic valve, or **aortic stenosis**, is also associated with sudden death.

Most cardiac deaths are preceded by an interval of congestive heart failure, or failure of the heart to pump blood effectively. Virtually all the diseases known to affect the heart can eventually lead to heart muscle insufficiency, including long-standing hypertensive heart disease, long-standing valvular dysfunction, and intrinsic disease of the heart muscle (**cardiomyopathy**). Heart failure presents certain signs and symptoms of strain on the circulatory system, discussed in the next section, and can be treated—but not reversed—with pharmaceutial agents that reduce the work of the heart or increase its contractility. Congestive heart failure is not a diagnosis in itself, however, but the manifestation of end-organ damage incurred by some other pathophysiologic process.

Symptoms, Signs, and Tests

Myocardial infarcts (MIs) typically cause severe, persistent chest pain that is often described as "squeezing" and that may radiate to the left shoulder, arm, neck, or jaw. Although these are the classic symptoms of MI, it often presents atypically, especially in women. Many people have no symptoms at all, may experience vague and nonspecific ones such as fatigue or shortness of breath, or may suffer sudden cardiac death or heart failure without any prior symptoms. The term *angina pectoris* refers to transient chest pain brought on by exercise or emotional stress and relieved by rest or vasodilator drugs. Angina pectoris is caused by transient hypoxia to the heart resulting from spasm of atherosclerotic coronary arteries.

Congestive heart failure manifests as fluid buildup in the lungs and other tissues. When fluid backs up in the venous system, it leaks across capillaries into pulmonary alveoli, pleural and peritoneal cavities, and soft tissues of the limbs. Patients therefore experience shortness of breath because of **pulmonary edema** causing poor oxygenation of blood in the lungs and restriction of lung movement by pleural fluid, swelling of the abdomen secondary to accumulation of fluid in the peritoneal cavity (**ascites**), and swelling of the legs (**peripheral edema**).

Physical examination can easily detect such fluid accumulation. The amount of fluid in the venous system can be assessed by examining the fullness of neck veins while the patient is seated or lying down. Pleural fluid can be detected by auscultation, or listening with the stethoscope over the thoracic cavity. Movement of air through the air spaces sounds muffled and far away if there is fluid in the pleural space, and there may be rales or crackles caused by fluid-filled alveoli opening during inhalation. Percussion of the chest yields a dull thump rather than a bright, hollow sound if the chest is filled with fluid. Ascites can be detected by noticing a wave of fluid roll over the belly of a reclining patient when the abdomen is gently tapped on one side. Edema in the soft tissues is assessed by firmly pressing the skin of the ankle or leg with a fingertip and noticing how long the dimple remains. Pressure forces fluid out of the soft tissue, and it takes a few minutes for it to fill in again. Nonedematous soft tissue springs back within a few seconds.

Other important aspects of the cardiac physical examination include listening for heart valve murmurs, estimating heart size, measuring blood pressure, and checking the pulse for the rate and regularity of its rhythm. Heart **murmurs** are abnormal sounds of the heart heard with the aid of a stethoscope. They are caused by abnormal flow of blood through the heart valves or major vessels. A heart murmur may be functionally unimportant or may indicate serious underlying disease. Heart size is assessed by feeling for the point of major impact of the heart against the chest wall during systole. This is normally close to the midaxillary line, between the fourth and sixth ribs, on the left side. If it is deviated to the left, the heart is likely enlarged. The pulse is most easily assessed by palpation of the radial artery in the wrist.

Arterial blood pressure is measured using a sphygmomanometer. This device is a cuff with an attached pressure gauge that can be applied to a limb and inflated above arterial pressure. By listening over an artery distal to the cuff, one can hear the pulse when the pressure drops below the systolic pressure, and the pulse sound disappears when the blood pressure drops below the diastolic pressure. The pressures at which the pulse begins and ceases to be heard are recorded as systolic and diastolic pressures, respectively.

Procedures and laboratory tests used in the evaluation of heart disease include chest x-ray, echocardiogram, electrocardiogram (ECG or EKG), serum enzyme levels, and cardiac catheterization. Chest x-ray may give an indication of the size and shape of the heart, but it is not a very sensitive test. **Echocardiography** is a noninvasive procedure that provides an image of the heart based on ultrasound waves that are reflected at tissue interphases. This very valuable tool allows for assessment of size and function of various aspects of the heart, including the heart walls and the cardiac valves, and also depicts abnormal structures, such as abnormal growths on heart valves or holes through the atrial or ventricular septum. When coupled with Doppler analysis, the path and velocity of blood flow through the heart can be charted.

Electrocardiography records electrical activity at electrodes placed at standard locations on the body surface. The electrical activity of the heart can be inferred from electrical activity recorded at these sites. Results usually require interpretation by an experienced physician. ECG is most often used in the diagnosis of myocardial infarcts, either recent or old. It is also used to define rhythm disturbances (arrhythmias) and to monitor the course of a disease or the effect of therapy.

The **stress test** determines the effectiveness of oxygen delivery to myocardial tissue. An ECG taken after a patient walks on a treadmill or is given a medication that mimics the effect of exercise on the heart can detect evidence of myocardial ischemia. The blood may also be injected with a radioactive substance during the stress test. Areas of the heart that are not receiving adequate blood supply do not take up the radioactive substance, so an x-ray of the heart can show a defect in the area of poor perfusion.

Specific enzymes released from dying muscle can be measured in the blood and are helpful in determining if and when an acute myocardial infarct has occurred (**Figure 9–6**). Cardiac **troponins** and **creatinine phosphokinase (CK)** have peak elevations at different times following onset of a myocardial infarct. Testing the blood

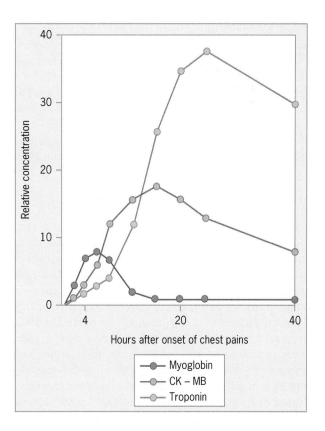

FIGURE 9–6 Temporal pattern of cardiac enzyme elevations after a myocardial infarction.

for these enzymes can give an indication of whether myocardial injury has occurred and how old, or established, the injury is. Myoglobin may also be a useful marker for early diagnosis of myocardial injury. **Brain natriuretic peptide (BNP)** is released from the heart when it is excessively stretched, as occurs in congestive heart failure. Its levels in the serum can help determine the presence of congestive heart failure and are often monitored to determine the effectiveness of medical therapy for congestive heart disease.

Cardiac catheterization is used for more extensive evaluation of serious cardiac problems. Catheters are flexible tubes that can be threaded through the vessels and into the heart to measure pressures in various chambers and to allow injection of radiopaque dyes. X-rays taken following injection of radiopaque dyes into the vascular system are called **angiograms**. Angiograms reveal the anatomy of the heart chambers and blood vessels, and thus can detect abnormalities in the route of blood flow. Radiopaque dyes can even be injected directly into the coronary arteries to outline atherosclerotic plaques.

Specific Diseases
Genetic/Developmental Diseases

Developmental abnormalities of the heart are almost all embryonic anomalies and collectively are called **congenital heart disease**. Of all the organs, the heart and great vessels are the most common sites of congenital defects, and the defects are likely to have serious consequences. Early diagnosis and surgical correction of a defect can dramatically alter life expectancy. Ventricular septal defects account for 30% of congenital heart diseases. The variety of other types each account for less than 10%. A few classic types are briefly presented in this section to illustrate the variety of blood flow disturbances that can occur with congenital disease of the heart and great vessels.

Bicupsid Aortic Valve

The most common congenital heart defect is a bicuspid aortic valve. The aortic valve usually has three cusps, but occasionally babies are born who have a two-cusped valve. This may present in infancy or childhood in the form of easy fatigability or chest pain but is often not detected until adulthood. Flow across the bicuspid valve is irregular, so the valve becomes deformed and scars. Extensive scarring of the valve leads to fusion of the valves along their edges and stenosis (**Figure 9–7**). The heart undergoes hypertrophy to generate the force necessary to open the valve during systole. Alternatively, the valve may become **incompetent**, allowing for the backflow of blood during diastole. This also eventually leads to left heart failure, because the heart has to pump an increased

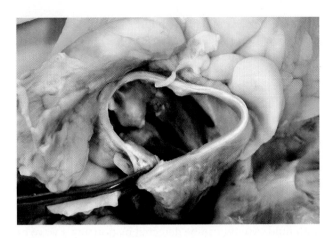

FIGURE 9–7 Stenosis of congenitally bicuspid valve. The aorta has been cut across and you are looking down the aorta on to the aortic valve. There are only two cusps, and these are thick and solid rather than thin and filmy. A large calcified vegetation bulges over the fixed, slitlike lumen.

volume of blood with each contraction. Most cases of aortic stenosis involve bicuspid valves.

BOX 9–1   Bicuspid Aortic Valve
Causes
Embryonic anomaly
Lesions
Aortic valve with two (rather than three) cusps
Manifestations
Often none until adulthood
Easy fatigability
Murmur of aortic stenosis
Heart failure

Atrial and Ventricular Septal Defects

During the fetal period, there is a hole, called the **foramen ovale**, in the septum between the right and left atria. The foramen ovale usually closes shortly after birth. If this septal defect remains open and is large (**Figure 9–8**), blood may flow from the left atrium to the right atrium, causing increased workload on the right side of the heart.

A hole in the interventricular septum (**Figure 9–9**) is more serious than an atrial septal defect because there is a greater pressure difference between the two ventricles than between the two atria. Blood is pushed from the left ventricle, in which the pressure is high, to the right ventricle, where the pressure is lower. Both ventricles therefore have to pump the same blood more than once. Over a number of years, the added workload leads to left and/or right heart failure.

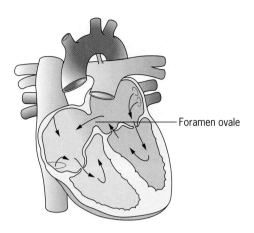

FIGURE 9–8 Atrial septal defect.

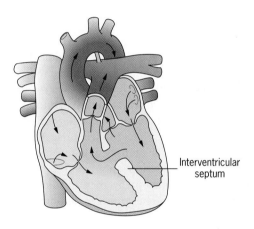

FIGURE 9–9 Ventricular septal defect.

Tetralogy of Fallot

The **tetralogy of Fallot** is the most common cause of cyanotic congenital heart disease. **Cyanosis** refers to the blue color of the skin imparted by poorly oxygenated blood. In cyanotic heart disease, blood is pumped from the right heart to the systemic circulation rather than to the lungs. Because it largely bypasses the lungs, blood is not adequately oxygenated. The four anatomic changes of the tetralogy (**Figure 9–10**) are (1) shift in position of the aorta so that both ventricles empty into it, (2) narrowing of the pulmonary outflow tract, (3) a ventricular septal defect shunting blood from the right ventricle into the left ventricle, and (4) right ventricular hypertrophy caused by the increased resistance to right ventricular emptying. Life expectancy is variable, depending on the severity of the defects and their amenability to surgery.

Coarctation of Aorta

Coarctation of aorta is a narrow fibrous constriction in the thoracic aorta (**Figure 9–11**). Proximal to the coarctation the blood pressure is usually elevated, and distal to the coarctation it is decreased. Decrease in the femoral artery pulse in a child may lead one to suspect the presence of this defect, and a marked difference in blood

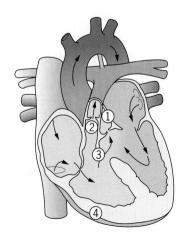

FIGURE 9–10 Tetralogy of Fallot. See text for explanation of numbers.

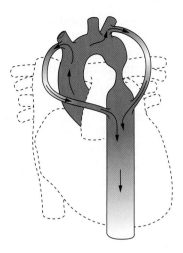

FIGURE 9–11 Coarctation of aorta.

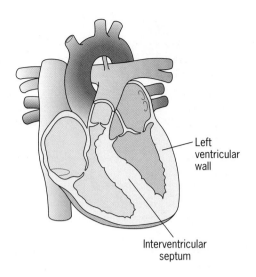

FIGURE 9–12 Hypertrophic cardiomyopathy

pressure in the arm versus the leg strengthens the suspicion. Surgical correction usually is curative if the disease is diagnosed early. The disease may easily go undetected, however, and, if so, the high blood pressure proximal to the coarctation eventually leads to left ventricular hypertrophy and heart failure.

BOX 9–4   Coarctation of Aorta
Causes
Embryonic anomaly
Lesions
Stenosis of descending aorta in thorax
Manifestations
Decreased femoral pulse
Hypertension in upper extremity
Murmur
Heart failure (late)

Hypertrophic Cardiomyopathy

Hypertrophic cardiomyopathy is one of three forms of cardiomyopathy, or diseases intrinsic to the heart muscle. The cardiomyopathies are discussed as a group later in this chapter. We single out hypertrophic cardiomyopathy for discussion here because it is a genetic disease. Numerous mutations can cause it. It is usually inherited in an autosomal dominant manner, but it can also occur sporadically. The mutation can affect any of the numerous proteins that make up the contractile apparatus of the heart muscle cells, such as myosin or troponin. How this leads to the manifestation of hypertrophy is not known, but with this mutation, the heart muscle, particularly the interventricular septum, becomes so thick that it encroaches on the lumen of the left ventricle and obstructs its outflow (**Figure 9–12**). Diastolic

filling is impaired because the volume of blood the left ventricle can accommodate is severely reduced, and consequently the stroke volume is reduced as well. In addition, the increased bulk of the heart requires increased oxygen, which the coronary arteries cannot necessarily supply even in the absence of atherosclerosis. The muscle may therefore undergo ischemia. Also because of the increased bulk, the muscle is electrically unstable, and patients may develop spontaneous arrhythmias. Hypertrophic cardiomyopathy may insidiously lead to heart failure, but it often comes to dramatic attention by causing sudden death in patients who were not aware that they had a cardiac condition. In fact, hypertrophic cardiomyopathy is one of the most common causes of death in young athletes.

BOX 9–5   Hypertrophic Cardiomyopathy
Causes
Genetic mutation (autosomal dominant)
Lesions
Severely thickened interventricular septum
Manifestations
Sudden death
Arrhythmia or infarction in septum

Inflammatory/Degenerative Diseases

Degenerative and inflammatory diseases of the heart cause more morbidity and mortality than any other disease in the United States. They are of diverse causes, but the outcome is similar in that they cripple this vital organ. Hypertensive heart disease is not really a primary heart disease but is discussed here because of its deleterious effect on the heart.

Coronary Artery Atherosclerosis

Atherosclerotic plaques are three-dimensional patches of lipid, fibrous tissue, and inflammatory cells that form on the inside of blood vessels. Here, we are concerned with how these small plaques may kill or severely disable an individual. Atherosclerosis of the coronary arteries is currently the major cause of morbidity and mortality in the United States.

Simplistically, you can imagine that atherosclerotic plaques narrow the lumens of the coronary arteries, thus reducing blood flow to heart muscle and to the conduction system of the heart (**Figure 9–13**). In practice, the correlation between the number and size of plaques and significant damage to the heart is not so simple, because the patterns of circulation vary considerably depending on *anastamoses*, or connections, between the right and left coronary arteries. Collateral blood vessel formation, or the development of a vascular network that bypasses the original coronary arteries and their main branches, occurs with recovery from a myocardial infarct and with aging, thus offering greater protection from subsequent myocardial infarcts. For these reasons, a single strategically placed plaque may kill one person at a young age, whereas another person may gradually develop complete occlusion of both coronary arteries and survive to old age.

In fact, it appears that gradual occlusion of an artery by atherosclerotic plaque induces the growth of protective collaterals and anastamoses, so this kind of atherosclerotic disease is not as fatal as you would think. Most myocardial infarcts resulting in sudden death are actually caused by *sudden disruption* of an atherosclerotic plaque. Exposure of collagen in the plaque induces formation of a thrombus, which can rapidly and suddenly occlude the vessel (**Figure 9–14**). Also, the contents of the ruptured plaque can flow downstream and occlude the coronary artery lumen distal to the site of the plaque. Alternatively, there can be spontaneous bleeding into the plaque such that the plaque is forced to bulge into the lumen, or the plaque may induce critical narrowing of the vessel as a result of vasospasm. Finally, marginally adequate blood flow may suddenly become inadequate when there is an increased need for oxygen by the myocardium because of exercise or emotional stress.

Chronic insufficiency of coronary artery blood flow causes pain accentuated by exertion (angina pectoris) because of the increased need of the myocardium for oxygen. Vasodilator drugs such as nitroglycerin (taken sublingually for quick action), or drugs used to treat high blood pressure, usually relieve the pain. Definitive interventions are usually not undertaken unless the patient is severely disabled by the pain or the pain begins to occur even when the patient is resting. The latter is called *unstable angina* and is a sign that an atherosclerotic plaque may be deteriorating.

The results of sudden insufficiency of coronary artery blood flow are arrhythmia, infarct, or both. Persons who

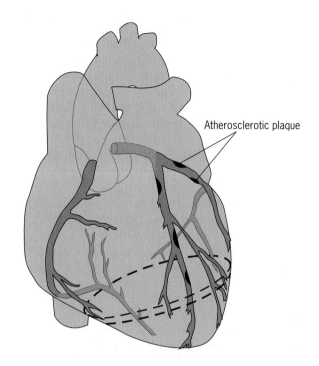

FIGURE 9–13 Coronary artery atherosclerosis.

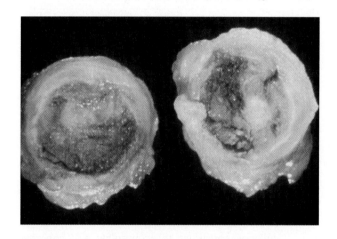

FIGURE 9–14 Thrombus in coronary artery. The artery is cut in cross section. The yellow material in the lumen of this artery is atherosclerotic plaque. The red, granular material is thrombus that has formed over the plaque and is occluding the lumen.

die suddenly of "heart attacks" actually die of an arrhythmia resulting from failure of propagation of the electrical impulse that times the pump. If a lethal arrhythmia does not occur, the person develops a myocardial infarct. Arrhythmias are potentially reversible and infarcts can heal, so emergency resuscitation can be effective if provided in time. The goal of therapy is to restore blood flow to the underperfused area. This is done by administration of drugs that lyse or destroy clots, such as tissue plasminogen activator, or by surgical interventions such as angioplasty, stenting, or cardiac bypass surgery. Any attempt to rescue the myocardial cells must be undertaken within hours of the onset of ischemia to be effective.

The most commonly used procedures to accomplish patency of coronary arteries are balloon angioplasty, stenting, and bypass grafting. In **angioplasty**, a catheter with a small, inflatable balloon on its tip is inserted into the coronary artery. The balloon is inflated when the catheter tip is at the area of atherosclerotic narrowing. Inflation of the balloon compresses the plaque, thereby rendering the vessel lumen patent. A **stent** is a wire cast that is placed inside the artery to brace the lumen open. Placement of a stent is usually preceded by angioplasty. **Coronary artery bypass graft (CABG)** uses a segment of either an artery (usually the internal thoracic artery) or vein (usually the saphenous vein) to divert blood flow around the diseased portion of the coronary artery. Which method is used to reestablish blood flow depends on the number of vessels that are diseased, the size of the plaque and degree of encroachment of the lumen, whether the occlusion is acute or chronic, and various functional characteristics of the patient him/herself, such as the individual's ability to withstand the stress of open heart surgery.

When an area of myocardium dies, the lesion is called a *myocardial infarct* and the process is called *myocardial infarction*. Once an area of muscle is killed by lack of oxygen, the following sequence of changes occurs:

1. For 12 to 18 hours, the heart appears normal both grossly and microscopically.
2. During days 1 to 5, there is progressive softening and disintegration of the dead muscle fibers (**Figure 9–15**). Microscopically, an inflammatory reaction sets in at the edge of the necrotic area (**Figure 9–16**).
3. Healing begins around day 5 with the ingrowth of granulation tissue (fibroblasts and capillaries), which replaces the dead muscle and begins to elaborate collagen.
4. By 2 weeks, sufficient collagen has been laid down to give new strength to the injured area, and the collagen continues to accumulate and contract for weeks to months. The end result is a dense, tough scar not unlike that which grows in the skin to heal a cut.

Complications can develop at any stage of the process of myocardial infarction and repair. Arrhythmias, such as ventricular fibrillation, may occur. Ventricular fibrillation causes sudden death unless medical care is immediately available. Sudden death occurs in up to one-third of individuals having acute myocardial infarcts. Artificial maintenance of heart contraction and breathing by cardiopulmonary resuscitation may be successful in keeping the patient alive until normal electrical activity can be reestablished. Another possible immediate complication is heart failure resulting from loss of function of a large area of myocardium. Heart failure causes venous congestion in the lungs with subsequent seepage of fluid into the pulmonary

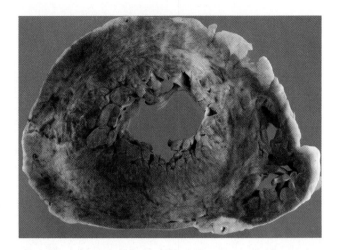

FIGURE 9–15 Myocardial infarct. The heart has been cut in the transverse plane. The right ventricle is seen in cross section on the right side of the image and the left ventricle on the left side. Notice that the muscle of the left ventricle is more than three times as thick as that on the right: the left ventricular wall is hypertrophic. This is a reflection of underlying heart disease and not caused by the infarct itself. The pale areas in the lateral wall of the left ventricle (far left) and the anterior (top) portion of the muscle represent recently infarcted tissue.

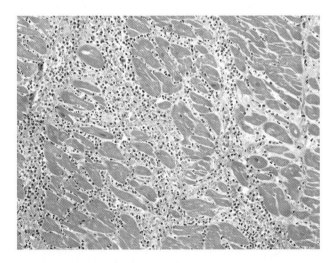

FIGURE 9–16 Myocardial infarct, microscopic image. Neutrophils are diffusely infiltrating necrotic myocytes.

air spaces (pulmonary edema). When more severe, there may be an inability to maintain the arterial blood pressure. Heart failure in the first few days after a myocardial infarct is more common in persons whose heart has already been weakened by previous myocardial infarcts.

Several other complications can occur after an infarct. The area of damage may extend further due to continuing inadequacy of the blood supply. A major reason for insisting on bed rest for patients undergoing a myocardial infarction is to prevent additional demand on the heart through physical exertion. Extension of the infarct may tip the patient into heart failure or cause a fatal arrhythmia. If the patient survives the myocardial infarction, s/he may still develop heart failure in the long run. This is because the viable muscle cells must undergo hypertrophy to take over the function of the muscle cells that were lost. Eventually, the hypertrophied cells no longer can respond to increased demand, and this leads to heart failure. Hypertrophy is a late complication of myocardial infarction because it requires time to develop.

Three less common complications of large infarcts are rupture, ventricular aneurysm, and endocardial thrombus formation. **Myocardial rupture** occurs when blood tears across an area of myocardial necrosis. If the rupture occurs across the lateral wall, blood floods the pericardial space, with resultant compression of the heart and sudden death. If the rupture involves a necrotic papillary muscle, the bicuspid (mitral) valve, which is tethered to the muscle, suddenly becomes incompetent, resulting in backflow of blood into the left atrium and pulmonary edema. Rupture occurs at the time of maximum softening of necrotic tissue, about four to seven days after the infarction occurred.

Aneurysms are saclike outpouchings of the heart or vessels. A **ventricular aneurysm** is an outward bulging of the scar of a large, healed left ventricular infarct. Scar tissue is not as strong as the original myocardial tissue, so the high pressure in the left ventricle can cause the scar to balloon outward. The aneurysm tends to impair the pumping activity of the left ventricle because the blood is not effectively moved out of it. **Mural** (wall) **thrombosis** is the formation of a blood clot on the endocardium overlying an infarct. Sometimes material breaks loose from a mural thrombus, resulting in a free-floating embolus that is carried through the arterial circulation and lodges at distant sites, producing infarcts in those tissues. The brain, intestines, and limbs are most commonly affected. Thus, it can happen that a patient recovering from a myocardial infarct suddenly develops a stroke because thrombotic material has embolized from the heart to cerebral vessels, causing an infarct in the brain.

Symptoms and signs of myocardial infarction are quite variable. Most patients have no symptoms prior to their first myocardial infarct, although a few may experience angina pectoris. Angina pectoris is more frequent in persons who have had one or more previous myocardial infarctions and have a marginally adequate blood supply to the heart. Although pain, particularly severe, "crushing" pain experienced just underneath the sternum and radiating down the left arm, is the classically described symptom of myocardial infarction, infarcts may be asymptomatic and heal without the patient being aware of them. Some patients may even present with heart failure resulting from advanced ischemia-induced loss of myocardial tissue without suspecting that they ever had a myocardial infarction in the past.

The diagnosis of myocardial infarction is made on the basis of elevated serum enzymes and an abnormal ECG. Treatment consists of giving thrombolytic agents to digest any blood clots that might be plugging coronary vessels and vasodilators, such as nitroglycerin, to reduce the amount of blood returning to the heart and increase the amount of blood that can get through stenotic coronary vessels. In addition, oxygen is given to maximize the oxygen carried by the blood, and morphine is given for pain control, which additionally reduces anxiety and therefore oxygen consumption elsewhere in the body. Aspirin and/or warfarin are given to prevent further development of thromboses. Other treatments address the possible complications.

BOX 9–6   Coronary Artery Atherosclerosis

Causes

Atherosclerosis

Hypertension

Lesions

Narrowing of coronary arteries

Myocardial infarct

Manifestations

Angina pectoris

Abnormal electrocardiogram

Myocardial infarct:

    Pain

    Elevated enzymes

    Abnormal ECG

    Shock or heart failure

Long-term complications

Rheumatic Heart Disease

Rheumatic fever is an uncommon hypersensitivity disorder that occurs in a small percentage of persons following a streptococcal infection, usually pharyngitis (strep throat). The protein of group A hemolytic streptococci is similar to the proteins in the heart and other connective tissues of susceptible individuals so that the antibodies that develop against the streptococci attack not only the bacteria but also the host tissue, especially the heart and joints. The inflammatory reaction is usually mild or asymptomatic but may produce a full-blown illness called *rheumatic fever*, characterized by myocarditis and arthritis. The illness is not usually serious in the acute stages and may gradually resolve without apparent residual effects. One or more episodes of rheumatic fever, however, can result in inflammation of the heart valves, which leads to scarring and deformity of the valves. **Figure 9–17** diagrams the changes that occur in the heart with scarring and dysfunction of the valves. The bicuspid (mitral) valve is usually more affected than is the aortic in rheumatic heart disease.

Valve dysfunction can manifest at any time after a known or presumed acute illness. The valve opening

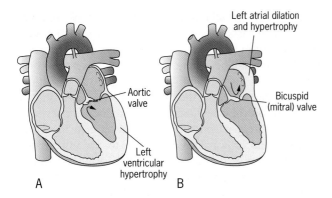

FIGURE 9–17 A. Aortic stenosis. **B.** Mitral stenosis.

BOX 9–7 Rheumatic Heart Disease

Causes

Hypersensitivity disorder

Cross-reaction of antibodies to group A streptococcus with antigens on heart valves

Repeated infection with group A streptococcus (strep throat)

Lesions

Scarring of heart valves (primarily bicuspid/mitral)

Bicuspid (mitral) valve regurgitation

Aortic valve stenosis

Manifestations

Murmurs

Left atrial dilation and hypertrophy

Pulmonary edema

Heart failure

Infective endocarditis (complication)

---

may be narrowed, or stenotic, and/or the valve may not be able to close completely, or be incompetent. Valvular stenosis and insufficiency result in distinctive murmurs. Fibrosis of the bicuspid (mitral) valve causes left atrial dilation and backup of blood into the lungs because of either obstruction of blood flow through the stenotic valve or **regurgitation** or backflow from the left ventricle if the valve is rendered incompetent. Patients may therefore present with symptoms of pulmonary edema. Stenosis of the aortic valve also causes left heart failure. In this case, the pump failure is caused by increased workload on the left ventricular myocardium because it has to generate more force to get the blood through the stenotic valve. Surgical replacement of damaged valves is often indicated.

In addition to inducing heart failure, valves damaged by rheumatic disease may become secondarily infected, causing *infective endocarditis* (discussion follows). Thus, rheumatic fever itself is less serious than its potential sequelae, heart failure and infective endocarditis.

To prevent the long chain of events of rheumatic heart disease, pharyngitis caused by group A hemolytic streptococci should be treated with antibiotics. Rapid and accurate diagnosis of group A hemolytic streptococci and treatment with antibiotics are effective in preventing rheumatic fever and its sequelae.

Infective Endocarditis

Endocarditis means inflammation of the inner lining of the heart, the endocardium, which also covers the heart valves. In fact, endocarditis preferentially involves the heart valves. In contrast to rheumatic valvulitis, **infective endocarditis** is caused by organisms living on the heart valves and producing an inflammatory reaction. The inflammatory reaction results in the buildup of a mound of fibrin, inflammatory cells, and infectious organisms on the heart valve, called a **vegetation**, and destruction of the delicate valvular architecture (**Figure 9–18**).

Bacteria are the most common cause of infective endocarditis. Most cases occur on previously damaged

valves—for example, those scarred by rheumatic heart disease or with congenital deformities, such as tricuspid aortic valves. The causative bacteria are usually normal residents of the mouth and throat. If they gain access to the bloodstream, they can adhere to the damaged valve and initiate infection. Alpha hemolytic streptococcus (*Streptococcus viridans*), a normal resident of the throat, is the most common offending organism. Because alpha hemolytic streptococci are very weak pathogens, they produce a smoldering infection on the heart valve, which gradually destroys the valve. In contrast, when a more virulent organism such as *Staphylococcus aureus* lodges on a heart valve, an acute infection ensues, which can rapidly destroy the valve. In either case, pumping of the

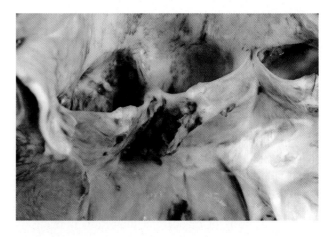

FIGURE 9–18 Destruction of cusps of the aortic valve by infective endocarditis.

blood is compromised by abnormal blood flow across the damaged valve, and the heart will rapidly fail. Also, organisms can be dislodged from the vegetations and carried in the bloodstream to other organs, such as kidneys or brain, resulting in multiple abscesses and rapid death.

Many cases of infective endocarditis could be prevented by preventing rheumatic fever because rheumatic valvulitis is the most common predisposing factor to the development of infective endocarditis. Those persons who already have damaged or congenitally abnormal heart valves can be protected with antibiotics from the bacteremia resulting from manipulative procedures such as dental extractions. The people most at risk for developing infective endocarditis, however, are intravenous drug users because the use of contaminated needles introduces bacteria directly into a vein, through which the offending organisms are carried directly to the heart. In these cases, right-sided valves are infected, whereas the bicuspid (mitral) valve is most commonly infected in infective endocarditis resulting from other causes.

Early diagnosis of infective endocarditis is essential to prevent its complications. Antibiotics must immediately be administered to prevent further damage to the valve, and in severe cases, surgical correction of valvular deficiency is required to prevent deterioration to heart failure.

BOX 9–8   Infective Endocarditis

Causes

Damaged valve from rheumatic or congenital heart disease

Bacteremia

IV drug use

Lesions

Inflammatory exudate containing causative organism on previously damaged heart valve

Manifestations

Fever

Leukocytosis

Murmur

Positive blood culture

Emboli to other organs

Heart failure

Myocarditis

Inflammation of the myocardium can be caused by viruses, bacteria, fungi, parasites, drugs, and immunologic disorders. Most cases are caused by viruses, with coxsackievirus being the most important. The onset of **myocarditis** may be abrupt or insidious. Chest pain similar to that caused by a myocardial infarct is a common symptom. Inflammation impairs the ability of the myocardium to contract, so heart failure and arrhythmias ensue. If the cause is viral, there is usually no specific treatment. Antiviral medications may be effective if it is known what type of virus is causing the inflammation. Supportive therapy, or decreasing the strain on the heart so that it can better heal itself, is the mainstay of treatment. In addition, medications that stabilize myocardial function are administered. These include drugs that enhance myocardial contractility, such as digitalis; drugs that decrease the workload of the heart by diminishing the volume of blood that it has to pump (vasodilators allow blood to pool in the venous system, and diuretics promote excess fluid excretion through the kidneys); and drugs that inhibit arrhythmias from developing. Steroids may also be given to decrease the inflammation in the heart muscle.

Hypertensive Heart Disease

Systemic blood pressure varies with the individual; however, generally, a systolic pressure of greater than 120 mm Hg and a diastolic pressure greater than 80 mm Hg are considered abnormal. High blood pressure (hypertension) leads to an increased workload on the heart, which leads to cardiac hypertrophy and eventually heart failure (**Figure 9–19**).

BOX 9–9   Hypertensive Heart Disease

Causes

Systemic hypertension

Lesions

Left ventricular hypertrophy

Manifestations

High blood pressure

Enlarged heart

Left heart failure

Pulmonary edema

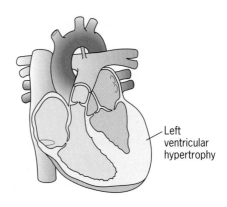

Left ventricular hypertrophy

FIGURE 9–19 Effect of systemic hypertension: left ventricular hypertrophy.

Hypertension can also occur in the pulmonary arterial system as a result of diffuse pulmonary disease or long-standing failure of the left heart. Pulmonary hypertension leads to right ventricular hypertrophy and eventually to right heart failure (**Figure 9–20**). Right heart failure caused by chronic lung disease is called *cor pulmonale*.

Cardiomyopathy

Cardiomyopathy refers to disease intrinsic to the heart muscle. There are three classes of cardiomyopathy: dilated, hypertrophic, and restrictive. These terms refer to an anatomic or functional derangement of the heart. The causes of these derangements are myriad and range from genetic diseases (hypertrophic cardiomyopathy, discussed in the section titled "Genetic/Developmental Diseases" earlier in this chapter) to toxins to aging processes. **Table 9–1** lists common causes of cardiomyopathies. In dilated cardiomyopathy, the heart muscle becomes so thinned out that the contractile filaments within cells no longer align properly and therefore cannot contract effectively. In restrictive cardiomyopathy, the heart muscle becomes stiff and cannot accommodate the usual volume of blood during diastole.

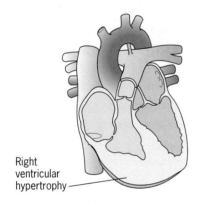

Right ventricular hypertrophy

FIGURE 9–20 Effect of pulmonary hypertension: right ventricular hypertrophy.

TABLE 9–1	Common Causes of Cardiomyopathy

Hypertensive
- Genetic defect of proteins of contractile apparatus

Restrictive
- Radiation fibrosis
- Amyloidosis
- Deposition of metabolic by-products of inborn errors of metabolism
- Deposition of iron in hemosiderosis

Dilated
- Alcohol toxicity
- Pregnancy-associated
- Genetic
- Diffuse ischemic injury

Cardiomyopathies often come to medical attention when the patient has already developed signs and symptoms of heart failure. The most dramatic presentation, however, is sudden death in high school and college athletes with undiagnosed hypertrophic cardiomyopathy. The other two forms of cardiomyopathy come to attention mainly in older adults.

Atrial Fibrillation

Fibrillation refers to uncoordinated contraction of the heart muscle, so the heart quivers rather than beats. Fibrillation of the atrial myocardium can lead to two harmful effects: (1) irregular transmission of the electrical impulse generated in the right atrium to the ventricles, so the pulse becomes irregular and the patient experieces faintness, dizziness, weakness, palpitations, and/or chest pain, and (2) incomplete emptying of the chamber so that the blood stagnates, clots, and then sheds bits of the clot into the vascular system, where it can travel to the brain and cause a cerebrovascular accident (stroke). **Atrial fibrillation** can also cause congestive heart failure if not treated and left to persist.

Atrial fibrillation increases in frequency with age and is more common in men. It is estimated that about 2% of men will have this condition by the age of 65 years, and 8% by the age of 80 years. Not all patients are symptomatic: the condition is often discovered when an ECG is performed for some other reason. Treatment is aimed at controlling the rate at which the ventricles respond to the uncoordinated stimuli generated in the right atrium, eradicating the source(s) of the aberrant rhythms, and anticoagulation to prevent the formation of thrombi.

Hyperplastic/Neoplastic Diseases

Neoplasms of the heart, whether benign, malignant, or metastatic, are rare. Metastatic lesions are more common than are primary ones, but the heart is usually a late receptacle for metastatic emboli. The cancer is often widespread in the body before it begins to grow in the heart. Even more rarely, metastases may interfere with the electrical conduction system and lead to arrhythmias or even death.

Organ Failure

Inadequacy of the cardiac pump may take two forms: cardiogenic shock or congestive heart failure. Shock is inadequate perfusion of tissues so that the metabolic demands of the cell—for delivery of oxygen and removal of waste products—are not met. Congestion is distention of veins caused by increased pressure within them. Shock, whether the result of heart damage or other conditions such as blood loss, is a serious acute condition. If blood pressure is not quickly restored, the patient will die. Congestion, in contrast, usually develops gradually and is less life threatening.

Cardiogenic shock refers to shock that is caused by failure of the heart. Essentially, the heart cannot maintain cardiac output adequate for perfusion. This condition is often the result of extensive myocardial infarction and rapidly leads to death in the majority of patients. Drugs given to constrict the vascular bed, which results in more blood returning to the heart, and others that improve the force of contraction of the heart are sometimes effective in controlling cardiogenic shock.

Congestive heart failure means the heart is unable to pump the blood that is returned to it. As a result, blood "backs up" into the pulmonary and/or systemic veins, with consequent leakage of fluid into the pulmonary alveoli and other tissues. Congestive heart failure, like cardiogenic shock, is most commonly the result of myocardial infarction but also occurs in the later stages of other forms of heart disease discussed in this chapter, including hypertensive heart disease, rheumatic valvular disease, severe myocarditis, or cardiomyopathies. It is important to recognize that congestive heart failure is not a diagnosis but a manifestation of some other underlying disease. When a patient presents in congestive heart failure, it is important to determine what is causing it because the cause may be treatable or even curable. Treating heart failure with diuretics and digoxin alleviates symptoms and improves heart function, but does not address the underlying condition.

Congestive heart failure is characterized as "left" or "right" sided depending on which ventricle is compromised in its function. Commonly, left- and right-sided failure occur together. The most common cause of right heart failure is left heart failure. This is because increased blood pressure transmitted into the lungs from left heart failure eventually has an adverse effect on the ability of the right side of the heart to pump blood into the lungs. **Left heart failure** causes increased venous pressure in the lungs as result of backup of blood because the left ventricle is no longer capable of pushing all the blood it receives into the systemic circulation. It usually manifests as shortness of breath (**dyspnea**) resulting from transudation of fluid into pulmonary alveoli (**Figure 9–21A**). Physical examination detects changes in the resonance of the thorax during auscultation, as well as the presence of rales during inspiration. **Right heart failure** causes enlargement of the liver and spleen (**hepatosplenomegaly**) as a result of congestion; edema, particularly noticeable in the ankles because of their dependent position; and distention of neck veins caused by increased venous pressure (**Figure 9–21B**).

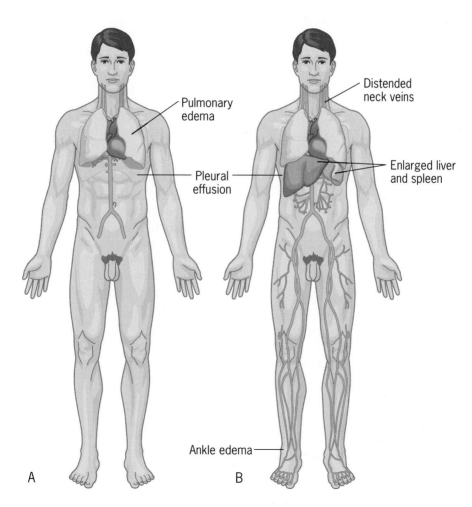

FIGURE 9–21 A. Left-sided congestive heart failure. **B.** Right-sided congestive heart failure.

The severity and duration of congestive heart failure vary. At its worst, it rapidly leads to death. In its mild forms, it may be controllable for many years with drugs, such as digitalis (digoxin), which improves myocardial contractile force; diuretics, which promote renal excretion of excess fluid; angiotensin-converting enzyme (ACE) inhibitors; and beta blockers. Various grading systems have been proposed that classify the degree of functional impairment, ranging from no symptoms (but laboratory or clinical evidence of heart muscle impairment) to severe heart disease requiring maintenance by mechanical pumps or heart transplantation.

Damage to the heart muscle, no matter what its cause, is not reversible. There is increasing research evidence that by "patching" the damaged heart with a plug of viable myocardial cells or by providing it with new stem cells, functional tissue could be restored. At this time, however, it is not clinically possible to restore damaged myocardium, and when the organ fails, the only option is to replace it. Mechanical pumps, called **left ventricular assist devices**, siphon blood from the left ventricle and pump it into the aorta through a tube. Although they are capable of sustaining blood flow for several months, they are used as temporizing measures—buying time, so to speak, until a donor heart becomes available. Mechanical hearts are becoming increasingly sophisticated but are still used experimentally. Definitive treatment is **heart transplantation**, which is limited by availability of donors and complicated by the side effects of lifelong immunosuppressant therapy.

Practice Questions

1. The most common injury to heart muscle is
   A. metastatic disease.
   B. hypertrophic cardiomyopathy.
   C. related to atherosclerosis.
   D. genetic or developmental defects.
   E. immunologic.
2. *Congestive heart failure* refers to which of the following?
   A. Sudden cardiac death
   B. Failure of the heart to pump effectively
   C. Peripheral edema and dilated neck veins
   D. Cardiac injury resulting from repeated myocardial infarctions
   E. Right heart failure resulting from lung disease

3. A 68-year-old competitive bicyclist has an abnormal stress test, though he denies ever having had anginal symptoms. Subsequent cardiac catheterization and angiogram reveal severe occlusion of one of his coronary arteries. Which of the following statements is most likely correct?
   A. He has had prior episodes of myocardial infarction.
   B. His heart is protected by numerous collaterals.
   C. He is at very high risk for sudden cardiac death.
   D. He will show ascites and peripheral edema on physical exam.
   E. He has unstable angina.
4. Which of the following statements comparing rheumatic heart disease and infective endocarditis is correct?
   A. Rheumatic heart disease affects myocardium, whereas infective endocarditis affects the endocardium.
   B. Rheumatic heart disease more commonly affects left-sided valves, whereas infective endocarditis more commonly affects right-sided ones.
   C. Rheumatic heart disease is caused by infection of valves by streptococci, and infective endocarditis is caused by infection of the valves by staphylococci.
   D. Both can result in embolization of bacteria from vegetations.
   E. Rheumatic heart disease is immunologically mediated, whereas infective endocarditis is infectious.
5. A 62-year-old man with signs and symptoms of endocarditis has an echocardiogram that reveals normal chamber sizes and function and a vegetation on the aortic valve. Which of the following complications is the patient not at risk for?
   A. Stroke
   B. Mesenteric ischemia
   C. Pulmonary embolism
   D. Splenic infarction
   E. Myocardial infarction

Hematopoietic System

OUTLINE

OBJECTIVES

1. Name and describe the origin and function of the major cellular components of the hematopoietic system.
2. Name and describe the most common types of diseases of the hematopoietic system.
3. Describe the clinical manifestations of anemia, polycythemia, thrombocytopenia, and leukopenia.
4. Define hematocrit, hemoglobin, red blood cell count, MCV, MCHC, and reticulocyte count, and describe how these laboratory parameters and the morphology of red blood cells on blood smears reflect the cause of anemia.
5. Describe the laboratory parameters by which white blood cells and platelets are assessed (white blood cell count, differential white blood cell count, and platelet count), and give normal ranges for these parameters.
6. Know the purpose of a bone marrow or lymph node biopsy.
7. Become familiar with other tests that are used to detect abnormalities of red and white blood cell structure and function (e.g., hemoglobin electrophoresis, sickle cell preparation, red cell fragility test, serum iron, serum ferritin and serum iron binding capacity, Coombs test, flow cytometry).
8. Define anemia and list the major categories of anemia according to (1) laboratory findings and (2) pathogenesis.
9. Define and list the major causes of leukocytosis, leukopenia, and thrombocytopenia.
10. Describe some of the major infections affecting blood cells.
11. Define polycythemia, and differentiate between primary and secondary polycythemia.
12. Describe the broad general classifications of leukemias (acute versus chronic, cell lineage) and lymphomas (Hodgkin versus non-Hodgkin).
13. Compare and contrast the etiology, lesions, and manifestations of leukemias, lymphomas, and multiple myeloma.
14. Describe the causes and effects of bone marrow failure.
15. Define and be able to use in context the words and terms in bold print in this chapter.

KEY TERMS

anemia
anemia of chronic disease
aplastic anemia
band
basophil
bilirubin
biopsy
blood smear
buffy coat
differential white blood cell count
ecchymosis
eosinophil

Epstein-Barr virus (EBV)
erythropoiesis
erythropoietin
ferritin
flow cytometry
folic acid deficiency
genetic analysis
glucose-6-phosphate dehydrogenase (G6PD) deficiency
granulocyte
granulocytosis
hematocrit

hematopoietic system
hemoglobin
hemoglobinopathy
hemolytic anemia
hereditary spherocytosis
Hodgkin lymphoma
human immunodeficiency
    virus (HIV)
hypersplenism
idiopathic
    thrombocytopenic
    purpura (ITP)
infectious mononucleosis
iron-deficiency anemia
leukemia
leukopenia
leukocytosis
lymphocyte
lymphocytosis
lymphoma
macrocytic, normochromic
    anemia
MCHC
MCV
megakaryocyte
microangiopathic hemolytic
    anemia
microcytic, hypochromic
    anemia
monocyte
monocytosis

mononuclear phagocytic
    system
multiple myeloma
myelophthisic anemia
neutrophil
normocytic, normochromic
    anemia
pernicious anemia
petechiae
plasma
platelet count
platelets
polycythemia vera
red blood cells
    (erythrocytes)
Reed-Sternberg cell
reticulocyte
reticulocytosis
serum
serum iron-binding capacity
sickle cell anemia
spherocyte
stem cell
thalassemia
thrombocytopenia
thrombocytosis
vitamin B$_{12}$–deficiency
    anemia
white blood cell (leukocyte)
white blood cell count

Review of Structure and Function

The major functional components of the hematopoietic (he-ma-to-poy-e'-tic) system are blood, bone marrow, lymphoid tissues, the mononuclear phagocytic system, and the immune system. Unlike other systems, these components are located within several organs and have overlapping functions. The major organs where these functional components reside are the bone marrow, blood vessels, spleen, lymph nodes, and thymus. This chapter concentrates on the blood and its cellular components and the bone marrow with brief mention of lymphoid tissues and the mononuclear phagocytic system.

The blood consists of plasma, the liquid component of blood and cells. Outside blood vessels, blood rapidly clots because fibrinogen in the plasma is rapidly converted to fibrin. If the fibrin is removed, the remaining fluid is called serum. The cells in the blood include red blood cells, which fall to the bottom of a tube of blood upon standing, and the platelets and white blood cells, which form a thin white layer between the serum and red blood cells called the buffy coat.

The stem cells of the hematopoietic system are produced by the yolk sac early in embryonic life, by the fetal liver from the third to sixth months of gestation, and then by the bone marrow. The bone marrow becomes the only production site after birth, and the cells live their mature lives at other sites: in the blood and in lymphoid and mononuclear phagocytic tissues. In the bone marrow, common precursor cells produce offspring that mature along any one of several pathways to produce erythrocytes, platelets, granulocytes, lymphocytes, and monocytes.

Mature erythrocytes live their 120-day life span in the blood carrying out the highly specialized function of oxygen transport. When senile, they are removed in the spleen and other mononuclear phagocytic tissues and their chemicals are returned to the body pool.

Red blood cells (erythrocytes) (Figure 10–1) are specialized cells that have no nucleus and whose hemoglobin-filled cytoplasm is shaped like a biconcave disk. The principal function of red blood cells is oxygen transport. The amount of oxygen that can be transported by the blood is determined by the number of red cells in circulation and the amount of hemoglobin in them.

Millions of old red blood cells are removed from the circulation each hour by mononuclear phagocytes in the spleen, liver, and, to a lesser extent, other sites. The most important product of the breakdown process is the iron portion of the hemoglobin molecule, which must be stored by the mononuclear phagocytic system for later production of new red blood cells. Proteins from the degraded red cells are returned to the body's protein pool. The major product of red blood cell breakdown, which requires excretion, is bilirubin. Bilirubin is derived from the non-iron-containing portion of the heme molecule. Bilirubin is carried by the blood to the liver, conjugated by liver cells, and excreted into the intestine through the bile duct. Serum bilirubin levels may rise if there is increased breakdown of red blood cells, if the liver is diseased, or if the bile duct is obstructed.

Platelets (Figure 10–1) are actually fragments of a bone marrow cell, the megakaryocyte. The megakaryocyte

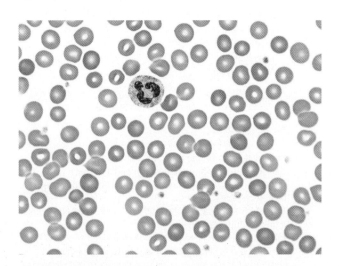

FIGURE 10–1 Normal peripheral blood smear: numerous red blood cells and a neutrophil toward the top of the field. The small blue dots between the cells are platelets. (Courtesy of Dr. David Yang, Department of Pathology and Laboratory Medicine, University of Wisconsin School of Medicine and Public Health.)

remains in the bone marrow, but its cytoplasmic fragments enter the blood where they are ready to participate in the blood clotting system when needed. Platelets are short lived and must be replaced continuously.

White blood cells (leukocytes) consist of **granulocytes** (**neutrophils** [Figure 10–1], **eosinophils**, and **basophils**), lymphocytes, and monocytes. Granulocytes also live their short lives (one day or less for neutrophils) in the blood where they are ever ready to participate in an inflammatory reaction; they are removed in the same manner as are red blood cells.

After leaving the bone marrow, **lymphocytes** (**Figure 10–2**) undergo further maturation. Some differentiate in the thymus to become T lymphocytes and become involved in cell-mediated immunity. Others differentiate in other lymphoid tissues to become B lymphocytes that are capable of further transforming into plasma cells for antibody production. Non-B, non-T lymphocytes have still other functions.

Monocytes (**Figure 10–3**) are the most widespread of the bone marrow–derived cells. Some circulate in the blood ready to participate in an inflammatory reaction; others undergo further specialization and reside in tissues, particularly the sinusoids of liver, spleen, lymph nodes, and bone marrow, but also in practically every tissue of the body. In tissues, they are referred to by many names: macrophages, histiocytes, reticuloendothelial cells, and Kupffer cells (in the liver). Tissue macrophages carry out the scavenger function of removing debris, including foreign materials and the body's own dead cells, and are referred to as the **mononuclear phagocytic system** (previously called the reticuloendothelial system). Macrophages also play a major role in cellular immune responses and in tissue repair by secreting cytokines.

The bone marrow consists of specialized connective tissue through which flows many capillaries. Filling the tissue are immature, intermediate, and mature forms of the various blood cells (**Figure 10–4**). Red blood cell intermediate forms are called rubricytes or normoblasts up until the time that the nucleus is extruded to form a red blood cell. Immature red blood cells retain basophilic material in their cytoplasm and are called **reticulocytes**. An increase in reticulocytes in the blood is an indication of early release from the bone marrow, and thus suggests accelerated red blood cell production. Red blood cells proliferate in clusters that are recognized by the small, round, dense nucleus of normoblasts in the cluster. The manufacture of erythrocytes is called **erythropoiesis**.

Granulocytes mature from myeloblasts to myelocytes to mature granulocytes. The **band**, an immature form of neutrophil, occurs at a stage just before the lobes of the nucleus become separated by a thin strand. When found in increased numbers in the blood (more than 6%), band neutrophils indicate increased production and early

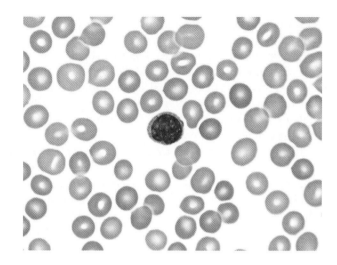

FIGURE 10–2 Normal peripheral blood smear: a lymphocyte is in the center of the field. (Courtesy of Dr. David Yang, Department of Pathology and Laboratory Medicine, University of Wisconsin School of Medicine and Public Health.)

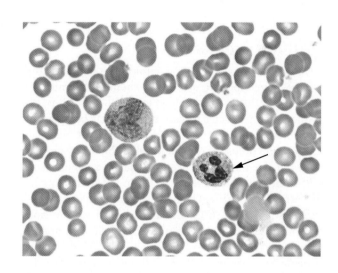

FIGURE 10–3 Normal peripheral blood smear with a monocyte and a neutrophil (arrow). (Courtesy of Dr. David Yang, Department of Pathology and Laboratory Medicine, University of Wisconsin School of Medicine and Public Health.)

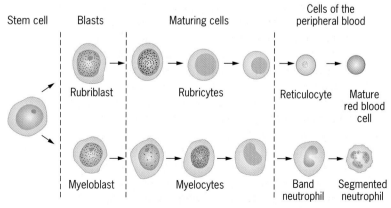

FIGURE 10–4 Maturation sequence of red blood cells and polymorphonuclear leukocytes.

release of neutrophils from the bone marrow. The characteristic neutrophilic, basophilic, or eosinophilic granules are acquired in the later stages of myelocyte differentiation. Granulocytic cells are spread diffusely throughout the bone marrow; their normal concentration is about two to four times that of red blood precursor cells. Monocytes develop from monoblasts and are mixed in with the granulocytes.

The bone marrow serves as a storage site for red and white blood cells that can be released when needed. The bone marrow can increase its production of blood cells in response to increased demand. Under normal circumstances erythrocytes live 120 days and neutrophils 12–24 hours. **Erythropoietin** is a hormone, released from the kidney, that stimulates erythropoiesis. When there are too few erythrocytes in circulation, more hormone is released to accelerate production of new cells. The production of neutrophils is mediated by GM-CSF (granulocyte-monocyte colony-stimulating factor).

Most Frequent and Serious Problems

Overall, the most common clinical problem relating to the hematopoietic system is **anemia**. Anemia is a decrease in the circulating red blood cell mass. Thus, it is a finding rather than a disease *per se*. It may be the result of decreased production of red blood cells or increased destruction or loss of red blood cells. The most common types of anemia are (1) iron-deficiency anemia resulting from dietary deficiency, (2) iron-deficiency anemia resulting from chronic bleeding from the uterus or gastrointestinal tract, (3) anemia associated with various chronic diseases, and (4) vitamin B_{12}–deficiency anemia (pernicious anemia) and folic acid–deficiency anemia. Anemia may be serious in itself if severe; otherwise, it is often a clue to the discovery and treatment of its underlying cause.

Most disorders of white blood cells are secondary effects of other diseases rather than primary in the hematopoietic system. For example, most infections are associated with an increased need for white blood cells and thus cause **leukocytosis**. If the infection is severe or prolonged, myeloid and/or lymphoid hyperplasia results.

Two of the top 10 leading causes of death in developing nations are infections of blood cells. *Malaria* is endemic in parts of the Americas, Asia, and Africa and kills an estimated 1–3 million people every year. The parasite responsible for malaria infects red blood cells and causes their periodic destruction. Infection with the **human immunodeficiency virus (HIV)** is a pandemic infection, meaning it is present everywhere in the world. It also kills an estimated 3 million people every year. The virus infects lymphocytes and destroys them at a rate that exceeds the ability of the body to replace them. Patients eventually succumb to infections.

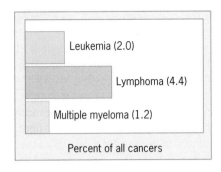

FIGURE 10–5 Relative frequency of primary hematopoietic cancers.

Primary cancers of the hematopoietic system are leukemias, lymphomas, and multiple myeloma. These cancers of white blood cells and their derivatives account for 6% of all cancers and most of the deaths from primary disease of the hematopoietic system (**Figure 10–5**).

Symptoms, Signs, and Tests

Most symptoms of hematopoietic system disease are nonspecific; they can be caused by diseases of other systems. The symptoms of anemia vary from no symptoms to heart failure. Heart failure occurs when there are insufficient amounts of red blood cells and, therefore, insufficient oxygenation of the tissues of the body, including the heart. Nonspecific symptoms of anemia include headache, easy fatigability, loss of appetite, heartburn, shortness of breath, edema of the ankles, and numbness and tingling sensations.

Physical examination may detect enlargement of lymph nodes (lymphadenopathy), spleen (splenomegaly), and liver (hepatomegaly), which can result from a wide variety of hematopoietic and nonhematopoietic diseases. The occurrence of tiny, pinpoint hemorrhages in the skin (**petechiae**) or on mucosal surfaces is an important finding that suggests a decrease in the number of circulating platelets. Other types of hemorrhage, such as nosebleeds or **ecchymoses** (large areas of hemorrhage into the skin), may be associated with decreased platelet count or a coagulation disorder. Pallor of the skin is found with severe anemia but is an unreliable sign for mild anemia.

Laboratory tests for hematopoietic disease include analysis of blood cells, biopsy of lymph nodes or bone marrow, and special tests for specific diseases. Analysis of blood cells is used for screening and diagnostic purposes. The most commonly used tests in this category are the hematocrit, hemoglobin, red blood cell count, white blood cell count, white blood cell differential count, red blood cell morphology, platelet count, and reticulocyte count.

The hematocrit, hemoglobin, red blood cell count, and blood smear are used to indicate the presence or absence of anemia and to characterize it as microcytic (small cells), normocytic, or macrocytic and as normochromic (normal amount of hemoglobin) or hypochromic. Anemia is defined as a decrease in circulating red

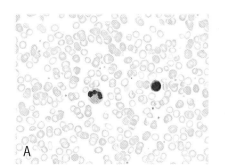
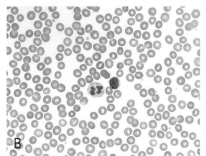
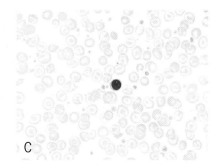

FIGURE 10–6 Classification of red blood cells by size and hemoglobin content as visualized on a blood smear. **A.** Hypochromic, with some microcytic forms. **B.** Normochromic, normocytic. **C.** Macrocytic. Lymphocytes in each frame are for size comparison. (Courtesy of Dr. David Yang, Department of Pathology and Laboratory Medicine, University of Wisconsin School of Medicine and Public Health.)

cell mass as measured by a low hematocrit, hemoglobin, or red blood cell count. **Hematocrit** is the volume of the red blood cells, expressed as a percentage, compared with other blood elements. When blood is centrifuged, the red cells form the sediment. The hemoglobin determination is a measurement of the amount of hemoglobin in grams per deciliter (g/dL). The red blood cell count, performed by counting the cells in a small chamber, is the number of red blood cells per cubic millimeter of blood.

The size and hemoglobin concentration of red blood cells can be estimated visually by placing a blood smear under a microscope or may be calculated from the hematocrit, hemoglobin, and red blood cell count. The **blood smear** is a useful, rapid means of classifying red blood cells as macrocytic, normocytic–normochromic, or microcytic–hypochromic (**Figure 10–6**). Other changes in red blood cell morphology may also be present and may give more specific clues to the cause of the anemia. The mean corpuscular volume (**MCV**), or mean red blood cell size, is calculated by dividing the hematocrit by the red blood cell count. The mean corpuscular hemoglobin concentration (**MCHC**) is calculated by dividing the hemoglobin by the hematocrit. These values are more useful than the smear itself in characterizing the size and hemoglobin concentration of red blood cells. **Table 10–1** gives the normal values for measurements of red blood cells and interpretations of high and low values.

The **white blood cell count** and **differential white blood cell count** are used to evaluate white blood cells. Blood cell counts are performed by automated cell counting instruments. The differential count involves identifying consecutive white blood cells on a smear and calculating the percentage of each type present. Absolute counts can be calculated from the percentages of each cell type and the total count. Absolute counts are of more value than are the relative percentages, because the numbers of specific types of leukocytes may vary independently of each other. **Table 10–2** gives the normal values and names applied to increases and decreases.

Platelets are evaluated by the **platelet count**, expressed as thousands per cubic millimeter. Normal values are between 150,000 and 400,000 per cubic millimeter. A platelet decrease is called **thrombocytopenia** and an increase is **thrombocytosis**.

The reticulocyte count is a measure of the percentage of immature red blood cells in circulation. Values greater than 2% are referred to as **reticulocytosis** and indicate an increased rate of production and release of new red blood cells.

Biopsy of the bone marrow is performed by boring a needle into bone (typically, the iliac crest, but other sites can be used) to obtain bone marrow tissue. The tissue can be smeared on a slide and stained or embedded in paraffin and sectioned. Bone marrow examination is used in the diagnosis of hematopoietic cancers and selected other hematopoietic diseases. Lymph node biopsy is most often used to evaluate the presence or absence of lymphoma, but it is also used to diagnose rare types of chronic infections.

TABLE 10–1 Measurements of Red Blood Cells

Test	Normal Values	Name of Low Value	Name of High Value
Hematocrit	Male: 40–54% Female: 37–49%	Anemia	Polycythemia
Hemoglobin	Male: 14.1–18.0 g/dL Female: 12.3–16.2 g/dL	Anemia	Polycythemia
Red blood cell count	Male: 4.7–6.1 million/mm³ Female: 4.2–5.6 million/mm³	Anemia	Polycythemia
MCV	82–97 μm³	Microcytosis (microcytic anemia)	Macrocytosis (macrocytic anemia)
MCHC	32–36 g/dL	Hypochromia (hypochromic anemia)	Hyperchromia (rarely occurs)

TABLE 10-2 Measurements of White Blood Cells

Test	Normal Values	Name of High Value	Name of Low Value
WBC count	4,300–11,600/mm^3	Leukocytosis	Leukopenia
WBC differential count Neutrophils	42–81%	Granulocytosis or neutrophilic leukocytosis	Granulocytopenia or neutropenia
Lymphocytes	10–47%	Lymphocytosis	Lymphopenia
Monocytes	0–10%	Monocytosis	Not applicable
Eosinophils	0–7%	Eosinophilia	Not applicable
Basophils	0–1%	Basophilia	Not applicable

Examples of special hematology tests include hemoglobin electrophoresis to evaluate genetic abnormalities in the hemoglobin molecule, insolubility of hemoglobin S in sodium hydrosulfite to test for the abnormal hemoglobin molecule in sickle cell anemia, and red cell fragility test to detect spherical red blood cells (**spherocytes**), which burst when exposed to hypotonic solutions. Iron concentrations may be measured in serum. Diseases that are the result of antibodies against red or white cells are evaluated by flow cytometry.

Flow cytometry is a technique by which cells can be tested for antigenic composition as well as size and cytoplasmic granularity. Cells flow through the cytometer in a single stream and are subjected to a laser beam; analysis of scattered light from the beam is used to determine the cell's physical properties. Application of fluorescent-tagged antibodies to the cells reveals the antigens on the cells and is, thus, very useful in categorizing leukemias and lymphomas. **Genetic analysis** is often undertaken to elucidate characteristic changes, such as mutations or translocations, of various lymphomas and leukemias.

Specific Diseases

Genetic/Developmental Diseases

Several important hereditary defects cause anemia, including sickle cell disease, thalassemia, hereditary spherocytosis, and glucose-6-phosphatase deficiency. For clarity, they are discussed in the following section with the other types of anemia.

Inflammatory/Degenerative Diseases

This section deals with anemias, disorders of white blood cells, disorders of platelets, and certain inflammatory disorders that characteristically affect the mononuclear phagocytic and lymphoid tissues. Many of these conditions are indirect results of injury, inflammation, and repair. Others, included in this section for convenience, are better classified as genetic disorders, metabolic disorders, or both.

The terminology used to describe diseases of blood cells is quite confusing, and unfortunately there is no way around this but simply memorizing definitions.

These disorders are initially categorized as to whether there is an excess or deficiency in circulating numbers of mature cells. More specific categorizations then follow depending on the etiology. In general, the suffix -*osis* refers to increased numbers and the suffix -*penia* refers to decreased numbers. The suffix -*emia* refers to blood. As with all terminology in medicine, these terms are not consistently used and names in and of themselves are often vague or ambiguous. For example, *leukemia* refers specifically to a neoplasm of white blood cells and not just to the presence of white blood cells in blood, *anemia* refers specifically to decreased red blood cells and not to the absence of blood in general, and excessive red blood cells can be called *erythrocytosis* or *polycythemia*.

Anemias in General

Anemia may be a finding in many diseases, including primary diseases of red blood cells and diseases that secondarily involve the hematopoietic system. A pathogenetic classification, or classification according to causal mechanisms, is given in **Table 10–3**. Anemia may be caused by either removal of red blood cells at a rate that exceeds the replacement capacity of the bone marrow (blood-loss anemias and hemolytic anemias) or decreased production of red blood cells by the bone marrow. Blood-loss anemia involves loss of blood from the vascular system, either externally to the body or internally. **Hemolytic anemia** involves destruction of red blood cells within the vascular or mononuclear phagocytic systems. When the mononuclear phagocytic system removes red blood cells before their normal life span is up, it is called extravascular hemolysis. If the red blood cells are actually destroyed in the bloodstream, it is called intravascular hemolysis.

A laboratory-oriented approach to the classification of anemia is based on common laboratory findings that help separate the most frequently encountered types of anemia in an efficient manner. Evaluation of red blood cell size and hemoglobin concentration gives three major categories of anemia. **Microcytic, hypochromic anemia** occurs with iron deficiency, with some cases of anemia of chronic disease, and with a few other rare diseases. **Macrocytic, normochromic anemia** is

TABLE 10–3 Classification of Anemia
Blood-loss anemias
• Acute blood-loss anemia
• Chronic blood-loss anemia
Hemolytic anemias
• Sickle cell anemia
• Thalassemia
• Hereditary spherocytosis
• Glucose-6-phosphate dehydrogenase deficiency
• Immune hemolytic anemia
• Hypersplenism
• Microangiopathic hemolytic anemia
Anemias with decreased red blood cell production
• Deficiency anemia
• Iron deficiency
• Vitamin B_{12} deficiency (pernicious anemia)
• Folic acid deficiency
• Anemia of chronic disease
• Myelophthisic anemia
• Aplastic anemia

usually the result of vitamin B_{12} or folic acid deficiency. **Normocytic, normochromic anemia** is a feature of most other types of anemia (Figure 10–6). The reticulocyte count helps separate anemias of decreased production (normal or low reticulocyte count) from those of increased destruction or loss (elevated reticulocyte count). The laboratory approach to classification must be applied with care, for there are some ambiguities. For example, chronic blood loss is not associated with an elevated reticulocyte count because the mechanism by which chronic blood loss produces anemia is iron deficiency. Thus, chronic blood-loss anemia is both a blood-loss anemia and an anemia caused by inefficient production of red blood cells. Another example is thalassemia. In thalassemia, there is both inefficient production of red blood cells because of the defective hemoglobin and increased extravascular hemolysis because the resulting cells are defective and consequently more subject to removal.

The classification of anemia is obviously very important because incorrect interpretation may result in failure to diagnose the underlying disease or apply the proper treatment. We suggest that you consider each type of anemia in terms of its pathogenetic mechanism, laboratory classification, and the context in which it is likely to occur.

Blood-Loss Anemias

Acute blood loss produces anemia within a few hours because of hemodilution, a process that allows replacement of blood serum before the bone marrow can replace lost cells. The red blood cells remaining in the anemic blood are normochromic and normocytic. Within a few days, an elevated reticulocyte count heralds the stepped-up production and release of new cells from the bone marrow. The bone marrow is capable of replacing a large

amount of lost blood. For example, a blood donor who gives 1 pint of blood suffers no ill effects. Blood lost need not be replaced unless the amount is such that hemodynamic effects, such as shock, occur.

Chronic blood loss is the slow loss of small amounts of blood over a period of time, most commonly the result of excessive menstrual bleeding and bleeding from the gastrointestinal tract. The bone marrow has sufficient capacity to replace this type of blood loss. Anemia occurs late in the course of chronic blood loss because of failure to recycle the iron from the lost red blood cells. Thus, chronic blood-loss anemia is a subcategory of iron-deficiency anemia. Chronic blood loss is discovered by taking a menstrual history or checking the feces for blood. Other forms of chronic blood loss are usually obvious from the patient's history.

BOX 10–1   Blood-Loss Anemia
Causes
Acute bleeding
Chronic bleeding
Lesions
Hyperplasia of bone marrow (compensatory)
Decreased iron stores
Manifestations
Normochromic normocytic anemia
Reticulocytosis
Hypochromic microcytic anemia
Decreased serum iron

Hemolytic Anemias

In hemolytic anemias, red blood cells are prematurely destroyed by mononuclear phagocytosis (extravascular hemolysis) or within the bloodstream (intravascular hemolysis). Extravascular hemolysis is more common. Hemolysis may be caused by the bone marrow producing defective red blood cells that are destined to a short life or by events that affect normal cells after they are released from the bone marrow.

In hemolytic anemia, there is an increased production of bilirubin as macrophages degrade the dead red blood cells. The transportation of this pigment to the liver for excretion is often manifested by an elevation of serum bilirubin and by mild jaundice. The bone marrow, which is stimulated by the anemia to produce more erythrocytes, becomes hyperplastic and releases more immature erythrocytes than normal, causing a reticulocytosis. With intravascular hemolysis, there also is free hemoglobin in the blood and urine and a decrease in serum haptoglobin, a serum protein that binds free hemoglobin. Patients with hemolytic anemia do not become depleted of iron because iron from the destroyed cells reenters the body's iron pool. In fact, increased absorption of iron and transfusion therapy can lead to iron overload, with excessive iron deposition in tissues, in these patients.

The mechanisms of hemolytic anemia include hereditary defects in red blood cells that decrease their life span, antibodies to red blood cells that cause their destruction or premature removal by the mononuclear phagocytic system, premature removal of red blood cells by the spleen as a result of chronic passive congestion (hypersplenism), and mechanical injury to red blood cells by rough surfaces in the bloodstream (**microangiopathic hemolytic anemia**) (**Figure 10–7**). Important diseases that illustrate these mechanisms are discussed.

Sickle cell anemia is one of several genetic abnormalities of hemoglobin structure caused by an altered sequence of amino acids in the globin molecule. The diseases produced by these genetic defects are called **hemoglobinopathies**, and the abnormal hemoglobin is designated by a letter or name of a place where it was first described. Sickle cell anemia occurs in persons with two genes for hemoglobin S (the homozygous state). Persons with one hemoglobin S gene (the heterozygous state) are said to carry the sickle trait and can be identified by hemoglobin electrophoresis. Identification of the trait is quite useful for purposes of genetic counseling. Hemoglobin S is a genetic abnormality predominantly of black people; overall, about 10% are heterozygous carriers and about 1% are homozygous persons with the disease. The abnormal hemoglobin results in some red blood cells becoming sickle (crescent) shaped under situations of low oxygen tension (**Figure 10–8**). The sickle cells are not only more susceptible to rupture and premature death, but also tend to sludge and obstruct small blood vessels. Vascular obstructions are particularly common in the spleen and bone, where they produce multiple small infarcts over a period of years. Patients with sickle cell anemia often live reasonably well with their anemia except during periods of so-called crisis, when more cells become sickled, leading to abdominal and bone pain from small infarcts and jaundice from the increased breakdown of red blood cells. Leg ulcers are a common complication of long-standing disease.

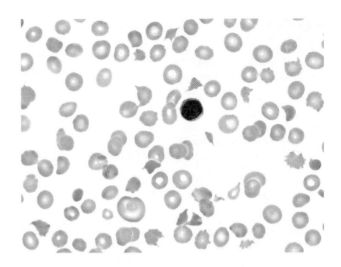

FIGURE 10–7 Peripheral blood smear of microangiopathic hemolytic anemia with fragmented red cells. (Courtesy of Dr. David Yang, Department of Pathology and Laboratory Medicine, University of Wisconsin School of Medicine and Public Health.)

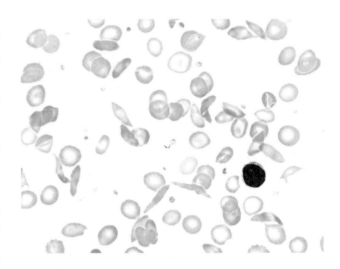

FIGURE 10–8 Sickle cell anemia, peripheral blood smear. Note the red blood cells with pointy ends and half-moon shapes. (Courtesy of Dr. David Yang, Department of Pathology and Laboratory Medicine, University of Wisconsin School of Medicine and Public Health.)

Thalassemia (**Figure 10–9**) is a genetic defect affecting the rate of synthesis of normal hemoglobin (hemoglobin A) resulting from a deficient production of alpha or beta globin. There is a compensatory increase in a type of hemoglobin found in the fetus (hemoglobin F) or in a type of hemoglobin found normally in small amounts (hemoglobin A2). Thalassemia is most common in Mediterranean countries and some parts of Africa and Southeast Asia. Thalassemia-major occurs in homozygous individuals, with severe anemia developing in infancy and leading to death in childhood or adolescence. There is a decrease in production of red blood cells because of increased destruction of immature red blood cells in the bone marrow.

BOX 10–2   Sickle Cell Anemia

Causes

Recessive genetic abnormality of hemoglobin S

Lesions

Sickled red cells

Vascular occlusions with infarcts

Hyperplasia of bone marrow

Manifestations

Crises of anemia and pain from vascular occlusion

Sickled red cells

Hemoglobin S

Occurs predominantly in black people

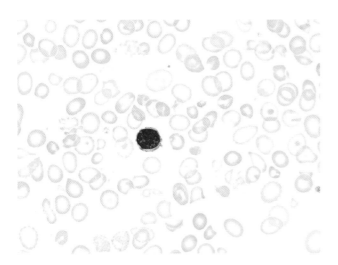

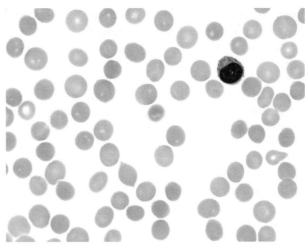

FIGURE 10–9 Thalassemia, peripheral blood smear. Many of the red blood cells are misshapen. (Courtesy of Dr. David Yang, Department of Pathology and Laboratory Medicine, University of Wisconsin School of Medicine and Public Health.)

FIGURE 10–10 Hereditary spherocytosis with red blood cells that lack central lucency because of their spherical shape. (Courtesy of Dr. David Yang, Department of Pathology and Laboratory Medicine, University of Wisconsin School of Medicine and Public Health.)

cell membrane and produce hemolysis. Discontinuance of the drug and normal replacement by young red blood cells end the hemolytic episode. The genetic abnormality is sex-linked and is present in 10–15% of black persons. Males are much more prone to develop anemia because

BOX 10–3   Thalassemia

Causes

Genetic defect of hemoglobin synthesis

Lesions

Severe anemia resulting from decreased production and increased destruction of red blood cells

Manifestations

Anemia

Hemoglobin F

Occurs in persons of Mediterranean, African, or Southeast Asian descent

BOX 10–4   Hereditary Spherocytosis

Causes

Dominant genetic defect

Lesions

Spherocytic red blood cells

Splenomegaly

Bone marrow hyperplasia

Manifestations

Spherocytes

Increased red blood cell fragility

Splenomegaly

BOX 10–5   Glucose-6-Phosphate Dehydrogenase Deficiency

Causes

Sex-linked recessive genetic defect

Lesions

None except biochemical abnormality

Manifestations

None unless given certain oxidant drugs

Enzyme deficiency

More common in African and Mediterranean descent

Hereditary spherocytosis (**Figure 10–10**) is a genetic defect of the red blood cell membrane with an autosomal-dominant inheritance pattern. The abnormal red blood cells are spherical rather than the normal flat, biconcave disks. As they filter through the spleen, they are more easily removed than are normal cells. The anemia is usually mild and often not discovered until adulthood. The spleen is enlarged because it traps the abnormal red blood cells. Removal of the spleen reduces anemia and alleviates symptoms. This is an example of a dominant disease that is perpetuated because its relatively mild nature and prolonged course allow persons with the disease to reach maturity and reproduce.

Glucose-6-phosphate dehydrogenase (G6PD) deficiency is a genetic enzyme defect that becomes manifest only when persons with the defect are exposed to fava beans or certain oxidant drugs such as antimalarial drugs, sulfas, nitrofurantoin, aspirin, and other analgesics. These patients have a mutant enzyme that becomes deficient in older red blood cells, allowing oxidants to damage the most affected females are heterozygous carriers. The disease can be prevented by screening high-risk individuals (black males) for the defect and then avoiding exposure to oxidant drugs.

Immune hemolytic anemia may be associated with antibodies that activate complement and lyse, or break, the red blood cell in the bloodstream or with antibodies that facilitate removal of the red cell by the spleen. Transfusion of blood with a major incompatibility between the donor's and recipient's ABO systems and severe cases of hemolytic disease of the fetus and newborn (formerly called erythroblastosis fetalis) are examples of causes of intravascular hemolysis. Certain drugs may induce antibodies to red blood cells and thus cause immune hemolytic anemia. In many cases of immune hemolytic anemia, the source of the antigen is the patient's own red cell antigens; thus, the anemia is classified as autoimmune hemolytic anemia. The Coombs test or flow cytometry detects the presence of antibodies attached to the surface of red blood cells and therefore is the test used to detect immune hemolytic anemias.

Hypersplenism is most commonly caused by chronic passive congestion of the spleen, a condition where the venous pressure is increased because of obstruction of the portal venous system, usually resulting from cirrhosis of the liver. The venous congestion causes the spleen to remove more blood cells than normal, thus producing a type of extravascular hemolytic anemia. The condition is suspected in a patient with cirrhosis and enlarged spleen and who often has **leukopenia** (decreased white blood cells) and thrombocytopenia (decreased platelets) along with anemia.

Microangiopathic hemolytic anemia (Figure 10–7) is caused by rough surfaces in the bloodstream as sometimes produced by prosthetic heart valves, rough atherosclerotic plaques, and disseminated intravascular thrombosis. The blood smear will show the fractured cells, called schizocytes or helmet cells.

BOX 10–6   Hemolytic Anemias

Causes

Genetic red cell defects

Antibodies to red cells

Hypersplenism

Lesions

Hyperplasia of bone marrow (compensatory)

Splenomegaly

Manifestations

Usually normocytic normochromic anemia

Reticulocytosis

Special tests of red blood cell survival and for specific conditions

---

Anemias with Decreased Red Blood Cell Production

The bone marrow may fail to put out enough red blood cells if it has an inadequate supply of nutrients to produce red blood cells, if its function is suppressed by the presence of chronic disease, or if the bone marrow tissue is insufficient in amount. The blood smear and red blood cell indices (MCV, MCHC) are used in initial screening because deficiency of iron produces a microcytic, hypochromic anemia, and deficiency of either vitamin B_{12} or folic acid produces a macrocytic anemia. Most other types of anemias are normocytic and normochromic.

Iron-deficiency anemia (**Figure 10–11**) is a common type of anemia. It may be caused by loss of iron or inadequate intake of iron. Loss of iron most commonly results from chronic blood loss, as has been discussed. Inadequate intake of iron occurs in infants fed on a milk and fruit diet without meat or supplemental iron; in women during the menstrual years (a combination of inadequate intake and increased loss); during pregnancy, when iron must be provided to the fetus; and in chronic intestinal diseases associated with malabsorption of iron. In iron-deficiency anemia, the red blood cells produced are smaller than normal and the area of central pallor is larger than normal because there is less hemoglobin per cell (microcytic hypochromic anemia). The anemia is often mild and unrecognized by the patient. Because iron stores are depleted, the serum iron is decreased and the proteins that bind iron in the serum are increased (elevated serum iron-binding capacity). Administration of iron causes an elevation of the reticulocyte count in a few days and an increase in hemoglobin after about 10 days.

Vitamin B_{12}–deficiency anemia is caused by failure to absorb vitamin B_{12} from the intestinal tract. Dietary vitamin B_{12} (extrinsic factor) must combine with a

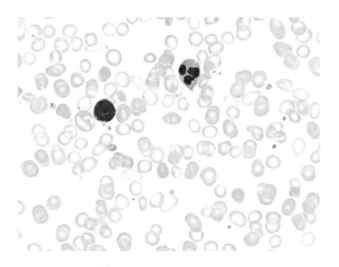

FIGURE 10–11 Iron-deficiency anemia. The majority of red blood cells are hypochromic. (Courtesy of Dr. David Yang, Department of Pathology and Laboratory Medicine, University of Wisconsin School of Medicine and Public Health.)

protein produced in the gastric mucosa (intrinsic factor) and be carried to the distal small intestine before it can be absorbed and carried to the bone marrow or body storage sites. Atrophy of the gastric mucosa, occurring mostly in persons older than age 60, with resultant insufficiency of intrinsic factor, is the most common cause of vitamin B_{12} deficiency. The disease produced is called **pernicious anemia**. Vitamin B_{12} deficiency causes disordered synthesis of DNA, resulting in accumulation of large, abnormal red blood cell precursors (megaloblasts) in the bone marrow. The maturation of red blood cells is delayed, and the red cells released into the bloodstream are larger than normal (macrocytic) (Figure 10–6C). The basic defect also affects other blood cells to a lesser degree. Pernicious anemia may be associated with permanent destruction in the spinal cord, which results in loss of coordination. Pernicious anemia is suspected when a macrocytic anemia with megaloblasts in the bone marrow is found, and it is confirmed by low serum levels of vitamin B_{12}. The Schilling test, which measures the degree of absorption of vitamin B_{12} from the intestine, is also a useful diagnostic test. Injections of vitamin B_{12} cure the anemia and are continued at regular intervals to prevent recurrence of the disease.

Folic acid deficiency also results in impaired DNA synthesis and produces a macrocytic anemia similar to pernicious anemia, except that the spinal cord degeneration does not occur. Folic acid deficiency results from inadequate diet such as is common in alcoholics, from increased need such as occurs in pregnancy, and from chronic intestinal diseases that produce malabsorption. Folic acid levels in the serum are used to distinguish folic acid deficiency from vitamin B_{12} deficiency.

Anemia of chronic disease has many causes and is diagnosed in patients with mild to moderate anemia in association with obvious chronic disease. It is the most common type of anemia and is unresponsive to therapy. Associated diseases include long-standing infections, cancer, chronic inflammatory diseases such as rheumatoid arthritis, and chronic renal disease. Approximately 10–15% of hospitalized patients may exhibit this type of anemia. Differentiation from mild iron-deficiency anemia is a particular problem because both types of anemia may be borderline microcytic with borderline serum iron levels and both may be present at the same time. The pathogenesis of the anemia is unclear, although there is suppression of red blood cell reproduction, reluctance of mononuclear phagocytic cells to release stored iron for production of new cells, and a mildly shortened red blood cell survival time. Diagnosis rests on a history of chronic disease in addition to laboratory studies that show normocytic, normochromic (or sometimes mildly microcytic, hypochromic) red blood cells, normal to slightly low serum iron and serum ferritin levels, and normal serum iron-binding capacity. Soluble transferrin receptor assay (sTfR) also is used to establish the diagnosis. **Ferritin** is a protein that binds free iron. Measurement of serum ferritin reflects total iron body stores. These are usually normal in anemia of chronic disease, in contrast to iron-deficiency anemia in which there is low total body iron and therefore low serum ferritin. For the same reason, **serum iron-binding capacity**, a test that measures the amount of the protein that carries iron in the blood, may be normal in the anemia of chronic disease but is elevated in iron-deficiency anemia. Also in contrast to iron-deficiency anemia, mononuclear phagocytic cells in the bone marrow contain abundant iron.

Myelophthisic anemia refers to anemia caused by replacement of the bone marrow by diseased tissue such as cancer or fibrous tissue. Cancer is the most common cause. Leukemias, lymphomas, multiple myeloma, and metastatic carcinoma from lung, breast, or prostate cancer can replace the bone marrow so that normal blood cells are produced in subnormal numbers. In addition to the anemia, there will be leukopenia and thrombocytopenia. Replacement of the bone marrow by fibrous tissue is called myelofibrosis. It may be the result of irradiation or drugs or of unknown cause. To compensate for bone marrow destruction, hematopoietic cells may take up residence in other sites, such as spleen, liver, and lymph nodes, a process called myeloid metaplasia or extramedullary hematopoiesis.

Aplastic anemia is an atrophy of the bone marrow, usually of unknown cause, but sometimes caused by chemical poisons such as benzene, drugs such as anticancer agents, and radiation. As in myelophthisic anemia, all blood cell elements may be reduced. Bone marrow biopsy is useful in distinguishing myelophthisic anemia from aplastic anemia, the former displaying the disease replacing the bone marrow and the latter displaying only a hypocellular bone marrow.

BOX 10–7 Anemia with Decreased Production

Causes

Iron deficiency

Vitamin B_{12} deficiency, folic acid deficiency

Chronic disease

Bone marrow replacement

Bone marrow atrophy

Thalassemia

Lesions

Usually normal bone marrow

Manifestations

Microcytic hypochromic anemia (iron deficiency)

Macrocytic anemia (vitamin B_{12} or folic acid deficiency)

Normochromic anemia (bone marrow replacement)

Normal or low reticulocyte count

Disorders of White Blood Cells

Degenerative and inflammatory disorders involving white blood cells are almost always secondary to disease of some other system. **Granulocytosis** is characteristic of acute inflammation; **lymphocytosis** and **monocytosis** occur with some chronic inflammations; and eosinophilia is characteristic of parasitic infections and some types of allergy. Neutropenia and lymphopenia occasionally occur with some types of infections. The white blood cell count may be decreased by excessive removal with hypersplenism or insufficient production in association with myelophthisic or aplastic anemia.

Disorders of Platelets

Thrombocytopenia is more common and more significant than is thrombocytosis. Mechanisms of thrombocytopenia include increased platelet destruction and decreased platelet production. Causes of increased destruction include antibodies to platelets, increased utilization of platelets such as occurs in some blood coagulation disorders, and hypersplenism. Causes of decreased production of platelets include myelophthisic and aplastic anemia. If necessary, in the short term, patients can be transfused with packets of platelets. Occasionally, treatment with any of a variety of drugs may be associated with the development of antibodies to platelets.

Idiopathic thrombocytopenic purpura (ITP) refers to thrombocytopenia without evident cause. This condition is believed to be the result of antibodies to platelets in most instances. It occurs as a short-lived disorder in children following infections. It also occurs in adults, especially young women, without a precipitating episode and with a prolonged course. In chronic cases, removal of the spleen often results in remission because the spleen can no longer remove the antibody-coated platelets. Corticosteroid drugs may cause a temporary rise in platelets.

Regardless of its cause, a markedly depressed platelet count is associated with bleeding from small blood vessels to produce petechiae. Thrombocytosis is associated with a few uncommon diseases and usually produces no ill effects.

Infections

As mentioned previously, infections frequently cause a secondary hyperplasia of myeloid, lymphoid, and mononuclear phagocytic tissues. A few types of infections, mostly chronic types, have their major effects in the hematopoietic system. Malaria is caused by small protozoa that live in red blood cells and cause episodes of red cell destruction manifested by fever and anemia. **Infectious mononucleosis** is caused by the **Epstein-Barr virus (EBV)** and produces enlargement of lymphoid tissue, including lymph nodes, pharyngeal lymphoid tissue, and spleen. The disease usually occurs in young persons in the second and third decades of life and runs a prolonged course, producing weakness, sore throat, and lymphadenopathy. Atypical reactive lymphocytes in the blood and a positive mono spot test for antibodies to the virus are the means of diagnosis.

Another serious infection involving blood cells is human immunodeficiency virus (HIV), infecting lymphocytes and leading to AIDS. AIDS and malaria are among the leading causes of death worldwide.

Granulomatous diseases such as tuberculosis and systemic fungal infections have a strong tendency to localize in organs with much mononuclear phagocytic tissue, including lymph nodes, spleen, liver, and bone marrow. Sarcoidosis is an idiopathic granulomatous disease that also produces widespread granulomatous lesions in the mononuclear phagocytic tissues.

Hyperplastic/Neoplastic Diseases

The diseases called **leukemias** are white blood cell cancers characterized by extensive bone marrow replacement with neoplastic white blood cells. Leukemias can be either granulocytic or lymphocytic. **Lymphomas** are also white blood cell cancers and are characterized by involvement of sites other than the bone marrow or blood, often with production of mass lesions, and mostly of lymphocytic origin. **Multiple myeloma** is a cancer of plasma cells, usually arising in the bone marrow and usually unassociated with leukemia.

Phenotypic studies using flow cytometry and immunohistochemical staining have contributed greatly to the differential diagnoses and classification of these diseases. Without treatment, hematopoietic malignancies are uniformly fatal. Establishment of the curative potential of various chemotherapeutic regimens and/or radiation therapy, plus the introduction of bone marrow transplantation, have made the classification of these diseases based on cell type much more important. Treatment in the future will depend on even more sophisticated classifications based on differences in genes between subtypes of neoplasms and the proteins produced by the genes.

BOX 10–8   Thrombocytopenia

Causes

Antibodies to platelets

Coagulation disorders

Hypersplenism

Bone marrow replacement

Bone marrow atrophy

Lesions

May be splenomegaly or bone marrow damage

Manifestations

Petechial hemorrhages

Thrombocytopenia

Only a general outline of this complicated subject is presented here.

Polycythemia

Polycythemia is an increase in red blood cells as a result of persistent overproduction. It is a form of hyperplasia that may be primary and idiopathic (of unknown cause) or secondary to some other, underlying disease. Primary polycythemia is called **polycythemia vera**. Secondary polycythemia is mediated by increased production of erythropoietin, a hormone that stimulates development and maturation of erythrocytes. The main causes of excess erythropoietin production include (1) hypoxia caused by chronic lung disease, cyanotic heart disease, or living at a high altitude, and (2) excess production of erythropoietin by any one of several rare neoplasms. Athletes, especially cyclists, occasionally take erythropoietin illegally to increase their oxygen-carrying capacity.

Secondary polycythemia resulting from hypoxia is necessary to sustain oxygenation of tissue. Polycythemia increases the viscosity (thickness) of the blood, which may lead to thrombosis and hemorrhage. Polycythemia vera is much less common than secondary polycythemia and appears to be a primary proliferative disease of bone marrow. Polycythemia vera can be treated by myelosuppressive therapy and phlebotomy to reduce the risk of thrombosis. White blood cells and platelets may also be increased in conjunction with polycythemia vera, and the disease may lead to myelofibrosis. In rare cases, leukemia develops.

BOX 10–9 Polycythemia

Causes

Unknown

Chronic hypoxia

Rare neoplasms secreting erythropoietin

Lesions

Hyperplasia of bone marrow

Manifestations

Thromboses and bleeding

Polycythemia

Leukemias

Leukemias comprise several types of malignant neoplasms of white blood cells that originate and spread diffusely in the bone marrow and usually produce high white blood cell counts in the peripheral blood. Leukemic cells often diffusely infiltrate other organs, such as the spleen, liver, and lymph nodes.

Leukemias are usually classified by the type of white cell involved and the chronicity of the disease. The degree of differentiation of the leukemic cells relates closely to the likely duration; thus, acute leukemias have poorly differentiated cells and a rapid course, whereas chronic leukemias have well-differentiated cells and a slow course. Most leukemias involve either lymphocytes or granulocytes (mostly neutrophils). Monocytic leukemia is less common, while basophilic and eosinophilic leukemias are rare. Acute lymphocytic leukemia is the most common type of childhood leukemia and is rapidly fatal unless treated very aggressively with multiagent chemotherapy. Successful therapy may lead to long-term survival and cure. Chronic lymphocytic leukemia is a much different disease; it occurs in older adults and runs a prolonged, indolent course, with many patients dying from other causes before the leukemia has time to kill them. Both acute and chronic granulocytic (myelogenous) leukemia occur predominantly in adults and are less likely to be cured than is leukemia in children.

Acute leukemias (**Figure 10–12**) are composed of more primitive or less well-differentiated cell types called *blasts*; chronic leukemias are composed mainly of mature cells with a limited number of primitive blast forms. Acute leukemias have an abrupt onset with bleeding resulting from thrombocytopenia, anemia, fatigue, fever, and weight loss. The white blood count may be normal or elevated. In chronic leukemia, the symptoms, although similar, appear gradually, and by the time they develop the white blood count may be very high, and organs, such as the spleen, liver, and lymph nodes, enlarged by leukemic infiltrates. Diagnosis is made by examination of the blood smear and bone marrow, and patients are often referred to major centers for treatment, which usually is chemotherapy.

BOX 10–10 Leukemias

Causes

Unknown

Benzene

Topoisomerase treatment

Lesions

Bone marrow replacement by neoplastic cells

Leukemic cells in blood

Organ infiltrates

Manifestations

Weakness

Anemia

Bleeding

Infections

Leukemic cells in blood and bone marrow

Lymphomas

Lymphomas comprise several types of malignant neoplasms of lymphocytes and histiocytes that originate in lymphoid tissues outside of the bone marrow, most

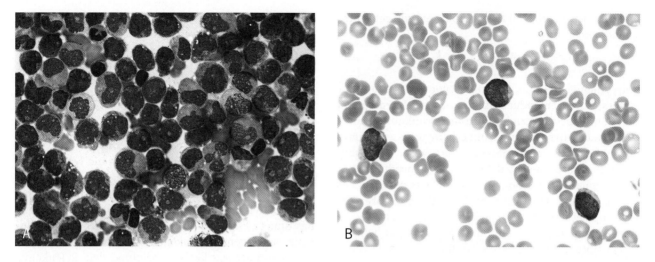

FIGURE 10–12 Acute myeloid leukemia. **A.** Bone marrow biopsy. The hematopoietic elements are virtually replaced by a population of myeloid blast cells. **B.** Blasts are present in the peripheral blood. (Courtesy of Dr. David Yang, Department of Pathology and Laboratory Medicine, University of Wisconsin School of Medicine and Public Health.)

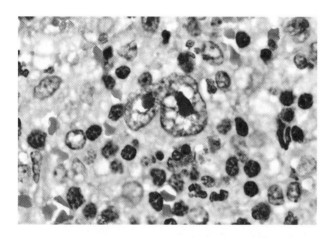

FIGURE 10–13 A Reed-Sternberg cell has a large, "owl-eyed" bilobate nucleus with prominent nucleoli. This is one of the diagnostic histologic findings in Hodgkin lymphoma. (Courtesy of Dr. David Yang, Department of Pathology and Laboratory Medicine, University of Wisconsin School of Medicine and Public Health.)

often in lymph nodes. Lymphomas usually produce mass lesions, in contrast to leukemias, in which disease is concentrated within the bone marrow. Further, lymphomas usually do not spill malignant cells into the bloodstream; that is, they are aleukemic.

The classification of lymphomas is based on cell type and is very complex. The World Health Organization (WHO) classification is the most widely used current classification. Major categories include Hodgkin lymphoma and non-Hodgkin lymphoma. **Hodgkin lymphoma** is characterized by a large, malignant cell with a multilobed nucleus containing prominent nucleoli that is known as a **Reed-Sternberg cell** (**Figure 10–13**). Unlike most malignancies, Hodgkin lymphomas contain many benign cells, including lymphocytes, histiocytes,

neutrophils, eosinophils, and fibroblasts; these additional cells are used for subclassification and their presence or absence relates to prognosis. Non-Hodgkin lymphomas are classified on the basis of cell size (small versus large), immunologic markers (T cell, B cell, or neither), histologic pattern (follicular versus diffuse), and details of cell structure.

The ultimate purpose of trying to subclassify disease is to estimate prognosis better and to provide optimal therapy; considerable progress has been made with regard to lymphomas. The survival from Hodgkin disease, once considered to be zero, is greatly improved for all types with aggressive radiation therapy and/or chemotherapy, and long-term survival or even cure is now expected in many patients with the less malignant types of disease. Follicular lymphomas have a long median survival without therapy but are not cured by chemotherapy. In contrast, patients with diffuse large cell lymphoma can be cured or live greatly prolonged periods by aggressive chemotherapy, but they have a short survival without therapy.

Diagnosis and classification of a lymphoma are made by biopsy. Patients are often referred to major centers for therapy, which usually consists of radiation and/or chemotherapy.

BOX 10–11   Lymphomas

Causes

Unknown

Lesions

Neoplastic masses in lymph nodes or other organs

Manifestations

Lymphadenopathy or other mass

Lymphoma by biopsy

Multiple Myeloma

Multiple myeloma is a malignant neoplasm of plasma cells. For unknown reasons, it arises in the bone marrow and grows to replace bone marrow, with localized destruction of surrounding bone. Another characteristic feature is the production of immunoglobulins, which can be detected in the blood and urine. Multiple myeloma is a disease of middle-aged and older adults that presents with anemia, infection, multifocal destructive bone lesions, and sometimes renal failure from immunoglobulin precipitates in renal tubules. Although chemotherapy has prolonged survival, the ultimate prognosis is poor.

BOX 10–12 Multiple Myeloma

Causes

Unknown

Lesions

Plasma cell neoplasm in bone marrow and bone

Manifestations

Bone pain

Anemia

Immunoglobulins in blood and urine

Malignant plasma cells by bone marrow biopsy

Organ Failure

Bone marrow failure has been discussed previously as myelophthisic anemia and aplastic anemia, conditions associated with replacement or atrophy of the bone marrow. The results of bone marrow failure are anemia, leukopenia, and thrombocytopenia. These effects, in turn, lead to increased likelihood of infection and bleeding. Failure of the lymphoid system is associated with immune deficiency. Failure of the mononuclear phagocytic system is not clearly defined but results in greater susceptibility to infection.

Practice Questions

1. A 36-year-old woman complains to her physician of chronic lethargy. She also admits to excessive blood loss during her menstrual periods for several years. Laboratory examination reveals a low hemoglobin level and small erythrocytes. Which of the following types of anemia does she most likely have?
   A. Sickle cell
   B. Hemolytic
   C. Iron-deficiency
   D. Thalassemia

2. In a large laboratory, routine review of test results at the end of a day reveals a patient with a white blood cell count of 72,000—93% of which are lymphocytes with many immature forms. The diagnosis in this patient is almost certainly which of the following?
   A. Leukemia
   B. Lymphoma
   C. Granulocytosis
   D. Polycythemia

3. In a patient with severe shortness of breath and pallor, you notice petechiae on the skin of her neck and arms. Which of the following would be the most important laboratory tests to order first?
   A. Hemoglobin, white blood cell count, and platelet count
   B. Bone marrow biopsy and hemoglobin
   C. Reticulocyte count and platelet count
   D. Platelet count and serum immunoglobulin level

4. A peripheral blood examination in a 43-year-old man with neurologic symptoms reveals a low hematocrit, low hemoglobin, and a strikingly high MCV. Which of the following is the most likely diagnosis?
   A. Sickle cell anemia
   B. Hereditary spherocytosis
   C. Pernicious anemia
   D. Folic acid deficiency

5. An acute inflammatory process, such as bacterial pneumonia, would most likely result in increased numbers of which type of cells?
   A. Erythrocytes
   B. Granulocytes
   C. Lymphocytes
   D. All of the above

Bleeding and Clotting Disorders

OUTLINE

OBJECTIVES

1. Describe the roles of vessels, platelets, and plasma coagulation factors in hemostasis.
2. Provide an overview of the coagulation cascade, including the concepts of the intrinsic and extrinsic pathways of activation, the concept of a cascade, the most important enzymes and reactions in the cascade, the end product, and how clots are eventually dissolved.
3. Understand the most common and serious manifestations of disorders of bleeding and clotting (trauma, thrombocytopenia, hereditary coagulation disorders, deep vein thrombosis and pulmonary embolism, disseminated intravascular coagulation).
4. Understand that bleeding or thrombosis may be a manifestation of underlying diseases or a side effect of medications, and gain an appreciation for the wide range of diseases that can manifest in this manner.
5. Recognize physical signs that reflect a hemorrhagic diathesis.
6. Describe laboratory tests that can aid in the workup of a bleeding or clotting disorder—in particular, the platelet count, activated partial thromboplastin time, prothrombin time (INR), and fibrin-split products/D-dimer.
7. Relate the function of factors V, VII, VIII, IX, X, XII, and XIII to the coagulation deficit caused by their absence, and name diseases associated with these defects.
8. List and describe some of the vascular, platelet, and coagulation disorders leading to abnormal bleeding (hemorrhage).
9. Understand how heparin and warfarin (Coumadin) are used therapeutically, how they work at the molecular level, what risks are associated with their use, and how their doses are monitored.
10. Understand how the elements of Virchow's triad relate to thrombosis.
11. List and describe some of the vascular, platelet, and coagulation disorders leading to abnormal clot formation (thrombosis).
12. Define and use in context all terms in headings and in bold print in this chapter.

KEY WORDS

activated partial thromboplastin time (aPTT)
adhesion
aggregation
amyloid
antithrombin
aspirin
bleeding time
blood clotting
blood coagulation
clotting cascade

coagulopathy
consumption coagulopathy
disseminated intravascular coagulation (DIC)
embolus
epistaxis
extrinsic pathway
factor V Leiden mutation
factor XII
factor XIII
family history
fibrin

fibrin degradation
    products/D-dimer
fibrinogen
fibrinogen assay
fibrinolytic system
hematochezia
hematoma
hematuria
hemolytic uremic syndrome
    (HUS)
hemophilia A
hemophilia B
hemorrhagic diathesis
hemorrhagic disease of the
    newborn
hemostasis
Henoch-Schönlein purpura
heparin
hypersplenism
idiopathic
    thrombocytopenia
    purpura (ITP)
International Normalized
    Ratio (INR)
intrinsic pathway
liver disease
lupus anticoagulant

megakaryocyte
menorrhagia
organized thrombus
petechiae
plasmin
platelet count
platelet function analyzer
prostacyclin
protein C
prothrombin time (PT)
pulmonary embolism
purpura
stasis
thrombin
thrombocytopenia
thrombocytosis
thrombosis
thrombotic
    thrombocytopenia
    purpura (TTP)
thrombus
tissue factor
uremia
Virchow's triad
vitamin K
von Willebrand disease
warfarin

Bleeding and clotting disorders are treated in this separate chapter because they involve both the vascular and hematopoietic systems. Bleeding and clotting chemistry is somewhat complicated, but oversimplification would not do justice to either the student or the subject.

Review of Structure and Function

Hemostasis is the process that prevents excessive bleeding following injury. The mechanisms of hemostasis involve a complex interaction of blood vessels, platelets, and chemical coagulation factors in plasma. Hemostasis is highly regulated by numerous activating and inhibiting mechanisms that allow the process to proceed rapidly but not excessively under normal conditions.

Blood vessels confine blood and allow it to circulate. The endothelial cells lining blood vessels normally prevent the activation of blood platelets and plasma coagulation factors, but when the endothelium is injured, platelets and the coagulation mechanism are activated to prevent leakage of blood from the vessel.

To begin with, blood vessels undergo spastic contraction in response to injury, thus aiding hemostasis by decreasing the blood flow to the injured area. Spasm of the smooth muscle of small arteries (arterioles) can occlude the vascular lumen and stop bleeding from an injured vessel within a few minutes. Shunting of blood to noninjured vessels provides collateral circulation, thus limiting injury to the tissue supplied by the vessel as well as allowing the injured vessel to heal itself. Spasm in medium-sized and larger arteries may aid in hemostasis by decreasing blood flow but is often not sufficient to stop bleeding entirely.

Platelets, also called thrombocytes, are cytoplasmic fragments of **megakaryocytes**, large cells that reside in the bone marrow. These fragments of cytoplasm that get pinched off the megakaryocytes contain numerous potent activators of inflammation and coagulation, but they do not contain nuclei and have only a rudimentary synthetic and respiratory apparatus. Normally, 150,000 to 400,000 platelets per microliter circulate in the blood with a life span of 8 to 10 days each. If they are not needed for hemostasis, they are removed by the mononuclear phagocytic system as they become senescent.

The major functions of platelets at the site of an injury are to physically obstruct blood flow, promote vasoconstriction, release chemicals that further the hemostatic process, and facilitate clot retraction in the healing phase. Platelets stick to any surface other than normal endothelium—a process called **adhesion**. Endothelial cells normally produce a potent inhibitor of adhesion and activation called **prostacyclin**. In addition, platelets normally travel in the center of the column of flowing blood, so they are only rarely in contact with the endothelium. However, minor injury to the endothelial layer that exposes underlying extracellular connective tissue components activates platelets and coagulation factors. Adhesion is accompanied by **aggregation** of platelets to each other as they form a platelet plug. In small vessels, the plug itself may be sufficient for hemostasis (**Figure 11-1**). Adhesion and aggregation are potentiated by collagen (exposed by the endothelial injury), epinephrine (released from adrenal glands during stress and from the platelets themselves), arachidonic acid (from platelets and other cells in the injured areas), ATP (adenosine triphosphate; released from platelets), and thrombin (an enzyme in the coagulation cascade; described later).

Chemicals released from platelet granules as they adhere and aggregate facilitate hemostasis and coagulation. These chemical mediators include vasoactive amines, which cause vascular smooth muscle contraction; epinephrine and arachidonic acid, which accelerate aggregation of additional platelets; and components of the platelet surface, which are a necessary ingredient for the coagulation cascade. Platelets are also integral to the repair process.

The process of converting plasma from a liquid to a solid is called **blood coagulation** or **blood clotting**. The solidification step in this process involves the conversion of **fibrinogen**, a large, soluble plasma protein produced by the liver, to fibrin monomer. Fibrin monomer polymerizes to form **fibrin**, a stringy, strong, insoluble protein. Fibrinogen may leak into tissues during inflammation and coagulate to form a fibrinous exudate. When the process occurs in a blood vessel it is called **thrombosis**, and the end result, the blood clot, a **thrombus**. Thrombi contain fibrin with entrapped red blood cells and platelets (**Figure 11-2**).

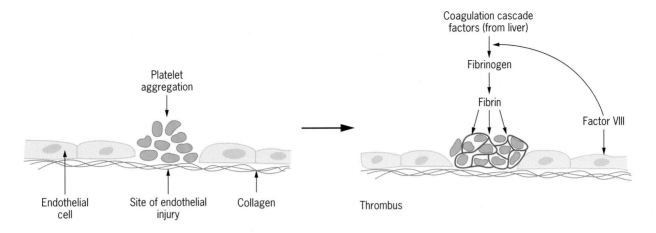

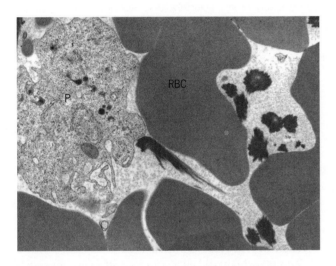

FIGURE 11–1 Platelets aggregate and stick to collagen at the site of endothelial injury.

FIGURE 11–2 Electron micrograph (20,750 magnification) of a thrombus with an entrapped platelet (P) and red blood cells (RBC). The dark spots are the fibrin that holds the thrombus together.

Thrombosis is a complex process involving a tightly regulated interaction between tissues, platelets, and plasma proteins called coagulation factors. The final step in the process, the formation of fibrin, occurs through a series of enzymatic steps referred to as the coagulation or **clotting cascade**. It is called a cascade because the product of each step catalyzes and augments the next step, and often even potentiates preceding steps so that the reaction accelerates rapidly. The reaction can be slowed or stopped by inhibitors, which are also serum proteins that are activated by injury or inflammation at the same time as the coagulation cascade itself. The factors involved in the coagulation cascade have been designated by Roman numerals and also often have a name. With well over a dozen factors and inhibitors—some acting on more than one other molecule in the cascade, and some having more than one name—the entire mechanism becomes extremely complex. It is not necessary for you to memorize the cascade in all its detail. The

following discussion is meant to introduce you to some of the most important chemicals and processes involved in the reaction. At least a rudimentary knowledge of it is needed to understand and diagnose bleeding and clotting disorders.

The coagulation cascade is presented in an abbreviated form in **Figure 11–3**. As mentioned, the end result is the conversion of fibrinogen to a stable fibrin clot and thereby conversion of blood from a liquid to a solid state. The conversion of fibrinogen to fibrin is dependent on two active enzymes. The first is the enzyme **thrombin**, which converts fibrinogen to fibrin monomer. The fibrin monomer is then acted on by a second enzyme (fibrin-stabilizing factor, or **factor XIII**), to be turned into a stable fibrin polymer.

The active enzymes that stabilize the fibrin clot, and indeed all others in the coagulation cascade, are derived from inactive precursors that circulate in the blood at all times. Thrombin is derived from an inactive precursor called prothrombin (factor II). The conversion of prothrombin to thrombin is dependent on the active form of factor X, in conjunction with its cofactor factor V, calcium ions, and phospholipids.

Looking at the coagulation cascade (Figure 11–3), you can see that factor X can be converted to its active form through two distinct pathways. In the first, called the **extrinsic pathway**, a molecule called **tissue factor**, which is present in extracellular fluid and blood, combines with factor VII. This complex of tissue factor and factor VII activates factor X. In the second, called the **intrinsic pathway**, factor X can be converted to factor Xa (activated factor X) by the activated form of plasma factor IX. Plasma factor IX also requires a cofactor (factor VIIIa) and calcium ions to facilitate its activity. Factor IX is, in turn, activated by factor XI or the tissue factor/factor VII complex; factor XI is converted to factor XIa by the active form of **factor XII**, or Hageman factor.

Note that some of the reactions in the coagulation cascade can be catalyzed by more than one active enzyme,

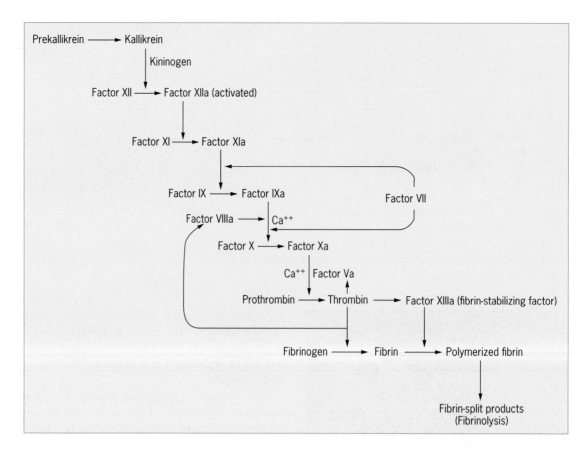

FIGURE 11-3 Chemical reactions (cascade) of blood coagulation and fibrinolysis.

and that thrombin itself activates several of the cofactors (factor V, factor XIII). Thrombin also activates several of the molecules involved in inflammation. Indeed, inflammation and coagulation are both called into play when tissue is injured, and thrombin is just one of the molecules that can "cross-talk" between the two processes. Finally, as excess thrombin is washed away from a site of injury, it actually activates some of the plasma inhibitors of coagulation—proteins that are as integral to the coagulation cascade as the procoagulants are. Thrombin is therefore critical to the body's reaction to injury in more than one way and regulates more than just the formation of a stable fibrin polymer.

Once a clot has formed, it is necessary to have a mechanism for its appropriate removal so that the tissue can repair. This removal is accomplished by the **fibrinolytic system**. This is similar to the coagulation cascade in that it is a sequence of enzymatic steps, each requiring an active enzyme produced from an inactive serum protein. The active enzyme **plasmin** is formed from plasminogen in the presence of a variety of activators, including tissue-derived plasminogen activator and urokinase. Plasmin breaks down the insoluble fibrin clot into soluble fragments called fibrin-split products. Some thrombi, particularly large ones, cannot be completely lysed, in which case they are replaced by granulation tissue and

eventually fibrosis. A thrombus converted to scar tissue is called an **organized thrombus**.

Patients who have had a stroke (cerebrovascular accident) or myocardial infarct as a result of a thrombus in a cerebral or coronary vessel can be treated with recombinant tissue plasminogen activator (tPA) or streptokinase. There can be a favorable outcome with these "clotbusters" if they are administered within approximately 3 hours after the onset of symptoms, or before there is permanent tissue damage.

Hemostasis is needed to prevent bleeding, but unregulated coagulation is not otherwise desirable. Several inhibitors of the coagulation mechanism have been identified that protect against the potentially devastating consequences of unchecked coagulation. As already mentioned, the endothelium produces prostacyclin, which is a potent inhibitor of platelet function. Other molecules are activated at the same time as the factors in the coagulation cascade. **Antithrombin** binds to and inactivates thrombin. **Protein C**, when activated in the presence of its cofactor, protein S, can inactivate the cofactors factor V and factor VIII. Also, tissue factor pathway inhibitor (TFPI) inhibits the factor VII/tissue factor complex. Many of these antithrombotic molecules are being discovered as patients present with unexplained problems relating to sporadic thromboses, such as myocardial infarcts, deep vein thromboses, and repeated pregnancy losses.

Most Frequent and Serious Problems

Trauma is the most common cause of hemorrhage: everyone experiences bleeding as a result of trauma. Minor traumatic hemorrhages, such as scraped knees or cut fingers, are controlled by the normal hemostatic mechanisms. However, injury to larger vessels may not result in hemostasis rapidly enough to prevent exsanguination. Access to medical facilities, where the lost blood volume can be replaced and excessive bleeding surgically controlled, is of the essence in such injuries. Bleeding caused by sudden rupture of a large artery is the most life threatening. For example, fatal hemorrhage may occur from a ruptured aortic aneurysm or from a bleeding peptic ulcer. In addition, trauma and surgical operations increase the likelihood of significant hemorrhage in patients with preexisting vascular disease.

Spontaneous bleeding may be anticipated when the platelet count drops below 10,000 per microliter or when platelets are defective. Typical causes of **thrombocytopenia** (decreased numbers of circulating platelets) include bone marrow failure and peripheral destruction of platelets. Bone marrow failure can be induced by many primary or secondary diseases, including leukemia or bone marrow metastases. It may also be induced by medical therapies, such as chemotherapy. In these cases, megakaryocytes disappear and platelet numbers drop rapidly as platelets are consumed. Peripheral destruction of platelets can occur in various disease states as well. For example, if the spleen becomes enlarged, it can sequester platelets so that they are not available to circulate in the blood. Antibodies may be induced against platelets, as in the disease idiopathic thrombocytopenic purpura (ITP), causing immune-mediated platelet destruction. Patients with temporary platelet deficiency, such as might be caused by cancer chemotherapy, can be treated with platelet transfusions; however, the underlying cause of thrombocytopenia should always be sought and treated.

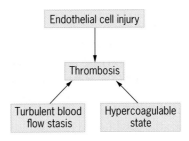

FIGURE 11–4 Virchow's triad. Hypercoagulability, abnormal blood flow, and endothelial injury contribute to thrombosis, individually or in combination. Of the three, endothelial injury is the most important.

Hereditary coagulation disorders, such as hemophilia, are rare, but people with these disorders require considerable medical care over many years. Acquired coagulation disorders are typically associated with other diseases or with some drugs in susceptible individuals. Anticoagulation therapy may be given to patients at increased risk of thrombosis, but this should be monitored very tightly so as to avoid uncontrolled and serious bleeding.

Thrombosis is usually secondary to some other condition. The father of pathology, the German scholar Rudolf Virchow, described the conditions leading to thrombosis. These are known as **Virchow's triad**: endothelial cell injury, stasis or turbulence of blood flow, and a hypercoagulable state (**Figure 11–4**). Table 11–1 lists various conditions that can contribute to endothelial injury, altered blood flow, or hypercoagulability. These are discussed later in the section on disorders characterized by thrombosis. Suffice it to say here that a piece of a thrombus can break off and travel through the bloodstream, only to get stuck eventually in a smaller vessel. This happens with **pulmonary embolism**: a thrombus forms in a vein, usually in the pelvis or legs, is dislodged, is carried via the right heart to the lungs, and gets stuck in pulmonary arteries. Given the long list of conditions predisposing individuals to thrombosis in Table 11–1, it is no wonder that deep vein thrombosis and pulmonary embolism are common, especially in hospitalized patients, and may even occur in persons who are otherwise perfectly healthy (e.g., pregnant women).

TABLE 11–1 Conditions Leading to Endothelial Injury, Altered Blood Flow, or Hypercoagulability		
Endothelial Injury	**Altered Blood Flow**	**Hypercoagulability**
• Trauma • Vasculitis • Cigarette smoke • Radiation • Atherosclerosis • Infarction • Turbulent blood flow • Bacterial endotoxins	• Bifurcation of arteries • Atherosclerosis • Aneurysm • Venous stasis (incompetent venous valves, bed rest)	• Increased estrogen (birth control pills, pregnancy) • Trauma • Surgery • Inherited coagulopathy • Cancer • Obesity

Disseminated intravascular coagulation (DIC) is a serious condition occurring in critically ill patients. Patients develop fibrin thrombi in small vessels throughout the body, where they cause microinfarcts and extensive tissue injury, and at the same time bleed extensively through other vessels, such as those in the mucosa of the gastrointestinal tract. Simultaneous clotting and bleeding make the condition very difficult to treat: giving anticoagulants aggravates the bleeding, while giving procoagulants aggravates the disseminated thrombosis.

Symptoms, Signs, and Tests

A patient with a tendency to bleed, whether known by a history of bleeding or by abnormal laboratory tests, is said to have a **hemorrhagic diathesis**. An abnormality in the coagulation mechanism leading to either excessive bleeding or excessive clotting is referred to as a **coagulopathy**.

A decrease or deficiency of platelets causes bleeding from small vessels in the skin and internal surfaces such as the nose, gastrointestinal tract, and urinary tract in the form of **petechiae** (small hemorrhages) (**Figure 11–5**), **epistaxis** (nosebleeds), **hematuria** (blood in the urine), or **hematochezia** (fecal blood). Women may present with prolonged, excessive menstrual bleeding (**menorrhagia**) or increased bleeding following delivery. Tissue bleeding, such as occurs with coagulation deficiencies, tends to occur at one site at a time with minor trauma and produces a localized collection of blood (**hematoma**). Typical sites are the joints, soft tissues, and brain. Larger collections of blood in the skin are referred to as **purpura** because of their red-purple color.

A history of previous bleeding, such as after circumcision or tooth extraction, and a **family history** of bleeding may provide the clues to diagnosis of a hereditary coagulation defect. Such a history is particularly important in patients scheduled for an operation because the history

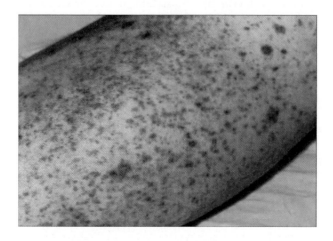

FIGURE 11–5 Petechiae. These small hemorrhages appeared on the skin of a patient after application of a tourniquet.

may call attention to a problem even while screening tests for bleeding disorders are normal.

Laboratory tests for bleeding disorders are used to determine the specific pathogenesis of the problem—that is, whether the disorder is attributable to abnormal function of vessels, platelets, or the clotting cascade. They are also used to monitor the effect of therapy and to preoperatively screen patients who are at high risk. Some of the more common tests are discussed here.

The **platelet count** is simple. It is performed on most hospitalized patients as a part of a complete blood count. Although the normal platelet count is 150,000 to 400,000 per microliter, spontaneous hemorrhage as a result of thrombocytopenia is rare if the count exceeds 10,000 per microliter. Abnormalities in platelet function are not identified by this test.

Bleeding time is no longer used to assess coagulation disorders but is of historical interest. Essentially, bleeding time was assessed by making a small cut (1 mm deep and 1 cm long) on the forearm and measuring how long it takes to stop bleeding. There were various methods used to ensure that the test was performed in a standardized fashion, but it was always difficult to administer and difficult to interpret—and, as you can imagine, not particularly popular with patients. It was a crude measure of how well platelets, vessels, and coagulation proteins interact with one another, but it did not point to where the problem was if the bleeding time was prolonged or shortened. For this reason, laboratories are now using more sophisticated tests that directly measure the activity of platelets *in vitro*. The **platelet function analyzer** (PFA-100) is an instrument that measures platelet-dependent coagulation under flow conditions. Blood is forced through an aperture in a membrane that is coated with the extracellular molecule collagen, which is a potent activator of platelets. The time it takes for a platelet plug to form that occludes the aperture is called closure time (CT). Closure time is very sensitive to qualitative and quantitative platelet defects. This test, however, does not distinguish between specific platelet disorders and therefore is followed by specific testing such as platelet aggregation studies or von Willebrand factor assays.

The **activated partial thromboplastin time (aPTT)** tests for deficiencies in the intrinsic pathway of the coagulation mechanism. A sample of the patient's blood is drawn into a container containing citrate. The citrate binds calcium, an essential ingredient in clotting, so that the blood will not clot in the vial on its way to the laboratory. At the start of the test three ingredients are added: calcium; a surface contact material, such as finely ground glass, to activate the coagulation system; and phospholipid as a substitute for platelets. Normally, fibrin solidifies the plasma in this test in about 30 seconds. The test is sensitive to defects in the intrinsic pathway, such as hemophilia, but less sensitive to prothrombin, fibrinogen, or factor VII deficiencies. Once it has been determined that a bleeding disorder is caused by abnormalities of the intrinsic pathway of coagulation, specific tests are available to assess the function of the individual factors that might be deficient.

The **prothrombin time (PT)** is used to assess disorders of the extrinsic pathway of coagulation—that is, defects in the proteins prothrombin, factor VII, factor V, and factor X. It is less sensitive to fibrinogen deficiency. Factor VII activates factor X when tissue factor and calcium are added to the citrated plasma. PT is usually expressed in terms of the **International Normalized Ratio (INR)**. The PT will vary from laboratory to laboratory based on the reagent used in the test. The INR compares the patient's PT to that of the "normal" population recorded by the same test in the same laboratory. The normal ratio is about 1, meaning the patient's PT is the same as that of the reference population. The INR is used to follow patients on warfarin therapy. Patients respond very differently to the same dose of warfarin, so the dose needs to be titrated very carefully for the drug to remain in the therapeutic range but not make the patient susceptible to spontaneous bleeding.

Because neither the partial thromboplastin time (PTT) or the PT is very sensitive to fibrinogen, the **fibrinogen assay** can be used to measure fibrinogen levels. Measurement of **fibrin degradation products/ D-dimer** reflects fibrinolysis *in vivo*. The test is particularly useful in the diagnosis of disseminated intravascular coagulation and for screening patients suspected of having deep venous thrombosis.

Specific Diseases

In this chapter, we vary from discussing diseases in terms of genetic/congenital, inflammatory/degenerative, and neoplastic derangements. Bleeding and clotting disorders are more easily understood when classified as to whether they cause hemorrhage or clotting, and at what level they affect the clotting system. Rare genetic diseases, such as hemophilia or von Willebrand factor deficiency, affect a specific component of the clotting mechanism, but very often hemorrhage or thrombosis occur secondary to some other altered physiologic process. A wide range of diseases can result in injury to vessels, disorders of platelet number or function, or derangements of the coagulation cascade, from autoimmune diseases to infections, degenerative and nutritional disorders, trauma, neoplasia, and liver or renal failure. **Table 11–2** lists conditions that result in hemorrhage resulting from injury to vessels. It is provided to illustrate the diversity of diseases that can predispose individuals to this complication. It is not intended to be essential material that you should memorize or master for the purposes of understanding basic physiologic processes. Because this amount of detail can become overwhelming to the reader of an introductory text, we have refrained from providing comprehensive lists for the rest of the disorders leading to hemorrhage or

thrombosis discussed subsequently. Instead, we briefly mention only a few of the diseases that result in bleeding or thrombotic complications to illustrate the basic pathophysiology involved and to emphasize the need for close evaluation of the patient so that the underlying problem is diagnosed and treated.

Disorders Characterized by Hemorrhage
Vascular Disorders

The most common vascular causes of hemorrhage (Table 11–2) are trauma and diseases that erode blood vessels. In some of these situations, the cause and effect are obvious and bleeding is controlled by the normal hemostatic process or mechanically by the patient or healthcare worker. The petechial or purpural lesions that often characterize a hemorrhagic diathesis are usually not in and of themselves life threatening. The underlying condition may very well be, however. Internal bleeding may result in significant morbidity and even mortality. For example, **amyloid** is a protein produced in a variety of diseases but commonly, for no apparent reason, with increasing age. It is an insoluble protein that tends to deposit in vessels. When amyloid precipitates in the vessels of the brain, these become weak and susceptible to spontaneous hemorrhage. Because space is limited in the cranium, even a relatively small volume of blood can exert severe, life-threatening pressure on the brain.

Bleeding from vascular disruption, as occurs with trauma or ruptured aneurysms, may be life threatening because of circulatory collapse, or shock. Large volumes of blood can be lost from even relatively small arteries and veins. Worse, some internal bleeds, such as ruptured aortic aneurysms, may go undetected until the patient suddenly decompensates because large volumes of blood can be lost into body cavities (other than the cranium) before the patient becomes symptomatic. Once detected, immediate consideration should be given to stopping the bleeding and replacing the blood volume. If the bleeding site is accessible, pressure, suture, or a tourniquet can be applied. This may staunch the flow of blood, but access to a hospital is critical for definitive management. If sufficient blood is lost, saline solution is used as a first choice in volume replacement in the emergency situation. Replacement of red blood cells usually is not needed because the patient has a considerable reserve capacity, but blood volume must be replaced immediately to prevent shock.

Even when bleeding is not so severe as to be life threatening, the underlying disease may wreak havoc in other organs. **Henoch-Schönlein purpura** is a condition affecting primarily children. It typically follows an infection by streptococcal organisms, such as "strep throat." Antibodies produced against the organism react with proteins in vessel walls, resulting in inflammation of the vessels and subsequent bleeding. The skin rash, a "palpable purpura," is

TABLE 11–2 Diseases of Vessels Causing Hemorrhage

Cause	Pathophysiology
Trauma	Mechanical disruption of vessel wall
Infections Meningitis caused by *Neisseria meningitides*	Bacterial toxins damage vessel wall
Endocarditis	
Sepsis	Disseminated intravascular coagulation
Abscess/bronchiectasis	Erosion of infectious process through vessel walls
Genetic/congenital Ehlers-Danlos syndrome	Genetic abnormality in the production of collagen
Hereditary hemorrhagic telangiectasia	Thin, weak, highly convoluted vessels in mucous membranes and skin that tend to bleed easily
Berry aneurysms	Aneurysmal dilation in vessels at base of brain, is susceptible to rupture
Immunologic Drug reactions (many drugs have been implicated, including antibiotics, anticonvulsants, and diuretics)	Circulating immune complexes deposit in vessel walls, inducing inflammation
Henoch-Schönlein purpura	
Takayasu and other forms of arteritis	Inflammation (many of these are idiopathic) causes weakening of vessel wall
Metabolic/nutritional/degenerative/endocrine disorders Vitamin C deficiency (scurvy)	Vitamin C is necessary for the formation of collagen
Aging	Nutritional requirements of aging may not be met; collagen becomes structurally weak with increasing age
Atherosclerosis	Atherosclerosis leads to aneurysm formation, weakening the vessel wall
Cushing syndrome	Excessive corticosteroid production consumes proteins necessary for maintaining vascular structure
Amyloidosis	Insoluble protein (amyloid) deposits in vessel walls, making them structurally unstable
Neoplasia Neoplasms of blood vessels	Neoplastic blood vessels are not as strong as normal ones
Other neoplasms	Tumor erodes into blood vessels (e.g., lung cancer)

often the first sign of this condition but usually causes no problems. The more significant problems are bleeding into the gastrointestinal tract, resulting in severe abdominal cramps, arthritis causing severe pain, and injury to glomeruli, resulting in acute renal failure. Renal failure may (rarely) progress to chronic dialysis dependence. Thus, though the initial manifestations of many of these diseases—particularly petechial and purpuric skin rashes—may look innocuous at physical exam, it is imperative that the underlying condition be rapidly diagnosed and treated.

Platelet Disorders

Thrombocytopenia (decreased numbers of platelets, variably defined as fewer than 150,000 or fewer than 100,000 per microliter) can lead to diffuse and spontaneous bleeding. However, it is infrequently seen if the count exceeds 10,000 per microliter. The decision to transfuse platelets prophylactically to a patient without active bleeding is highly individualized; however, usually platelets are not transfused if the count exceeds 30,000–50,000 per microliter. The most common manifestations of decreased platelet numbers are petechial hemorrhages, hematuria, and gastrointestinal hemorrhage. The cause of thrombocytopenia is either decreased production or increased destruction of platelets. Production problems are usually the result of bone marrow failure or destruction of the hematopoietic tissue. This can result from primary diseases of the bone marrow, such as myelodysplasia or myeloproliferative diseases, or be secondary to numerous medical, iatrogenic, or neoplastic conditions.

A bone marrow examination can confirm decreased megakaryocytes in the case of primary or secondary bone marrow failure. With increased platelet destruction, however, megakaryocytes will be normal or increased in number. Causes of increased platelet destruction are varied. **Idiopathic thrombocytopenia purpura (ITP)** is an autoimmune disease in which the body makes antibodies to platelets. The "tagged" platelets are rapidly cleared by phagocytes of the liver and spleen. ITP may be a primary autoimmune disease or a manifestation of other disorders of immune regulation such as systemic lupus erythematosus or HIV/AIDS. **Thrombotic thrombocytopenia purpura (TTP)** and **hemolytic uremic syndrome (HUS)** use up platelets faster than the bone marrow can produce them. TTP is an idiopathic syndrome primarily affecting adults, while HUS primarily affects children and older adults following a gastrointestinal infection. Both cause widespread formation of thrombi in small vessels, which in turn causes extensive tissue damage as well as hemolysis (destruction of red blood cells, resulting in anemia). Disseminated intravascular coagulation also consumes platelets as microthrombi form in the vasculature, but the underlying problem appears to be one of coagulation rather than of platelet numbers. Diseases of the spleen can cause excessive sequestration of normal platelets so that decreased numbers are present in the peripheral blood although adequate or even increased numbers are released from the bone marrow. This condition is called **hypersplenism**. Again, the list of causes of hypersplenism is long and includes such diverse conditions as portal hypertension, sarcoidosis, lymphoma, genetic storage diseases, tuberculosis, and malaria.

Disorders of platelet function may be hereditary or acquired. Hereditary disorders are rare but interesting because they help the medical professions understand platelet function. Patients with **von Willebrand disease**, an autosomal dominant disease, lack the plasma factor called von Willebrand factor. This factor mediates platelet adhesion and needs to bind to factor VIII to become functional. Patients with this disease therefore have abnormal tests of both platelet function and coagulation function (aPTT). It is important to identify these patients because they may not manifest significant bleeding problems during their daily lives but experience severe problems when they have to undergo an operation. Other hereditary platelet disorders include a deficiency of platelet receptors for von Willebrand factor, a deficiency of platelet aggregation and clot retraction, and deficiency of the release of platelet components.

Like most of the conditions discussed in this chapter, numerous acquired disorders can interfere with platelet function. They range from iatrogenic to genetic and metabolic (e.g., liver or kidney failure). Two examples are provided here: uremia and aspirin intake. In severe renal failure, waste products accumulate in the blood, a condition called **uremia**. Uremia induces abnormalities of platelet function, including impaired adhesion and impaired activation of platelets. The exact mechanism is not known. One pathway may involve circulating toxins that poison the platelets. **Aspirin** interferes with platelets' ability to synthesize the prostaglandin thromboxane A_2. This is one of the first chemical products to be released from platelets when they are activated and facilitates platelet aggregation and adhesion. If aspirin is taken occasionally for a small pain, the inhibition of thromboxane A_2 does not cause any problem. If it is taken chronically for pain, such as arthritis, it can cause serious damage to the gastrointestinal mucosa and result in ulcers, which are not only painful but also have a propensity to bleed. However, taken at small doses on a daily basis, aspirin does not cause gastrointestinal hemorrhage and can prevent the formation of thrombi in critical vessels such as the carotid or coronary arteries. This is the rationale for administration of a daily "baby aspirin" (81 mg) to older patients or those at risk for coronary or cerebral events.

Coagulation Disorders

Coagulation disorders may also be hereditary or acquired. Hereditary disorders have greatly enhanced the medical professions' understanding of the role of the various coagulation factors. Hemophilia is the most common of the hereditary coagulation disorders, and both forms of it are sex-linked. The genes for the two most common forms of hemophilia are present on the X chromosome, so males are affected while females require two defective genes to manifest the disease. Though this can occur, it is extremely rare. **Hemophilia A**, or classic hemophilia, is a deficiency of factor VIII and occurs in about 1 of 5,000 males. Twenty percent of these appear to be new mutants—that is, there is no family history of the disease. This was a prevalent disease among European royalty. Queen Victoria was a carrier of the defective X chromosome and passed it on, via one of her sons and two of her daughters, to the royal houses of Spain, Russia, and Prussia. **Hemophilia B**, or Christmas disease, is a deficiency of factor IX and is about one-tenth as common as hemophilia A. Persons with hemophilia bleed into joints, muscle, and soft tissues and can bleed excessively from minor operations such as circumcision or tooth extraction. The diagnosis is based on the history of bleeding, screening tests that indicate a coagulation factor defect (platelet count, PT, and PTT), and specific tests for factors VIII and IX. Hemophiliacs suffer lifelong bleeding problems and typically become crippled by bleeding into joints, leading to degenerative arthritis. Factors VIII and IX are available commercially for lifelong replacement and emergency therapy, but they are expensive.

Other hereditary coagulation disorders are autosomally transmitted, much rarer, usually less severe, and lack specific treatment. Fresh-frozen plasma may be used to provide the missing factor in emergencies or prior to an operation.

Acquired coagulation disorders are much more common than are inherited ones. These can be caused by inadequate production of coagulation factors, excessive destruction of coagulation factors, or drugs that inhibit coagulation. All of the coagulation factors circulating in the plasma are produced in the liver (except for von Willebrand factor, which is a product of endothelial cells). Severe acute or chronic **liver disease** may be associated with bleeding because of deficiency of one or more of these factors. Some of the factors require **vitamin K** for their synthesis. Vitamin K is a fat-soluble vitamin produced by bacteria in the intestines, so reduction of the bacteria with antibiotics or malabsorption of fats can lead to a hemorrhagic diathesis as a result of vitamin K deficiency. Newborns, who lack intestinal flora, are given vitamin K parenterally to prevent **hemorrhagic disease of the newborn.**

Coagulation factors may be consumed rapidly by excessive coagulation, thus paradoxically superimposing a hemorrhagic diathesis on top of a coagulation process. This has led to the term **consumption coagulopathy**, which, in its most severe form, is disseminated intravascular coagulation. Another form of destruction of coagulation factors occurs when hemophiliacs who have received many transfusions of exogenous coagulation factors develop antibodies to them.

Potent pharmacologic anticoagulants are available to inhibit plasma proteins involved in thrombosis. Warfarin and heparin are the two most common ones. **Warfarin** reduces the amount of vitamin K available for use by the liver enzymes that produce coagulation factors. **Heparin** enhances the function of antithrombin, which in turn inactivates not only thrombin but also other molecules in the coagulation cascade. The two drugs are used in different clinical settings. Warfarin is used by outpatients who are at high risk for clot formation. It can be taken orally, takes a long time to reach therapeutic levels, and has a long-term effect. Heparin is used acutely to prevent clot formation in high-risk, hospitalized patients. Its half-life is only 90 minutes, and it is administered intravenously or subcutaneously. The doses of warfarin and heparin have to be titrated very carefully so as to prevent the development of a hemorrhagic diathesis while still maintaining an effective anticoagulant effect. Heparin is monitored by aPTT, while warfarin is monitored by the INR. Protamine is used to treat an overdose of heparin; an overdose of warfarin is treated by administration of vitamin K.

Disorders Characterized by Thrombosis

Figure 11–4 illustrates Virchow's triad, the factors predisposing to thrombus formation. Vascular disorders, abnormal blood flow, and coagulation disorders all can lead to aberrant clot formation. Sometimes there is injury at all three levels, but an abnormality in just one can result in abnormal clotting. As with causes of hemorrhage, numerous underlying diseases lead to injury of the vessels, abnormal blood flow, or coagulation disorders (Table 11–1). The following discussion is not meant to be exhaustive, but rather to provide a rational scaffolding with which to think about these diseases.

Unregulated thrombosis is pathogenic in several ways. In small vessels, when there is critical or complete obstruction to blood flow, thrombosis causes ischemic injury to the tissue supplied by that vessel. This is the mechanism of injury in cerebral and coronary infarcts (cerebrovascular accident and myocardial infarction, respectively). Thrombi can cause diffuse tissue injury if they form extensively in very small vessels. This occurs in the thrombocytopenia purpura states (discussed earlier) and diffuse intravascular coagulation (DIC). Thrombi occurring in larger arteries or in veins usually do not cause injury by occlusion. Although they may be occlusive in large veins, there are usually sufficient venous anastamoses to drain affected areas adequately. Instead, large thrombi are pathogenic because pieces of them may break off and travel to other sites in the body. These bits of thrombi traveling in the circulation are called **emboli**. Thrombi forming in the heart over an area of infarcted myocardium may give rise to emboli that get carried into the systemic circulation and get wedged into small arteries of the kidneys or spleen. Emboli from the heart or carotid arteries are a very common cause of cerebral infarct (stroke). Embolism is the most common cause of renal and splenic infarcts. Thrombi forming in veins of the legs or pelvis may break off and travel via the right side of the heart to the lungs. This potentially catastrophic event, pulmonary embolism, has already been mentioned in other settings.

Once thromboses have formed, it is imperative to prevent their complications. Fibrinolytic agents, such as streptokinase or tissue plasminogen activator (tPA), can be given to attempt to dissolve clots before tissue injury has occurred. Equally as important is the need to determine what caused the clot in the first place. Every patient should be carefully evaluated for the presence of risk factors for thrombosis, because if the underlying disease is not addressed, the patient runs the risk of developing recurrent thromboses. If the underlying disease cannot be reversed and the patient is at risk because of constitutional factors, such as inherited mutations, s/he should be put on anticoagulant therapy. This may be a simple "baby aspirin" (81 mg), to interfere with platelet function, or warfarin, which requires close follow-up with serial INR measurements.

Vascular Disorders

Endothelial injury exposes extracellular molecules to platelets and coagulation proteins. These extracellular substances, such as collagen and tissue factor, are potent activators of platelets and the coagulation cascade. Injury to the endothelium is therefore a potent cause of thrombosis. Damage to the endothelium can occur at sites of infarction or vasculitis. The former is a common cause of thrombus formation in the heart. In fact, intraventricular thrombosis is one of the dreaded complications of myocardial infarction. Thrombosis can also occur at the site of an atherosclerotic plaque. If this occurs in small arteries, occlusion by thrombus can cause infarction of the tissue supplied by that artery. This is one of the mechanisms by which myocardial infarction occurs. Vasculitis more commonly affects smaller vessels. Remember that there is a lot of cross-talk between the inflammatory and coagulation cascades, so inflammation alone, in addition to exposure of tissue in the vessel wall, can potentiate coagulation.

Note that endothelial cells do not necessarily need to be denuded from the basement membrane to initiate thrombosis. Endothelial cells constitutively express anticoagulant molecules, such as prostacyclin, nitric oxide, or thrombomodulin. Any shift in the relative levels of pro- and anticoagulant substances can potentially lead to thrombosis. A number of factors appear capable of inducing such a shift, including increased pressure in the blood vessel, turbulent flow of blood in the vessel, bacterial endotoxins, toxins in cigarette smoke, radiation, and even circulating substances such as increased cholesterol.

The second element of Virchow's triad, abnormal blood flow, contributes to thrombosis in several ways. One, already mentioned, is that it can cause endothelial injury. Another is that when blood flow is turbulent, as for example over an atherosclerotic plaque or at the bifurcation of an artery, platelets are forced away from the center of the stream of blood, where they usually travel, to the periphery. This brings them into contact with endothelial cells and thereby increases the likelihood that they will become activated. The third is that when the flow of blood is turbulent, blood pools in some areas. Pooling or slower-than-normal flow of blood is called **stasis**. Stasis occurs, for example, in aneurysms, or pathologic outpouchings of a vessel wall. When blood becomes stagnant, platelets and coagulation factors are not carried away at a sufficient rate to prevent clot formation. Indeed, aneurysms, whether in cardiac ventricles, the aorta, or smaller vessels, invariably contain clots. Stasis also appears to be one of the mechanisms of clot formation in the veins of the legs and pelvic veins. If the valves in veins become incompetent or the action of surrounding muscles is reduced, the blood in the veins does not return to the systemic circulation as rapidly as normal. Sluggish blood flow or even complete stasis of the blood then facilitates clot formation.

Platelet Disorders

Abnormalities of platelet number or function are not common causes of thrombosis. **Thrombocytosis** (excessive platelets defined by platelet counts exceeding 500,000 per microliter) may induce thrombosis or, paradoxically, bleeding. Causes include idiopathic thrombocythemia, bone marrow hyperplasia secondary to loss or destruction of red blood cells, cancer, splenectomy, and inflammatory diseases. More common is the transient increase in platelets that follows trauma, operations, and childbirth, which, along with venous stasis caused by bed rest, has been incriminated as a predisposing cause of deep leg vein thromboses and subsequent pulmonary embolism.

Coagulation Disorders

Disseminated intravascular coagulation (DIC) is a clinical syndrome caused by diffuse, systemic coagulation. Multiple thrombi plug small vessels throughout the body. These rarely lead to ischemic complications. Instead, the clinical manifestations are dominated by bleeding resulting from consumption of coagulation factors and platelets by the microthrombi. Diffuse oozing from mucous membranes can result in tremendous blood loss and hemodynamic instability. Coagulation tests reveal many abnormalities and fibrin degradation products are elevated. DIC can be activated through either the intrinsic or extrinsic pathways of coagulation, but it is not a primary disease. It is precipitated by serious underlying disease such as massive trauma, shock, septicemia, or cancer, but it also can occur as a complication of pregnancy because of tissue factors entering the maternal bloodstream from the placenta. Treatment includes transfusion with fresh-frozen plasma and platelets to restore all the depleted factors. However, the most important therapy in DIC is treating the underlying cause of the coagulopathy.

Rare hereditary deficiencies of antithrombin III, protein C, or protein S cause spontaneous thrombosis. These proteins are inhibitors of the coagulation cascade; if they are deficient, thrombosis is not regulated very well. Spontaneous thrombosis may also be associated with a common inherited mutation in the factor V molecule, called the **factor V Leiden mutation**. This mutation causes a structural deformity in the cofactor factor V, making it resistant to inactivation by protein C. People who carry even one copy of this mutated gene (heterozygotes) may be afflicted with recurrent thromboses, usually deep vein thromboses. Homozygotes usually experience more complications. It is difficult to assess the prevalence of the mutated gene in the population because not everyone carrying it will develop complications or be tested, but it is estimated to be around 5% in the Caucasian population and much less in other races. The presence of the allele may come to attention when a young patient without risk factors develops recurrent thromboses or experiences repeated pregnancy loss. These manifestations prompt testing for the mutation. The co-presence of factor V Leiden and other inherited thrombophilic mutations, such as **lupus anticoagulant**, has a more than additive effect on the development of thromboses.

As with platelets, coagulation factors are increased after trauma, operations, and childbirth, thus contributing to the tendency to form thrombi under these conditions.

Practice Questions

1. Which of the following accurately states the difference between hemostasis and coagulation?
   A. Hemostasis refers to the pathologic stagnation of blood in vessels, whereas coagulation refers to the solidification of plasma.
   B. Hemostasis primarily involves endothelial cells, whereas coagulation primarily involves platelets.
   C. Hemostasis refers to the formation of a thrombus, whereas coagulation refers to activation of the clotting cascade.
   D. Hemostasis refers to cessation of blood flow through an injured vessel, whereas coagulation refers to solidification of plasma.
   E. Hemostasis and coagulation are synonymous terms.

2. Proteins of the coagulation cascade, and their inhibitors, are primarily produced by
   A. enzymes in the liver.
   B. stem cells in the bone marrow.
   C. reticuloendothelial cells in the spleen.
   D. endothelial cells lining blood vessels.
   E. the coagulation cascade.

3. Factor IX is activated by
   A. tissue factor/factor VII complex.
   B. activated factor XI.
   C. activated factor X.
   D. thrombin.
   E. calcium.

4. A 64-year-old woman with hypersplenism runs the risk of spontaneously bleeding into her joints when the platelet count drops below which level?
   A. 100,000 per microliter
   B. 50,000 per microliter
   C. 25,000 per microliter
   D. 10,000 per microliter
   E. 5,000 per microliter

5. Of the following genetic conditions discussed in this chapter, which is the result of an inherited problem with platelet function?
   A. Hemophilia A
   B. Hemophilia B
   C. Von Willebrand disease
   D. Gaucher disease causing hypersplenism
   E. Factor V Leiden deficiency

Lung

OUTLINE

OBJECTIVES

1. Review the anatomy and physiology of the lung and describe the structures and molecules that contribute to ventilation.
2. Become familiar with the concepts of restrictive and obstructive lung diseases, and describe how they differ in terms of etiology, lung function, and manifestations.
3. Describe the deleterious effect of smoking on the health of the lung, and identify the diseases with which smoking is most strongly correlated.
4. List the most common and serious lung diseases.
5. Describe physical symptoms and clinical signs of altered lung function and laboratory tests that can be done to further define pulmonary diseases.
6. Describe the causes, manifestations, and treatment of congenital and genetic diseases affecting the lung (respiratory distress syndrome of the newborn, cystic fibrosis, and alpha-1 antitrypsin deficiency disease).

7. Describe similarities and differences among lobar, broncho-, and interstitial pneumonia in terms of cause, location, manifestations, predisposing conditions, causative organism, and treatment.
8. Understand the natural history of tuberculosis, in particular the difference between primary and secondary tuberculosis.
9. List some of the more common granulomatous diseases of the lung.
10. List the four types of obstructive pulmonary diseases.
11. Describe the causes, manifestations, and treatment of asthma.
12. Define chronic obstructive pulmonary disease and its relationship to chronic bronchitis and emphysema, and describe how chronic bronchitis and emphysema differ clinically and histologically.
13. List the most important acute and chronic interstitial lung diseases and describe the causes, manifestations, and treatment of each.
14. Describe the causes, manifestations, and treatment of various vascular disorders affecting the lung, such as pulmonary embolism, pulmonary hypertension, and pulmonary infarct.
15. Describe the clinical and histologic classification of pulmonary neoplasms, and become familiar with the staging system for lung cancer.
16. Describe the causes, manifestations, and treatment of lung cancers.
17. Define, describe, and be able to use in context all the words in bold print in this chapter.

KEY TERMS

abscess
acidosis
acute respiratory distress
   syndrome (ARDS)
alpha-1 antitrypsin
   deficiency disease
alveolus
anthracosis

apnea
asbestosis
Aspergillus
asthma
atelectasis
Blastomyces
bronchiectasis
bronchoscopy

chronic bronchitis
chronic obstructive
    pulmonary disease
    (COPD)
Coccidioides
Cryptococcus
cyanosis
cystic fibrosis
diffuse alveolar damage
    (DAD)
diffuse idiopathic
    pulmonary fibrosis
diffusion
diffusion capacity
dyspnea
elastin
emphysema
empyema
granuloma
hemoptysis
Histoplasma
honeycomb lung
hyaline membrane disease
hypercapnia
hypersensitivity
    pneumonitis
hypoxemia

mucociliary escalator
mycobacteria
non-small cell carcinoma
obstructive lung disease
orthopnea
perfusion
pleural effusion
pneumoconiosis
pneumonia
pneumonitis
pulmonary edema
pulmonary embolism (PE)
pulmonary hypertension
pulmonary infarct
restrictive lung disease
sarcoidosis
silicosis
small cell (neuroendocrine)
    carcinoma
spirometry
surfactant
tachypnea
tuberculin test
tuberculosis
vasculitis
ventilation

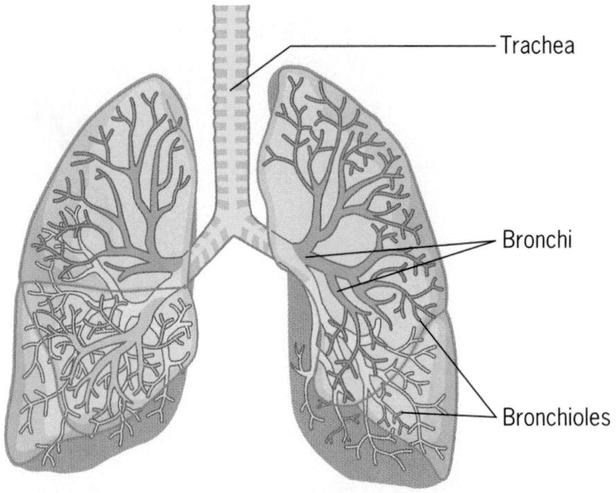

FIGURE 12–1 Gross anatomy of the trachea and lungs. The left lung has two lobes and the right lung has three. The trachea branches into bronchi, which in turn branch into bronchioles of decreasing diameter.

Review of Structure and Function

The main function of the lungs is to transfer oxygen from the atmosphere to the blood and carbon dioxide from the blood to the atmosphere. The lungs also serve as a filter of air and blood, and, like the kidney and liver, they are involved in the detoxification and excretion of certain toxins and metabolites.

To carry out its main function, air must be moved from the atmosphere to the terminal units of the lung, a process called **ventilation**, and gas must pass across tissue from air to blood or from blood to air, a process called gas exchange or **diffusion**. **Perfusion** refers to blood flow through the pulmonary capillary bed.

The ventilatory pathway is treelike, with the trachea as the trunk and branching bronchi as limbs. Bronchi occupy only a small fraction of the lung space compared with the air spaces (**Figure 12–1**). Movement of air in the tracheobronchial tree is brought about by muscular movement of the rib cage and diaphragm and elastic recoil of the lungs. Smooth muscle in the bronchial wall controls the diameter of the bronchi and thus the resistance to air flow.

The functional units for gas exchange are thin-walled, wide-mouthed sacs called **alveoli** (**Figure 12–2**). A cluster of alveoli with their associated respiratory bronchioles form an *acinus*. Alveolar walls, the structures across which diffusion takes place, are very thin. They consist of capillaries, a scant amount of connective tissue, and epithelial lining cells called *Type I pneumocytes*. Type I pneumocytes have very thin cytoplasm, much like an endothelial cell, and make up most of the inner lining of the alveolus. The endothelium of the capillary and

epithelium of the Type I pneumocyte share basement membranes in areas, providing a very short distance for gases to move across.

Two other very important cells reside within alveoli. One is the *Type II pneumocyte*, which secretes **surfactant**, a phospholipid that lowers the surface tension of the alveolar lining fluid, preventing the alveolus from collapsing during exhalation. Surfactant is not produced by the lungs until late in fetal life. This is one reason why premature infants are at risk for pulmonary failure: though the lung tissue is adequately developed, the alveoli cannot fully open without surfactant, and the neonate's blood can therefore not be adequately oxygenated. The other cell in the alveolus is the *macrophage*, which scavenges foreign particles that are aspirated into alveoli. Macrophages are also present within the connective tissue of the lung—for example, around bronchioles.

The pulmonary connective tissue contains a molecule that is particularly essential to its function, called **elastin**. Elastin is a tightly coiled protein that can stretch under pressure. Once the pressure is released, elastin recoils to its original state. This property affords the lung considerable elasticity: as the alveoli become distended with air during inspiration, the elastin fibers stretch, and their recoil helps propel the air out of the lung.

Although the skin, mouth, and intestines are more exposed to gross environmental contamination, the lung is more vulnerable because the lining of the distal air sacs is designed for gas exchange, not for dealing with foreign substances. Protection of the air spaces is provided by a specialized epithelial lining of the bronchial tree proximal to the acinus, called the **mucociliary escalator**. This epithelium is composed of columnar cells, some containing cilia on the lumenal surface and others producing mucus. The mucus traps inhaled

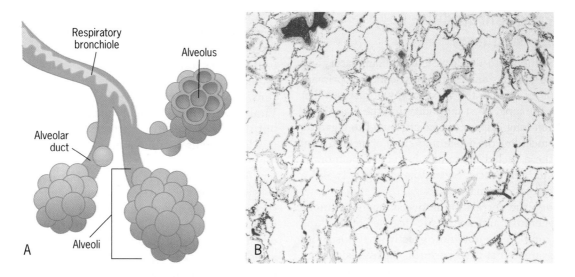

FIGURE 12–2 Histology of the lung. **A.** The acinus is composed of a respiratory bronchiole, alveolar duct, and the cluster of alveoli that receive air from that duct. **B.** The structure of the acinus is not easily seen on histology. Instead, the lung looks like a sheet of polygonal spaces enclosed by very thin alveolar walls.

particles, and the cilia convey the mucus upward toward the mouth, from whence it is swallowed or expectorated (spit out). When excessive material accumulates in the bronchi, the cough reflex helps expel it. Particulate material that does get into the alveoli is scavenged by alveolar macrophages.

Functional diseases of the lung can be classified as to whether they cause restriction or obstruction to air flow. **Restrictive lung diseases** are those that destroy the lungs' elastic property. These may be inflammatory diseases that adhere the lung to the chest wall so that it cannot fully deflate during exhalation because it is tethered to the rib cage, or muscular diseases that inhibit the action of the diaphragm or chest muscles so that the lungs cannot fully expand, or diseases affecting the connective tissue of the lung and destroying its elasticity, such as pulmonary fibrosis. **Obstructive lung diseases** are those that prevent the outflow of air through the bronchial tree so that air becomes trapped within the distal branches. Examples of obstructive lung diseases are chronic obstructive pulmonary disease, in which the bronchi are obstructed by thick mucus, and asthma, in which narrowing of the bronchi occurs through contraction of bronchial smooth muscle.

Before we turn our attention to descriptions of diseases, a few definitions are in order. The following conditions are not diseases in themselves but manifestations of other processes in the lung. **Atelectasis** refers to collapse of the lung. The lung can collapse for two reasons (**Figure 12–3**). Either there is external pressure on the lung causing it to deflate, or there is obstruction of a bronchus with secondary resorption of the air distal to the obstruction. External pressure can be applied to the lung from substances accumulating in the pleural cavity. Air, transudative or exudative fluid, lymph, and blood

can fill and distend the pleural space in various medical and traumatic conditions. **Bronchiectasis** is dilatation of a bronchus distal to a site of obstruction, with subsequent inflammation, bronchial destruction, and possibly abscess formation. It can occur in a variety of conditions—for example, following viral pneumonia, cystic fibrosis, tuberculosis, or aspiration of a foreign body. Bronchiectasis results in an obstructive pattern of lung function. The treatment of bronchiectasis requires removal of the offending agent, treatment of the underlying cause, antibiotics or anti-inflammatory medications, and, if it is confined to a single location and the inflammation does not clear, surgical removal of the affected segment of lung.

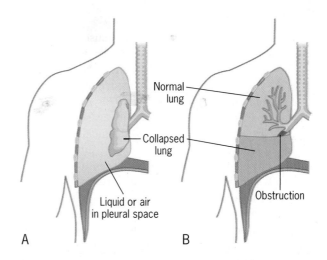

FIGURE 12–3 Atelectasis, or collapse of the lung, can be caused by external compression by liquid or air in the pleural space (**A**), or by bronchial obstruction and secondary resorption of the air distal to the site of obstruction (**B**).

Most Frequent and Serious Problems

The lung is subject to a wide variety of inflammatory and destructive diseases and is the most common primary site of cancer. Despite the wide variety of diseases that can affect the lung, most morbidity and the majority of deaths from lung disease can be attributed to cigarette smoking, including the deleterious effect of second-hand smoke. These include chronic obstructive pulmonary disease and lung cancer. Second-hand smoke is also a potent trigger of asthma.

Although the correlation between cigarette smoke and degenerative and neoplastic diseases of the lung is very strong, we do not know exactly what it is about cigarette smoke that is so harmful. Cigarettes contain thousands of different chemicals. It may be just a few that are toxic, or it may be a combination of some of them. Moreover, it is not just in the lung that tobacco smoke is harmful: smoking contributes to coronary artery disease, gastric and peptic ulcers, kidney and bladder cancer, pancreatic cancer, miscarriage, and low birth weight, among others. The cost to society for health care and time lost from work resulting from the negative health effects of cigarette smoking is exorbitant. The American Cancer Society estimates that smoking costs the nation $157 billion and causes 440,000 premature deaths every year. In the United States, laws that prohibit smoking in most public places and antismoking campaigns have changed general attitudes toward smoking. In the mid-1960s, about 40% of adults in the United States smoked, while by 2007, smoking prevalence had decreased to 20%. In other countries, especially those in which there is virtually no regulation of the content of cigarettes, their sale to minors, or smoking in public, and where up to 70% of the male population smokes (as in some Southeast Asian countries), the ravages of cigarette smoke on the population will be devastating.

In the United States, lung cancer causes more than one-third of cancer deaths in men. The lag time between onset of smoking and the development of cancer is about 30 to 40 years, so the current incidence of lung cancer reflects smoking trends from the 1970s and 1980s. In the early part of the 20th century, it was socially unacceptable for women to smoke, and the incidence of lung cancer in women was correspondingly quite low. This attitude changed in the first half of the century so that by the 1960s smoking prevalence among women was nearly that of men. Consequently, the incidence of lung cancer in women has also gone up, to the point that currently, lung cancer accounts for more deaths in women than breast cancer does. In contrast, in some nations, such as Scandinavian countries, the social "ban" on women smoking (at least in public) during the same time period has been quite strong, and consequently the incidence of lung cancer in women is low.

The lung is also the site of several important diseases that are not necessarily related to cigarette smoking. **Pneumonia** is infection of the lungs. It is most often caused by bacterial or viral organisms. Bacterial pneumonias commonly occur terminally in debilitated persons. Most pneumonias respond readily to antibiotics. Viral and mycoplasmal pneumonias are fairly common but rarely cause death. The term **pneumonitis** is used in a less specific sense to indicate inflammation of the lung usually limited to the interstitium. Pneumonitis may result from a viral infection, but it may also be a hypersensitivity reaction to inhaled organic dusts, such as mold particles or bird droppings, or a reaction to radiotherapy or drugs such as certain antibiotics or chemotherapeutic agents. Pneumonitis affects the alveolar walls, causing them to swell, and thereby hinders diffusion of gases across them. In chronic cases, pneumonitis can result in irreversible scarring and severe restrictive lung disease. **Chronic obstructive pulmonary disease** (**COPD**) is the combination of chronic bronchitis and emphysema that occurs almost exclusively in smokers, causes significant morbidity and disability, and is one of the most common reasons for lung transplantation. **Asthma** is a nondestructive lung disease that is most common in children and young adults. The smooth muscle of bronchioles constricts, impeding the flow of air from the lungs. Asthma may be an allergic reaction to inhaled pollens or dusts, but it may also be triggered by cold, exercise, or cigarette smoke. It requires considerable medical attention. Acute episodes are often severe enough to require emergency treatment. Deaths resulting from irreversible asthma are fortunately quite rare. **Cystic fibrosis** is the most common genetic disease in the white population. In the lungs, the genetic aberration results in the production of thicker than normal mucus in the airways. This tenacious mucus not only is resistant to clearance by the mucociliary escalator but also is an excellent culture medium for bacteria. Children with cystic fibrosis suffer repeated episodes of bacterial pneumonias, which eventually destroy the lung.

Symptoms, Signs, and Tests

Difficulty with breathing is called **dyspnea**, and lack of breathing is called **apnea**. **Orthopnea** refers to difficulty breathing while in a recumbent position. A person who is not getting enough oxygen breathes faster (**tachypnea**) and may often become frightened and anxious. A person not getting rid of enough carbon dioxide will be somnolent (carbon dioxide narcosis) and may even be unaware of danger. Partial obstruction of major airways produces noisy breathing, heard in severe cases even without a stethoscope as wheezing and rales.

Cough is caused by irritation of bronchi or accumulation of material, usually mucus, in the bronchi that needs to be cleared. The mucoid material coughed up from the lungs is *sputum*. **Hemoptysis**, the coughing up of blood, suggests serious destructive disease such as cancer or tuberculosis.

Physical examination involves observation of the rate and type of breathing. Tachypnea occurs in response to increased oxygen need, whether it be from lung disease or an increased metabolic rate, as occurs with fever. **Cyanosis** refers to blue mucous membranes or skin resulting from inadequate oxygen saturation of the blood. Percussion (tapping on a finger placed against the chest) may reveal dull or low-pitched sounds suggestive of underlying pulmonary consolidation or pleural effusion. Listening to the chest with a stethoscope can yield a cacophony of sounds. Bubbly sounds, called rales, are created by turbulent air–fluid mixtures and indicate transudate or exudate in the lung, as might be caused by heart failure or pneumonia. Wheezes reflect airway obstruction, as occurs in asthma or chronic obstructive pulmonary disease. Diminished normal breath sounds suggest consolidation or pleural effusion.

Spirometry, or pulmonary function testing, is the standard test for measuring the functional capacity of the lung. It measures the volume of air flowing into and out of the lungs during forced inspiration and expiration in relation to time. In **Figure 12–4**, compare resting *tidal volume*, the amount of air moved into and out of the lungs during normal respiration, to *forced vital capacity (FVC)*, the maximum amount of air that can be taken in and exhaled under strenuous effort. Forced vital capacity is decreased in restrictive lung diseases, which inhibit complete expansion or recoil of the lung tissue. Another informative measure is the forced expiratory volume in one second, or FEV_1, which is the volume of air that can be moved out of the lungs under maximal effort in 1 second. This measure is reduced in diseases that impede the flow of air out of large and medium-sized bronchi. Comparison of FEV_1 to FVC allows differentiation between restrictive and obstructive diseases: in restrictive disease, both FVC and FEV_1 are decreased, while in obstructive disease, FEV_1 is decreased out of proportion to FVC.

Diffusion capacity, or the facility with which gases cross the alveolar walls, is another measure of pulmonary function. Diffusion capacity is decreased in diseases causing inflammation, destruction, or fibrosis of the alveolar walls, such as pneumonitis, pneumoconiosis, or pulmonary fibrosis.

The ultimate measure of pulmonary function is the oxygen and carbon dioxide content of arterial blood. This is an indirect measure of problems with diffusion or perfusion. Whether gas exchange is impaired or the lungs receive inadequate blood flow, the concentration of gases in the blood is abnormal while the ventilatory rate may still be normal. Low blood oxygen is **hypoxemia**, and high blood carbon dioxide is **hypercapnia**.

Visualization of the lung tissue can be achieved by radiography: chest roentgenogram (x-ray) or CT scan. This is particularly useful to look for mass lesions in the lung, such as cancers, or diffuse processes that distort the normal architecture, such as pneumonia, pulmonary edema, or pulmonary fibrosis. Usually, the radiographic appearance is diagnostic, for example, of pneumonia or pulmonary edema. However, it may be necessary to determine whether a particular process or mass is inflammatory, neoplastic, or infectious. Sputum can be obtained for culture and cytology (microsopic examination of cells in body fluids). Biopsy of the trachea, bronchi, and lung can be taken during **bronchoscopy** (endoscopic examination of the trachea and bronchi). Fluid or tissue can be obtained from the pleural cavity or pleura for culture or cytology. If these techniques fail, open lung biopsy and histologic examination of the lung tissue may be necessary to establish the nature of the disease.

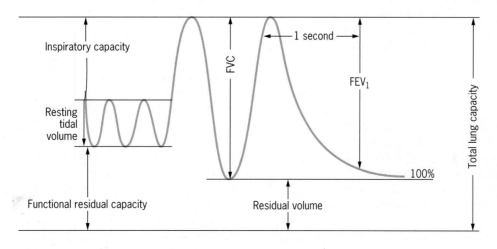

FIGURE 12–4 Pulmonary function test.

Specific Diseases

Genetic/Developmental Diseases

Congenital anomalies of the lung are rare. They include hypoplastic lobes, lobes with a separate blood supply (pulmonary sequestration), and cysts. At birth, pulmonary function suddenly becomes critical. **Hyaline membrane disease**, or respiratory distress syndrome of the newborn, may develop at this time if the lungs are not sufficiently mature. Cystic fibrosis is a genetic disease that slowly destroys the lungs as a result of repeated superimposed infections. Another classic genetic disease affecting the lungs is **alpha-1 antitrypsin deficiency disease**, which causes emphysema as a result of destruction of alveolar walls by uninhibited inflammatory enzymes. This disease is discussed in the section on chronic obstructive pulmonary disease because it is illustrative of the changes occurring with pure emphysema.

Respiratory Distress Syndrome of the Newborn (Hyaline Membrane Disease)

The importance of pulmonary alveolar surfactant is nowhere more evident than at birth. If sufficient surfactant is present, the alveoli will not just inflate but will stay open, allowing the diffusion of gases; otherwise, the alveoli collapse and are severely resistant to opening again. Surfactant production usually begins at about 20 weeks of gestation, but it is not present in sufficient amounts to sustain alveolar ventilation until very late in the fetal period. Surfactant is excreted into the amniotic fluid *in utero*, where it can be measured in samples obtained by amniocentesis. This is sometimes necessary when the mother's life is in danger and the fetus needs to be delivered as rapidly as possible. If there is insufficient surfactant in the amniotic fluid, surfactant production can be stimulated by administration of glucocorticoids to the mother before delivery is induced. Babies born before 28 weeks are at highest risk of developing hyaline membrane disease.

Hyaline membrane disease results not just from collapse of air spaces, but also from secondary injury to alveolar lining cells. Inflammatory exudate consisting of edema fluid and blood floods the alveolar spaces, and a proteinaceous precipitate rich in fibrin builds up in dilated bronchioles and alveolar ducts (**Figure 12–5**). This "hyaline" (pink and acellular) membrane further interferes with the exchange of gases across the already damaged alveolar walls. Oxygen therapy, which is essential in this situation, unfortunately causes additional injury to the alveolar lining cells at high concentrations. Thus, with treatment of the disease, the cycle of injury and hyaline membrane formation may continue. Exogenous (synthetic or animal) surfactants can be administered directly into the lungs. This reduces the severity of the disease and has reduced mortality by 40%. Ultimately,

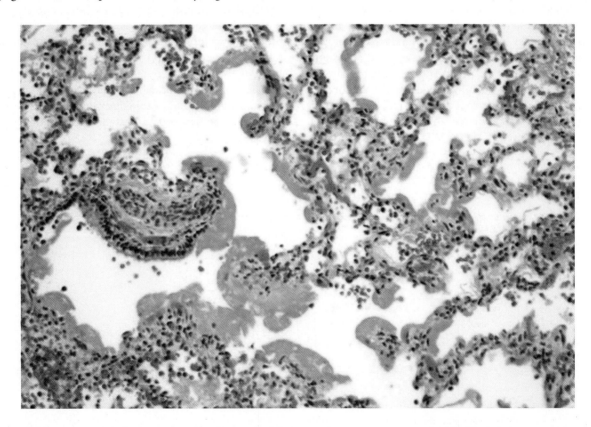

FIGURE 12–5 Hyaline membrane disease of the newborn. Dense pink, "hyaline" membranes line alveolar walls, which are additionally infiltrated by chronic inflammatory cells and have lost their lining of pneumocytes. (Courtesy of Dr. Michael Fritsch, Department of Pathology, University of Wisconsin School of Medicine and Public Health.)

however, the cure comes from nature itself: the lungs will begin to produce surfactant on their own if the infant can be kept alive long enough.

Improved management of this condition over the past two decades, including improved ventilation techniques and the ability to provide exogenous surfactant, has resulted in increased survival and has lowered the age and birth weight at which prematurely born infants can survive. Currently, mortality from respiratory distress syndrome of the newborn averages about 10%: it is higher in more premature infants and lower in those who are closer to term. Despite recent advances in management, however, respiratory distress syndrome is still the leading cause of death of premature infants, and infants who do survive may require prolonged oxygen supplementation because of permanent lung injury.

BOX 12–1   Respiratory Distress Syndrome (Hyaline Membrane Disease)

Causes

Lack of surfactant because of premature birth

Lesions

Inflammation (edema, hemorrhage)

Hyaline membranes lining alveolar walls

Manifestations

Tachypnea

Labored respirations

Cyanosis

Cystic Fibrosis

Cystic fibrosis is the most common genetic disease in people of European heritage. It is estimated that 1 in 20 white people carry the gene (it is very rare in black and Asian people). Cystic fibrosis is an autosomal recessive disease occurring in about 1 of every 2,000 white people, and about 1,000 people are diagnosed with this disease in the United States every year. Cystic fibrosis is caused by a mutation in the CFTR gene on chromosome 7, which codes for a protein regulating the movement of chloride ions across cell membranes of the sweat glands, bronchi, and pancreas. Exactly how this abnormality results in the clinical manifestation of thick mucus is not known. The pathophysiology appears to involve electrical and osmotic forces that draw sodium and water out of secretions to counter the effect of decreased chloride ions. In any case, the end result is plugging of various ducts and body passageways with thick mucus.

The earliest pulmonary manifestation of cystic fibrosis is a productive cough. The thick mucus in the airways promotes bacterial growth, and over time, the affected child suffers repeated bouts of pneumonia. The organisms that cause pulmonary infection in cystic fibrosis are *Staphylococcus aureus*, *Pseudomonas aeruginosa*, and *Burkholderia cepacia*. The last bacterium does not usually cause pneumonia in people without cystic fibrosis. As the disease progresses, additional manifestations of pulmonary injury occur: bronchiectasis, hemoptysis as the inflammatory process erodes blood channels, atelectasis caused by leakage of air into the pleural space through damaged pulmonary tissue, and eventually pulmonary fibrosis and pulmonary hypertension. **Figure 12–6** illustrates some of these changes. Patients with cystic fibrosis are also vulnerable to the development of an allergic reaction to a ubiquitous fungus, *Aspergillus*. In later stages, diffusion is hampered, so patients become dyspneic and hypoxic. Also, the altered architecture of the lung causes pulmonary hypertension to develop, so patients can eventually develop cor pulmonale.

It should be remembered that other organs are affected by cystic fibrosis as well. The thick mucus blocks sinus and nasal passages, resulting in chronic sinusitis. It can cause malabsorption and failure to thrive because of decreased release of pancreatic enzymes into the intestinal tract. Historically, the earliest sign described for this condition was salty-tasting skin. Though the disease affects the sweat glands, resulting in increased salt excretion via the sweat, this effect does not cause illness. Increased salt in sweat is the basis of one of the preliminary tests for cystic fibrosis, the sweat chloride test. Also, the manifestations of cystic fibrosis are variable: some people have primarily pancreatic disease, some have only pulmonary disease, and some cases of chronic sinusitis without pulmonary or pancreatic manifestations may be caused by an abnormal cystic fibrosis gene.

The treatment of pulmonary cystic fibrosis revolves around prevention and management of infection. Mechanical maneuvers to improve clearance of mucus, immunization against common childhood respiratory infections, administration of bronchodilators that increase the diameter of airways to facilitate mucus clearance, avoiding exposure to individuals with pulmonary infections, maintaining hydration to prevent further

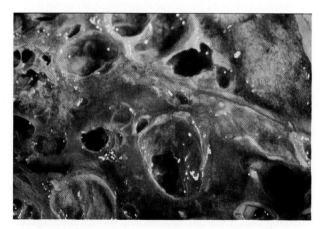

FIGURE 12–6 Cystic fibrosis. This is a close-up of the cut surface of the lung, showing large cystic lesions formed as a result of repeated bouts of infection, with resulting bronchiectasis and abscess formation.

thickening of mucus, use of prophylactic antibiotics, and prompt antibiotic treatment when infection does occur are the mainstays of treatment. Children with cystic fibrosis need to be frequently and carefully monitored. The care team usually comprises physical therapists, nurses, social workers, education specialists, and psychologists and includes support, education, and counseling for the entire family. With aggressive management, the development of end-stage pulmonary disease can be delayed, but not entirely prevented. Whereas half a century ago most people with cystic fibrosis died in childhood, now they mostly survive into their 30s. A genetic cure for the disease has not yet been found. Lung transplant, which is associated with high mortality, is reserved for people whose lungs are no longer able to maintain adequate blood oxygenation even with maximal medical therapeutic intervention.

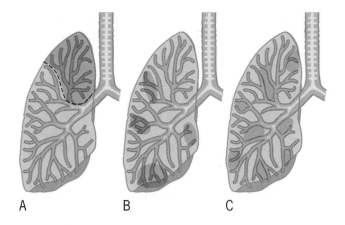

FIGURE 12–7 Comparison of lobar (**A**), broncho- (**B**), and interstitial (**C**) pneumonia in terms of their distribution in the lung.

BOX 12–2   Cystic Fibrosis

Causes

Autosomal recessive genetic defect

CFTR gene mutation (chloride ion channel)

Lesions

Mucus plugging of bronchi, sinus tracts, and pancreatic duct

Manifestations

Repeated bouts of pneumonia

Abnormal sweat chloride test

Bronchiectasis, hemoptysis, pneumothorax, pulmonary fibrosis

Extrapulmonary: failure to thrive, chronic sinusitis

Inflammatory/Degenerative Diseases

We group inflammatory/degenerative diseases into four categories: infections, chronic obstructive pulmonary diseases, acute and chronic noninfectious interstitial diseases, and vascular diseases.

Infections

Pneumonia

Pneumonia, or infection of the lungs, can be classified into three broad categories according to its distribution. *Lobar pneumonia* involves a discrete area of lung, often a single lobe, as the name suggests; while *bronchopneumonia* is a multifocal process, usually centered on bronchi, involving multiple areas of one or both lungs; and *interstitial pneumonia*, also called *pneumonitis*, is a diffuse process affecting the alveolar walls (**Figure 12–7** and **Table 12–1**). Histologically, lobar pneumonia and bronchopneumonia show alveolar spaces flooded by acute inflammatory cells, edema fluid, and fibrin (**Figure 12–8**). Pneumonitis, affecting the alveolar walls, demonstrates fewer inflammatory cells within the alveoli but thickening of the alveolar walls

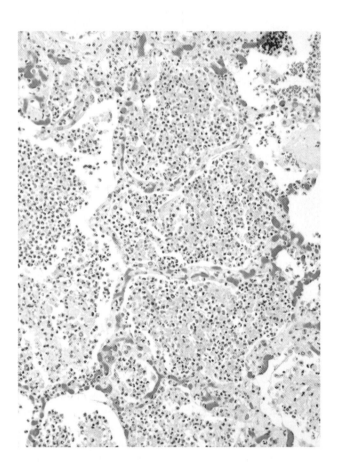

FIGURE 12–8 Acute pneumonia. Alveoli are filled with neutrophils and fibrin, and alveolar capillaries are congested.

as a result of the inflammation. The causative organisms and risk factors of these three patterns of pneumonia are different.

Lobar pneumonia is most commonly caused by *Streptococcus pneumoniae* (pneumococcus), a common resident of the mouth and throat that usually does not cause illness. Lobar pneumonia used to be the most common form of pneumonia and involved relatively

TABLE 12–1 Comparison of Lobar Pneumonia, Bronchopneumonia, and Interstitial Pneumonia

	Lobar Pneumonia	Bronchopneumonia	Interstitial Pneumonia
Most common organism(s)	• *Streptococcus pneumoniae*	• Gram-negative rods • Anaerobes • *Staphylococcus aureus* • *Pseudomonas aeruginosa* • Fungi	• Viruses • *Mycoplasma pneumoniae*
Symptoms/signs	• Dyspnea • Fever • Leukocytosis	• Dyspnea • Fever • Leukocytosis	• Upper respiratory tract infection • Mild symptoms
Radiography	• Diffuse consolidation of a single lobe	• Patches of consolidation throughout one or both lungs	• Diffuse lines and nodules in an "interstitial" pattern
Underlying condition	• Extremes of age, underlying illness	• Debilitation • Postsurgical state • Muscular diseases • Immunosuppression	• None
Histology	• Acute inflammatory cells and inflammatory exudate in alveoli	• Acute inflammatory cells and inflammatory exudate in alveoli	• Inflammation of alveolar walls

healthy as well as debilitated people. The bacteria and resulting inflammatory reaction spread through alveolar pores in a wavelike fashion, eventually involving the entire lobe of the lung. This form of pneumonia is diagnosed by the classic symptoms of respiratory distress, fever, and leukocytosis. Chest x-ray reveals lobar density (**Figure 12–9**). Examination of the sputum shows

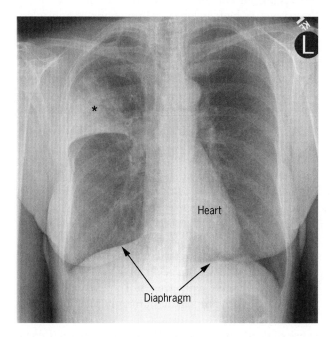

FIGURE 12–9 Chest x-ray of lobar pneumonia in the right upper lobe of an adult woman. Note the sharp demarcation of the pneumonia (asterisk) along the inferior edge of the upper lobe. (Courtesy of Dr. Donald Yandow, Department of Radiology, University of Wisconsin School of Medicine and Public Health.)

Gram-positive diplococci and sputum culture grows *S. pneumoniae*. Pneumococci are very susceptible to antibiotics such as penicillin, and the disease responds dramatically to treatment. In addition, the pneumococcal vaccine is an effective preventative.

Bronchopneumonia is caused by obstruction of small bronchi by mucus, aspirated gastric contents, neoplasms, or foreign objects. Organisms get trapped distal to the obstruction, multiply, and produce foci of infection. The location and extent of the infection depend on the underlying cause of the obstruction, the health status of the affected individual, and the nature of the causative organism. Many different kinds of bacteria and nonbacterial organisms can cause bronchopneumonia. In debilitated patients and those with abdominal infections, Gram-negative intestinal organisms, including anaerobic bacteria, are commonly the cause. In patients with chronic illnesses such as chronic lung disease or obstructing cancers, the bacteria causing the pneumonia are likely to be normal residents of the upper respiratory tract. Circulating bacteria in septic patients may seed the lung and cause multifocal pneumonia. Fungal organisms, such as *Aspergillus*, can also cause bronchopneumonia, primarily in immunocompromised individuals.

Two distinct forms of bronchopneumonia are aspiration pneumonia and Legionnaire disease. *Aspiration pneumonia* occurs when particulate material carrying bacteria, usually from the mouth or stomach, is inhaled and settles in the lower, more dependent lobes. This occurs most often in postoperative and debilitated persons and is enhanced by lack of full expansion of the lungs. The postoperative patient wants neither to breathe deeply nor to cough because both actions hurt, but both are important to facilitate the action of the mucociliary escalator. Debilitated and intoxicated patients and patients with intrinsic muscular diseases such as multiple sclerosis have difficulty "protecting" the airway; that is, the pharyngeal reflexes that normally prevent particulate material, such as food, from slipping into the trachea are weakened or defective. These patients are also at risk of developing aspiration pneumonia. *Legionnaire disease* is a bronchopneumonia caused by inhalation of the bacterium *Legionella pneumophila*, which lives in water storage tanks and cooling systems. The foci of inflammation can rapidly become confluent and affect large areas of the lung (**Figure 12–10**). This disease can be fatal if not treated in time.

Bronchopneumonia is more difficult to diagnose and treat than lobar pneumonia. It may require multiple sputum cultures to identify the causative organism, the pneumonia may be masked by underlying disease, and x-ray changes are less distinctive. Nevertheless, it must be detected quickly and treated effectively because it is a very significant cause of death in debilitated and bedridden patients with chronic diseases. It is also one of the most common causes of death in immunosuppressed patients, such as those with AIDS, those undergoing bone marrow transplantation, and organ transplant recipients. The organisms causing bronchopneumonia in these patients are usually harmless to persons with normal defense mechanisms. They include protozoa (*Pneumocystis jiroveci*), viruses (cytomegalovirus), fungi (*Aspergillus, Mucor, Cryptococcus*), and bacteria (*Staphylococcus,* Gram-negative bacteria).

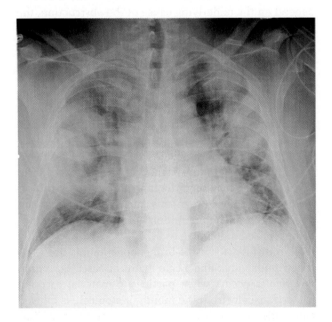

FIGURE 12–10 Chest x-ray of bronchopneumonia caused by *Legionella*. Note the fluffy, white infiltrates in all lobes of both lungs. (Courtesy of Dr. Donald Yandow, Department of Radiology, University of Wisconsin School of Medicine and Public Health.)

If bronchopneumonia is adequately treated, it usually resolves without any residual damage to the lung. In some cases, small scars may form at the periphery of the lung, but these are merely incidental findings and do not cause impairment of lung function. In severe cases **abscesses** can form. These are localized areas of suppuration and necrosis of underlying tissue. Abscesses can occur secondary to aspiration, obstruction of a bronchus by neoplasm, superinfection of an infarcted area of lung tissue, or sepsis, when bacteria circulating in the blood take up residence in the lung. Another dreaded complication of pneumonia is **empyema**, which is pus in the pleural cavity. This can occur if the bacteria spread from the lung to the pleural surface, or if an abscess erodes through the pleural surface and spills its contents into the pleural cavity. Abscess and empyema require surgery and drainage for cure.

Unlike in lobar pneumonia and bronchopneumonia, the inflammation of interstitial pneumonia or infectious pneumonitis affects the alveolar walls (rather than the alveolar spaces), and histologically there is a less pronounced acute inflammatory reaction. Interstitial pneumonias are often associated with an upper respiratory infection. They can vary in severity from mild and unnoticed by the patient to severe with cough, fever, and malaise. The most common cause of interstitial pneumonia is viral: influenza viruses, respiratory syncytial virus, rubeola (measles), and rhinovirus are well-known causative agents. *Mycoplasma pneumoniae*, a bacteria-like organism, is the most common causative agent, however. *Mycoplasma* is the cause of so-called walking pneumonia, or pneumonia that does not necessarily put the patient to bed, as lobar or bronchopneumonias do. The course of mycoplasma pneumonia can be shortened with antibiotic therapy. Antibiotics are, of course, not useful against viral pneumonitis, which is best treated with supportive measures such as rest and fluids. There is always the possibility, however, that inflammatory foci may become secondarily infected by bacteria, resulting in bronchopneumonia or abscess formation and necessitating antibiotic therapy.

Tuberculosis

In the latter part of the 20th century, **tuberculosis** (TB) came to be considered a relic of the past: it was treatable and hopes were high that it could be eradicated worldwide. However, the disease persisted with high prevalence rates in poor and crowded areas of the world, and in the 1980s the bacterium began to develop resistance to the common drugs used to treat it. Today, tuberculosis is again a major scourge of the human population. Along with HIV infection and malaria, it is the most common cause of death in the world. The problem of TB is compounded by its resistance to eradication by pharmaceutical intervention. Treatment of even non-drug-resistant TB requires a minimum of 6 months of therapy with at least four different drugs. These drugs have serious and often intolerable side effects, including hepatic toxicity. Drug-resistant TB requires treatment with additional antibiotics for longer periods of time. It is no wonder, then, that effective treatment is hampered by poverty, lack of access to drugs, and lack of access to health care. Moreover, incomplete eradication of the infection, resulting, for example, from premature termination of the treatment regimen, allows for the development of even more drug resistance in the bacteria.

Tuberculosis in humans is caused by *Mycobacterium tuberculosis* or *Mycobacterium bovis*. The former is more common and spreads from human to human via inhalation of aerosolized bacteria. It is the causative agent of pulmonary tuberculosis. The latter is transmitted by drinking infected cow's milk. It causes intestinal tuberculosis and is not transmissible from one person to the next. Pasteurization of cow's milk kills the bacterium, thereby preventing infection.

The natural history of pulmonary tuberculosis is very well known. The initial or primary infection is usually asymptomatic. To clear the infection, alveolar macrophages engulf the bacteria, but these are resistant to degradation by lysosomal enzymes. The tubercle bacilli not only survive but even replicate within the macrophages. Macrophages aggregate to form granulomas, which seal the bacteria off from the surrounding tissue, thus preventing them from spreading (**Figure 12–11**). Granulomas are most commonly found in the periphery of the lung and sometimes also in hilar lymph nodes (**Figure 12–12A**).

The bacteria may gain access to the bloodstream during the primary infection and be carried to other organs, including the brain, fallopian tubes, spleen, bone, or kidneys. Here they can lie dormant in granulomas for a very long time or cause slow and imperceptible—until extensive—destruction of the organ. Tuberculous meningitis is usually fatal, even if treatment can be initiated. Tubercular infection of the spine can cause repeated pathologic fractures and severe bowing of the vertebral column, a condition known as Pott disease. Infection of the fallopian tubes is a leading cause of infertility worldwide. If dissemination of the bacterium is extensive, many tiny granulomas form in multiple organs. This form of TB is called *miliary tuberculosis* (the individual granulomas look like small grains of millet—hence the name).

More ominous than the primary infection and its potential spread to other organs is the injury caused by reactivation of the infection in the lung. If the patient becomes immunosuppressed (old age or malnutrition may be enough to suppress the immune system sufficiently), or if the patient is reexposed to the bacteria, secondary infection occurs. Secondary infection is quite different from primary infection in terms of severity, location, and amount of tissue destruction. Because of previous exposure, lymphocytes now recognize the tubercle bacilli as foreign, resulting in a more rapid inflammatory reaction and greater amount of necrosis. The disease is usually

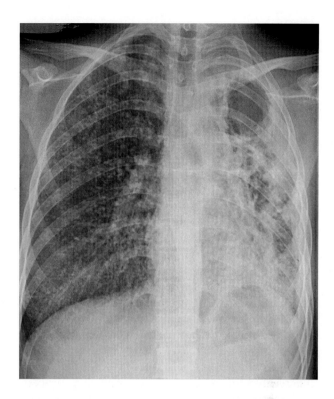

FIGURE 12–11 Chest x-ray of a person with tuberculosis. Numerous punctate and coalescing white nodules in both lung fields are granulomas. (Courtesy of Dr. Donald Yandow, Department of Radiology, University of Wisconsin School of Medicine and Public Health.)

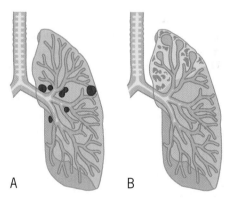

FIGURE 12–12 A. Solitary peripheral primary granuloma and secondary granulomas in hilar lymph nodes.
B. Advanced pulmonary tuberculosis with cavities connecting to bronchi, granulomas, and scarring of lung and pleura.

found in the apices (top) of the lungs because the organisms presumably grow better in the higher oxygen concentrations present there. The necrosis caused by the exuberant inflammatory reaction not only destroys lung tissue but may also involve and destroy bronchial walls. This allows necrotic debris to be sloughed out through the bronchi, leaving a cavity in the area of necrosis (**Figure 12–12B**).

Cavitary lesions are a hallmark of reactivated tuberculosis. Subsequent to the inflammation, the lung attempts to repair the damage, resulting in extensive scar formation. By the time the disease has run its course, the lungs are completely devastated by the combined inflammatory and fibrous processes.

In secondary or reactivated tuberculosis, the tubercle bacilli multiply unchecked within the areas of necrosis and are present in large numbers in the sputum and expectorated necrotic debris. It is during the stage of secondary infection that patients are most infectious. Moreover, during this stage the bacteria may again enter the bloodstream and disseminate to other organs. Patients with active tuberculosis may not experience any symptoms until fairly late in the course of the disease. Fever, night sweats, and weight loss are common complaints. These appear to be the result of release of cytokines such as tumor necrosis factor (TNF) and interleukins, which stimulate the acute-phase reaction. The cachexia for which tuberculosis was historically called "consumption" is also caused by the release of the acute-phase reactants.

Screening for tuberculosis is a multistep process. Initial exposure to the bacteria stimulates a delayed-type hypersensitivity reaction in the host. This is the basis of the **tuberculin test**: instillation of a small amount of inactive *Mycobacterium* antigen under the skin produces a large wheal in patients who have previously been infected with the bacterium. The test does not distinguish those with active disease from those in whom the disease is latent, however. Patients with a positive tuberculin test need to be further screened by chest x-ray. An irregular, spiculated lesion, especially in an upper lobe, is highly suggestive of tuberculosis, even in an asymptomatic adult. Definitive diagnosis must follow. **Mycobacteria** grow very slowly in culture: it may take 6 weeks or more for the culture to become positive. Newer molecular tests, which probe for specific DNA sequences present only in mycobacteria, yield results much more quickly. These are especially important in cases of multi-drug-resistant TB. Formerly, it took several weeks to confirm mycobacterial infection by culture, and several more weeks to determine which antibiotics the bacteria were sensitive to. Now, even the latter step can be done with probes for certain genes that are known to confer drug resistance.

Mycobacteria other than *M. tuberculosis* and *M. bovis* can cause serious infection in humans. *M. leprae* causes leprosy, which usually does not affect the lungs. In immunocompromised patients, bacteria of the *M. avium complex (MAC)* can cause serious infections. In the lung, MAC causes destruction similar to that caused by *M. tuberculosis*. MAC can also cause disseminated infection. In patients who are adequately treated for HIV, MAC can manifest as infection limited to the lymph nodes.

BOX 12–3 Tuberculosis

Causes

Mycobacterium tuberculosis

Lesions

Granulomas in lung and hilar lymph nodes

Secondary apical lesions with granulomas, cavities, and fibrosis

Isolated tuberculous lesions in brain, bone, fallopian tube, kidney, other

Miliary TB

Manifestations

Positive skin test

Apical lung lesions by x-ray

Coughing, including hemoptysis if severe

Dyspnea

Cachexia if advanced

Fungal Pneumonia

Most of the fungal organisms that can infect the lung are not primary human pathogens but rather grow in the soil or in bird or bat droppings. They are restricted geographically to the environment in which they can grow. *Histoplasma* occurs predominantly in the central United States, *Blastomyces* in the southeastern and midwestern United States, and *Coccidioides* in the southwestern United States, while *Cryptococcus* is found wherever there are pigeons, their primary host, and *Aspergillus* is present in soil around the world. These are the most common fungal organisms that infect the lung.

Primary infection with fungi may be asymptomatic but may also cause a flu-like illness, with fever, cough, rash, and muscle pain. The severity of the body's response to the organism is dependent on the amount of fungus that was inhaled. If the inoculum was very large, the primary infection can be life threatening. The characteristic pattern of symptoms that accompanies primary infection with *Coccidioides* is called San Joaquin Valley fever. It usually occurs in people who have a sudden, large exposure to aerosolized dust from soil, such as archaeologists who do not take precautions while digging in the Southwest. Once inhaled, fungal organisms can disseminate throughout the body and infect other organs. *Histoplasma*, for example, is notorious for infecting the eye, and *Cryptococcus* can infect the meninges, causing serious and life-threatening meningitis. Dissemination and its sequelae are more common, extensive, and serious in immune-compromised individuals.

What happens to the fungus after it has infected the lungs depends on the host's immune response and the type of fungus involved. The response to *Histoplasma* is granulomatous. Like mycobacteria, macrophages cannot entirely kill *Histoplasma* organisms, so they form granulomas around them. Over time, these become calcified, and small granulomas can also develop in lymph nodes, mimicking tuberculosis. The acute response to *Coccidioides*, *Blastomyces*, and *Cryptococcus* is usually an acute, neutrophilic pneumonia, but eventually necrotizing granulomas develop in response to these organisms as well. Over time, there can be destruction of the lung tissue by continued inflammation, cavitary lesions, bronchiectasis, and/or fibrosis.

The host's response to *Aspergillus* is most varied. The organisms can form tightly packed colonies, called fungus balls, inhabiting a preexisting space in the lung, such as an abscess cavity in an alcoholic patient who had prior bouts of aspiration pneumonia. These fungus balls, dramatic as they may appear, usually do not elicit much of a host reaction and are therefore clinically silent until they erode into an artery or bronchus. The host may develop a hypersensitivity reaction to *Aspergillus* antigens, however. This is called allergic bronchopulmonary aspergillosis. In severely immunocompromised individuals, the *Aspergillus* organism can become invasive, directly breaching vessel walls and embolizing to distant tissues (**Figure 12–13**). The host response to disseminated infection is very brisk, and the patient can easily succumb to a septic-shock-like illness.

The fungus can be seen in tissue biopsies with special stains; however, definitive diagnosis must be made in the microbiology laboratory. Antifungal medications are available. Some work better for different types of organisms, but therapy is usually prolonged and associated with toxicity. It is not necessary to treat latent infection, for example, of *Histoplasma*, because the likelihood that it will reactivate and lead to serious complications is very low. Unfortunately, antifungal medications may not be effective rapidly enough in immunocompromised patients, in whom fungal infections are serious and often deadly.

Obstructive Pulmonary Diseases

Obstructive disease of the lung occurs when there is partial impediment of the flow of air through bronchi, leading to inadequate ventilation. Obstructive conditions include chronic bronchitis, emphysema, asthma, and bronchiectasis. The term *chronic obstructive pulmonary disease* (COPD) has come to mean the combination of chronic bronchitis and emphysema that develops almost exclusively in smokers. In this section, we discuss asthma, chronic bronchitis, and emphysema. Bronchiectasis is a complication of underlying disease, such as cystic fibrosis, and the obstructive symptoms of bronchiectasis are usually present along with other manifestations of the disease, such as infection and restriction resulting from pulmonary fibrosis.

Blockage of air flow through bronchi results in similar symptoms regardless of the underlying disease. Wheezing as a result of turbulent air flow through partially blocked bronchi, cough as a result of excessive production of mucin, and dyspnea and tachypnea as gas exchange is impeded are common findings. Spirometry indicates a near-normal FVC but a markedly decreased FEV_1 because of the resistance to air flow out of the bronchi. Chest x-ray may not reveal any changes.

Asthma

Asthma results from spasm of bronchi. It is episodic: certain triggers cause bronchospasm, and removal of the trigger usually resolves the bronchial obstruction. The patient appears normal between episodes. During an asthmatic attack, the patient experiences "tightness" in the chest, is short of breath, wheezes with inspiration and/or exhalation, coughs, and may be quite anxious and frightened. There is also excessive mucus formation during an attack, which the patient coughs up during

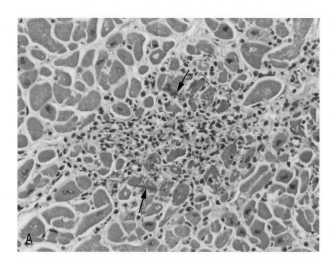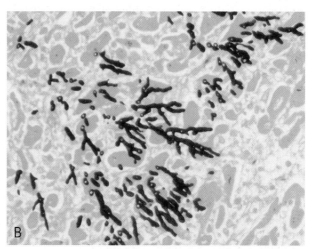

FIGURE 12–13 Invasive *Aspergillus*. These photomicrographs are from the heart of a patient who died of disseminated *Aspergillus* infection. **A.** H&E stained section. The fungi (arrows) have invaded the heart muscle and elicited the formation of microabscesses. **B.** Gomori methenamine silver stains the walls of the fungal hyphae black. The myocardiocytes are green. This stain highlights many more organisms than were appreciated on the original H&E stained sections.

recovery. There is no permanent damage to the lung, but in severe, chronic cases histologic changes, such as bronchial muscle hypertrophy and hyperplasia of mucous glands, do occur. The diagnosis of asthma is not made histologically, however: its diagnosis rests on the clinical demonstration of airway obstruction by spirometry and its reversibility by administration of bronchodilators.

Unlike chronic bronchitis and emphysema, asthma is reversible. Removal of the stimulus causing the attack reverses the bronchospasm, and numerous bronchodilating and anti-inflammatory drugs relieve and even prevent symptoms. The reversibility of the airway obstruction differentiates asthma from other causes of obstructive lung disease and is one of the characteristic diagnostic findings.

The pathophysiology of asthma involves external allergens or irritants, increased reactivity of the bronchi, and inflammation. Two different and not entirely understood mechanisms underlie the bronchospasm and inflammation of asthma. One is a type-1 hypersensitivity (allergic) reaction. This is called *extrinsic* or *atopic* asthma. The other is mediated by intrinsic hyperreactivity of the airways to irritants that do not trigger an immunologic response. Examples of such triggers are stress, cigarette smoke, exercise, cold, and viral infection. Most people with asthma are sensitive to irritants in both categories. Irrespective of the nature of the stimulus, the same medications reverse the bronchoconstriction and ameliorate the inflammation.

Atopic asthma is the most common type. It begins in childhood in patients who manifest other symptoms of allergy, such as rhinitis or eczema. The triggering agent is usually a common environmental antigen, such as pollens, house dust (cockroach droppings and animal danders are potent stimuli), and certain foods (e.g., milk). The antigen stimulates the release of histamine from mast cells and activation of T lymphocytes. The resultant release of cytokines results in inflammation with extensive bronchial edema and mucus production, and spastic contraction of the smooth muscle and bronchial walls.

The pathophysiology of nonatopic, or intrinsic, asthma appears to involve either direct stimulation of parasympathetic nerve fibers by the irritant or altered inflammatory responses in the bronchial wall. Certain drugs (e.g., aspirin) and chemicals used in occupational settings (e.g., epoxy resins, formaldehyde) can trigger asthmatic attacks after repeated exposure, through as yet unknown mechanisms.

If the trigger is known, avoiding exposure to it is sufficient to prevent asthmatic attacks. This is not always feasible, however, especially when the antigen is ubiquitous in the environment, such as ragweed pollen in the summer. Desensitization by repeated exposure to minute quantities of the antigen so that the body develops a protective antibody-mediated response to it may prevent the asthmatic attacks. If the trigger is not known, skin testing, which involves instilling a small amount of antigen subcutaneously and observing the size of the resultant wheal, can be performed. In cases of atopic asthma, skin testing often uncovers sensitivity to more than one antigen. In many cases, the allergen or irritant is identified simply by observation over many asthmatic attacks, as for example those caused by cold air or exercise.

Treatment is directed at reducing the reactivity of the bronchial muscles and mucous glands. The intensity of treatment required to control attacks is the basis of the clinical classification of asthma into mild, moderate, and severe. Some people can be treated simply with bronchodilators—agents that relax smooth muscle—administered at the onset of an episode of wheezing and tightness. Most cases of atopic asthma in children can be treated this way. In addition, most cases of atopic asthma in children become less severe with age. In more recalcitrant cases, patients may have to use bronchodilators continuously, as a prophylactic measure. Even small children can use a simple spirometer that measures the amount of air that can be forcefully exhaled to tailor when bronchodilators should be administered. This is a very effective tool that prevents asthmatic attacks and frequent hospitalization. Anti-inflammatory agents such as steroids may have to be added to the treatment regimen in severe cases.

"Brittle" asthma refers to severe asthma with persistent tightness, coughing, or wheezing between attacks, despite maintenance medication, and frequent, sudden exacerbations. Patients with brittle asthma require intensive medical control and are often hospitalized. A prolonged attack is called *status asthmaticus*. In the past, before effective management strategies were worked out, status asthmaticus was a not uncommon and dreaded development in asthmatics. In this condition, respiration is so compromised that gas exchange fails and the patient becomes severely hypoxic. Status asthmaticus is a fatal condition if it cannot be promptly reversed.

BOX 12–4   Asthma

Causes

Allergens

Viral infection

Other irritants: cold, exercise, drugs, occupational vapors

Lesions

Bronchial spasm

Inflammation

Increased mucus production

Manifestations

Wheezing

Dyspnea

Cough

Chronic Obstructive Pulmonary Disease: Chronic Bronchitis and Emphysema

Chronic bronchitis has a clinical definition: persistent cough with sputum production for at least 3 months in at least 2 consecutive years. Emphysema is defined morphologically: there is permanent enlargement of air spaces resulting from destruction of their walls (**Figure 12–14**). Chronic obstructive pulmonary disease (COPD) refers to the combination of chronic bronchitis and emphysema that occurs virtually exclusively in smokers. Not all smokers develop it, and some are affected more seriously than others. In some, chronic bronchitis may be the predominant manifestation; in others, emphysema may predominate. It is very unusual to find one without the other, however. The two conditions can occur in people who have never smoked, and there are certain diseases that may result in only one pattern of obstruction. Patients with cystic fibrosis, for example, may very well have chronic bronchitis as it is defined clinically because of repeated pulmonary infections. Patients with alpha-1 antitrypsin deficiency develop very severe emphysema, but without the chronic bronchitis.

Although chronic bronchitis is defined clinically, over time histologic changes do occur secondary to prolonged inflammation. Bronchial mucous glands become hypertrophic, reflecting the increased mucus production that occurs with chronic irritation of the bronchi. This mucus is responsible for the airway obstruction. Some degree of muscular spasticity also plays a role because the symptoms of COPD may be ameliorated with bronchodilators, as in asthma. Patients with chronic bronchitis tend to have frequent respiratory infections, because the air passages distal to the mucus plugs are not properly cleared. Cigarette smoke is thought to contribute to the disease in various ways. It appears to be the irritant that stimulates excessive mucus production by the bronchial mucous glands, and it inhibits the action of the cilia in the mucociliary escalator. In addition, irritation from the chronic smoke exposure and inflammation can cause metaplasia and dysplasia of the bronchial mucosal lining. Chronic bronchitis is treated with bronchodilators, antibiotics, and steroids, if necessary, but it is not reversed completely unless the patient stops smoking.

Emphysema is an obstructive disease because loss of the alveolar parenchyma causes reduction in the amount of elastin in the lung and consequently loss of the elastic recoil that keeps airways open. It is presumed that a toxin in cigarette smoke interferes with the balance of enzymes and free radicals in the lung so that these cause damage and eventually destruction of the alveolar walls. This is the mechanism of injury in alpha-1 antitrypsin deficiency disease. In this genetic disease, neutrophilic proteases are not scavenged when released into the tissue by the normally resident alpha-1 antitrypsin enzyme, and they procede to digest the lung parenchyma. Patients develop very severe emphysema at a young age, and the course of the disease is hastened by smoking. A similar process is thought to occur in the pathogenesis of emphysema related to cigarette smoke: cigarette smoke causes inflammation and thereby attracts neutrophils (or activates neutrophilic enzymes and free radicals directly), and the resident antiproteases in the lung cannot scavenge the released neutrophilic enzymes rapidly enough to prevent damage.

Emphysema can be classified as central, panacinar, paraseptal, and bullous, depending on the distribution of the involved air spaces. These different types tend to correlate with different etiologies—smoking causes central emphysema, or destruction of the alveoli immediately around the terminal bronchi with sparing of distal ones, while alpha-1 antitrypsin deficiency disease causes destruction of both central and peripheral alveoli, or panacinar emphysema. For practical purposes, however, regardless of etiology, the end result is destruction of the alveoli in all portions of the lung. *Bullous emphysema* refers to the formation of blebs or grossly visible bubbles. These develop most commonly in the subpleural portion of the lung, and they are very susceptible to rupture. When they rupture, air rushes into the pleural space, causing pneumothorax, atelectasis, and the sudden onset of dyspnea. This is one of the causes of death in COPD. Severe bullous disease can be treated by surgical excision of the bullae.

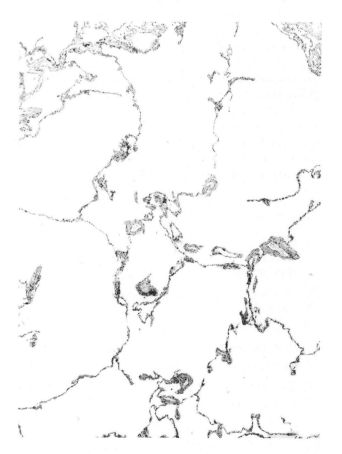

FIGURE 12–14 Emphysema. Compare the dilated air spaces in this micrograph with the size of normal alveoli in Figure 12–2B.

Both emphysema and COPD cause problems with ventilation. Essentially, air is trapped distal to the site of obstruction. This means that oxygen-poor, carbon dioxide-rich air is not exchanged effectively with fresh air. The total size of the lungs increases because of the trapped air, but despite the increased volume, most of the air in the lungs is "dead"—it does not contribute to gas exchange. The thorax becomes visibly expanded, hence the moniker "barrel chest." Radiography demonstrates not only a flattened diaphragm and increased space occupied by the lungs but also radiolucency of the lungs because of the increased air/tissue ratio (**Figure 12–15**).

Normally, the concentration of carbon dioxide in the blood regulates breathing by the respiratory center in the brain stem. Retention of carbon dioxide stimulates the respiratory center to increase the rate of breathing. With chronically elevated carbon dioxide levels, however, the respiratory center becomes used to the high carbon dioxide levels, and low blood oxygen becomes the stimulus for breathing. At this stage of the disease, oxygen therapy may kill a patient because it removes the stimulus for breathing.

Pure chronic bronchitis and pure emphysema have different clinical appearances. Chronic bronchitis presents as productive cough, recurrent pulmonary infections, and severe hypoxia, manifested as a blue tinge to the skin and mucous membranes. Patients with emphysema usually have more of a barrel chest as a result of the excessive air trapped in the enlarged air spaces. They use accessory muscles of respiration (chest wall muscles, for example) and sit hunched over to help elevate the diaphragm and compress the chest during expiration. The increased rate of breathing and use of accessory muscles consume a large amount of energy, and emphysematous patients are accordingly often quite thin. These characteristic appearances have inspired the clinical descriptors "blue bloater" and "pink puffer" to patients with primarily chronic bronchitis and emphysema, respectively.

Treatment of COPD involves a combination of supportive, medical, and surgical interventions. Smoking cessation is critical to treatment. Although it may not reverse the disease, it prevents further injury and is associated with decreased disability. Steroids decrease inflammation, bronchodilators help keep airways open, supplemental oxygen can be given, antibiotics are used to treat infection, and surgery may be necessary to remove areas of bronchiectasis or bullae or reduce the volume of lung that traps dead air and consequently prevents other portions of the lung, which are not quite so damaged, from expanding fully. Despite these interventions, COPD causes severe morbidity and mortality: it is the third leading cause of death in the United States, and death is usually preceded by many years of disability. Death in COPD is usually the result of severely compromised air exchange with severe hypercapnia and resulting **acidosis** (increased acidity of the blood, which is incompatible with the physiologic function of cells), cor pulmonale, congestive heart failure, or pneumothorax.

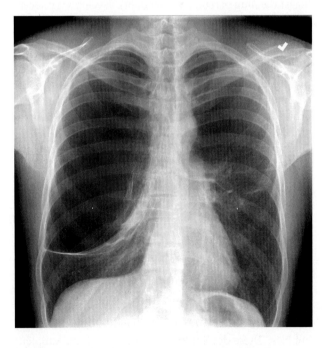

FIGURE 12–15 Chest x-ray of chronic obstructive pulmonary disease. The lung fields, particularly on the right side, are very radiolucent because of the decreased tissue (emphysema), and the diaphragm is pushed downward bilaterally because of the increased lung volume. (Courtesy of Dr. Donald Yandow, Department of Radiology, University of Wisconsin School of Medicine and Public Health.)

BOX 12–5   Chronic Obstructive Pulmonary Disease

Causes

Smoking

Alpha-1 antitrypsin deficiency

Lesions

Destruction of alveolar walls with coalescence of alveoli

Increased mucus production

Bullae

Bronchial spasm

Manifestations

Dyspnea, tachypnea

Barrel chest

Chronic bronchitis

Pulmonary infection

Increased work of breathing

Pneumothorax

Noninfectious Interstitial Diseases

Diseases of the interstitium—the alveolar walls—effect a restrictive pattern of lung injury. As the alveolar walls become infiltrated by an inflammatory process, edema fluid, or fibrosis, they become stiff and move poorly. This causes a decrease in the total volume of air that is moved in and out of the lungs with respiration as well as a decrease in the FEV_1. The symptoms of interstitial disease are similar to those of obstructive disease: dyspnea, tachypnea, and eventually cyanosis as the blood is no longer adequately oxygenated. Patients are also susceptible to the development of pulmonary hypertension, cor pulmonale, and pulmonary infection.

Interstitial lung diseases can be acute or chronic. The acute forms are pulmonary edema and diffuse alveolar damage. These two conditions are serious and potentially fatal and require intense medical management. They are not usually considered in the group of restrictive lung diseases, which classically refers to chronic, smoldering conditions that require very different interventions. Nevertheless, for the sake of illustrating how interstitial diseases cause ventilatory disturbances, we discuss the acute interstitial diseases here as well as the chronic ones.

Pulmonary edema is rarely a primary lung disease. It occurs when the body's fluid-handling mechanisms are overloaded or capillaries in the lung become damaged. In congestive heart failure, for example, the inability of the heart to move blood through the circulatory system results in pooling of fluid in venous channels and its seepage across capillary walls secondary to increased hydrostatic pressures. In the lung, the fluid leaks into the interstitium and then into alveoli, causing difficulties with ventilation as the interstitium becomes inflexible and the fluid in the air spaces restricts the diffusion of gases. In the setting of congestive heart failure, pulmonary edema usually develops slowly and insidiously. Patients generally complain of dyspnea when lying down, a condition called orthopnea. They may put several pillows under their head when sleeping: this causes the fluid to gravitate to lower portions of the lung, leaving the upper ones relatively dry and more capable of gas exchange. Pulmonary edema can also develop suddenly, as often happens with damage to the capillaries. Smoke, certain drugs or chemicals, and aspirated gastric contents are among the agents that can cause damage to the capillary endothelium and subsequent leakage of fluid into the interstitial space.

The damage incurred by acute injury to the alveolar walls induces acute respiratory distress syndrome (ARDS) as it is called clinically; histologically, it is characterized by diffuse alveolar damage (DAD). This condition is morphologically identical to respiratory distress syndrome of the newborn: inflammation of the alveolar walls and injury to the alveolar lining cells causes the alveoli to fill with edema fluid and red blood cells, and hyaline (proteinaceous) precipitates line the alveoli (Figure 12–5). The list of factors capable of causing DAD is unfortunately very long (Table 12–2). The most common causes are septic shock, diffuse pulmonary infection, aspiration, and head injury. Diffuse alveolar damage is usually global and in both lungs. The accumulated

TABLE 12–2	Short List of Conditions That Are Known to Cause Diffuse Alveolar Damage (Acute Respiratory Distress Syndrome)

Infection
- Overwhelming bacterial pneumonia
- Viral pneumonia
- Fungal pneumonia
- *Pneumocystis jiroveci* pneumonia
- Bacteremia
- Septic shock

Trauma
- Burns
- Near-drowning
- Lung contusion
- Head injury
- Fat or air embolism

Aspiration/inhalation
- Gastric contents
- Smoke
- Oxygen at high concentrations
- Corrosive chemicals

Iatrogenic
- Drugs
- Transfusion of blood products
- Radiation
- Contrast material
- Lung surgery
- Cardiopulmonary bypass

Metabolic or systemic conditions
- Uremia
- Pancreatitis
- Disseminated intravascular coagulation

Other
- High altitude
- Collagen vascular disease

Idiopathic

inflammatory cells and debris in the alveolar walls cause the lungs to become excessively heavy and stiff. At autopsy, they feel firm and rubbery rather than light and fluffy. ARDS is a very serious condition and fatal in more than 50% of cases. It usually develops very rapidly and requires admission to an intensive care unit. Treatment must involve removal of the offending substance, if known and if possible, and supportive measures, such as oxygen administration and mechanical ventilatory support, while the lung heals itself. The patient may recover completely, with no residual evidence of the injury, or may develop varying degrees of fibrosis, a condition known as organizing DAD.

Chronic diffuse interstitial disease develops slowly and often imperceptibly in patients who have repeated exposure to certain irritants. Often, the cause of the fibrosis is not known. These conditions all have in common fibrosis of the alveolar walls, which leads to restrictive disease of variable severity. Physical examination reveals dyspnea and tachypnea, with some abnormal breath sounds but no evidence of airway obstruction. Chest x-ray reveals normal lung sizes but diffuse shadows, nodules, or irregular lines throughout the lung fields, known as "ground glass opacities". Whereas in early stages there may be histologic variation in the appearance of the various diseases causing pulmonary fibrosis, by the time they have run their course the lungs all look the same: large air spaces are separated from one another by fibrous bands, leading to the name honeycomb lung (Figure 12–16), with superimposed infection and abscess formation. Replacement of the thin, delicate, and flexible alveolar walls by thick bands of stiff fibrous tissue results in the restrictive pattern of pulmonary function that eventually leads to dyspnea, cyanosis, pulmonary hypertension, cor pulmonale, and death. In addition, these lungs are susceptible to superinfection by bacteria (notably tuberculosis), fungi, and viruses.

Various conditions cause chronic, diffuse interstitial injury. Most of these diseases can be diagnosed clinically, on the basis of a history of exposure to a known irritant, characteristic radiographic appearances, serum tests for antibodies (collagen vascular diseases), and pulmonary function tests. Open lung biopsy may provide ancillary information but is not always necessary. Often, the cause of the restrictive disease is not discovered and the patient is treated supportively—in other words, with the goal of slowing down or ameliorating the disease process rather than providing a cure. Of the diseases causing chronic, diffuse interstitial lung injury, pneumoconiosis, hypersensitivity pneumonitis, sarcoidosis, and idiopathic pulmonary fibrosis are the most common. These are the ones we discuss in this section.

Pneumoconiosis refers to environmentally induced pulmonary fibrosis resulting from inhalation of particulate matter. Macrophages in the alveoli usually scavenge airborne particles that are small enough to escape entrapment in the mucociliary escalator and gain entry into alveolar spaces. If the load of inhaled dust is severe and/or chronic, however, the ability of macrophages to eliminate it is overwhelmed. Dust particles infiltrate the alveoli and set up a chronic inflammatory process that results in scarring, and activation of macrophages results in continuous chronic inflammation and resultant fibrosis. Pneumoconioses usually develop in the occupational setting: miners of coal, people who work with silica (glass cutters, sand blasters), and people who work with asbestos (a potent fire-retardant often used in insulation) are at risk of developing this disease. However, pulmonary fibrosis develops in only a fraction of exposed persons.

Anthracosis is carbon accumulation in the lungs and its draining lymph nodes. It is more severe in city dwellers, factory workers, and coal miners, who inhale carbon from pollution or coal dust on a more or less daily basis. Anthracosis is generally harmless because carbon by itself elicits very little fibrous reaction. It is often merely a startling finding at autopsy: coal-black lines and nodules criss-cross the pleural surface, stud the parenchyma, and darkly stain the hilar lymph nodes. In contrast, coal miners may develop progressive fibrosis after many years in the mines. Why coal should simply accumulate in patches of macrophages in one person and cause massive pulmonary fibrosis in another is not known. It may be that factors other than the coal dust itself, such as the concomitant inhalation of other, more pathogenic dusts and the person's innate inflammatory response to the dust, play a role.

Silicosis is caused by inhalation of crystalline forms of silica, such as quartz. These are potent inducers of fibrosis. The mechanism appears to involve recruitment of increasing numbers of inflammatory cells by cytokines released by macrophages that have engulfed silica particles. Lungs are initially involved with small nodules of scar tissue, which eventually coalesce to cause end-stage lung (Figure 12–17).

Asbestosis, a condition caused by the inhalation of fibrous silicates, can also lead to interstitial pulmonary fibrosis. Unlike carbon and silica, asbestos is a known carcinogen: both lung cancer and mesothelioma, malignancy of the pleura, are strongly linked to asbestos exposure. The effects of asbestosis are unpredictable, because many people harbor the fibers without obvious deleterious effect.

Another environmental and possibly occupational disease that can lead to end-stage lung is **hypersensitivity**

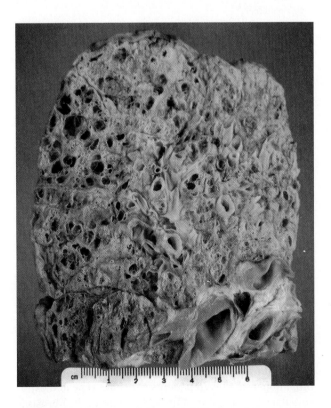

FIGURE 12–16 Honeycomb lung. This is the upper lobe of a lung of a patient who died of pulmonary fibrosis. No normal-appearing lung parenchyma is present. Spaces of varying sizes are surrounded by bands of fibrosis.

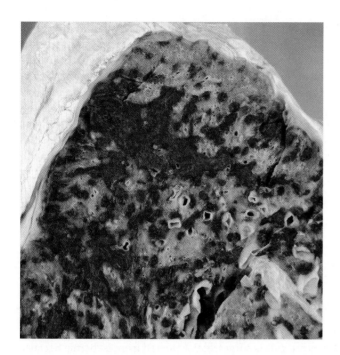

FIGURE 12-17 Close-up photograph of a lung affected by silicosis. The sharply delineated, black areas are coalescing areas of fibrosis that are stained dark by anthracotic pigment, possibly derived from coal dust.

pneumonitis. As the name implies, this disease involves a delayed-type hypersensitivity response to inhaled irritants. The irritant is usually an organic dust, such as molds (in hay or the soil used to grow mushrooms) or animal feces (the term "pigeon breeders lung" refers to this disease developing in people who are exposed to bird droppings). The list of dusts that can elicit hypersensitivity pneumonitis is very long (**Table 12-3**). It is imperative that patients who present with a restrictive lung disease be asked about their history of exposure to organic dusts in great detail because effective treatment of hypersensitivity pneumonitis requires strict avoidance of further exposure to the irritant. If such exposure cannot be avoided (e.g., in farmers who prefer to suffer aggravation of the disease because of repeated exposure

to hay rather than stop farming), the development of end-stage pulmonary fibrosis may not be preventable even with pharmaceutical intervention. The inflammation caused by repeated or continuous exposure to the organic dust affects the alveolar walls. Lymphocytes and loose granulomas infiltrate the interstitium, and the continuous, low-grade inflammation eventually results in diffuse scarring of the lung tissue. The end result is honeycomb lung, indistinguishable from end-stage lung caused by other interstitial lung diseases.

Sarcoidosis is a generalized, noncaseating granulomatous disease of unknown cause and with varying clinical manifestations. The organs most commonly involved are lung and lymph nodes. In some individuals, pulmonary fibrosis is the dominant process: these patients have a worse prognosis than others with predominantly lymph node disease. In disseminated disease, noncaseating granulomas can be seen in virtually any organ, including the heart, liver, skin, and eye. In the lung, small foci of granulomatous inflammation (**Figure 12-18**) eventually coalesce and result in scarring of the parenchyma. The disease may regress spontaneously or with steroid therapy; only a minority of patients develop end-stage pulmonary fibrosis. Sarcoidosis is most common in young adults and is more common in women, black people, and residents of the southern United States. The disease appears to result from the combination of an immunologic predisposition and exposure to an as yet unidentified, but possibly infectious, antigen.

Diffuse idiopathic pulmonary fibrosis is the clinical term that refers to a distinct pattern of lung injury whose cause is not known. In this form of interstitial lung disease, the fibrosing process begins at the periphery of the lung and moves inward to the hilar region. This pattern is readily detected by CT imaging of the lungs. Different

TABLE 12-3	Partial List of Dusts Known to Cause Hypersensitivity Pneumonitis

Agricultural Products
Hay, grain, barley, sugarcane, maple bark, soil used to grow mushrooms, compost, peat moss, cheese casings, grapes

Water (mist)
Humidifiers, air conditioners, saunas, hot tubs, indoor pools

Animals
Bird droppings or feathers, mollusk shell dust

Chemicals
Heavy crack use, plastics, paints, resins, beryllium

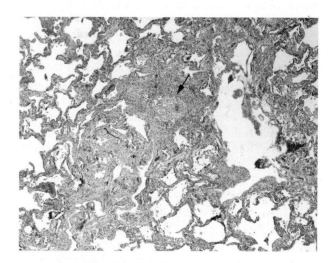

FIGURE 12-18 Sarcoidosis. The arrow points to a granuloma. There is increased fibrosis and the alveolar walls in the vicinity of the granuloma are thick and rigid in comparison to those in a normal lung (see Figure 12-2B).

areas of the lung show inflammatory and fibrosing lesions of different ages—that is, some areas are minimally affected while others are already severely fibrotic. The course of the disease is unpredictable and often fatal, despite administration of anti-inflammatory agents. Idiopathic pulmonary fibrosis is the third most common reason for patients to undergo a lung transplant in the United States (following COPD and cystic fibrosis).

BOX 12–6   Chronic Interstitial Lung Diseases

Causes

Inorganic dusts (coal, silica, asbestos)

Organic dusts (mold, feces)

Unknown

Lesions

Focal and diffuse fibrosis of the lung

Manifestations

Dyspnea

Pulmonary hypertension, cor pulmonale

Emphysema, tuberculosis, other infection

Vascular Conditions

Pulmonary edema results from left heart failure with resultant backup of fluid and increased venous pressure in the pulmonary veins. When severe or prolonged, fluid passes through the alveolar walls into alveoli and finally into the pleural space, producing a **pleural effusion**. Both interstitial fluid and pleural effusion cause restriction of pulmonary function.

Pulmonary embolism (PE) is a potentially fatal condition (this condition is also discussed in the "Vascular System" chapter). It results when thrombi in the leg or pelvic veins are carried to the right heart and pumped into the pulmonary arteries. Pulmonary emboli are sometimes apparent clinically but are much more often found at autopsy. In fact, it is notoriously difficult to diagnose PE clinically. Its presentation is variable but usually involves some degree of dyspnea of sudden onset, and there may be accompanying pleuritic chest pain. Especially when a large embolus occludes the pulmonary arteries at their bifurcation (called a "saddle embolus" because it sits astride the bifurcation point), PE can cause sudden death. If they are small and carried to the periphery of the lung, emboli often resolve without producing significant injury. Various conditions can predispose to the formation of pulmonary emboli, including prolonged immobility or bed rest, recent surgery, leg or pelvic fractures, pregnancy, obesity, underlying malignancy, airplane rides, or an underlying (and often unsuspected) coagulopathy.

Pulmonary hypertension has already been mentioned as developing in the setting of COPD and end-stage pulmonary disease and leading to cor pulmonale. Various other diseases, such as recurrent pulmonary embolism and autoimmune diseases, can also lead to pulmonary hypertension. The hallmark lesions of pulmonary hypertension are atherosclerosis—fatty streaks and plaques—in the intima of the larger-caliber arteries and, microscopically, thickening of the pulmonary arteriolar walls. Pulmonary hypertension is defined clinically as pressure in the vasculature of the lungs exceeding one-quarter that in the systemic circulation. The right side of the heart has to generate a much greater force to push blood against this resistance, and eventually right heart failure ensues. This can be caused by acute or chronic conditions. For example, acute cor pulmonale may result from pulmonary emboli, and chronic cor pulmonale is associated with emphysema and fibrotic lung lesions.

Pulmonary infarcts are rare because the lung receives its blood supply from two richly interconnected sources: the pulmonary arteries arising directly from the pulmonary trunk and the bronchial arteries arising from the thoracic aorta. Because of the collaterals between the two, lung tissue is somewhat protected from ischemia because even if one artery is occluded, the tissue is still perfused by the other. Nevertheless, especially in critically ill patients who suffer a pulmonary embolism in a medium-sized artery, infarcts can occur. They are based on the pleural surface and may cause pleuritic chest pain when they become inflamed in the course of the infarction.

Finally, various **vasculitic** conditions can affect the arteries of the lungs. Wegener granulomatosis, microscopic polyangiitis, and Churg-Strauss syndrome are poorly understood autoimmune conditions that cause inflammation of arteries and/or capillaries with subsequent ischemic damage of the pulmonary parenchyma. They are too infrequent to be discussed in detail here.

Hyperplastic/Neoplastic Diseases

Cancer of the lung is the most common cause of cancer death in the United States. Its relation to smoking has already been discussed in the opening section of this chapter. Benign lung neoplasms are rare and even less rarely cause any functional disturbance. They may present as incidentally found lesions on radiography, and be removed out of concern that they harbor cancer.

Most lung cancers arise from stem cells in the bronchial epithelium—hence the alternate term *bronchogenic carcinoma*. The pathologic classification of lung cancer involves determination of the type of cell the malignant ones resemble. The most common histologic variants are squamous cell carcinoma and adenocarcinoma. This classification is not very useful clinically, however. For the purposes of treatment and prognostication, cancers are classified as small cell and non-small cell carcinoma, of which non-small cell carcinoma is more common. This division is useful clinically because, in general, non-small cell carcinomas are potentially curable by surgery while small cell carcinomas, though they respond initially to chemotherapy, are not curable surgically and are rapidly fatal.

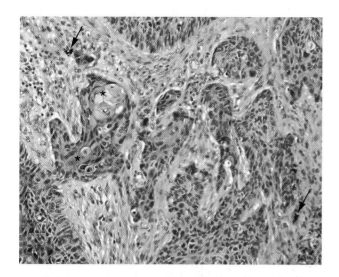

FIGURE 12–19 Squamous cell carcinoma. Malignant cells form irregular sheets of cohesive cells that recapitulate the epidermis, complete with keratin formation (asterisks). Mitotic figures (arrows) are frequent.

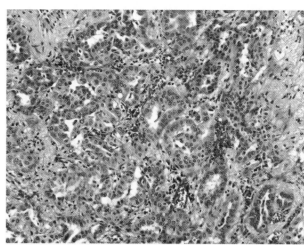

FIGURE 12–20 Adenocarcinoma. Malignant cells form irregular, haphazardly arranged glands.

There are numerous histologic variants of **non-small cell carcinoma**, some of which have a predilection for arising in certain areas of the lung. For example, squamous cell carcinoma (**Figure 12–19**) is more often central (hilar), while adenocarcinoma (**Figure 12–20**) often arises in a scar in the periphery of the lung. These carcinomas extensively invade adjacent tissues, such as the pleura, chest wall, and mediastinal structures. Some symptoms of the cancer can be related to direct extension of the tumor, such as hoarseness from involvement of the recurrent laryngeal nerve. Others are related to obstructive symptoms, as the cancer grows into and

occludes bronchi: dyspnea, pneumonia, and hemoptysis. Spread to lymph nodes of the hilar region is common, as is hematogenous spread to many organs. Metastasis to the brain and bone is notorious for producing clinical problems, and liver metastasis is pretty much universal in the terminal stages. The diagnosis may be suggested by x-ray but must be confirmed by sputum cytology and/or lung biopsy.

Staging criteria (**Table 12–4**) include the size of the primary lesion, the extent to which it has spread locally, and, of course, whether it has spread by the lymphatic or hematogenous route to lymph nodes or distant organs. As with

TABLE 12–4 Simplified Staging Criteria and Prognosis for Non-small Cell Lung Carcinoma

Stage	Description	5-Year Survival
Stage IA	• Tumor no larger than 3 cm, confined to the lung	80%
Stage IB	• Tumor size between 3 and 5 cm, confined to the lung, or • Tumor that extends to the main bronchus or invades the visceral pleura, or • Tumor that is associated with atelectasis or obstructive pneumonia distal to the site of obstruction	60%
Stage IIA	• Any tumor that qualifies for Stage IB and also has metastasized to regional lymph nodes on the same side as the cancer, or • Tumor size between 5 and 7 cm, confined to the lung	40–50%
Stage IIB	• Tumor between 5 and 7 cm, with metastasis to regional lymph nodes on the same side as the cancer, or • Tumor larger than 7 cm, confined to the lung, or • Tumor that invades structures beyond the lung (the chest wall, diaphragm, pericardium), or • Tumor that is associated with atelectasis or obstructive pneumonia involving the entire lung, but without nodal or distant metastasis, or • Tumor of any size with a separate tumor nodule in the same lobe	
Stage IIIA	• Any tumor qualifying for Stage IIB, with metastasis to lymph nodes on the same side as the cancer but more distant than the hilar region	25–30%
Stage IV	• Tumor of any size, with any degree of lymph node involvement, and with spread to distant organs (metastatic disease)	10%

all cancers, it is preferable to detect the carcinoma while it is still small and confined to the lung because surgical cure can be achieved. Most non-small cell lung cancers are detected in Stage III, however, when spread has already occurred and the lesion is no longer resectable. Screening for lung cancer is notoriously difficult. The malignant cells in invasive carcinoma destroy the surrounding parenchyma and cause fibrosis as they grow. This forms a discrete nodule by direct examination and a circumscribed shadow on chest x-ray (**Figure 12–21**). Radiography (chest x-ray or high-resolution CT) can detect small nodules, but this is neither specific nor cost-effective as a screening tool. Even if only high-risk individuals (smokers) were screened, radiography would detect far too many inconsequential nodules that would have to be followed with additional tests, thereby overloading the already creaky medical system with unnecessary follow-up testing. In addition, previous studies have shown that screening does not reduce mortality from the disease: in other words, although some cancers may be detected at an earlier stage, this does not necessarily translate into a survival benefit. Treatment of non-small cell carcinoma involves a combination of chemotherapy, surgery, and radiation therapy.

Small cell (neuroendocrine) carcinoma is morphologically and clinically distinct from non-small cell carcinoma.

Morphologically, it consists of sheets of poorly cohesive cells with scanty cytoplasm and numerous mitotic figures and areas of necrosis (**Figure 12–22**). Clinically, it is almost always detected when it has spread widely in the chest cavity and beyond. Surgical cure is impossible: chemotherapy and radiotherapy can prolong life but are not curative. This kind of cancer is most strongly associated with smoking. Some small cell carcinomas become manifest because they produce hormones in an unregulated fashion. The most common hormone produced by small cell lung cancer is ACTH, so patients might present with Cushing syndrome.

Small cell carcinomas are derived from the neuroendocrine cell lineage. A few other tumors of neuroendocrine derivation occur in the lung. The cells of these lesions resemble small cell carcinoma except for the blatantly malignant features. Well-differentiated neuroendocrine tumors, formerly called *carcinoid tumors*, usually do not metastasize and are essentially benign lesions that are cured with excision. The notion of a continuum of neuroendocrine tumors is reflected in the newer terminology, in which typical carcinoids are "well-differentiated neuroendocrine carcinomas," and small cell carcinoma is "poorly differentiated neuroendocrine carcinoma." Well-differentiated neuroendocrine tumors can develop in nonsmokers, and they tend to grow into the lumen of

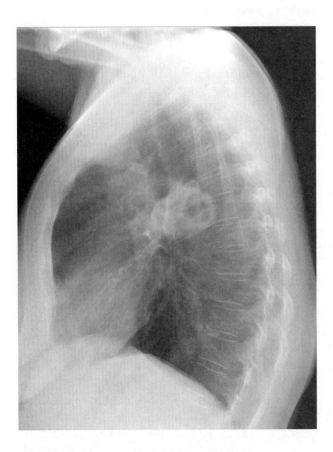

FIGURE 12–21 Lateral chest x-ray of an older adult woman showing a discrete nodule of carcinoma in the right upper lobe. (Courtesy of Dr. Donald Yandow, Department of Radiology, University of Wisconsin School of Medicine and Public Health.)

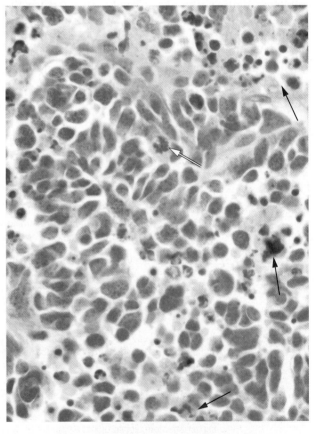

FIGURE 12–22 Small cell carcinoma. The white arrow is pointing to an atypical mitotic figure, and the black arrows are pointing to necrotic and apoptotic cells.

bronchi, causing obstructive symptoms including cough and pneumonia distal to the site of obstruction. They may also produce vasoactive amines, resulting in episodes of flushing, diarrhea, and cyanosis. This is called the "carcinoid syndrome".

The reason non-small cell carcinoma is not simply called large cell carcinoma is that "large cell carcinoma" occurs in both the non-small cell and small cell groups of cancer. This is where terminology gets incredibly confusing and it is not necessary to get into a discussion of these variants here. If someone speaks of "large cell carcinoma," they are most likely referring to large cell neuroendocrine carcinoma, which is a high-grade variant of neuroendocrine carcinoma.

Finally, the lung is the most common site of *metastatic cancer* spreading by the bloodstream from other sites. Microscopic tumor emboli can be carried to the pleura or to small vascular channels in the fibrous connective tissue of the lung. Here they may grow as linear streaks or nodules on the pleural surface or as expanding, usually multiple, circumscribed nodules within the lung parenchyma. The most common tumors to spread to the lung are the most common tumors in general: breast, prostate, and colon cancer. Also, because sarcomas preferentially spread via the bloodstream, the lung is a characteristic site of sarcoma metastasis as well.

BOX 12–7   Lung Cancer

Causes

Unknown

Smoking

Asbestosis

Lesions

Masses of squamous, glandular, neuroendocrine, or undifferentiated cells, usually arising from a bronchus

Manifestations

Dyspnea

Weight loss

Pneumonia

Hemoptysis

X-ray appearance

Organ Failure

Lung failure results when air exchange across the alveolar walls is compromised to such an extent that oxygen saturation of the blood is insufficient to maintain cellular respiration and/or carbon dioxide is elevated to such an extent that it causes acidosis of the extracellular environment, which is incompatible with life. Numerous diseases can result in lung failure. For heuristic purposes, they can be thought of as conditions that interfere with gas exchange across the alveolar wall and diseases that prevent the alveoli from filling with fresh air. Diseases of the alveolar wall include all the restrictive diseases mentioned

previously, including acute (ARDS, pulmonary edema) and chronic ones that lead to end-stage pulmonary fibrosis. In addition, diseases of the chest wall such as severe bowing of the vertebral column, rib fractures, or neuromuscular degeneration causing weakening of the muscles of respiration can result in inadequate ventilation. Atelectasis is another example of a restrictive lung injury that can ultimately prove lethal. Diseases of the alveolar spaces include obstructive diseases as well as various forms of trauma that prevent air from getting into the lungs (drowning, aspiration of foreign objects, or strangulation). Some medical conditions that do not primarily affect the lungs can lead to altered lung function and death. Decreased activity of the respiratory center caused by trauma or opiate toxicity can decrease the respiratory drive, for example.

Manifestations of lung failure can be sudden death, as occurs with large pulmonary emboli or atelectasis of both lungs; severe illness of short duration leading to death, as occurs with acute respiratory distress syndrome; or, in most cases, a long and inexorable diminution of lung function. In the latter case, respiratory failure is usually accompanied by the development of cor pulmonale and symptoms of right heart failure, including fluid accumulation in the legs and abdomen, cirrhosis of the liver, and portal hypertension. Death may also be hastened by superimposed pneumonia. Lung cancer may cause death by diverse mechanisms including infection, obstruction, and cachexia.

Practice Questions

1. Resistance to the flow of air through the bronchial tree is controlled by
   A. bronchial smooth muscle.
   B. the rate of production of mucus.
   C. surfactant.
   D. Type I pneumocytes.
   E. elastin.
2. Which of the following statements best characterizes the difference between restrictive and obstructive lung disease?
   A. Restrictive lung disease is reversible, whereas obstructive lung disease is not.
   B. Restrictive lung disease refers to restriction of the lungs' movement, whereas obstructive lung disease is caused by inability of the lung to inflate completely.
   C. Restrictive lung disease is characterized by a decrease in peak flow as measured by spirometry, whereas obstructive lung disease is characterized by an increase in the total lung volume.
   D. Restrictive lung disease is caused by destruction of the lungs' elastic property, whereas obstructive lung disease is caused by obstruction of the flow of air out of the air passages.
   E. Restrictive lung disease is more commonly caused by smoking, whereas obstructive lung disease is more commonly caused by infection.

3. What do cystic fibrosis, hypersensitivity pneumonitis, and idiopathic pulmonary fibrosis have in common?
   A. They are genetic diseases.
   B. They lead to the development of end-stage lung.
   C. They are the three most common reasons for lung transplantation in the United States.
   D. They are strongly associated with cigarette smoking.
   E. They begin in childhood.

4. *Miliary tuberculosis* refers to
   A. tuberculosis of the spine.
   B. disseminated granulomas in several organs.
   C. tuberculosis developing in military recruits.
   D. tuberculosis of the spleen.
   E. latent tuberculosis.

5. A 24-year-old woman presents to the doctor with shortness of breath, cough, and a low-grade fever. The symptoms began shortly after she moved in with her boyfriend, who lives in a three-bedroom house filled with exotic birds. She had asthma as a child, but the symptoms "are not like that." She most likely is suffering from which of the following conditions?
   A. Asthma, whose symptoms have changed as she has gotten older, triggered by bird feathers
   B. A conversion disorder because she feels neglected by her boyfriend who prefers the company of the birds
   C. Hypersensitivity pneumonitis, triggered by exposure to dusts generated by the birds
   D. Diffuse alveolar damage, which can be triggered by many things
   E. Sarcoidosis, which is unrelated to the birds or the boyfriend

6. A 26-year-old pregnant woman is confined to her bed because she fractured her leg in several places in a skiing accident. What condition should her physician be most worried about her developing?
   A. Bronchopneumonia
   B. Hyaline membrane disease of the newborn
   C. Pulmonary embolism
   D. Pulmonary infarct
   E. Acute respiratory distress syndrome

7. Which of the following statements about lung cancer is correct?
   A. Lung cancer is the leading cause of cancer death in men and women in the United States.
   B. Non-small cell cancer is not related to smoking.
   C. Lung cancer rarely metastasizes.
   D. Lung cancer can be detected in early stages with the recommended screening protocol.
   E. Women have a lower rate of lung cancer because they are protected by estrogens.

CHAPTER 13

Oral Region, Upper Respiratory Tract, and Ear

OUTLINE

OBJECTIVES

1. Identify the structures of the head and neck, their function, and the most common diseases of each.
2. Recognize the common symptoms of head and neck diseases, tools for visual inspection of deep organs, radiographic techniques, and other specialized tests to assess the structure and function of head and neck organs.
3. Compare and contrast cleft lip and cleft palate and identify their etiology, complications, and treatment.
4. Define dental caries and periodontal disease and identify what causes them, how they can be prevented, and their complications.
5. Identify the one bacterial causative agent of upper respiratory tract infections that it is necessary to identify and treat to avoid serious injury to other organs.
6. Identify the most common complications of upper respiratory tract infections in children, adults, and older adults.
7. Define sinusitis, identify its causes, and recognize the rationale for its treatment in the acute and chronic phases.
8. Define otitis media and describe its epidemiology, clinical recognition and management, and potential complications.
9. Distinguish between sensorineural and conductive hearing loss and compare and contrast the causes of hearing loss in the neonatal, pediatric, adult, and older adult populations.
10. Identify the most common malignant neoplasm of the head and neck region, and identify the risk factors that are implicated in its development.
11. Identify the complications that result from failure of the organs and structures of the head and neck.
12. Define and be able to use in context all words and terms in bold print throughout the chapter.

KEY TERMS

acute necrotizing ulcerative gingivitis	epiglottis
allergic rhinitis	eustachian tube
aphthous stomatitis	gingiva
audiometer	herpes stomatitis
cochlea	influenza
conductive hearing loss	laryngoscope
croup	larynx
deafness	leukoplakia
dental caries	malocclusion
dental plaque	Ménière disease
ear	mucoepidermoid carcinoma
	mumps

nose
obstructive sleep apnea
oral cavity
ossicles
otitis media
otosclerosis
otoscope
parotitis
periodontal disease
pharynx
pleomorphic adenoma
positive-pressure ventilator
presbycusis
pulpitis
salivary glands

sensorineural hearing loss
sinus
sinusitis
Sjögren syndrome
squamous cell carcinoma
tinnitus
tonsils
tracheostomy
tympanic membrane
undifferentiated
    nasopharyngeal
    carcinoma
upper respiratory infection
vertigo
vestibular apparatus

Review of Structure and Function

The importance of the head and neck organs is reflected in the number of specialists involved in taking care of the diseases arising in them. These include dentists, dental subspecialists, otolaryngologists, otologists, plastic surgeons, head and neck surgeons, and speech pathologists, to name just a few.

The head and neck, small as they are in comparison to the rest of the body, contain numerous structures that lie in very complicated and intricate relationships to one another (**Figure 13–1**). The oral cavity, including the teeth, tongue, and walls of the mouth, is part of the digestive system (mastication and swallowing of food), respiratory system (a secondary pathway for breathing), neurologic system (taste), and phonetic box for speech. The salivary glands (parotid, submandibular, lingual, and minor salivary glands of the oral mucosa) provide moisture to soften and add carbohydrate-digesting enzymes to food.

The nose is crucial to respiration, moisturizing air and filtering large particles from it as it passes through the nasopharyngeal passages to the trachea. Its upper portion contains the sense organ for smell. Bordering it on all sides are sinuses or air pockets in the bone. These are lined by respiratory mucosa that is continuous with that of the nose and trachea. The pharynx serves as a passageway for air, provides the musculature for swallowing, and contains the openings of the eustachian tubes, which serve as pressure equalizers for the middle ears. The pharynx also contains abundant lymphoid tissue, including the tonsils, which aid in the recognition of antigens such as foreign materials and microorganisms that enter the body via the air or food. The larynx is a major air passage to the lungs and contains the vocal cords. Lying over the opening to the larynx is a thick flap of tissue called the epiglottis, which folds over the larynx during swallowing to prevent aspiration into the trachea.

The ear detects sound and also contains in its inner portion the vestibular apparatus, which is a sensory organ for body equilibrium. The tiny bones, or ossicles, of the auditory apparatus lie in the middle ear. The canal leading to the middle ear from the environment, or the external ear, conducts vibrations in the air toward the tympanic membrane, which separates the middle from the external ear. Vibrations striking against the tympanic membrane are converted by the ossicles into fluid waves, which in turn get transmitted into the snail-shaped cochlea in the inner ear, where neural impulses are generated and transmitted via the auditory nerve to the brain. The vestibular apparatus consists of fluid-filled sacs lying at right angles to one another.

The neck contains large vascular channels that bring blood to and from the head and brain, large muscles that stabilize the head and cervical spine and control the head's movements, the thyroid gland, and numerous lymph nodes. The lymph nodes lie primarily in chains along the vessels in the neck. They are frequent sites of metastasis from carcinomas in the head and neck (e.g., larynx and thyroid) and chest (lung and breast), and they also frequently enlarge secondary to lymphomas and infections. The diseases affecting lymph nodes are not addressed in this chapter, nor are diseases of the arteries, veins, and muscles. In this chapter, we concentrate on the diseases that affect the organs in bold print in the previous paragraphs.

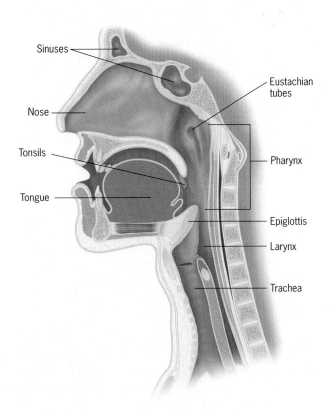

Sinuses

Nose

Tonsils

Tongue

Eustachian
tubes

Pharynx

Epiglottis

Larynx

Trachea

FIGURE 13–1 Anatomy of the head and neck organs.

Most Frequent and Serious Problems

Dentist's visits, the "cold" or "flu," earaches in children, sinus infections, and allergies are so common that people often do not even think of them as diseases. Because they do not cause much morbidity or disability, let alone death, people think of them more as a nuisance than a serious condition. However, together they account for a sizable portion of healthcare expenditure, for most doctor office visits, and for the most amount of time lost from school and work resulting from health issues.

Dental care provided by dentists represents about 5% of the total U.S. healthcare expenditure. The actual expenditure on teeth is much greater than the preceding statistic suggests, because that number does not include expenses for toothpastes, brushes, flosses, dental rinses and washes, and cosmetic products or the dental care provided in hospitals in the form of orthognathic (jaw) surgery. The central concern of dentists is avoidance and control of **dental caries**, or holes in the teeth created by bacteria, and **periodontal disease**, or inflammation of the gums that can lead to tooth loss.

Although people often do not even consider dental care as part of their overall health care, **upper respiratory infections** are not ignorable. The symptoms they produce stand out of proportion to the damage they cause to the body. They are estimated to be the cause of 40% of time lost from jobs and are one of the most common causes of visits to doctors for acute conditions. By far the majority of upper respiratory tract infections resolve on their own, but complications do occur. The most common is **sinusitis**, which results in continuous nasal discharge, headache, and facial pain. The infection can also spread into the lungs and even become complicated by a superimposed bacterial infection, resulting in bronchitis or pneumonia. An upper respiratory tract infection caused by the **influenza** virus can be fatal, especially in children, older adults, and people with an underlying medical condition. The influenza epidemic of 1918–1919, in which globally up to 100 million people perished, demonstrates just how deadly this disease can be. Epidemiologists are constantly on the alert to detect new, virulent viruses and develop and implement containment strategies before outbreaks can occur.

Otitis media, or inflammation of the middle ear, is often a very painful condition primarily affecting infants and small children. It is estimated that otitis media results in approximately two clinic visits per child per year. Hearing loss, or **deafness**, increases in incidence with age. It can be caused by a number of factors, from genetic abnormalities to degenerative diseases that destroy the middle or inner ears or the auditory nerves. A gradual diminution of acuity is the most common cause of hearing loss, affecting 30–35% of adults between 65 and 75 years of age.

Allergies, or inflammation of the respiratory mucosa and ocular conjunctiva secondary to environmental antigens, are also very common. Control of allergic symptoms, such as itching, swelling, and increased secretions in the eyes, nose (**allergic rhinitis**), sinuses, and throat, accounts for a large amount of healthcare dollars. Though it can be a considerable nuisance, allergic rhinitis is not life threatening.

Life-threatening disorders affecting the head and neck are relatively rare. Cancers of the head and neck account for only 3–5% of all cancers in the United States. Their incidence (excluding thyroid cancers) is approximately 20% that of lung cancer. The most common cancer in this region is **squamous cell carcinoma**, which usually develops in the oral cavity (gums and palate), on the tongue, or in the pharynx or larynx. Like lung cancer, it is strongly linked to cigarette smoking. Complete excision can be curative if the cancer is caught at an early stage, but treatment is often associated with significant morbidity, including difficulties with eating, swallowing, talking, and breathing.

Symptoms, Signs, and Tests

Physical examination of the head and neck includes visual inspection as well as palpation. Most dental caries are asymptomatic and detected by dentists and their assistants by careful visual examination of the teeth. Caries are holes dug into the tooth enamel by bacteria. If these holes penetrate deeply into the tooth to affect the nerve, they can cause very severe pain, but they can usually be visualized before they have caused that much destruction. Dentists also examine the tongue and sides of the mouth for evidence of inflammation or neoplasia. The ear is examined with an **otoscope**, which allows inspection of the external ear and external surface of the tympanic membrane. Fluid and pus in the middle ear can be seen reflected against the tympanic membrane. Palpation of the face and neck detects masses, such as enlarged lymph nodes or nodules in the salivary glands.

Visual examination of the nasal passages, pharynx, and larynx is not undertaken routinely, but prompted by the patient's symptoms. These may include nasal stuffiness, fullness, hoarseness, a tickling or lump in the throat, or difficulty or pain with swallowing. Specialized instruments such as mirrors or **laryngoscopes**, which employ fiber-optic technology to access the curved nasopharyngeal passages, are used to visualize the mucous membranes of the upper respiratory tract. Other instruments can be used to assess the function of the vocal cords.

Radiographic techniques are used to further delineate pathologic processes. X-rays are taken routinely in dentists' offices to detect caries in locations that are not readily seen by inspection and to guide their treatment. Computed tomography (CT) scans are useful to assess the severity of sinus inflammation and to trace the extent of tumors. Magnetic resonance imaging (MRI) is particularly useful in evaluating the soft tissues in the head and neck region. Fluoroscopy is used to assess the swallowing apparatus. This technique takes a radiographic video so that the relationships of anatomic structures can be observed while they are in motion.

Function tests for hearing employ **audiometers**, or devices that generate auditory stimuli. Auditory acuity is assessed by asking the patient to respond when he or she hears the tone generated by the machine, which is manipulated in pitch and intensity by the specialist administering the test.

Microbiology may be required for detection and identification of organisms causing infection. This is particularly important in cases of sore throat, when the healthcare practitioner does not want to miss identifying a streptococcal throat infection because of the risk of the development of rheumatic heart disease or poststreptococcal nephritis. Tissue biopsies are taken to determine the etiology of certain inflammatory processes (e.g., fungal infection of the sinuses) or to detect the presence of hyperplasias or neoplasias.

Specific Diseases

Genetic/Developmental Diseases

Various rare types of genetic or developmental abnormalities occur in the oral and ear structures that may either be isolated or occur in conjunction with defects of other organs. Cleft lip and cleft palate are two of the more common congenital abnormalities of the head and neck region, and are discussed in the next subsection. Various forms and degrees of improper dental development may also have a congenital basis. The most common is **malocclusion** (improper contact between upper and lower teeth). About half the cases of deafness in children are genetic; the other half are the result of congenital conditions such as intrauterine rubella infection. Bizarre abnormalities of facial structure may occur in children with severe mental retardation.

Cleft Lip and Cleft Palate

Cleft lip, a defect on either side of the midline of the upper lip (**Figure 13–2**), occurs with or without cleft palate, a defect in the roof of the mouth that normally separates the oral cavity from the nasal cavity. These failures of late embryonic development can usually be easily surgically corrected within the first 2 years of life. Until then, infants may have problems with feeding and, because the eustachian tube may not open properly into the pharynx, may develop repeated ear infections. Surgery corrects or improves phonation, mastication, and cosmetic appearance and restores proper eustachian tube function. The defect may be induced by teratogens but is most commonly sporadic. It is the result of failure of development of tissues that normally converge and fuse in the midline of the face.

BOX 13–1   Cleft Lip and Cleft Palate
Causes
Embryonic anomaly
Lesions
Defect in the upper lip on either side of the midline (cleft lip)
Defect in the roof of the mouth (cleft palate)
Manifestations
Abnormal appearance
Speech difficulties
Difficulties with feeding

Inflammatory/Degenerative Diseases

Most health problems of the oral region, upper respiratory tract, and ear are acute or chronic infections. The most significant inflammatory diseases of these regions are discussed, followed by several less frequent but significant degenerative conditions of the ear.

Dental Caries

Dental caries is a microbial disease in which the calcified portion of teeth (enamel and dentin) becomes demineralized. Disease activity is greatest in childhood, and caries are the predominant cause of tooth loss in persons younger than 35 years of age. Bacteria adhere to the tooth surface in the form of a tenacious, nonvisible mass called **dental plaque**. As the bacteria metabolize sugars, they produce acid that erodes the tooth enamel. Daily removal of the plaque through brushing and flossing and reduction of sugar in the diet reduce the incidence of caries. When fluoride ion is incorporated into the crystalline structure of the dental enamel, the susceptibility of teeth to the formation of caries is greatly reduced. Introduction of

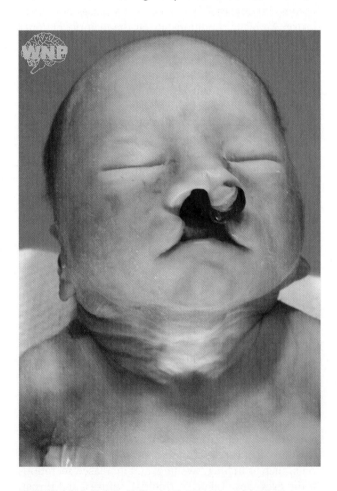

FIGURE 13–2 Cleft lip/cleft palate in a near-term fetus that was live born but had multiple other anomalies that were incompatible with life. Note the tissues in the middle of the upper lip (philtrum), nose (nasal column), and palate have not fused. (Courtesy of Dr. M. Shahriar Salamat, Department of Pathology and Laboratory Medicine, University of Wisconsin School of Medicine and Public Health.)

fluoride into drinking water and toothpaste has reduced the incidence of caries by more than 75%.

Caries may erode into the central connective tissue core of a tooth or *dental pulp*, causing infection and necrosis of the pulp. Complications of **pulpitis** include tooth loss, periapical abscess, periapical granuloma, and periapical cyst. Abscess is the most acute and destructive complication. A periapical granuloma is not really a granuloma but rather a low-grade inflammation that stimulates abundant granulation tissue formation. Periapical cysts form from islands of epithelium that are trapped in a periapical granuloma and proliferate to form a squamous epithelial-lined cavity. Root canal therapy can prevent tooth loss caused by pulpitis.

BOX 13–2   Dental Caries

Causes

Dental plaque

High-carbohydrate diet

Poor dental hygiene

Lesions

Caries (cavities)

Inflamed dental pulp (late)

Manifestations

Gross cavity, or hole in tooth enamel

Defect in enamel on x-ray

Pain

Loss of tooth (late)

Pulpitis and its complications

Periodontal Disease

Periodontal disease refers to a usually painless, chronic, low-grade inflammation of the supporting tissues of teeth, or **gingiva** (gums). It increases in prevalence with age and is the major cause of tooth loss in adults. As with caries, dental plaque is the major etiologic factor. Accumulation of plaque between the tooth and gingiva

---

BOX 13–3   Periodontal Disease

Causes

Dental plaque

Poor dental hygiene

Lesions

Gingivitis

Periodontitis

Manifestations

Gingival changes by inspection

Bleeding

Resorption of bone by x-ray

Tooth loss (late)

---

causes persistent, low-grade inflammation. This can be recognized by changes in color, texture, and amount of gingival tissue, as well as an increased propensity for the gingivae to bleed. If allowed to progress, the inflammation can extend to underlying bone, causing it to be resorbed and teeth to become loose. Daily removal of plaque by brushing and flossing is an effective means of preventing and reducing periodontal disease.

Halitosis

Halitosis is the medical name for bad breath. It can be caused by certain pungent foods, such as garlic, but the most common cause is bacterial breakdown of amino acids, which produces foul-smelling sulfide gases. The bacteria reside on the gums, in dental plaque, and on the back of the tongue. A particularly severe manifestation, associated with ulcerated and bleeding gingivae, is called **acute necrotizing ulcerative gingivitis** (Vincent's disease, trench mouth). It is caused by fusiform and spirochetal bacteria that are normally present in the mouth. Poor dental hygiene or underlying disease that lowers host resistance can allow these bacteria to overgrow and their waste products to accumulate. Treatment of this severe form includes peroxide rinses and antibiotics. Less severe forms are usually adequately treated with thorough oral hygiene.

Herpes Stomatitis (Cold Sores)

Herpes simplex type I is a very prevalent virus of humans. Following primary infection, herpes simplex virus (HSV) has the ability to lie dormant in nervous tissue. HSV-1 lies dormant in facial nerves. Its favorite site of activity is in and around the mouth: at the mucocutaneous border of the lips, on the gums or hard palate. It produces painful blisters that eventually ulcerate and crust over (**Figure 13–3**). Primary infection usually occurs during childhood and may be associated with more severe symptoms, such as pharyngitis and lymphadenopathy. Reactivation usually occurs under conditions of stress, such as trauma, sudden and intense sun

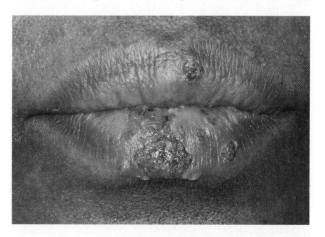

FIGURE 13–3 Herpes stomatitis. There are several weeping ulcers and blisters on the upper and lower lips. (Courtesy of Yale Residents' Slide Collection, Dermatology Department, Yale University School of Medicine.)

exposure, immunosuppression, or fever from another viral illness. HSV-1 is easily transmitted among family members. Genital herpes is caused by a different virus (HSV type II).

Aphthous Stomatitis (Canker Sores)

Aphthous means spot, and *stoma* means mouth, so aphthous stomatitis is a painful inflammatory spot in the mouth. These spots are very discrete, shallow, painful ulcers that gradually heal in 7 to 10 days (**Figure 13–4**). The lesions are similar to herpes stomatitis in that they are activated periodically, but they differ from herpes in their discrete appearance and occurrence on different areas of the oral mucosa. There are many putative causative agents, including citrus fruits, trauma to the gums, nutritional deficiencies, certain drugs, and some autoimmune diseases. Treatment is symptomatic, though if an underlying condition such as iron deficiency is present, it should be treated.

Upper Respiratory Infection

The term *upper respiratory infection* (URI) refers to a clinical presentation of sore throat (pharyngitis), nasal discharge (rhinitis), headache, fever, and fatigue. Other symptoms, such as muscle aches, cough, or sinus pain, may also be present. Any of these symptoms may predominate over the others, or even occur in the absence of the others.

Upper respiratory infections are usually self-limiting. They run a course of a few days to a week, often prostrating the patient for a part of this time. URIs are contagious. The causative agent is transmitted through aerosolized droplets—in other words, through sneezing and coughing. Transmission can be reduced by the patient covering his or her nose and mouth when sneezing or coughing, and by thorough and frequent washing of hands or use of antiseptic gels. There is no cure for the common cold, though more and more sophisticated drugs that counteract the symptoms stock the pharmacy shelves. The putative effect of vitamin C, echinacea, or zinc in reducing the duration of a cold has not been proved in well-designed randomized, controlled studies.

Viruses are the most common cause of URIs, and many different kinds of viruses have been implicated.

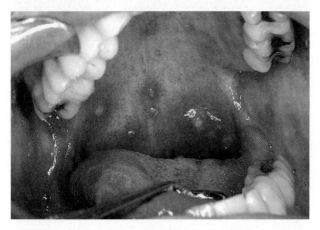

FIGURE 13–4 Aphthous stomatitis. (Courtesy of Sol Silverman, Jr., DDS/CDC.)

Rhinovirus, coronavirus, adenovirus, and respiratory syncytial virus are some of the more common ones. The influenza virus causes symptoms similar to the common cold, but of much greater severity. Bacteria such as group A streptococci, *Bordatella pertussis*, and *Haemophilus influenzae* can also cause URIs. Some of these infectious agents were the scourge of children before the advent of vaccinations and antibiotics. Immunizations have greatly reduced the incidence of these diseases in areas where immunizations are readily available and routinely given. Effective immunizations are difficult to develop for the more common viruses causing URIs because there are so many of them and their antigenic makeup is so variable. The same is true for the influenza virus. Every year, a vaccine is developed against those flu viruses that scientists predict will be most prevalent in the coming year, based on detailed global epidemiologic studies. Because the vaccine is developed against only a few strains of the virus, and because the virus can readily and easily shift its antigenic makeup, the flu shot is not entirely preventive.

Most of the time, there is no reason to identify the agent causing the URI definitively, because this knowledge would not alter its treatment. Only those cases caused by group A beta hemolytic streptococci should be identified and treated with antibiotics. Antibiotic treatment against group A strep does not reduce the length of the illness very significantly, but it does reduce the infectious period and it virtually eliminates the development of harmful sequelae of infection, such as rheumatic fever, poststreptococcal nephritis, meningitis, or scarlet fever. Strep throat can be identified by microbial culture, which takes 24–48 hours, or by a *rapid strep test*, which detects a carbohydrate produced by strep and not by other organisms. Although the rapid strep test can easily be performed in a doctor's office and may give a positive result in 15 minutes or less, it is not very sensitive (it will not detect all cases of strep throat), so a negative test result still needs to be followed up with a microbial culture. Physical examination is not sufficient to determine whether a URI is caused by streptococcal or viral organisms. There is no correlation between the amount of redness and exudate in the throat and the presence of streptococci. The degree of elevation of leukocytes in the blood does not correlate with cause, either. Only the rapid strep test or microbial culture can confirm strep throat, and only when strep throat has been confirmed should antibiotics be given. Other bacteria causing URIs run a self-limited course and do not cause sequelae, so there is no reason to detect them specifically or treat them with antibiotics.

By far the majority of cases of URI are minor illnesses that cause discomfort for less than a week and then go away entirely. However, especially in children and older adults, they may have serious complications. In children, swelling of the lymphoid tissue of the nasopharynx (adenoids) and the pharyngeal tonsils in response to inflammation of the respiratory tract can cause blockage of the openings of the eustachian tubes, which in turn predisposes the children to otitis media (described later). Enlarged tonsils may also partially obstruct breathing, which results in poor sleep and irritability. A common reason for the removal of tonsils and adenoids in pediatric patients is repeated URIs exacerbated by these complications. Upper respiratory infections predominantly involving the larynx can cause laryngeal edema, partial airway obstruction, and difficult inspiration. In children, this causes **croup**, a laryngeal spasm characterized by a loud, high-pitched inspiratory sound. Patients have the feeling that they cannot breathe, which is very anxiety provoking, and labored respirations. Swelling of the nasal mucosa may cause obstruction of drainage from the sinuses, with resultant sinusitis. Pneumonia can also complicate a URI, if the inflamed tissues become secondarily infected with a bacterial organism. Pneumonia developing in the setting of a URI is a common cause of death in older adults. URI by itself very rarely leads to death, unless it occurs in patients with serious immune compromise or other underlying disease. Influenza is different from the common cold in this respect. The flu kills an estimated 36,000 people in the United States every year. Most deaths occur in the pediatric and older adult age groups.

BOX 13–4   Upper Respiratory Infections

Causes

Several types of viruses, including influenza virus

Group A streptococci

Other bacteria (rare)

Lesions

Redness of mucosa of nasopharynx

Swelling of tonsils or adenoids

Inflammatory exudate over tonsils

Manifestations

Rhinitis, pharyngitis, tonsillitis, laryngitis

Fever, fatigue, muscle aches

Cough

Complications: otitis media, sinusitis, pneumonia, croup, rheumatic heart disease, poststreptococcal nephritis, death (influenza)

Sinusitis

Inflammation of the respiratory mucosa lining sinus cavities and obstruction of the openings that drain them result in accumulation of fluid within the sinuses. Obstruction to drainage of the sinuses can be anatomic, as when the nasal septum is deviated, or it can be secondary to occlusion of the sinus tracts by edematous thickening of the respiratory mucosa during inflammation. The edema that occurs with inflammation may be severe enough that it causes polypoid thickening of the mucous membranes of the nose and sinuses, and these polyps can also occlude the sinus openings. Inflammation can be the result of an infectious agent, usually viral and accompanying a URI, or it can be allergic. Although inflammation and fluid accumulation are enough to trigger the symptoms of sinusitis, the accumulated fluid or mucus can also become infected by bacteria or fungi.

Sinusitis is clinically defined as *acute* if it lasts less than 1 month and is self-limited, and as *chronic* if it persists or is recurrent. Symptoms of sinusitis are nasal congestion, headaches, facial pain (particularly over the affected sinuses), thick and discolored mucoid discharge from the nose, and postnasal drainage. Radiologic studies demonstrate opacification of the sinuses by fluid (**Figure 13–5**). Because most cases of sinusitis occur in the shadow of a viral URI or seasonal allergies, they are not treated with anything other than drugs that give symptomatic relief: saline sinus washes, decongestants, and pain medications. Most cases do resolve spontaneously. However, if superimposed infection occurs, symptoms persist and become more severe. In these cases, antibiotics or antifungal agents should be administered. Fungal sinusitis is more common in diabetic or immunocompromised patients.

Chronic sinusitis is often difficult to treat. Antibiotics and/or antifungals cannot always clear the infection. Inflammation may be reduced by steroid therapy, but this carries its own risks and side effects. Sometimes,

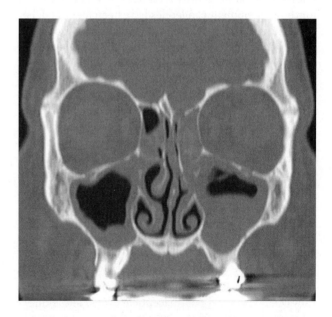

FIGURE 13–5 Sinusitis, CT scan, coronal plane. The skull bones are highlighted in white, and the nasal turbinates make curlicues in the middle of the face. Both maxillary sinuses, especially the left one, contain a homogenous gray shadow, with stranding across the empty (black) space that remains of the sinus cavity. The gray shadow represents an acute inflammatory exudate composed of fluid, inflammatory cells, mucus, and edematous respiratory mucosa. The same gray shadow extends up to and obliterates the ethmoid sinus on the left side and also involves the ethmoid sinus on the right. (Courtesy of Dr. Michael Hartman, Department of Neuroradiology, University of Wisconsin School of Medicine and Public Health.)

surgery can be helpful, for example, by removing polyps that obstruct the sinus outflow tracts, repairing a deviated nasal septum, or enlarging the sinus drainage tracts. In chronic cases that fail to respond to maximal medical management, the respiratory mucosa may be surgically stripped from the sinuses in an effort to eliminate the inflammation.

Allergic Rhinitis (Hay Fever)

"Hay fever" is a misnomer—the condition is rarely if ever triggered by hay and does not cause fever. *Allergic rhinitis* is a better descriptor: this is an allergic response to environmental antigens and it causes symptoms similar to a common cold, including a runny nose (rhinitis), scratchy throat, and itchy eyes. Especially in children, it is often seen in conjunction with an allergic rash (eczema) or asthma.

There are numerous known triggers for allergic rhinitis. In the Midwest of the United States, it is most often seasonal. Tree pollens, crop pollens, grass, and certain wildflowers such as ragweed are well-documented antigens. Others are household dusts, such as animal dander and the excrement of mites and cockroaches. These cause perennial symptoms.

The peak incidence of allergies is in early school-age children, and a smaller peak occurs in the young adult years. Symptoms rarely begin in adulthood, and they rarely diminish in severity with age. Several risk factors for the development of allergies have been identified. For example, allergies are more common in urban than rural areas, more common in males than in females, more common in children who were bottle rather than breast fed, and tend to run in families.

Allergic rhinitis is not a serious or fatal condition, but it can cause significant discomfort and morbidity. Sinusitis is a frequent complication. Some specialists prefer the term *rhinosinusitis* because rhinitis and sinusitis so often occur together. The boggy, swollen nasal mucosa may form polyps, which obstruct breathing and require surgical removal. Constant nasal stuffiness, runny nose, itchy eyes, and scratchy throat result in irritability and fatigue. It has been documented that people who suffer from allergic rhinitis have cognitive impairment, including decreased learning and memory, during allergy season, and feel psychologically and socially impaired. This morbidity translates into billions of dollars of direct (physician visits and pharmaceutical drugs) and indirect (absenteeism from school and work) costs every year in the United States.

Many different kinds of medications are available that help alleviate the symptoms of allergies. Antihistamines, which block the release of histamine from mast cells and thereby greatly reduce the swelling of the mucous membranes and production of secretions, are very effective but often have intolerable side effects, such as profound drowsiness or cognitive delay. Decongestants such as pseudoephedrine also reduce rhinitis but may have equally unpleasant side effects. Steroids injected onto the mucosal surface of the nasal passages reduce the activity of leukocytes, particularly eosinophils, which play a prominent role in allergic reactions. Eye drops are available that reduce inflammation of the conjunctivae. *Desensitization therapy*, or allergen injection immunotherapy, is useful if the specific allergic trigger can be identified. This involves exposing the patient repeatedly to ever-increasing doses of the identified allergen. Over time, this controlled exposure alters the immune system so that it does not overreact when the allergen is encountered naturally. Often, more than one of these agents has to be used to reduce symptoms effectively. The best medicine is, of course, prevention, though this may not be achievable if it entails getting rid of a beloved pet or moving to area with a more arid environment.

Otitis Media

Otitis media is inflammation of the middle ear. It is most common in infants and young children as a consequence of upper respiratory infections. Pharyngeal edema causes obstruction of the eustachian tube, with resultant loss of air in the middle ear space, development of negative pressure, and seepage of fluid into the middle ear from surrounding membranes. In addition, the viruses causing URIs, such as the rhinoviruses, can infect the lining of the eustachian tube and middle ear, causing both swelling and subsequent blockage of the tube and increased secretions. The fluid that accumulates in the middle ear provides a fertile culture medium for bacteria. Culture of the fluid for bacteria is usually not performed because of the inaccessible location of the middle ear behind the eardrum.

Even in the absence of bacterial infection, the accumulated fluid causes severe pain. The child can be irritable and inconsolable and is often also feverish. Inspection through an otoscope reveals a swollen, red eardrum (**Figure 13–6**). Pain medications such as acetaminophen rapidly reduce the discomfort. Whether or not to treat all earaches in children with antibiotics, at what time to begin administering them, what signs or symptoms are more closely related to and therefore predictive of bacterial infection, and the role of tubes inserted across the tympanic membrane to help drain the middle ear are all hotly contested topics in the pediatric literature. Suffice it to say here that, just as not all cases of URI or sinusitis require antibiotic therapy, so also otitis media, which is most often seen in the setting of a viral URI, does not always require antibiotic therapy. Nevertheless, the potential complications of otitis media are severe, so considerable care should be exercised to avoid them.

With suppurative otitis media, the eardrum can rupture, resulting in drainage of pus from the external ear. The infection may spread into the skull bone, in particular to the thick peg of bone behind the ear, the mastoid process. This is particularly serious because it may lead

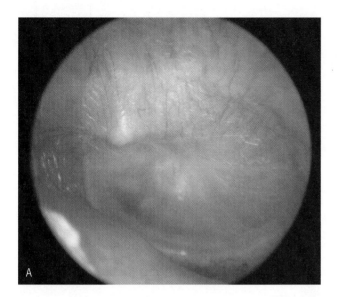 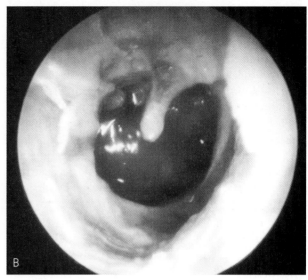

FIGURE 13–6 Otitis media. **A.** Normal tympanic membrane as seen by otoscopy. The membrane is thin and translucent. (© CNRI/Science Source) **B.** Eardrum that has been destroyed by otitis media. The middle ear is red and swollen and an inflammatory exudate covers the external ear canal. (© BSIP/Science Source)

to permanent hearing loss or spread of infection into the brain. Repeated bouts of otitis media can result in hearing impairment. Even in the absence of permanent hearing loss, children with frequent otitis media may have delayed speech and language development. Chronic low-grade otitis media may lead to the formation of a mass of keratinized tissue within the middle ear, called a *cholesteatoma*, which can become infected or erode the structures of the middle ear, resulting in hearing loss.

Otitis media is very rare in adults. As the head and neck grow, the eustachian tube straightens out so that gravity can facilitate drainage of the middle ear. Adults may still get fluid accumulation in the ears during a URI, with the feeling of fullness or popping in the ear, but the severe pain and fever that characterize otitis media in children rarely happen in adults.

BOX 13–5   Otitis Media

Causes

Obstruction of eustachian tube

Viruses

Bacteria

Allergies

Lesions

Inflammation of the middle ear

Accumulation of fluid in the middle ear

Manifestations

Pain

Swollen, red eardrum

Fever

Complications: mastoiditis, tympanic membrane rupture, hearing loss, speech and language development delay, cholesteatoma

---

Hearing Loss

Hearing loss can be caused by a wide variety of insults, from genetic to infectious to degenerative and traumatic, and unfortunately it is often iatrogenic—that is, a side effect of medical treatment (e.g., aminoglycoside antibiotics or chemotherapeutic treatment). Different etiologies are more common at different ages. Hearing loss can generally be classified as to whether it is **sensorineural**, meaning that the cochlea and/or auditory nerve are damaged, or **conductive**, meaning that the external or middle ear, which conduct sound waves through the air and translate them into fluid waves, are damaged. Often, hearing loss is both sensorineural and conductive.

In children, hearing loss is most often congenital or infectious. The causes of congenital hearing loss are myriad: malformation of the bones of the auditory canal or middle ear; uterine infection such as cytomegalovirus (CMV), rubella, or toxoplasmosis; various genetic conditions that can be autosomal dominant, autosomal recessive, X-linked, or even mitochondrial; a teratogenic insult; or prematurity. The most common infectious process in infants and children that can result in hearing loss is otitis media and its complications (discussed earlier).

Hearing loss occurring with increasing age is called **presbycusis**. This is a very common and strikingly undertreated condition. When systematically screened, 60% of patients older than the age of 73 years have hearing loss; of these, only 20% will purchase a hearing aid, and of those, only about 75% consistently use it. Underrecognition of this condition is detrimental, because hearing loss in older adults is a significant cause of low self-esteem, social isolation, and depression and probably also contributes to dementia.

Hearing loss associated with aging usually begins in the high frequencies and is usually symmetrical. It is associated with **tinnitus**, or the sensation of ringing in the ears. Its cause is generally attributed to nonspecific degeneration of the hearing apparatus caused by the cumulative effects of lifetime exposure to noise, medications, infections, and reduced blood flow that results from age-related changes to arteries. Presbycusis may have a genetic basis, and it is more commonly seen in the setting of other underlying diseases or conditions, such as diabetes mellitus, cerebrovascular disease, and hypertension. Smoking is also a risk factor.

The treatment for hearing loss is a hearing aid. External aids are often avoided by patients because they are uncomfortable, unsightly, and rapidly fill with cerumen (ear wax); also, the batteries are costly. In addition, many patients complain that the hearing aid does not make speech any clearer to recognize but simply increases the loudness of background noise. Implanted hearing aids, or cochlear implants, conduct sound through the skull bone rather than through the air passages of the external and middle ears. Implantation is quite safe and rarely complicated by infection, but implants are generally not used to treat presbycusis unless the hearing loss is very severe.

Ménière disease, or endolymphatic hydrops, is a degenerative disease of the vestibular apparatus. The triad of symptoms of Ménière disease consists of sudden bouts of **vertigo** (dizziness or spinning), tinnitus, and hearing loss. The vertigo usually lasts at least 20 minutes and often an entire day. It is very severe, often induces vomiting, and debilitates the patient. The hearing loss is sensorineural and fluctuates: it is more severe during episodes of vertigo than in between flares. What causes Ménière disease is not known, and there are no tests that are specific for this disease. Its symptoms can be caused by a variety of other conditions, from cerebrovascular accidents to tumors growing on the auditory nerve. Diagnosis therefore entails carefully excluding all other possible causes of the symptoms. Often, the patient suffers repeated episodes before the diagnosis is made. Even then, there is no effective treatment. It is thought that the symptoms result from swelling or distention of the fluid-filled sacs making up the vestibular apparatus. Reduction of the fluid with diuretic drugs and antihistamines and avoidance of vasoconstrictive agents such as tobacco, caffeine, or chocolate may prevent episodes. In very severe cases, the inner ear is surgically destroyed, resulting in permanent hearing loss on that side but dramatic relief of symptoms.

Another cause of hearing loss is **otosclerosis**, which is growth of new bone in the middle ear that can impede the vibration of the ossicles, resulting in a mechanical loss of hearing. The condition occurs most frequently in young women, hearing loss is gradual in onset, there are usually no associated symptoms, and the eardrum appears normal. Patients with otosclerosis have excellent inner ear function, so they benefit from the use of hearing aids. Surgery to reestablish the ossicular chain by replacing the involved bone with a prosthetic device has a very high rate of success.

Other known causes of deafness in persons of all ages include cholesteatoma, neoplasms, psychogenic causes, and toxins.

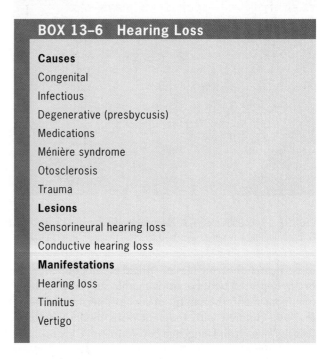

BOX 13–6   Hearing Loss

Causes

Congenital

Infectious

Degenerative (presbycusis)

Medications

Ménière syndrome

Otosclerosis

Trauma

Lesions

Sensorineural hearing loss

Conductive hearing loss

Manifestations

Hearing loss

Tinnitus

Vertigo

Degenerative Diseases of the Salivary Glands

Inflammatory and degenerative conditions of the salivary glands are rare, but there are many of them. **Mumps**, an infectious disease caused by a virus, was formerly—and still is in many areas of the world—one of the most common childhood diseases. It causes painful swelling of the parotid gland, or **parotitis**, and is often accompanied by inflammation of other tissues. Vaccination is highly effective in preventing this disease. Stones, or *sialoliths*, can form in salivary glands and cause obstruction of ducts, also resulting in pain and swelling. This occurs most commonly in the setting of infection of the submandibular gland.

One of the more common autoimmune diseases, **Sjögren syndrome**, causes immune-mediated destruction of the cells that produce tears in the lacrimal gland and saliva in the salivary glands. Patients with Sjögren syndrome have persistent dry eyes and dry mouth. Sjögren syndrome is commonly seen in association with rheumatoid arthritis. The symptoms of dry eyes and dry mouth are extremely uncomfortable and the lack of tears and saliva can cause considerable damage to the eyes and the teeth. Tears keep the conjunctival surface moist and wash away extraneous substances that may have adhered to the surface of the eye, and saliva is to some extent protective against bacterial decay of tooth enamel. With adequate preventative and symptomatic treatment, serious damage can be averted.

Hyperplastic/Neoplastic Diseases

Squamous Cell Carcinoma

The most common primary neoplasm of the head and neck region is squamous cell carcinoma, which can affect the mouth, tongue, pharynx, tonsils, or larynx. In these locations, it is strongly associated with a history of tobacco exposure, including chewing tobacco. The combination of tobacco and alcohol seems to potentiate the development of carcinoma in these areas. Squamous cell carcinoma can also occur on the lip and earlobe, in which case it is associated with lifetime sun exposure. In these locations, it is very easily cured by excision, sometimes followed by radiation therapy, because it usually does not grow very invasively or metastasize.

Unlike the carcinomas on the lip and earlobe, squamous cell carcinoma of the oral cavity, pharynx, and larynx is associated with significant morbidity and mortality. Complete excision usually leaves a loss of function, ranging from difficulty swallowing and loss of taste sensation, to loss of voice, depending on the location of the cancer. Excision may be curative if the cancer is small; larger lesions need to be followed with radiation therapy, which can cause severe, painful inflammation of the mucous membrane lining of the oropharynx. Prognosis is related to the size of the cancer at the time it is detected, lymph node involvement, and distant metastases. As with all cancers, early-stage disease is associated with a better prognosis (around 80% 5-year survival) in comparison to late-stage disease (around 20% 5-year survival).

The symptoms of squamous cell carcinoma relate to the site at which it is growing. When it is seen, either on easily visible surfaces such as the lip or tongue, or with a laryngoscope or mirror in the pharynx or larynx, it presents as an expanding, ulcerating, encrusted lesion (**Figure 13–7**). On the tongue, it may first be detected as a white plaque, called **leukoplakia**. If it is growing on the palate, it may cause obstruction of the nasopharyngeal passages. Deeper in the throat, it can cause hoarseness, pain, or difficulty with swallowing. Palpation of the neck may detect enlarged lymph nodes if the cancer has already metastasized. Imaging studies, particularly MRI, are performed to assess the extension of the tumor into the surrounding soft tissues.

Some of the head and neck cancers are associated with viruses. One of these is human papillomavirus (HPV), which in some studies is implicated in up to 90% of squamous cell carcinomas of the head and neck region. The strain of HPV seen in these cancers is one of the high-risk strains known to cause squamous cell carcinoma of the cervix, and oral sex is a strong risk factor. The association of high-risk sexual activity, tobacco, and alcohol seems to be more than additive in initiating and promoting this cancer. Other viruses that have been implicated in squamous cell carcinoma of the head and neck region are HSV and human immunodeficiency virus (HIV).

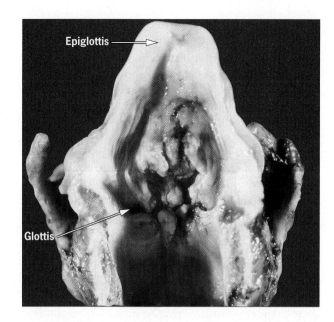

FIGURE 13–7 Gross appearance of squamous cell carcinoma of the larynx. The larynx is opened from the posterior, revealing a fungating and polypoid mass that has destroyed the right and left vocal folds (glottis) and extends into the epiglottis.

Epstein-Barr virus (EBV), the virus causing mononucleosis, has long been known to be the etiologic agent of **undifferentiated nasopharyngeal carcinoma**. This particularly aggressive tumor is very rare in developed nations but prevalent in Asia and Africa. In some areas of China, it accounts for 18% of all cancers. EBV is very prevalent even in developed countries. Up to 90% of adults will have acquired EBV during childhood and adolescence. Why, in the face of such high prevalence, nasopharyngeal carcinoma occurs more commonly in some geographic areas and not in others is currently not understood. Its development is apparently not caused by the presence of EBV alone but requires potentiation by some other, presumably environmental, factor. Although nasopharyngeal carcinoma is aggressive clinically and poorly differentiated microscopically, it is quite sensitive to radiotherapy, and remissions can be achieved with this modality alone.

Salivary Gland Tumors

Tumors of the salivary glands are very rare, but there is a bewildering array of them. Most salivary gland neoplasms arise in the parotid gland, and the majority are benign. The so-called mixed tumor, or **pleomorphic adenoma**, is the most common, accounting for about half of all neoplasms of the salivary glands. It is called mixed, or pleomorphic, because of its appearance under the microscope: it is composed of both epithelial and stromal elements, in widely varying proportions. The most common malignant neoplasm of the salivary glands is **mucoepidermoid carcinoma**. The only known risk factors for the development of neoplasms of the salivary glands are a history of radiation exposure and smoking. Most cases are idiopathic.

Organ Failure

Loss of the ability to masticate (chew) occurs with loss of teeth, fractures of the mandible, extensive cancer operations, and severe congenital abnormalities. Patients may still be able to swallow very soft foods and liquids, but maintaining adequate caloric intake can be very difficult.

The same holds with impairment of swallowing, or deglutition. The muscles used in swallowing may be compromised with neuromuscular diseases such as multiple sclerosis, poliomyelitis, a cerebrovascular accident, severe debilitation, or extensive surgery for cancer of the oral cavity, tongue, or pharynx. The swallowing apparatus also protects the airway from aspiration of food and gastric contents. Thus, when the muscles of deglutition are weakened, not only is caloric intake impaired, but the risk for aspiration is greatly increased. Aspiration results in chemical injury to the air passages and aspiration pneumonia.

Obstruction of the pharyngeal passages by enlarged tonsils can cause loud snoring as a result of turbulent flow of air. More severe and potentially life-threatening is **obstructive sleep apnea**. This is a debilitating condition in which patients repeatedly stop breathing for as long as 1 minute during their sleep. The resultant hypoxia interrupts their sleep as they awaken or semi-awaken to resume breathing. They have very poor sleep quality because of the frequent interruptions, become chronically sleep deprived, and suffer impairment of daytime functioning. The cause of obstructive sleep apnea is thought to be collapse of the pharyngeal passages when the patient is relaxed and supine. It is more common in obese people. Removal of excess tissue in the nasopharynx, such as the tonsils, and treatment with an external device that keeps the pharynx open during sleep, called a **positive-pressure ventilator**, can relieve the symptoms.

Sudden obstruction of the air passages by a foreign object, such as a piece of food, can lead to asphyxiation. Extensive obstruction or surgery of the larynx may necessitate placement of a **tracheostomy**, or opening into the trachea directly through the anterior portion of the neck.

Diseases of the larynx that cause loss of voice are most commonly cancers that overgrow and paralyze the vocal folds, which are eventually permanently removed by surgery. Patients can regain speech by learning to force air through the upper esophagus into the mouth.

There are many salivary glands in the head and neck region and it is uncommon for all of them to fail, except with Sjögren syndrome. Even with complete destruction of the affected glands, preventive and symptomatic treatment usually averts severe damage. More worrisome than damage to the lacrimal and salivary glands is concomitant damage to internal organs from advanced autoimmune destruction.

Loss of the ability to hear is the most common organ failure of the diseases of the head and neck. Any person with a detectable hearing impairment may be described as relatively deaf, although the essence of deafness as the word is generally used is the inability to hear and understand the spoken voice. The prevalence and magnitude of the problem of hearing loss were discussed earlier in this chapter.

Practice Questions

1. Which of the following is the most common cancer of the head and neck region in the United States?
    A. Nasopharyngeal carcinoma
    B. Pleomorphic adenoma
    C. Squamous cell carcinoma
    D. Mucoepidermoid carcinoma
    E. Cholesteatoma

2. A laryngoscopic exam will most likely identify the cause of which of these patients' problems?
    A. A 43-year-old man who had numerous middle ear infections and now complains of pain in his ears when he swallows
    B. A 23-year-old man who developed a runny nose and itchy throat that are persistent since he moved to the Midwest 2 months ago
    C. A 33-year-old woman with chronic sinusitis who complains of persistent drainage in the back of the throat
    D. A 43-year-old man who is an alcoholic and heavy smoker and who complains of hoarseness and pain with talking
    E. A 43-year-old woman who complains of a persistent dry mouth that makes it difficult to swallow

3. Complications of dental caries include all of the following except which one?
    A. Periapical abscess
    B. Periapical granuloma
    C. Pulpitis
    D. Tooth loss
    E. Dental plaque

4. Which of the following is the least common cause of sinusitis?
    A. A fungal infection
    B. A bacterial infection
    C. Nasal polyps
    D. Allergies
    E. A viral infection

5. Complications of repeated otitis media include all of the following except which one?
   A. Speech and language delay
   B. Cholesteatoma
   C. Hearing loss
   D. Rupture of tympanic membrane
   E. Blockage of eustachian tube

6. Presbycusis is caused by which of the following?
   A. Intrauterine infection with rubella
   B. Lifetime exposure to noise, medications, and trauma
   C. Toxicity of medications
   D. Repeated otitis media in childhood
   E. Ménière disease

7. Which of the following is not a risk factor for development of carcinoma of the head and neck?
   A. The combination of alcohol and smoking
   B. Dental caries
   C. Oral sex
   D. Epstein-Barr virus infection
   E. Sun exposure

Gastrointestinal Tract

OUTLINE

OBJECTIVES

1. Review the structure and function of the organs of the gastrointestinal tract.
2. Identify the most common diseases of the gastrointestinal tract that cause mild discomfort and serious morbidity and the most common reasons for surgical intervention into the gastrointestinal tract.
3. Describe how hemorrhage, altered motility, and perforation of the gastrointestinal tract present, and name a few common causes of each of these.
4. List and describe common laboratory and radiographic techniques that are used to diagnose diseases of the alimentary tract.
5. List the four most common malformations of the gastrointestinal tract, and describe their complications.
6. Describe the causes, lesions, manifestations, and treatment of congenital pyloric stenosis and Hirschsprung disease.
7. Define gastroesophageal reflux disease and describe how it manifests, how it is treated, and what its potentially serious complications are.
8. Describe the relationship between gastritis and peptic ulcer.
9. List and describe some of the major causes of malabsorption.
10. Compare infectious diarrhea and food poisoning in terms of causative agents, likely situations for their occurrence, and timing of onset and recovery.
11. Describe inguinal hernia, its complications, and treatment.
12. Recognize why acute appendicitis is often misdiagnosed.
13. Compare and contrast ulcerative colitis and Crohn disease in terms of what parts of the gastrointestinal tract are involved, the pattern of inflammation, age of onset, complications, surveillance, and treatment.
14. Define pseudomembranous colitis and describe the patient who is susceptible to developing it.
15. Describe the causes, lesions, and manifestations of colonic diverticulosis.
16. Compare and contrast cancers of the gastrointestinal system in terms of incidence, risk factors, and prognosis.
17. Name the precursor lesions of colonic carcinomas, recognize how they are detected and diagnosed, and understand the reasoning behind surveillance colonoscopy.
18. Describe how deficient functioning of various segments of the gastrointestinal tract can be circumvented.
19. Be able to define and use in context all the words in bold print in the chapter.

KEY TERMS

acute appendicitis	bariatric surgery
adenoma	barium enema
adynamic ileus	Barrett's esophagus
antrum	botulism
anus	celiac disease
appendix	*Clostridium difficile*
autoimmune gastritis	colon

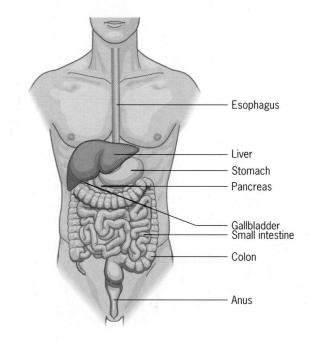

FIGURE 14–1 Anatomy of the organs of the alimentary tract.

Review of Structure and Function

The digestive or gastrointestinal system includes the oropharynx (mouth, salivary glands, pharynx), the alimentary tract (esophagus, stomach, small intestine, large intestine, including the vermiform appendix, and anus), and the pancreaticobiliary tract (liver, gallbladder, bile ducts, and pancreas) (**Figure 14–1**). Here, attention is on those structures primarily responsible for the digestion of masticated food, absorption of water and nutrients, and excretion of waste products of digestion. Digestion is the mechanical, chemical, and enzymatic process by which ingested food is converted into simple soluble substances suitable for assimilation into cells of the body for production of energy and synthesis of tissues.

The **esophagus** is a straight, muscular tube that conveys food from the pharynx to the **stomach**. The stomach is a distensible organ whose epithelial components vary in different locations. In the body or **fundus** of the stomach, mucosal cells secrete *hydrochloric acid* and *proteolytic enzymes*, which aid in digestion. The mucosa of the lower part of the stomach, or **antrum**, is lined by mucous cells that produce thick, basic mucus that protects the epithelial cells from the high acidic content of

the gastric juice. The extreme distal end of the stomach is called the **pylorus**. This is a muscular sphincter that controls the rate of emptying of the stomach into the small intestine. The **small intestine** is divided into the **duodenum, jejunum**, and **ileum**. The major function of the small intestine is absorption. Different nutrients are absorbed in different parts of the small intestine. For example, iron is absorbed in the duodenum, whereas vitamin B_{12} is absorbed in the terminal ileum. The large intestine, or **colon**, is also divided into segments, called the cecum, ascending colon, transverse colon, descending colon, sigmoid colon, and rectum. The **appendix** is a nonfunctional vestigial structure attached to the cecum. The colon is a storage reservoir for the wastes left over from digestion and also is the main site of water absorption. The **anus** is the termination of the digestive tract. It is a muscular sphincter, which allows for controlled evacuation of rectal contents.

In all segments of the gastrointestinal (GI) tract, the wall is made up of the same four layers, which are all continuous with one another from one segment to the next: the mucosa, submucosa, muscularis propria, and serosa (**Figure 14–2**). The mucosal layer, or **mucosa**, has three components: an **epithelium** lining the surface and forming glands that is supported by loose connective tissue called the **lamina propria** and a unique thin muscular layer called the **muscularis mucosae** (**Figure 14–3**). The cells making up the mucosal layer are varied in accordance with their specialized function at each level of the tract. The esophagus is lined by stratified squamous epithelium, which promotes easy gliding of masticated food from the mouth to the stomach. The stomach is lined by

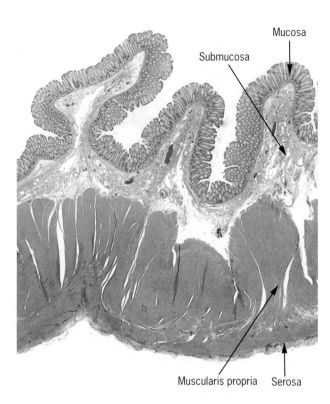

FIGURE 14–2 The layers of the wall of the gastrointestinal tract. The portion depicted here is from the colon.

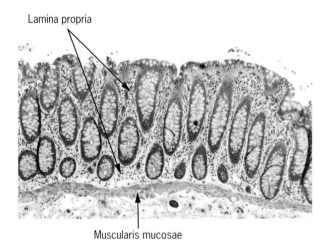

FIGURE 14–3 The mucosa of the colon comprises glands lined by epithelial cells (*), which also spread along the lumenal surface. The glands are separated by a lamina propria rich in inflammatory cells. The muscularis mucosae separates the mucosa from the submucosa.

a thick glandular mucosa, which provides acid and proteolytic enzymes to help break up food, and mucus to protect the stomach mucosa from the harmful effect of acid. The small intestinal mucosa has a villous structure, which provides a large surface area for active absorption, and the large intestinal mucosa is lined by abundant

mucus-secreting cells, which facilitate storage and evacuation of the feces.

Deeper than the mucosa is the **submucosa**, which provides structural support to the mucosa. It contains abundant lymphatic and vascular channels, which pick up absorbed nutrients and carry them to the liver for further processing. The deep muscle layer, called the **muscularis propria**, contracts rhythmically to move materials through the alimentary tract. The **serosa** is a thin, smooth membrane present on the outer surface of those parts of the alimentary tract that lie within the abdominal cavity. It is smooth and slippery and keeps the highly tortuous loops of bowel from becoming tangled up. The serosa is continuous over the **mesentery**, the connective tissue attachment of the bowel that contains blood vessels, lymphatics, and nerves.

For the intestinal tract to carry out its job of digestion, absorption, and excretion, the contents of the lumen must be propelled along the tract at an appropriate rate, and reverse movement prevented. Waves of muscle contractions, called **peristalsis**, carry a bolus of swallowed food down the esophagus, and a sphincter at the lower end of the esophagus prevents regurgitation. Contractions in the stomach emanate as waves from the body of the stomach and proceed toward the pylorus. They serve to mix the digesting food and push it into the duodenum. The greater the distention of the stomach, the stronger the contractions and the more rapid the emptying.

The muscle of the pylorus only partially closes the outlet from the stomach, so intestinal contents can regurgitate into the stomach, particularly when the small intestine is not emptying normally. Excessive distention of the stomach may result in vomiting, a process in which the esophageal sphincter opens and abdominal contractions forcibly propel gastric and small intestinal contents upward through the esophagus. Under normal conditions, movement of lumenal contents of the small intestine is most rapid in the upper small intestine and decelerates distally. Contents gradually pass from the ileum to the cecum, and reverse movement is partially prevented by the ileocecal valve. The rate of movement in the colon depends on the amount of solid material that remains and its water content. When the rectum becomes distended, an urge for voluntary relaxation of the anal sphincter to induce defecation occurs.

The digestive process begins in the mouth, where carbohydrate-splitting enzymes, called *amylases*, from the salivary glands mix with food during mastication. In the stomach, the proteolytic enzyme pepsin and hydrochloric acid are added to the ground-up food to facilitate the digestive process. The greatest volume of digestive enzymes is added in the duodenum. These originate in the pancreas. They include more amylases, proteolytic enzymes called *trypsins*, and fat-splitting enzymes called *lipases*. In addition, *bile salts*, the main constituent of bile produced by the liver, emulsify lipids into small water-soluble packets so that they can be transported and digested. The final phase of the digestive process occurs on the surface of small intestinal epithelial cells, where carbohydrate-splitting and protein-splitting enzymes are present. Complex endocrine and nervous mechanisms coordinate the timing of the secretion and storage of digestive enzymes, hydrochloric acid, and bile salts so that appropriate amounts are available when needed. For example, the sight of food induces salivation and gastric secretions via nervous stimulation; distention of the gastric antrum causes release of gastrin, a hormone that stimulates acid production and gastric emptying; and emptying of food into the duodenum causes secretion of the hormones secretin and pancreozymin, which, in turn, cause the pancreas to secrete more fluid and enzymes and the gallbladder to empty bile into the duodenum.

The human gastrointestinal tract is colonized by trillions of bacteria of about 500 different species. These begin to colonize the tubular gut immediately after birth, and within a few weeks after birth the **gut microfloral environment** is usually well established. Bacteria are present in highest concentration in the ileum and colon. The sheer numbers of bacteria are staggering: it is estimated that there are 10 times as many bacteria in the gut as there are cells in the body, and they make up more than half the dry weight of feces. Intestinal bacteria serve many important functions: they facilitate the digestion of certain carbohydrates, produce nutrients such as folate and vitamin K, influence the development and function of intestinal epithelial cells, influence the development and responsiveness of the gastrointestinal immune system, and metabolize certain drugs to active metabolites. Changes in the composition of the intestinal microbial flora may be implicated in diverse diseases such as food allergies, inflammatory bowel disease, and malabsorption syndromes.

Most Frequent and Serious Problems

The most common problem confronting patients is functional alteration of movement through the alimentary tract. **Constipation** refers to infrequent and/or difficult evacuation of feces. Constipation is frequently associated with a low-bulk diet and with aging. **Diarrhea** refers to abnormally frequent and liquid stools. Both constipation and diarrhea are symptoms, not diseases. Their underlying cause should always be determined and reversed, if possible. Worldwide, diarrhea is one of the most common causes of infant mortality. It is most often caused by a foodborne infectious agent or toxin. In the United States, enteritis causing severe or fatal diarrhea primarily is a significant health problem in rural or overpopulated areas. The most common functional alteration of the alimentary tract diagnosed by gastroenterologists in the United States is **irritable bowel syndrome**, which has no known organic cause and is treatable only with dietary modifications. Its symptoms are variable and include constipation, diarrhea, and crampy abdominal pain.

Many organic diseases of the alimentary tract cause temporary morbidity but are rarely fatal. It is difficult to accrue accurate statistics on the incidence or prevalence of many of these conditions because some, such as gastroesophageal reflux or "stomach flu," are not always severe enough to come to medical attention, and some, such as diverticular disease, may never cause the patient any problems and are not detected at all during their lifetime. Probably the most common of these illnesses is viral enteritis, commonly known as intestinal flu or stomach flu. Manifestations include nausea, vomiting, and diarrhea. When adequate care is administered, the course is self-limited. Acute overindulgence in alcoholic beverages produces an illness similar to viral enteritis, although muscle aches and pains and fever are less frequent and the duration is often shorter. Diverticulosis of the colon is common and rises in prevalence with increasing age but only occasionally causes symptoms.

Gastroesophageal reflux disease (GERD) is a very common problem in the United States. This occurs when highly acidic gastric contents slip back up into the end of the esophagus. The symptom this causes is commonly referred to as heartburn. GERD is one of the most common conditions for which people make visits to the doctor, and the overall costs of this disease (prescription drugs, over-the-counter drugs, and decreased productivity, or time lost from work) amount to an estimated $10 billion every year in the United States alone. Infection of the stomach by **Helicobacter pylori** is another common condition. *H. pylori* causes gastritis and ulcers of the stomach and duodenum. On a worldwide basis, distribution of *H. pylori* infection varies widely. In the United States, its prevalence rises with increasing age: about 20% of people younger the age of 40 years and 50% older than the age of 60 years have the bacteria in their stomach. In developing nations, the prevalence is much higher in younger individuals, and transmission appears to be related to crowded living conditions and consumption of contaminated food and water.

Diseases of the anus are another important source of discomfort to patients. Mild anal problems include itching in children caused by pinworms, simple itching in adults (pruritis ani), and **hemorrhoids**. More severe anal lesions include thrombosed hemorrhoids, fissures, abscesses, and pilonidal sinuses.

Polyps can grow anywhere in the gastrointestinal tract. They are discovered by endoscopic procedures, by which the mucosa of the gastrointestinal tract is directly visualized. In the colon, polyps can be precursors of carcinoma, and their timely removal prevents the development of colonic adenocarcinoma. For this reason, periodic colonoscopy is recommended as a screening tool for all individuals older than the age of 50 years.

Inguinal hernia is an outpouching of the abdominal cavity into the groin into which loops of bowel can slip and become entrapped. Preventive repair of inguinal hernias is one of the most common abdominal operations, performed about as frequently as cholecystectomies (removal of the gallbladder). **Acute appendicitis** is another common indication for operations on the alimentary tract. This occurs more frequently in children and adolescents than in adults. **Bariatric surgery**, or surgery to reduce the size of the stomach in an effort to curb the appetite, is becoming increasingly popular as the obesity epidemic rampages across developed nations. Because colon cancer is the most common carcinoma, and the first step in achieving cure is surgery, surgical removal of cancerous portions of the colon is another common operation. Finally, any surgical intervention in the abdomen, whether for removal of the appendix or the gallbladder, or even from a cesarean section, can result in adhesions between loops of bowel that can cause pain and obstruction of the alimentary canal. Lysis of abdominal adhesions is therefore another common reason for surgical incursion into the abdomen.

Common medical conditions that require more intensive health care include carcinomas, duodenal and gastric ulcers, and inflammatory bowel disease. Carcinoma of the colon is fatal about 40% of the time, but esophageal and gastric carcinomas are even more serious conditions: the 5-year survival for these is around 10–20% (Table 14–4). The incidence of gastrointestinal tract cancers is quite variable around the world: esophageal and gastric cancers are much more common in parts of Asia and Africa than in Western nations, while the incidence of colon cancer is up to 20 times lower. Duodenal and gastric ulcers can be fatal if they erode through the entire wall of the stomach or duodenum, causing rupture and chemical peritonitis, or if they erode into an adjacent artery, causing massive hemorrhage. Rupture of esophageal varices, infarction of the bowel resulting from occlusion of the mesenteric artery, and perforation with generalized peritonitis regardless of cause are also serious and often fatal conditions. The term *inflammatory bowel disease* refers to two diseases of unknown etiology presumed to have an autoimmune component, called **ulcerative colitis** and **Crohn disease**. They affect about 1 million people in the United States, cause lifelong suffering, and incur high costs of care, including immunosuppressive medications, hospitalizations for complications, and surgery.

Symptoms, Signs, and Tests

Many manifestations of alimentary tract disease can be related to hemorrhage, altered motility, and perforation. **Table 14–1** lists these complications, their manifestations, and common causes.

Hemorrhage manifests differently if it is mild or severe and if it occurs in the upper (esophagus, stomach, duodenum) or lower (small intestine, large intestine, rectum, anus) part of the tract. Severe hemorrhage from the upper alimentary tract leads to **hematemesis**, or vomiting of blood. Vomited blood is bright red if fresh, but has the appearance of coffee grounds if it has been in contact with acid in the stomach. Severe upper tract bleeding can also produce **melena**, or black, tarry stools, as a result of alteration of the blood as it passes down the tract. Severe bleeding from the lower alimentary tract produces bright red blood in the stool (**hematochezia**). Mild bleeding from the upper or lower tract will not be noticed by the patient or produce changes in the color of the feces but can be detected by chemical tests of the feces for hemoglobin. This is called the **occult fecal blood test**. Mild, prolonged bleeding leads to loss of iron and eventually to iron-deficiency anemia. Mild bleeding tends to be an early manifestation of gastrointestinal cancers, so fecal blood tests and blood counts constitute important routine screening tests for adults, and abnormal results should always be followed with an investigation for a source of bleeding.

Altered motility can refer to hyperactivity or hypoactivity of the bowel. It manifests as vomiting, diarrhea, and diminished or increased bowel sounds. Obstruction of the alimentary tract, which can be complete or partial, causes bowel proximal to the obstructed segment to contract forcibly in an attempt to overcome the obstruction. This causes sloshing of the liquid bowel contents, or increased bowel sounds, which can often be heard even without the aid of a stethoscope. The proximal portion of the bowel will also be distended, and if the obstruction is not relieved, gastrointestinal contents will be pushed out through the stomach and esophagus through vomiting. Partial obstruction can often spontaneously resolve if the bowel is allowed to rest by not introducing any food or liquid and allowing gases to escape through a tube threaded through the nose into the stomach. Complete obstruction usually requires surgical reduction, or removal of the obstructed segment.

Adynamic ileus refers to delayed movement and emptying of the gut caused by paralyzed gastrointestinal musculature rather than by a physical obstruction. Adynamic ileus occurs most commonly during the first few days after abdominal operations. When ileus is present, gastrointestinal contents can be vomited and aspirated, causing pneumonia. This is one of the reasons people are not allowed to eat in the first few days after an operation.

Vomiting, diarrhea, and constipation are most commonly functional—in other words, related to altered motility associated with generalized illness, central nervous system disease, or gastrointestinal diseases such as irritable bowel syndrome or gastroenteritis. Diseases causing structural alterations, such as pyloric stenosis, inflammatory bowel disease, or cancer, must be taken into consideration if these symptoms are severe or prolonged.

Perforation of the intestinal tract into the peritoneal cavity is life threatening. Because the peritoneum is essentially a large cavity, the irritating substance escaping from the perforated gut (acid, intestinal bacteria,

TABLE 14-1 Manifestations and Common Causes of Diseases of the Gastrointestinal Tract

	Symptoms/Signs	Common Causes
Hemorrhage	• Hematemesis • Melena • Hematochezia • Occult fecal blood test • Iron-deficiency anemia	• Peptic ulcer • Esophageal varices • Cancer at any level of the GI tract • Hemorrhoids
Altered motility	• Vomiting	• Gastroenteritis • Obstruction • Central nervous system disease • Pyloric stenosis
	• Diarrhea	• Gastroenteritis • Inflammatory bowel disease • Malabsorption • Irritable bowel syndrome
	• Constipation	• Low-fiber diet • Hirschsprung disease • Cancer
	• Obstruction	• Inguinal hernia • Adhesions • Adynamic ileus
	• Dysphagia	• Esophageal ulcers, strictures
Perforation	• Pain • Rigid abdomen • Leukocytosis • Fever	• Appendicitis • Diverticulitis • Infarction • Toxic megacolon • Cancer • Deep ulcer

or feces) can easily spread throughout the peritoneum, causing severe inflammation. Peritoneal inflammation, even in the absence of perforation, causes pain, muscle contraction leading to a rigid abdomen, and adynamic ileus. Infection of the peritoneal lining can rapidly lead to shock. Systemic manifestations of peritonitis include fever and leukocytosis.

Dysphagia is pain with swallowing. It may be caused by a variety of esophageal lesions, such as ulcers or strictures. The location, duration, and time sequence of pain may help identify the cause. Sudden, severe abdominal pain suggests the possibility of perforation or sudden twisting of bowel. Duodenal ulcers produce a chronic, nonradiating, burning, epigastric pain perceived as deep to the abdominal wall. The initial manifestation of appendicitis is pain in the umbilical region, which shifts to the right lower quadrant of the abdomen as it becomes more severe. Severe crampy abdominal pain is one of the symptoms of inflammatory bowel disease but also occurs with disorders of motility.

Because of the considerable variety of lesions that can produce the manifestations just described, it is usually necessary to search for specific causes using laboratory, radiologic, and endoscopic procedures. Measurement of acid in the stomach is called gastric analysis. It is used to demonstrate the absence of acid (achlorhydria) or, rarely, high acid output. Laboratory tests on gastrointestinal contents, blood, and urine may be used to evaluate absorption from the alimentary tract by calculating oral intake and output from feces and urine or rise and fall of blood levels of the nutrient under study. Several types of tests for carbohydrates and fat detect malabsorption. Examination of feces for ova and parasites is undertaken to find ameba and helminths in the gastrointestinal tract. Fecal culture is used to identify specific bacterial pathogens. Breath tests can also be used to detect malabsorption and certain pathogenic bacteria, such as *H. pylori*. Abnormal amounts of products of metabolism are excreted by the lungs when certain digestive enzymes are or are not present, and they can be measured in exhaled air. Finally, examination of tissue samples through the microscope is essential in the diagnosis of inflammatory, developmental, autoimmune, and neoplastic diseases at all levels of the gastrointestinal tract.

Numerous radiologic techniques are used to examine the bowel. In a conventional radiogram (x-ray), air appears dark and fluid appears white. The presence of contrasting air–fluid levels in the small intestine on radiograms can indicate intestinal obstruction. Similarly, air under the diaphragm is indicative of intestinal perforation. The radiologist can further outline the normal and abnormal anatomic features of most segments of the gastrointestinal tract by use of a radiopaque material, such as barium. Barium can either be swallowed, to highlight the upper alimentary tract, or instilled by enema, to highlight the lower GI tract. **Upper GI series** refers to radiologic examination of the esophagus, stomach, and upper small intestine. **Barium enema** refers to radiologic examination of the rectum and colon. Barium within the gastrointestinal tube highlights any filling defects, such as cancers that are growing into the lumen of the tube (Figure 14–18). A conventional computed tomography (CT) scan can detect large masses involving the gastrointestinal tract. **CT colonoscopy** uses CT imaging to build high-resolution images of the inside of the gut that are fine enough to detect even small growths, such as polyps, within the gastrointestinal tube. Radiologists call this a virtual endoscopy.

Endoscopy refers to the use of a tube or flexible scope to look inside a body passageway. Most endoscopes are equipped with biopsy forceps to obtain tissue for microscopic examination. **Sigmoidoscopy**, the most common endoscopic procedure, is used to visualize the rectum and lower sigmoid colon. **Colonoscopy** is used to visualize and biopsy lesions of the entire colon and distal ileum. Upper gastrointestinal endoscopy is used to visualize and biopsy lesions of the esophagus, stomach, and the first portion of the duodenum. Very thin, flexible tubes can also be pushed into the small intestine, primarily to look for sites of bleeding, as the small intestine rarely harbors polyps or cancers. The small intestine can also be visualized by **video capture endoscopy**. This entails the patient swallowing a small camera, about the size of a pill, that takes photographs as it is pushed through the gastrointestinal tract via normal peristalsis. It transmits the photographs to a recording device, from whence they are downloaded onto a computer and reviewed by a gastroenterologist.

Specific Diseases
Genetic/Developmental Diseases

Developmental abnormalities of the gastrointestinal tract are usually embryonic malformations that are surgically correctable. Their manifestations vary from being entirely asymptomatic, such as most cases of Meckel's diverticulum, to being incompatible with life if not surgically treated, such as severe pyloric stenosis or Hirschsprung disease. Often, malformations of the GI tract are associated with malformations in other organ systems. We discuss only the most common conditions here.

Malformations

Meckel diverticulum, or omphalomesenteric duct, is an outpouching of the ileum (**Figure 14–4A**) that results from failure of the embryonic connection with the yolk sac to disappear. It occurs in 2% of the population and is usually discovered at autopsy. In other words, it is an entirely innocuous structure that usually goes unnoticed during the life of the individual. The mucosa of a Meckel's diverticulum can contain epithelia from any portion of the gastrointestinal tract, including the pancreas and stomach. Gastric juices produced in a Meckel's diverticulum can cause erosion of the wall of the diverticulum, causing perforation and peritonitis. This is a rather rare indication for emergency abdominal surgery. Other degenerative processes in the diverticulum can cause hemorrhage or small intestinal obstruction.

Esophageal atresia is the absence of part of the esophagus so that the upper esophagus ends as a blind pouch (**Figure 14–4B**). Often, there is a connection of the trachea to the distal esophagus (tracheoesophageal fistula). This condition needs to be surgically corrected to establish continuity of the alimentary canal and prevent reflux of acidic and corrosive gastric juices into the lungs. **Congenital diaphragmatic hernia** is a hole in the diaphragm (**Figure 14–4C**), through which portions of the alimentary tract can slide into the thorax. This does not necessarily affect the function of the gastrointestinal tract, but the abnormally placed organs can compress the lungs and impair breathing. **Imperforate anus** is failure of the anus to connect with the rectum (**Figure 14–4D**). Abnormal pathways, or fistulae, develop between the rectum and adjacent organs, resulting in anomalous expulsion of fecal matter through the urinary bladder or vagina. This condition is also surgically correctable.

BOX 14–1   Malformations

Causes

Embryonic anomalies

Lesions

Remnant of embryonic structure (Meckel's diverticulum)

Incomplete tube (esophageal atresia, imperforate anus)

Abdominal wall defect with herniation (diaphragmatic hernia, inguinal hernia)

Manifestations

None

Hemorrhage

Perforation

Intestinal obstruction

Vomiting, absence of bowel movements

Aspiration

Impaired breathing

Intestinal incarceration

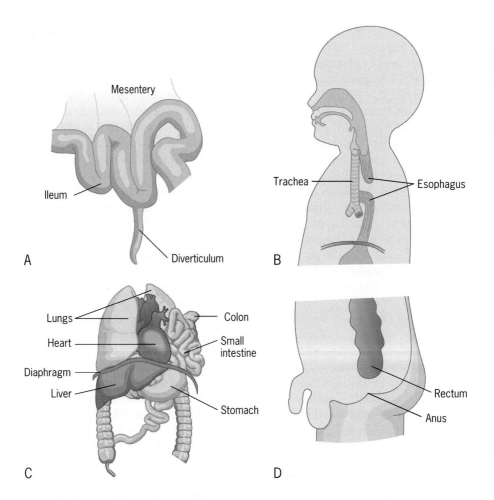

A

B

C

D

FIGURE 14–4 Malformations of the gastrointestinal tract. **A.** Meckel diverticulum. **B.** Esophageal atresia. **C.** Congenital diaphragmatic hernia. **D.** Imperforate anus.

Congenital Pyloric Stenosis

Congenital pyloric stenosis is narrowing of the outlet of the distal stomach as a result of hypertrophy of the pyloric muscle (**Figure 14–5**). The pyloric sphincter is often so thick that it can be felt as an olive-shaped mass on palpation of the upper abdomen. The cause is unknown, and for some reason, symptoms of projectile vomiting after feeding do not begin until 2 to 4 weeks after birth. Other than Meckel's diverticulum, this is the most common developmental abnormality of the alimentary tract. It occurs almost exclusively in boys. A simple operation to split the thickened pyloric muscle effects a cure.

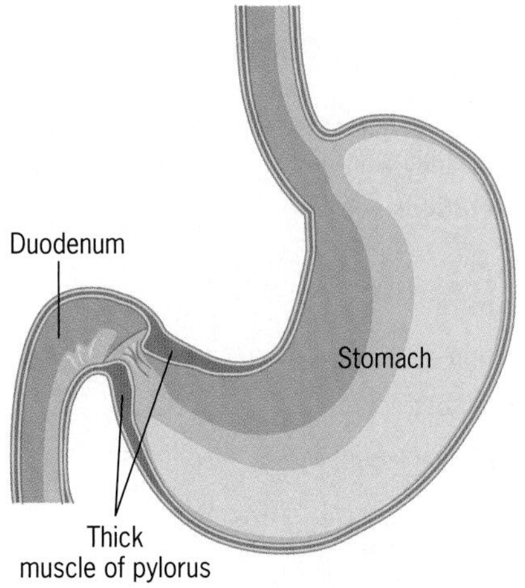

FIGURE 14–5 Congenital pyloric stenosis.

BOX 14–2   Congenital Pyloric Stenosis
Causes
Unknown
Lesions
Thickened muscle of pyloric sphincter
Manifestations
Onset at age 2 to 4 weeks
Usually in boys
Projectile vomiting
Dehydration and weight loss

Hirschsprung Disease

A rich plexus of nerves in the submucosa and muscularis propria of the entire gastrointestinal tract coordinates peristalsis and regulates the production of hormones that stimulate digestion and absorption. Lack of *ganglion cells*, or nerve cell bodies, in the rectum results in defective evacuation of feces, with consequent massive distention of the colon, or **megacolon** (**Figure 14–6**). This condition is called **Hirschsprung disease**. It is suspected in infants with chronic constipation and distended abdomen. Biopsy of the rectum, to demonstrate absence of ganglion cells, is necessary for diagnosis. Surgical removal of the aganglionic segment and reattachment of the normal bowel to the anus results in reestablishment of function of the distal colon with preserved anal control of defecation.

BOX 14–3   Hirschsprung Disease

Causes

Unknown

Lesions

No ganglion cells in a segment of rectum

Narrow rectum, distended colon

Megacolon

Manifestations

Constipation

Abdominal distention

Variable age of onset of symptoms

Inflammatory/Degenerative Diseases

The diseases discussed in this section illustrate the great variety of inflammatory and degenerative conditions that involve the alimentary tract. These diseases vary by location within the gastrointestinal tract, chronicity, manifestations, and degree of medical or surgical intervention required for control. Infections and degenerative and autoimmune processes can affect any segment of the gastrointestinal tract, but some infectious agents or inflammatory conditions have predilections for particular locations. In this section, we discuss the most common inflammatory or degenerative conditions in a sequential manner, beginning with the esophagus and ending at the anus. This discussion is not comprehensive. Some conditions, such as bowel infarction, volvulus (twisting of the bowel around its mesentery), irritable bowel syndrome, pinworm infection, hemorrhoids, and pilonidal cysts are not discussed in the interest of keeping the chapter to a reasonable length.

Reflux Esophagitis

Reflux esophagitis, also called gastroesophageal reflux disease (GERD), is irritation of the mucosa and submucosa of the lower esophagus by acidic gastric contents. It is caused by incompetence of the sphincter at the lower end of the esophagus. This is not an anatomic sphincter, like the pyloric muscle, but rather a functional one: the muscle at the distal end of the esophagus simply opens in response to food being propelled toward it from the oropharynx. In reflux esophagitis, the muscle dilates abnormally, allowing gastric juices to wash back up into the esophagus.

In many cases, there is an associated **hiatal hernia**, which allows the stomach to slide up through the diaphragm into the thorax (**Figure 14–7**). The diaphragm provides some of the tone of the esophageal sphincter, so release of the gastroesophageal junction from this anatomic relationship potentiates reflux. Hiatal hernia is a common finding that increases in frequency with age. Despite its strong association with gastric reflux, most hiatal hernias are asymptomatic and not associated with an incompetent lower esophageal sphincter. Other

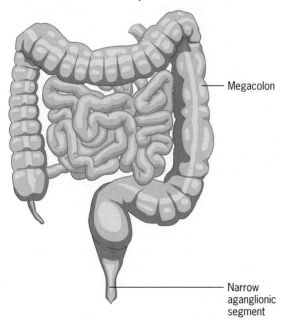

FIGURE 14–6 Megacolon in Hirschsprung disease.

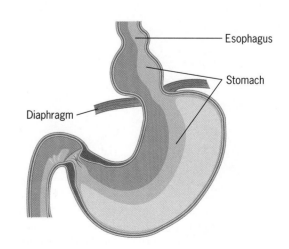

FIGURE 14–7 Hiatal hernia.

conditions associated with reflux esophagitis include alcohol, smoking, obesity, and pregnancy.

The occasional heartburn one might feel after a heavy meal does not usually cause any serious damage to the esophagus. Persistent, severe reflux, however, can cause secondary changes. Persistent inflammation induces metaplasia of the esophageal mucosa. The usual stratified squamous mucosa is replaced by gastric-type, mucus-secreting columnar mucosa, presumably in an attempt to protect the esophageal wall from chemical irritation and ulceration. The gastric mucosa can then undergo a second metaplastic alteration to intestinal-type epithelium, complete with intestinal absorptive and mucous cells (**Figure 14–8**). If this alteration extends more than 3 cm above the anatomic gastroesophageal junction, it is called **Barrett's esophagus**. Barrett's esophagus requires frequent monitoring by endoscopy and biopsy because it is a premalignant condition. Most adenocarcinomas of the esophagus arise from Barrett's esophagus.

In addition, severe and persistent inflammation can lead to ulceration and subsequent scarring. Contraction of the scar tissue causes stricture formation in the esophagus, which causes pain with swallowing and impairment of the ability to eat solid and, if severe, even liquid foods.

Reflux should be addressed well before any other complications develop. At the very least, patients should avoid foods that increase acidic reflux, such as chocolate, coffee, and alcohol, and take medications that reduce acid production by the gastric epithelium, such as proton pump inhibitors. Inflammation can be reduced if reflux is eradicated, but Barrett's esophagus is not considered to be a reversible condition. People with biopsy-proven Barrett's esophagus should be monitored with frequent endoscopy and biopsy so as to detect and treat dysplasia and carcinoma at a curable stage. Strictures can be released by surgical means.

GERD is very common. About 10% of the adult population of the United States suffers from reflux at least once a week, if not more frequently. It can occur in children and increases in frequency with age. It is one of the most common reasons for office visits, and an estimated one third of healthcare spending is for medications to control reflux. However, only about 10% of people with severe reflux develop Barrett's esophagus, and of those, only 1% will develop esophageal adenocarcinoma.

BOX 14–4   Reflux Esophagitis

Causes

Incompetent lower esophageal sphincter

Esophageal hiatal hernia

Alcohol

Smoking

Obesity

Pregnancy

Lesions

Inflammation of distal esophagus

Gastric metaplasia

Intestinal metaplasia (Barrett's esophagus)

Ulceration, stricture

Manifestations

Heartburn, chest pain, cough

Endoscopy: hernia, esophagitis, gastric and intestinal metaplasia

Dysphagia

Adenocarcinoma of esophagus

Gastritis

Acute injury to the gastric mucosa is caused by agents that compromise the protective mucous barrier lying over the epithelial cells, exposing them to damage by acidic gastric juices. The most common injurious agents are alcohol and nonsteroidal anti-inflammatory drugs (NSAIDs). The cells of the gastric epithelium normally are replaced every 2–6 days, so superficial injury heals rapidly if the offense is not repeated. Chronic ingestion of NSAIDs, chemotherapy and radiation therapy, and chronic alcohol use can cause more severe damage that results in destruction of the epithelium with resultant hemorrhage or even perforation. Symptoms of acute **gastritis** include nausea, vomiting, and epigastric pain.

There are two major forms of chronic gastritis: fundal, or autoimmune, gastritis and *Helicobacter* gastritis. **Autoimmune gastritis** involves the fundus, where the acid- and enzyme-producing cells are located. As the name implies, this is an autoimmune disease in which autoantibodies are produced against components of parietal cells, which are the cells that produce gastric acid. Over many years, parietal cells are destroyed, resulting in atrophy of the fundal epithelium. Autoantibodies

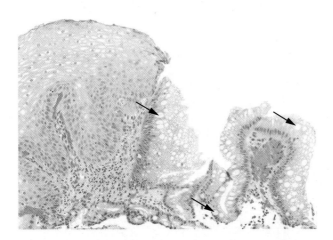

FIGURE 14–8 Intestinal metaplasia in the esophagus. The normal squamous epithelial lining of the esophagus on the left side of the picture changes abruptly to intestinal type epithelium with goblet cells (arrows) on the right side of the picture.

are also produced against **intrinsic factor**, a protein that is required for absorption of vitamin B_{12} in the ileum. Decreased levels of vitamin B_{12} eventually result in **pernicious anemia**. Nowadays, this type of anemia is discovered before it becomes pernicious, and is treated with vitamin B_{12} supplementation. Symptoms of full-blown pernicious anemia include neurologic signs such as tingling in the hands and feet, neuropathic pain, and mild cognitive impairment; symptoms of anemia such as fatigue, pallor, and rapid heart rate; thyroid hormone abnormalities; and, curiously, a grotesquely swollen, red tongue.

Helicobacter pylori is a curved bacterium that lives in the mucous layer of the gastric epithelial surface (**Figure 14–9**) and incites an acute as well as chronic inflammatory reaction most prominent in the antral part of the stomach. About 80% of people with acute *H. pylori* infection experience no symptoms at all. It is the chronic gastritis induced by long-standing *H. pylori* that comes to medical attention. More than 90% of chronic gastritis is caused by this organism. Symptoms, which again are not present in all patients, include gnawing, burning upper abdominal pain, and loss of appetite.

H. pylori is thought to be the most prevalent infective agent worldwide. Prevalence rates vary from 10% to 80%. In the United States, about 25% of adults are thought to harbor the organism. Infection becomes more frequent with age; infection rates are highest in poor, crowded, and rural areas; and prevalence rates vary by ethnicity and level of education. Based on these demographic and epidemiologic factors, it is thought that transmission occurs via infected food or water, but the exact mode of transmission has not been determined.

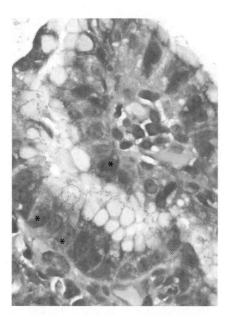

FIGURE 14–9 *Helicobacter pylori* organisms in the stomach. This portion of stomach, stained with a modified Giemsa stain rather than the usual H&E, is photographed at 400x magnification. Epithelial cell nuclei are marked by asterisks. This stain highlights the bacteria as small dark rods adherent to the surface of the gastric epithelial cells (inside the circle, and all along the layer of mucin through the center of the image).

Antibiotics in conjunction with proton pump inhibitors are highly effective in treating *H. pylori* infection. The medications have to be taken for a couple of weeks to ensure complete eradication of the organism, so compliance may be an issue. Repeated courses of therapy are sometimes necessary. Infection with *H. pylori* is a strong risk factor for the development of peptic and duodenal ulcers (discussed later) as well as for various malignancies. In fact, *H. pylori* has been proclaimed a carcinogen. People with *H. pylori* infection are six times more likely to develop gastric cancer than are those without such infection. *H. pylori* also stimulates the development of **MALT lymphoma**. The long-standing, smoldering inflammation in the stomach appears to stimulate the immune cells of the mucosa-associated lymphoid tissue (MALT) of the gastric epithelium to become relatively autonomous. Gastric MALT lymphoma is an indolent lymphoma that usually stays confined to the stomach, but it can spread to other organs in later stages of the disease. It is the only cancer that is treatable with antibiotics: eradication of the *H. pylori* infection causes regression of the tumor in its early stages. Unfortunately, the same is not true for gastric adenocarcinoma.

H. pylori gastritis can be diagnosed in a variety of ways. Antibodies produced against the bacterium can be detected in blood. Products of metabolism of the organism can be detected in a breath test or in gastric juices obtained during endoscopy. The organism can be seen in the epithelium of the stomach in gastric biopsies (Figure 14–9).

BOX 14–5 Acute and Chronic Gastritis

Causes

Helicobacter pylori

Autoimmune gastritis

NSAIDs, alcohol

Lesions

Inflammation of stomach mucosa

Manifestations

Nausea, vomiting

Upper abdominal pain

Loss of appetite

Bleeding

Propensity for development of gastric cancer, lymphoma (*H. pylori* infection only)

Peptic Ulcer

Peptic ulcers are most common in the first part of the duodenum but also occur in the stomach or in the esophagus in cases of long-standing GERD. The word *peptic* refers to the acidic digestive juice produced by the stomach, which is one of the contributing factors in the development of ulcers. The stomach mucosa is protected from these juices by a thick mucous coat, but the duodenum and esophagus do not have such an effective protective barrier. Increased acid secretion, usually in conjunction with some other factor that compromises the integrity of the epithelium, causes lethal injury to the epithelial cells. These slough, exposing the submucosa, with its rich plexus of blood vessels, to the further erosive activity of the gastric acid and digestive enzymes.

A peptic ulcer is a sharply punched-out area of epithelial cell loss, at the base of which is granulation tissue covered by an inflammatory exudate (**Figure 14–10**). Peptic ulcers come to medical attention when they cause pain or bleeding. Symptoms include nausea, vomiting, bloating, and gnawing or burning upper-abdominal pain that typically occurs about 1–3 hours after meals, is relieved by alkali or food, and is worse at night. Occasionally, the pain is referred to the chest or back, where it can be mistaken for a myocardial infarction. The pain may be so aggravating that it inhibits adequate caloric intake, resulting in weight loss. Bleeding can manifest as iron-deficiency anemia, detected on routine blood work, or resulting in fatigue and pallor, or as massive bleeding. The latter occurs when the ulcer erodes into a large vessel, usually an artery, which then spews blood into the gastric lumen. This is a surgical emergency, because large amounts of blood can be lost in a short amount of time. Endoscopic techniques are used to clamp or cauterize the bleeding vessel at the base of the ulcer. Another serious complication of ulcers is perforation, which occurs if the ulcer gnaws all the way through the gut wall, and which results in peritonitis.

Acid secretion can be increased by *H. pylori*, stress, and various medical conditions such as alcoholic cirrhosis or hypocalcemia. Additional epithelial injury is incurred by such things as NSAID use, smoking, or steroids. *H. pylori* is one of the biggest risk factors in the pathogenesis of peptic ulcers: about 75% of patients with peptic ulcers have *H. pylori* infection. By comparison, only 20% of people infected with *H. pylori* develop peptic ulcers.

The treatment of peptic ulcers revolves around decreasing acid secretion and eliminating the cofactors that led to the development of the ulcers in the first place, such as *H. pylori* or NSAID use. Although most duodenal ulcers heal with medical therapy or even spontaneously, recurrences are common. Some patients require surgical intervention. Operations can be performed to remove a nonhealing ulcer, to remove the gastric antrum, which secretes the acid-stimulating hormone gastrin, or to partially remove the gastric body and its acid-secreting glands. In addition, vagotomy (cutting the vagus nerve) reduces the nervous stimulation to acid production.

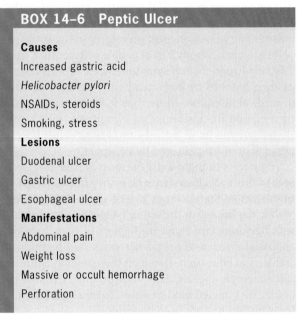

BOX 14–6   Peptic Ulcer

Causes
Increased gastric acid
Helicobacter pylori
NSAIDs, steroids
Smoking, stress
Lesions
Duodenal ulcer
Gastric ulcer
Esophageal ulcer
Manifestations
Abdominal pain
Weight loss
Massive or occult hemorrhage
Perforation

Malabsorption Syndromes

Failure to digest and/or absorb food is called **malabsorption**. Malabsorption can be caused by a variety of disease processes that impair enzyme activity and absorption of nutrients across the gastrointestinal epithelium. These include genetically based enzyme deficiencies; pancreatic insufficiency; infectious diseases, which alter intestinal microflora; autoimmune diseases; surgical reduction of a considerable length of the small intestine, which reduces the surface area available for absorption; or nonspecific degenerative changes in older adults.

There is considerable geographic variation in the prevalence of enzymatic deficiencies. In Asian countries, **lactase deficiency** affects about 90% of the population. Most infants are born with functioning lactase enzyme, but as they mature, their ability to digest *lactose*, a carbohydrate present primarily in dairy products, diminishes. When people with lactase deficiency eat dairy products, the bacteria in their colon ferment the lactose and produce abundant gases, which result in abdominal bloating, flatulence, and diarrhea. Lactase can be supplemented in the diet, but avoidance of lactose-containing foods also prevents symptoms. Reduction or absence of any other enzyme involved in digestion can result in similar symptoms.

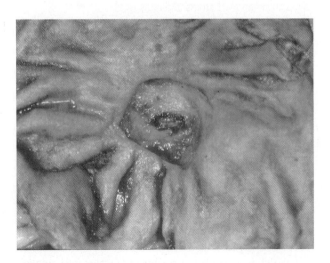

FIGURE 14–10 Peptic ulcer. The stomach mucosa is tan-orange and slightly granular. The ulcer is the punched-out defect in the center of the image. At the base of the ulcer is necrotic debris with some recent hemorrhage (dark red material) around the periphery.

Celiac disease is a prevalent malabsorption syndrome, affecting about 1–2% of the population, particularly individuals of northern European descent. In patients with celiac disease, *gluten*, a protein present in grains, induces injury to the mucosa of the small intestine. The injury is immune mediated: the body produces an antibody to a component of gluten, which elicits an inflammatory attack on the epithelial cells of the duodenum and jejunum. The villi, normally long, delicate, fingerlike projections, become short and stubby or even entirely flat (**Figure 14–11**). This dramatically reduces the surface area over which absorption can take place. Not only is caloric intake hindered, but also absorption of vitamins, calcium, and iron. Resulting symptoms are referable to the gastrointestinal tract, such as abdominal pain, diarrhea, flatulence, and fatty, foul-smelling stool (from decreased absorption of fats); to deficiencies of essential vitamins and minerals, such as impaired blood clotting (vitamin K deficiency), hyperparathyroidism (calcium deficiency), and iron-deficiency anemia; and to inadequate caloric intake. Avoidance of gluten in the diet, primarily foods made of wheat, reverses the inflammation and structural changes of the villi. Celiac disease often runs in families, suggesting that it has a genetic basis, and can be associated with other autoimmune diseases, such as diabetes mellitus type 1. If the inflammation is prolonged and untreated, adenocarcinoma or T-cell lymphoma can develop in the intestine. Diagnosis is suggested by histologic examination of duodenal biopsies and demonstration of anti-gluten antibodies in the serum. Definitive diagnosis is made when there is complete resolution of symptoms and reversal of duodenal injury after gluten is completely withdrawn from the diet.

BOX 14–7 Malabsorption Syndromes

Causes

Enzyme deficiency

Gluten sensitivity

Pancreatic insufficiency

Surgical reduction of gastrointestinal tract

Lesions

Mucosal inflammation and atrophy

Others related to underlying cause—for example, pancreatic atrophy

Manifestations

Bloating, flatulence, diarrhea

Large, bulky, foul-smelling stools

Weight loss, failure to thrive

Abnormalities of tests for fat and carbohydrate absorption

May be abnormal intestinal biopsy (celiac disease)

Secondary effects: iron-deficiency anemia, coagulopathy, hyperparathyroidism

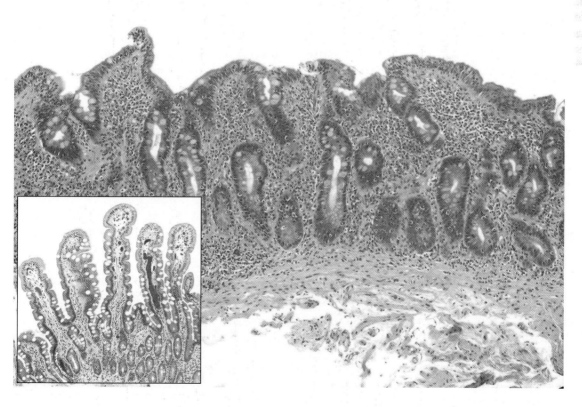

FIGURE 14–11 Celiac sprue. The inset shows normal duodenal mucosa with long, finger-like villi. The villi in celiac sprue are absent: the mucosa is flat and the lamina propria expanded by inflammatory cells.

Infectious Diarrhea and Food Poisoning

Intestinal infections are typically spread by the fecal–oral route. Most microorganisms that are ingested are destroyed by the acid in the stomach and pass through the gastrointestinal tract without causing harm. Highly virulent organisms can escape destruction in the stomach and invade the mucosa of the upper small intestine (viruses) or distal small intestine and colon (*Ameba, Shigella, Campylobacter*). Microorganisms that are less virulent or more susceptible to destruction in the stomach must be ingested in larger numbers to cause disease. Intestinal disease caused by microorganisms of low or intermediate virulence is typically associated with food poisoning. Entire colonies of pathogenic bacteria—for example, *Salmonella*—are ingested in contaminated food and by their sheer number overcome the host's defenses. The intestines may also serve as a portal of entry for organisms that cause systemic infections, such as typhoid fever or tuberculosis. And, of course, the intestines can harbor parasites such as the tapeworm, pinworm, and fluke that can cause malnutrition as well as symptoms referable to infection in other organs. In this section, we discuss only those infectious agents that cause diarrhea and food poisoning. **Table 14–2** compares some of the more common ones.

Viral enteritis (intestinal flu) is the most common type of gastrointestinal infection. *Rotavirus* and noroviruses (e.g., Norwalk virus) are the most common causes and account for the majority of childhood deaths resulting from diarrhea. Viral enteritis can be both seasonal, or epidemic, and sporadic. Children are more commonly involved than are adults. The virus is easily transmitted in institutional settings such as day care centers, schools, hospitals, and nursing homes. The virus grows in surface epithelial cells of the small intestine, leading in 1 to 2 days to nausea, vomiting, diarrhea, and malaise that last from one to several days. Diagnosis is presumptive, and treatment revolves around preventing excessive fluid loss from vomiting and diarrhea. Distribution of oral rehydration packets, promotion of breastfeeding, and increased attention to cleanliness of drinking water have reduced infant deaths resulting from diarrhea from the first to second leading cause of death in this age group worldwide.

Traveler's diarrhea refers to any acute diarrheal illness in travelers to foreign countries. Natives usually are immune or have low-grade involvement because of prior exposure. Entertoxin-producing *Escherichia coli* (ETEC) and *Campylobacter jejuni* are the most common causes of traveler's diarrhea. *E. coli* is a bacterium that normally colonizes the intestinal tract, usually within hours after an infant's birth. Various strains are pathogenic, however. ETEC produces a couple of toxins that induce chloride and water secretion and impair absorption in the intestine. The person affected by traveler's diarrhea may be mildly inconvenienced by diarrhea and abdominal cramps or completely incapacitated for one to several days. In either case, the affliction is self-limited and neither identification of the particular organism causing it nor antibiotic therapy is necessary. Prevention consists of avoidance of nonsterile fluids and raw or undercooked foods.

When several people who have eaten the same food become ill with vomiting and diarrhea, **food poisoning** should be suspected. Outbreaks of food poisoning are investigated by public health authorities, who search for the source of the contaminated food. This may be a food handler who does not know that s/he is infected but is capable of transmitting the organism to others or food that has been poorly refrigerated, such as chicken salads consumed at a picnic on a warm summer day.

TABLE 14–2　**Comparison of Infectious Diarrheas and Food Poisoning**

	Causes	Manifestations	Duration	Setting
Viral enteritis	*Rotavirus*, noroviruses most common	Acute-onset diarrhea, vomiting; may lead to dehydration	1–2 days	Epidemic, seasonal; day care centers, nursing homes
Traveler's diarrhea	Enterotoxin-producing *Escherichia coli* most common	Acute-onset diarrhea, abdominal cramps, malaise	About 1 week	Travel to foreign country
Food poisoning	Bacteria—for example, *Salmonella* enterotoxins	Acute onset, 1–4 hours after eating contaminated food	1–2 days	Usually several people who ate the same food are affected
Dysentery	Bacillary (*Shigella*) Amoebic (*Entamoeba histolytica*)	Profuse mucoid or bloody diarrhea	About 1 week; amoebic can be chronic	Epidemic or endemic; poor sanitation, infected water
Typhoid fever	*Salmonella typhi*	Fever, bloody diarrhea, delirium	4–6 weeks	Epidemic; asymptomatic carriers
Cholera	*Vibrio cholerae*	Profuse, watery diarrhea	Lethal within 24 hours	Epidemic

The pathogenic factor of food poisoning is either colonies of organisms such as *Salmonella* or *C. jejuni* that have grown in the food and are capable of causing damage to the intestinal epithelium, or **enterotoxins**, which induce vomiting and diarrhea. Enterotoxins are chemicals produced by bacteria that have detrimental effects on a host's cells. Examples include the enterotoxin B produced by *Staphylococcus aureus* growing in contaminated dairy products or processed meats, which stimulates a profound inflammatory response by activating immune cells; and the botulinum toxin, which is produced by *Clostridium botulinum* and is toxic to nerve cells. The former causes a self-limited disease that requires only supportive care during the time in which the toxin passes through the system and epithelial cells regenerate. **Botulism**, however, is a potentially deadly disease because it causes paralysis of muscles, including the muscles of respiration. Treatment requires supportive care, including mechanical ventilation, if necessary, until the body has cleared the toxin on its own.

All forms of food poisoning can be prevented by keeping food properly refrigerated, maintaining adequate hygiene, and using sterile canning procedures. Cooking contaminated food can kill bacteria, such as *Salmonella* (the typical culprit when enteritis is contracted after eating raw eggs), but it does not eliminate enterotoxins. Infant botulism is the most common form of botulism in the United States, and contaminated honey is the primary reservoir. *C. botulinum* can colonize the infant gut because the intestinal microflora are not mature until after the first year of life. Infants should therefore not be given honey or honey-containing foods before their first birthday.

Dysentery is severe diarrhea with mucus and/or blood in the feces. Bacillary dysentery is caused by *Shigella*, a bacterium transmitted by contaminated food and water. Amoebic dysentery is caused by the protozoan *Entamoeba histolytica*. *Shigella* is highly virulent: ingestion of just a few of the organisms can cause disease. However, it is also quite susceptible to gastric acid. As with most food- and waterborne illnesses, dysentery occurs most commonly in institutional settings (nursing homes, army barracks) and in poor, rural, or overcrowded living conditions. The diarrhea is accompanied by fever, chills, and abdominal pain. In case of *Shigella*, the infection is self-limited; however, *Entamoeba* can get into the bloodstream and travel to other parts of the body, setting up abscesses in distant sites. Liver abscess is the most common complication of *E. histolytica* infection. Amoebic infection requires antibiotics for eradication. Both organisms can be identified in stool, *Shigella* by culture and *E. histolytica* by direct examination of feces for the organism.

No discussion of enteritides is complete without mention of typhoid fever and cholera—two epidemic, lethal gastrointestinal infections. Typhoid fever, caused by *Salmonella typhi* or *S. paratyphi* (not to be confused with the *Salmonella* causing food poisoning), causes an illness of 4–6 weeks' duration, characterized by high fevers, gastrointestinal hemorrhage, and possibly even encephalitis. The mortality is about 20% if not treated. Survivors may harbor the bacteria in the liver and gallbladder and shed it asymptomatically, thus propagating transmission. Vaccination exists for travelers to areas of the world where the prevalence of the disease is still high.

Cholera is a diarrheal illness with a fatality of up to 60% if not treated. *Vibrio cholerae* produces an enterotoxin that alters the permeability of epithelial cells of the large intestine, resulting in profuse, watery diarrhea. The afflicted patient can lose 1 liter of fluid an hour and rapidly succumbs to dehydration within 24 hours. Antibiotics can eradicate the bacteria but usually not in time to save the victim's life. Oral rehydration cuts fatality to less than 1% if administered on time. Transmission occurs in epidemic fashion. In the 19th and 20th centuries, epidemics of cholera spread in waves across Europe and the United States from India, where it was endemic. After public health initiatives promoted public sanitation programs in most of the developed world, cholera outbreaks diminished. Today, they predictably occur in poor and overcrowded areas or in settings where civil strife or natural disasters destroy public sanitation infrastructures, such as in Haiti after the 2010 earthquake. An oral vaccine offering moderate protection is available, but the best means of preventing cholera outbreaks is through widespread implementation of proper sanitation and water purification systems.

Inguinal Hernia

Inguinal hernia, commonly referred to as a "rupture," is an outpouching of abdominal contents into the groin (**Figure 14–12**). Loops of bowel can become incarcerated, or caught, in the pouch so that they cannot move in unison with the rest of the intestine. Incarcerated hernias are susceptible to becoming twisted, occluded, or pinched off. This is called *strangulation* and is a medical

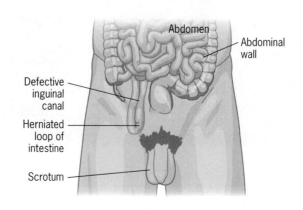

FIGURE 14–12 Inguinal hernia.

emergency because the loop of bowel will undergo necrosis, with subsequent perforation and/or peritonitis. It is obviously best to surgically repair the hernia before such complications occur. Inguinal hernia repairs are one of the most common operations performed in the United States.

Inguinal hernias are much more common in men than in women because in males, the peritoneum is normally carried into the inguinal region with the testes as these descend from the abdomen into the scrotum during fetal development. The path the testes take usually seals off on its own, but it is susceptible to being forced open again, especially subsequent to abdominal strain, such as is incurred by lifting heavy objects. Hernias can also occur in children and in women, and they can occur in other locations. The abdominal wall at the umbilicus, for example, is a weak spot that can tear and allow escape of abdominal contents underneath the skin. This occurs particularly in obese individuals. Surgical scars are also weaker than the native musculature and can tear, allowing abdominal contents to bulge through the abdominal wall.

BOX 14-8 Inguinal Hernia

Causes

Congenital weakness of abdominal wall in groin

Lesions

Peritoneal pouch extends through abdominal muscles

Manifestations

Pouch felt on physical exam; loop of bowel can be pushed back into abdomen

Strangulation, obstruction, infarction, perforation, peritonitis

---

Acute Appendicitis

The vermiform appendix is a vestigial outpouching of the proximal colon that has no known function but often becomes acutely inflamed (**Figure 14-13**). The bacteria

causing the inflammation are those normally present in the colon. Sometimes a calcified mass of feces (fecalith) blocks the lumen of the appendix, thus predisposing it to infection, but often an underlying reason for the inflammation is not discovered. Surgical removal of the acutely inflamed appendix is necessary to avoid complications such as abscess formation, perforation leading to peritonitis, and spread of the infection to the liver.

Appendicitis is more common in children and adolescents than in adults. It begins with pain, usually starting in the umbilical region and then moving to the right lower quadrant of the abdomen. The inflammation of the peritoneum causes tenderness to palpation, and the abdominal muscles become rigid in response to the irritation. Rebound tenderness is exacerbation of pain when the abdominal wall is suddenly released after deep palpation. The patient may also complain of abdominal pain when walking because the impact of the feet on the ground is referred to the abdomen. These signs are not always present, however, and not specific because diseases of adjacent organs, such as the right ovary and fallopian tube and distal ileum, can cause similar symptoms. The patient will usually have fever and anorexia, and the white blood cell count will be elevated. These are also nonspecific findings. CT scan can be instructive if the inflammation has already caused significant edema. Not even experienced surgeons are always right in predicting whether a patient's abdominal pain is truly caused by appendicitis; about 15–40% of appendices removed for the clinical impression of appendicitis are entirely normal when examined by the pathologist.

Acute appendicitis is a surgical emergency. The appendix can rupture and cause peritonitis leading to sepsis. Appendicitis is the most common indication for surgical intervention in the abdominal cavity. Nowadays, removal of the appendix can be achieved by laparoscopic surgery, in which instruments, including a video camera, are introduced and manipulated robotically via small holes in the abdomen. Recovery after such operations is very rapid.

BOX 14-9 Acute Appendicitis

Causes

Usually unknown

Fecalith

Lesions

Acute inflammation of appendix

Abscess, peritonitis if severe

Manifestations

Abdominal pain

Rebound tenderness

Anorexia

Fever

Leukocytosis

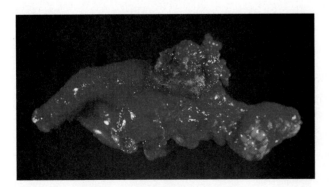

FIGURE 14-13 Acute appendicitis. The resected end of the appendix is on the left, the tip is on the right. The appendix is bright red, and in the mid-portion it is perforated. A mass of hemorrhagic and fibrinous debris exudes from the rupture site. The surrounding adipose tissue also is inflamed.

Inflammatory Bowel Disease

Inflammatory bowel disease refers collectively to two chronic inflammatory conditions of the intestinal tract called ulcerative colitis and Crohn disease. Their pathogenesis appears to involve a complex interaction of genetic, immune, microbial, and environmental factors. Both diseases cause diarrhea, hemorrhage, and abdominal pain. The symptoms can significantly interfere with a person's daily activities and cause severe pain and weight loss. The conditions are much more common in Caucasians (in fact, they have their highest prevalence among some Jewish populations) and most commonly appear in adolescence and young adulthood. They have a second peak in incidence in the 50- to 70-year age group.

Owing to the similarity of presentation, the specific diagnosis may not immediately be obvious. Even microscopically, the two diseases are so similar that it is not always possible to differentiate between the two on histologic findings alone. The diagnosis requires a thorough medical history, endoscopic exam, and microscopy documenting acute injury to the deep portions of the enteric mucosa, the intestinal crypts. The main discriminating factor between the two diseases is the pattern of injury (**Table 14–3**). Ulcerative colitis (UC) is confined to the mucosa of the colon, always involves the rectum, and extends proximally to variable extents (**Figure 14–14A**). It may affect the distal ileum if the inflammation extends as far as the cecum, but it does not extend to the small intestine, stomach, or esophagus. Crohn disease is patchy, involves all layers of the bowel wall, and occurs most commonly in the distal ileum (**Figure 14–14B**). It also often involves the colon (hence the confusion with UC), but its distribution is not continuous: patches of severe inflammation are separated by areas of entirely uninvolved mucosa. It rarely involves the rectum, but it can affect other areas of the GI tract including the esophagus and stomach.

Both diseases have serious long-term complications. Chronic inflammation can induce dysplasia in UC, which can further progress to carcinoma. Colon cancer begins to develop after about 10 years of involvement with the

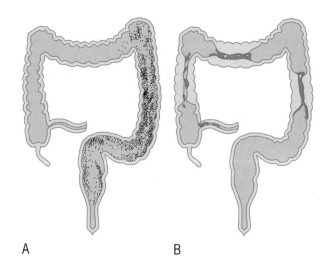

FIGURE 14–14 Distribution of ulcerative colitis (**A**) and Crohn disease (**B**) in the colon and terminal ileum.

disease. About 5% of patients with UC develop colon cancer, but the risk is higher if the entire colon is involved. UC patients should undergo periodic endoscopic evaluations, with extensive biopsies of the mucosa, to detect dysplasia before invasive cancer has developed. About 5% of patients with UC will develop *primary sclerosing cholangitis*, an inflammatory obliteration of the bile ducts in the liver, leading to obstruction of the outflow of bile and eventually cirrhosis and its complications. Complications of Crohn disease result from full-thickness inflammation of the bowel wall, which induces strictures and subsequent obstruction of the bowel, abscesses, and fistula tracts that tunnel through the bowel wall into adjacent tissues or organs. Perianal fistulae are particularly common. Crohn disease patients with colonic involvement should also have periodic endoscopies to evaluate for dysplasia and carcinoma, although the incidence of carcinoma in Crohn disease is not as high as in UC. Patients with inflammatory bowel disease can also develop symptoms of inflammation in other tissues of the body, such as the eye, skin, and joints.

TABLE 14–3	**Differences Between Ulcerative Colitis and Crohn Disease**	
	Ulcerative Colitis	**Crohn Disease**
Distribution in intestinal tract	Always involves rectum, proceeds proximally, may involve terminal ileum	Ileum and colon most common; stomach, esophagus, mouth can also be involved
Involvement of bowel wall	Mucosal involvement only	Transmural involvement
Involvement of mucosa	Continuous Broad, superficial ulcers	Discontinuous (patchy) Deep, sharp, longitudinal fissures and ulcers
Complications	Neoplasia Primary sclerosing cholangitis	Strictures, abscesses, fistula tracts Fat and vitamin malabsorption
Surgery	Curative in severe cases or cases with neoplasia	Contraindicated except to treat complications

Treatment of inflammatory bowel disease involves reducing enteric inflammation. Steroids, nonsteroidal anti-inflammatory drugs (e.g., aspirin enemas), chemotherapeutic agents that interfere with DNA synthesis in rapidly replicating cells of the immune system (e.g., methotrexate), and drugs that interfere with powerful signaling molecules in the inflammatory response are all of proven benefit. Total removal of the colon in severe UC that is not responsive to medical management or in which dysplasia has been histologically documented is curative. Resection of Crohn disease–induced strictures and surgical excision of fistula tracts are feasible, but the disease recurs virtually 100% of the time in the remaining GI tract and the medical anastamoses heal poorly. Control of the diseases also requires dietary management to prevent iron-deficiency anemia, vitamin deficiencies, and weight loss.

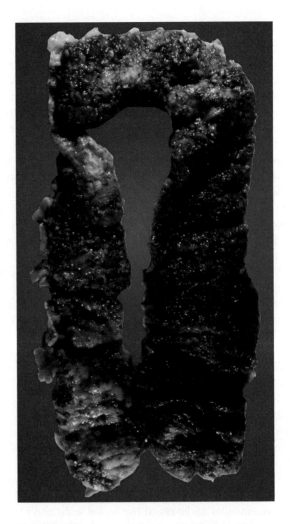

FIGURE 14–15 Pseudomembranous colitis. The bowel has been opened to expose the lumenal surface. A few areas of relatively normal, pink mucosa are visible, but most of the surface is covered by green to black patches of necrotic debris. This is the "pseudomembrane" composed of necrotic mucosa, acute inflammatory cells, fibrin, and bacteria.

BOX 14–10   Inflammatory Bowel Disease

Causes

Unknown

Lesions

Ulcerative colitis—diffuse chronic mucosal inflammation of colon

Crohn disease—localized inflammatory thickening anywhere in the alimentary tract, most commonly in the ileum

Manifestations

Chronic diarrhea

Chronic hemorrhage leading to anemia

Weight loss

Exacerbations and remissions

Interference with lifestyle

Cancer as late complication

Pseudomembranous Colitis

The *pseudomembrane* of **pseudomembranous colitis** consists of necrotic cells, mucus, fibrin, and acute inflammatory cells forming a sticky exudate on the mucosal surface of the colon (**Figure 14–15**). Pseudomembranous colitis occurs most commonly in the setting of prolonged antibiotic use. Antibiotics diminish the diversity of microbes living in the gut, which promotes overgrowth of the bacterium *Clostridium difficile*. *C. difficile* produces an enterotoxin that causes irreversible damage to the colonic epithelial cells. The dead cells, along with the other debris of inflammation, are discharged onto the surface of the denuded colonic wall. Manifestations are fever, abdominal pain, leukocytosis, and watery diarrhea, which can lead to dehydration. If severe, the inflammation can extend transmurally. This is usually associated with the life-threatening complication *toxic megacolon*. Toxic megacolon can occur with other diseases, such as UC or Hirschsprung disease. It is characterized by severe dilation and paralysis of a segment of the colon and can proceed to perforation, sepsis, and shock. If untreated, toxic megacolon has a fatality rate of about 20%. Pseudomembranous colitis should be suspected in any patient on antibiotics who develops sudden diarrhea.

BOX 14–11   Pseudomembranous Colitis

Causes

Antibiotics, allowing overgrowth of *C. difficile*

C. difficile enterotoxin

Lesions

Pseudomembrane overlying colonic surface, composed of dead cells and inflammatory debris

Manifestations

Abdominal pain, fever, leukocytosis, watery diarrhea

Toxic megacolon, sepsis, shock

Colonic Diverticulosis

Multiple outpouchings (sing., *diverticulum*, pl., *diverticula*) of the colon develop with increasing frequency with advancing age at points of weakness in the muscular wall of the colon, especially the sigmoid colon (**Figure 14–16**). About 50% of people older than 60 years have some degree of diverticulosis, but rarely are they symptomatic. Occasionally, a diverticulum becomes inflamed, possibly because its lumen is occluded by a fecalith. The symptoms of diverticulitis are pain, localized usually to the left side of the abdomen, fever, nausea, and a change in bowel habits. An abscess can develop in the area of the inflamed diverticulum and cause more severe symptoms. The inflamed diverticulum might also rupture, resulting in peritonitis. These complications require emergency surgical intervention and aggressive antimicrobial therapy. Once the inflammation subsides, the tissue can scar down, resulting in obstruction. This also requires surgical treatment. More rarely, an artery in the vicinity of a diverticulum can rupture as a result of erosion of the arterial wall, causing massive rectal bleeding.

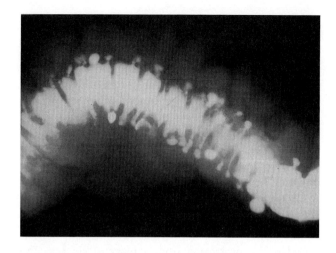

FIGURE 14–16 Diverticulosis. This is a radiograph of a barium enema. The barium, which is radiopaque and appears white, fills numerous diverticula, or outpouchings of the bowel wall.

BOX 14–12   Colonic Diverticulosis

Causes

Related to aging

Lesions

Outpouchings of colonic mucosa through bowel wall

Most common in sigmoid colon

Manifestations

Usually asymptomatic

Diverticulitis with pain, fever, and
  altered bowel function

Stricture and obstruction

Massive rectal bleeding

Hyperplastic/Neoplastic Diseases

Gastrointestinal tract cancers account for about 20% of all cancers. Colon cancer accounts by far for the majority of these. In this section, we discuss in detail only cancer of the colon and its precursors, and limit the discussion of cancers of the esophagus, stomach, small intestine, and anus to a few important points. **Table 14–4** compares the incidence, survival, stage at which most commonly detected, age at diagnosis, and risk factors for these carcinomas.

Etiologic factors for cancers of the esophagus and stomach (GERD, *H. pylori* infection) have already been discussed in other sections. There are many different types of cancers of the small intestine, each with its own risk factors and statistics, so it is difficult to give generalizations. Adenocarcinoma of the small intestine is virtually unheard of outside the setting of familial cancer syndromes or Crohn disease. Cancer of the anus arises from the squamous mucosa of the anal outlet and is strongly associated with the human papillomavirus (HPV), the same virus that causes cervical cancer. It is more common in homosexual men and in patients simultaneously infected with HIV. Because it occurs in a readily visible and palpable area of the body, cancer of the anus usually comes to attention when it is still localized and so can be cured with surgical excision.

TABLE 14–4   Comparison of Esophageal, Gastric, Small Intestinal, Colorectal, and Anal Carcinomas

	Incidence	5-Year Survival	Stage at Which Most Commonly Diagnosed	Median Age at Diagnosis	Risk Factors
Esophagus	4:100,000	20%	III and IV	68 years	Smoking, alcohol, GERD
Stomach	8:100,000	25%	III and IV	71 years	*H. pylori*, food preservatives, smoking, genetics
Small intestine	2:100,000	Very variable, depending on type	III	67 years	Genetics, Crohn disease
Colon/rectum	49:100,000	80%	I and II	71 years	Low-fiber diet, genetics, physical inactivity, obesity, smoking
Anus	2:100,000	60%	I	61 years	HPV, smoking

As with all cancers, stage is the most important predictor of survival, and survival decreases with increasing stage. The incidence of esophageal and gastric carcinomas varies widely around the world, presumably because of environmental factors, such as using nitrite preservatives in food (China, stomach cancer) or possibly drinking scalding hot tea (northern Iran, esophageal cancer). There are no screening procedures for esophageal or gastric cancer, so most of these cancers are diagnosed when they have already spread beyond the wall of the bowel. When advanced, cancers of the tubular gut come to attention by causing bleeding or obstruction.

Colonic Polyps

A *polyp* is a protrusion from a mucosal surface. The protrusion could be an inflammatory lesion, a benign neoplasm, or a malignant neoplasm. The nature of a polyp cannot be determined by visual examination during endoscopy. Diagnosis requires that the polyp be completely removed and examined under the microscope. In addition, polyps are usually asymptomatic. They do not cause bleeding or intestinal obstruction unless they are very large.

Hyperplastic polyps are small, raised exaggerations of normal mucosal crypts (**Figure 14–17**). It is not known why they arise, and they do not represent a precancerous lesion. **Adenomas** are worrisome because they harbor genetic mutations that are precancerous. If left in place, adenomas can develop into cancer over the course of several years. For this reason, colonoscopy with removal of any identified polyps is recommended on a periodic basis in all people 50 years and older. People with known familial cancer syndromes in which the risk of colonic adenocarcinoma is increased and people with inflammatory bowel disease should begin having endoscopies earlier and have them more frequently.

BOX 14–13   Colonic Polyps

Causes

Increased age

Low-fiber and high-fat diet

Lesions

Hyperplastic polyp

Adenoma

Manifestations

Discovered at endoscopy

Bleeding, altered bowel movements if large

Carcinoma of the Colon and Rectum

The rectum is lined by the same type of epithelium as the colon, and cancer of the rectum has the same risk factors and demographic profile as does cancer of the colon. For these reasons, cancers in these locations are considered together as colorectal **carcinoma**. Adenocarcinoma of the colon and rectum can occur in the setting of familial

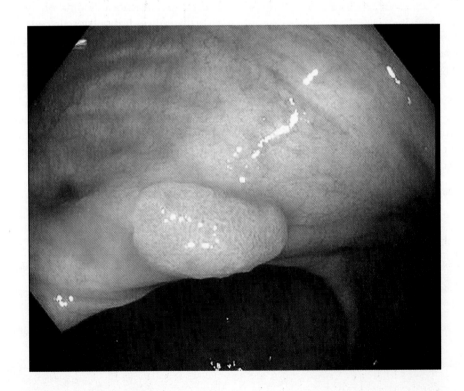

FIGURE 14–17 Colonic polyp, endoscopic image. A raised, pale lesion protrudes from the mucosal surface of the colon. (Courtesy of Dr. Mark Reichelderfer, University of Wisconsin Hospitals and Clinics.)

cancer syndromes such as *familial adenomatous polyposis* and as a complication of inflammatory bowel disease of long-standing duration. Most cases are sporadic, however. The association of diet with sporadic colorectal carcinoma is stronger than with any other type of cancer. Diets high in red meat, processed meats, and foods cooked at high temperatures (frying or grilling) are strong risk factors, while diets high in vegetables and fruits are protective. There is also considerable geographic variation in incidence: in general, colorectal cancer is very rare in developing nations in comparison to developed ones. Other risk factors include increasing age, physical inactivity, obesity, smoking, alcohol use, and type 2 diabetes mellitus. A common denominator to some of these risk factors is delayed colonic emptying. The long contact time of the feces with the colonic epithelium promotes mucosal injury, which over time could lead to the accumulation of cancer-causing mutations.

Early diagnosis of colorectal cancer is possible because it can be seen directly by endoscopy, which is safe (though uncomfortable) and can be done on an outpatient basis. Patients who cannot tolerate an endoscopic procedure can have a barium enema (**Figure 14–18**) or specialized CT colonography that detects masses. Surgical resection is curative if the cancer is still localized to the colonic wall. The cancer arises in the mucosa and gradually grows through the colonic wall to the serosa and simultaneously expands into the lumen (**Figure 14–19**). At any time after it has invaded beyond the mucosa, it can spread through lymphatic channels to the lymph nodes in the pericolonic and mesenteric fat. Cancer cells can gain access to the bloodstream by further spreading up the lymphatic system to the thoracic duct or by directly invading veins. Bloodborne metastases are most frequently found in the liver. **Table 14–5** describes the criteria by which colonic adenocarcinoma is staged and indicates 5-year survival by stage. Although surveillance endoscopy can detect cancers early, it is really only an option to patients who have access

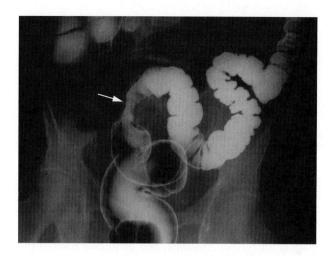

FIGURE 14–18 Barium enema illustrating a constricting colon cancer (arrow) with proximal dilation of the colon resulting from obstruction of the lumen by the cancer.

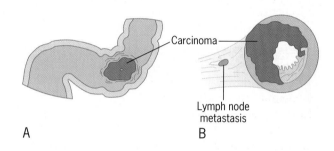

FIGURE 14–19 Carcinoma of the colon. **A.** Carcinoma spreading over the surface of the mucosa. **B.** Carcinoma extending through the layers of the bowel wall and eventually spreading to regional lymph nodes.

to specialized medical services. This is one of the reasons why many cancers are still detected at an advanced stage.

Manifestations, when they do occur, are related to the growth of the cancer into the bowel wall (**Figure 24–20**) and into the bowel lumen. Bleeding and altered bowel

TABLE 14–5	**Colon Cancer Staging and 5-Year Survival by Stage**	
	Stage Description	**5-Year Survival**
I	Cancer limited to submucosa or inner muscularis propria	93%
IIA	Cancer penetrating through full thickness of bowel wall	85%
IIB	Direct spread of cancer into adjacent organs or structures	72%
IIIA	Involvement of 1–3 lymph nodes by cancer that is growing in the submucosa or superficial muscularis propria	83%
IIIB	Involvement of 1–3 lymph nodes by cancer that is growing through the full thickness of the bowel wall, with or without direct growth into adjacent structures	64%
IIIC	Involvement of 4 or more lymph nodes by cancer growing to any depth in the bowel wall	44%
IV	Distant organ spread	8%

Data from the National Cancer Institute's SEER database of patients diagnosed with colon cancer between 1991 and 2000.

habits are the most common symptoms. Bleeding can be noted by the patient who sees frank blood in the stool, it can be detected by simple tests of fecal occult blood, and it can present in the form of iron-deficiency anemia detected by routine blood tests. Iron-deficiency anemia in an adult male is caused by colonic carcinoma until proven otherwise. Altered bowel habits resulting from colonic carcinoma can take the form of diarrhea, constipation, or narrow, pencil-shaped stools. Development of colonic obstruction or pain implies more extensive tumor growth.

Diagnosis requires histologic confirmation. Unless the carcinoma is already metastatic at the time of diagnosis, surgical resection is usually performed. Histologic examination of the resected colon is necessary for adequate staging for further treatment and prognostication. If the tumor has spread to the lymph nodes or distant sites, chemotherapy, radiation therapy, and additional surgical procedures (e.g., removal of metastases in the liver) may be necessary. Rectal carcinoma is often irradiated or treated with chemotherapeutic agents before surgery to minimize the tumor burden before resection is performed.

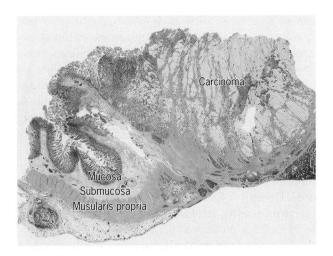

FIGURE 14–20 Carcinoma invading through bowel wall. Normal mucosa, submucosa, and muscularis propria are present on the left side of the image. On the right side, a highly disorganized growth of epithelial (mucosal) cells, producing abundant mucus, has obliterated the submucosa and muscularis propria and is proliferating on the serosal surface of the bowel (far right lower corner). It also is present as a tight wad of cells in the subserosal adipose tissue (far left lower corner). This carcinoma is very advanced, or of high stage.

BOX 14–14   Carcinoma of Colon and Rectum

Causes

Sporadic, related to risk factors (e.g., low-fiber diet, inactivity, obesity)

Familial cancer syndromes (e.g., familial adenomatous polyposis)

Inflammatory bowel disease of long duration

Lesions

Adenocarcinoma

Variable invasion of colonic wall and metastasis to lymph nodes, liver, and other organs

Manifestations

Often asymptomatic: detected by endoscopy, barium enema

Iron-deficiency anemia, occult fecal blood, frankly bloody stools

Change in bowel movements

Organ Failure

Acute failure of the absorption process can be tolerated for a number of days. Severe vomiting or diarrhea, however, may lead to fatal loss of fluids. Infants are most susceptible to fluid loss and much more frequently require intravenous fluid replacement or oral rehydration than do adults. Usually, serious morbidity attributable to diseases of the gastrointestinal tract result from complications of the disease process rather than from aberrations of digestion and absorption. Examples include perforation with peritonitis (e.g., toxic megacolon), massive gastrointestinal blood loss (e.g., peptic ulcer), and obstruction (e.g., stricture in Crohn disease).

Surgical resection of large parts of the tubular gut can be fairly well tolerated. For example, the esophagus can be entirely removed and the stomach pulled up into the thorax and connected to the esophageal stump just underneath the pharynx to maintain continuity of the gut. The stomach is made considerably smaller during bariatric surgery, which is performed to improve health by curbing the appetite and promoting weight loss in obese individuals. The entire colon is removed to control severe ulcerative colitis, and long pieces of the small intestine can be removed for obstruction, infarction (e.g., resulting from occlusion of the mesenteric artery), or Crohn disease. These operations require a change in food consumption, such as eating many small meals rather than a few large ones so that the shortened gut is not overburdened by a single large bolus of food, or consumption of dietary supplements, such as essential vitamins and minerals.

If the continuity of the proximal portion of the gut cannot be maintained or the patient is too debilitated to be able to swallow, **tube feedings** can provide calories and nutrients. A gastric tube conveys nutrients to the stomach through the nose if caloric supplementation is required only short term, while a *percutaneous endoscopic gastrostomy (PEG) tube* is inserted across the abdominal wall into the stomach if long-term supplementation is necessary.

Defecation can also be mechanically circumvented. If the colon or rectum need to be removed, or an interruption is made in the small intestine, the afferent loop of gut can be opened to the abdominal skin. This is called an **ileostomy** or **colostomy** depending on what part of the gut is interrupted. The opening is covered with a plastic bag to catch feces, which the patient can easily change himself or herself (Figure 14–21). An ileo/colostomy usually does not interfere with daily activities and patients can lead comfortable lives until the remaining parts of the GI tract can be reconnected.

The only defect in GI function that cannot easily be circumvented is chronic failure of absorption in the small intestine. If more than one-half to two-thirds of the small intestine is surgically removed, absorption is severely compromised. In cases of **short bowel syndrome**, where insufficient absorption takes place simply because the small intestine has been reduced in length, patients have profuse, fatty stool because of decreased absorption of fat and water and develop deficiencies of vitamins and minerals (calcium; the fat-soluble vitamins A, D, E, and K; magnesium; folic acid; zinc). In severe cases, they can suffer weight loss and malnutrition. The diet must be heavily supplemented with essential nutrients and calories to prevent secondary complications such as iron-deficiency anemia and coagulation disorders.

Total parenteral nutrition (TPN) or administration of carbohydrates, lipids, salts, proteins, and essential minerals and vitamins through the bloodstream, is necessary in some debilitated patients or patients with severely compromised small intestinal function. TPN can be administered chronically, though complications such as infection of the line or liver failure from fatty acid accumulation are common.

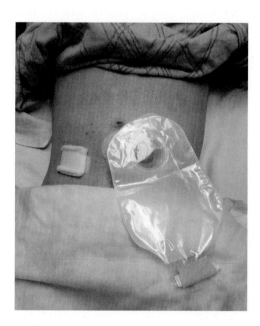

FIGURE 14–21 Ostomy in a patient with inflammatory bowel disease. A plastic bag is attached to the ostomy to the left of the umbilicus. (Courtesy of Lynette Scott, Nursing, University of Wisconsin Hospitals and Clinics.)

Practice Questions

1. The histologic layer that is composed of epithelial cells with specialized functions in different segments of the gastrointestinal tract is called the
   A. lamina propria.
   B. mucosa.
   C. muscularis propria.
   D. submucosa.
   E. mesentery.

2. The most common manifestation of gastrointestinal tract disease is
   A. functional alteration of gut motility.
   B. infant diarrhea.
   C. gastrointestinal flu.
   D. hemorrhage.
   E. gastroesophageal reflux disease.

3. The purpose of screening colonoscopy is to
   A. detect Barrett's metaplasia.
   B. detect dysplasia in Crohn disease.
   C. detect and remove polyps.
   D. detect diverticula.
   E. detect carcinoma.

4. A 76-year-old man with known colonic diverticulosis notices bright red blood in his stool. This is an example of which of the following?
   A. Melena
   B. Hematochezia
   C. Hematemesis
   D. Diarrhea
   E. Fecal occult blood

5. A 56-year-old man has long-standing gastroesophageal reflux disease. Which of the following is he not at risk for developing?
   A. Barrett's esophagus
   B. Strictures
   C. Gastric carcinoma
   D. Adenocarcinoma of the esophagus
   E. Ulcers

6. Complications of *H. pylori* infection include all of the following except which one?
   A. MALT lymphoma
   B. Gastric adenocarcinoma
   C. Peptic ulcer
   D. Barrett's esophagus
   E. Chronic gastritis

7. Three people who had lunch together in a restaurant all experience the sudden onset of vomiting and diarrhea 2–3 hours later. Their food was most likely contaminated with
   A. *Clostridium botulinum.*
   B. *Staphylococcus aureus.*
   C. norovirus.
   D. *Shigella.*
   E. *Vibrio cholera.*

8. Which of the following cancers is most common in the United States?
   A. Gastric
   B. Esophageal
   C. Small intestinal
   D. Colonic
   E. Anal

Liver, Gallbladder, and Pancreas

OUTLINE

OBJECTIVES

1. Review the structure and function of the liver, gallbladder, and pancreas, and name some of the major functions of hepatocytes.
2. Describe the most frequent diseases of the liver, gallbladder, and pancreas, and state which are likely to be fatal.
3. List some of the more common symptoms and signs of injury to the liver, gallbladder, or pancreas, and relate these to the underlying abnormality.
4. List some of the common laboratory tests that are used to detect liver disease.
5. Describe the role of imaging techniques and liver biopsy in the detection and management of diseases of the liver, pancreas, and gallbladder.
6. Name the causes of jaundice in neonates.
7. Describe the etiology, lesions, and manifestations of cystic fibrosis of the pancreas.
8. Name the hepatitis viruses and compare them in terms of their manifestations and the diseases or complications they cause.
9. Recognize the difference between dose-dependent and idiosyncratic drug reactions, and give examples of each.
10. Describe the patients who are vulnerable to developing fatty liver disease, and describe its complications.
11. Name the three most common forms of autoimmune disease of the liver.
12. Describe how gallstones form, manifest, and are cured.
13. Describe the causes, lesions, and manifestations of acute and chronic pancreatitis.
14. Define cirrhosis and describe how it develops.
15. List the complications of cirrhosis and relate them to the underlying hepatic dysfunction.
16. Be able to define and use in proper context all the terms in bold print in this chapter.

KEY TERMS

acinus
acute pancreatitis
albumin
alkaline phosphatase
ascites
aspartate aminotransferase (AST)
autoimmune hepatitis
bile
bile salts
biliary atresia
biliary colic
bilirubin
canaliculus
cholangiocarcinoma
cholecystectomy
cholelithiasis

chronic pancreatitis
cirrhosis
clotting factors
coagulopathy
common bile duct
cystic duct
cytochrome p450
enzymatic necrosis
ERCP
fulminant hepatitis
gallbladder
hepatic encephalopathy
hepatitis
hepatitis viruses (A, B, C, D, and E)
hepatocellular carcinoma
hepatocyte

hepatomegaly
idiosyncratic
islet of Langerhans
jaundice
Kupffer cell
liver
metabolic syndrome
micelle
pancreas
papilla of Vater
portal hypertension
portal triad
portal vein

primary biliary cirrhosis
primary sclerosing
   cholangitis
sinusoid
spontaneous bacterial
   peritonitis
steatohepatitis
steatorrhea
steatosis
urea nitrogen
varices

Review of Structure and Function

The **liver** and the **pancreas** are glandular organs with excretory ducts emptying into the second portion of the duodenum, usually at a common orifice called the **papilla of Vater (Figure 15–1)**. The excretory product of the liver is **bile**, which is transported from the liver via hepatic bile ducts. On its way to the duodenum, bile is stored in a reservoir called the **gallbladder**, which is connected to the bile ducts by the **cystic duct** and in turn drains to the papilla of Vater via the **common bile duct**. The excretory product of the pancreas is a fluid rich in enzymes that digest food once they are delivered to the small intestine.

Most of the blood from the abdominal organs is carried to the liver via the **portal veins** and filtered past the parenchymal cells of the liver, the **hepatocytes**, before being returned to the heart via the hepatic vein. Because portal blood has little oxygen left after passing through the abdominal organs, the liver has a second source of blood, the hepatic artery, that delivers oxygenated blood from the aorta. The bulk of the liver is composed of hepatocytes, aligned in cords or plates separated by **sinusoids** through which the blood from the portal vein percolates to the central vein **(Figure 15–2)**. Also within the sinusoids are resident mononuclear phagocytic cells called **Kupffer cells**, which phagocytose particulate matter present in the blood. Between the cell membranes of

adjacent hepatocytes are tiny **canaliculi** that carry bile produced by the hepatocytes to the portal area, where they empty into epithelial-lined bile ducts. Canaliculi are usually not visible by light microscopy.

Branches of the hepatic artery, portal vein, and bile ducts course together in the **portal triad** (Figure 15–2). Blood flowing into the liver through the portal vein filters into the sinusoids. Here, hepatocytes and Kupffer cells remove waste products and nutrients. Waste products are metabolized by the hepatocytes. The metabolites may be returned to the blood, stored in the hepatocytes, or converted to components of bile and excreted into bile canaliculi. The bile is carried through the canaliculi back to the portal areas for excretion via the bile ducts, while the blood itself drains into central (or hepatic) veins and eventually gets carried to the inferior vena cava and back to the heart.

The liver is very metabolically active and its functions are of vital importance (**Table 15–1**). Whereas mechanical or pharmacological replacement of heart, lung, or kidney function is to some degree feasible, as yet there has been no success in producing an artificial organ that is capable of replacing the liver. Of the many metabolic functions of the liver, five are briefly reviewed here: (1) production of bile salts, (2) excretion of bilirubin, (3) metabolism of nitrogenous substances, (4) production of serum proteins, and (5) detoxification of drugs and poisons. These five are not necessarily the most important, but they are the basis of common clinical and laboratory tests that give clues to the functional status of the liver.

The liver's main contribution to digestion is bile. Bile is composed of **bile salts**, which are bipolar molecules derived from cholesterol that aggregate into spherical masses or **micelles (Figure 15–3)**. Lipids are soluble inside the micelle, whereas the outer surface of the micelle is water soluble. Micelles can therefore solubilize lipids in the aqueous environment of the digestive tract. They prevent cholesterol from crystallizing and emulsify or dissolve dietary lipids so that they are more easily digested by lipases in the gastrointestinal tract. Bile greatly facilitates the digestion of fats, including the fat-soluble vitamins A, D, E, and K. If there is interference with the production or excretion of bile, the digestion of fats is greatly impaired.

Bile is also important in the clearance of **bilirubin**, a breakdown product of hemoglobin. Approximately 1 in 120 red blood cells dies every day. Whereas the iron in hemoglobin is scavenged for reuse and the globin portion of the molecule is broken down to amino acids, the iron-carrying portion of the molecule, bilirubin, is excreted. The liver cannot remove all of the bilirubin from the blood immediately, so in the normal state of equilibrium between bilirubin production and clearance there is about 1 mg/dL of bilirubin in the blood. After the liver cells remove bilirubin from the blood, they conjugate it with glucuronide molecules to make it water soluble for excretion into bile. Bilirubin is bright yellow. When it is

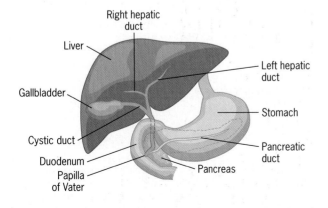

FIGURE 15–1 Anatomic relations of the liver, biliary tract, pancreas, and duodenum.

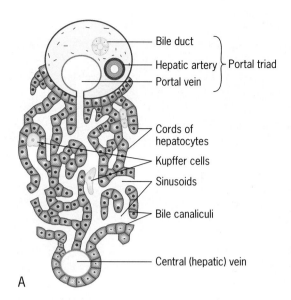

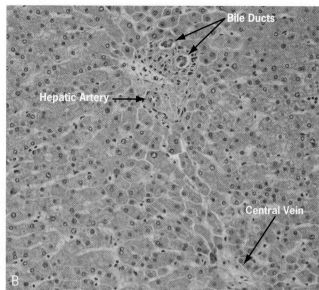

FIGURE 15–2 Basic histologic structure of the liver. **A.** Schematic. **B.** Photomicrograph.

present in excess, it imparts a yellow color, or **jaundice**, to the skin, eyes, and internal organs.

Another metabolic product of hepatocytes is **urea nitrogen**. The breakdown of dead cells produces nitrogenous products such as ammonia. Also, the breakdown

of protein by bacteria in the intestines produces ammonia, which is absorbed into the blood. The liver converts these nitrogenous products to urea nitrogen and returns the urea nitrogen to the bloodstream, from whence it is excreted by the kidney. Severe liver failure results in accumulation of ammonia in the blood and severe kidney failure results in accumulation of urea nitrogen in the blood.

The liver is one of the main sites of metabolism of drugs, including pharmaceutical agents, and poisons, including alcohol. Hepatocytes contain a rich array of enzymes by which potentially toxic substances are neutralized and cleared from the system. The most important of these is **cytochrome p450**, or CYP. This enzyme catalyzes the first step in the clearance of many drugs,

---

TABLE 15–1   Functions of the Liver

Nutrition
- Metabolism of fats
  - Production of bile to emulsify fats and aid in their intestinal absorption
  - Synthesis, storage, and metabolism of fatty acids and cholesterol
- Metabolism of carbohydrates
  - Production of glucose for immediate use by brain and red blood cells
  - Storage of carbohydrates
- Storage of vitamins and minerals
  - Vitamins D, E, and K
  - Vitamin B$_{12}$
  - Copper
  - Iron

Clearance of waste products
- Bilirubin
- Ammonia
- Pharmaceutical agents
- Environmental toxins
- Endogenous hormones
- Drugs of abuse

Regulation of blood volume
- Production of albumin

Hemostasis
- Production of serum protein clotting factors

Immune regulation
- Clearance of bacteria circulating in the bloodstream
- Antigen presentation by liver sinusoidal endothelial cells

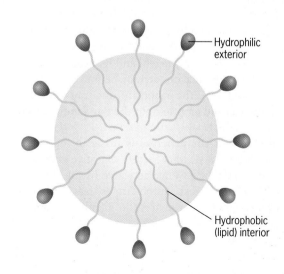

FIGURE 15–3 Schematic diagram of a micelle.

including acetaminophen, barbiturates, warfarin, and alcohol. There is some familial variation in the degree of CYP activity, and CYP activity can also be induced or impaired by the simultaneous administration of other drugs that are also cleared by this enzyme. In addition, some of the intermediates in the metabolic pathway are actually more toxic than the original agent was.

There are three clinically important implications for the manner in which toxins are cleared from the liver:

1. Individual variation in the clearance of drugs may make clinical response unpredictable, for example, to the drug warfarin. Some individuals require a much higher dosage than others do for a therapeutic effect, and some can suffer serious consequences if given drugs at a dose that has no effect on others.

2. Coadministration of drugs that are cleared by the same enzyme system, such as acetaminophen and barbiturates, can cause delayed clearance of the drugs and their intermediates.

3. If the enzyme clearance system is impaired, the accumulation of metabolic intermediates and reactive oxygen species can cause damage to cells. This occurs, for example, with sustained alcohol use.

The liver produces several important serum proteins. One of these is **albumin**, which maintains osmotic pressure and can carry nonsoluble molecules such as unconjugated bilirubin in the blood. Altered albumin levels may be indicative of underlying liver injury. Other proteins produced by the liver are the **clotting factors** of the coagulation cascade. Patients with severe liver disease often encounter problems with blood clotting and prolonged bleeding times. The liver is therefore integral to the regulation of blood volume and to hemostasis.

Whereas the liver has a large array of metabolic functions, only some of which are directly related to digestion, the pancreas has a much more limited range of operations. It has both exocrine and endocrine functions, and both of these are related to nutrition. The pancreas is a long, narrow glandular organ lying horizontally in the midabdomen behind the peritoneum. Its tail stretches toward the spleen on the left, and its head nestles in the curve of the proximal duodenum, behind the distal stomach (Figure 15–1). The pancreatic duct runs the length of the pancreas and empties into the duodenum after joining the bile duct.

The bulk of the pancreas is made up of glands, or acini (**Figure 15–4**), that secrete digestive enzymes into the pancreatic duct. When activated by intestinal juices, these enzymes digest carbohydrates, fats, and proteins. Scattered among the pancreatic glands are clusters of endocrine cells called the **islets of Langerhans** that produce insulin and other hormones. Insulin regulates the level of glucose in the blood. Destruction or removal of pancreatic tissue—as occurs, for example, in cystic fibrosis—causes insufficiency of pancreatic enzyme

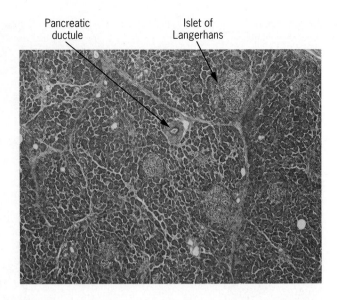

Pancreatic ductule   Islet of Langerhans

FIGURE 15–4 Histology of the pancreas. The bulk of the pancreatic tissue is made up of acini, which are organized into lobules separated by thin fibrous bands. The proteinaceous products of the acini are drained by the pancreatic ducts. Interspersed throughout the parenchyma are rounded collections of pale-staining cells, the islets of Langerhans, which are the endocrine units of the pancreas.

production and insufficiency of insulin production. Pancreatic enzymes can be replaced orally, so adequate nutrition can usually be maintained. Insulin must be replaced via injections.

Most Frequent and Serious Problems

The most common problem affecting the accessory digestive organs is the development of *choleliths*, commonly referred to as gallstones. In developed countries, these are most often precipitates of cholesterol crystals. Choleliths are usually asymptomatic but can produce serious complications such as obstruction of bile flow as a result of migration of stones into the common bile duct. It is estimated that 20-40% of adults in the United States have gallstones, and about 1–4% develop symptomatic **cholelithiasis** every year. The definitive cure for cholelithiasis is surgical removal of the gallbladder, or **cholecystectomy**. This is one of the most common surgical procedures performed in the United States.

The most common problem affecting the liver is inflammation, or **hepatitis**. There are many different causes of hepatitis, including infections, autoimmune diseases, drug reactions, alcohol, and obesity. Some forms of hepatitis are acute and resolve spontaneously, such as hepatitis caused by the hepatitis A virus, the most common cause of hepatitis in Africa and parts of Asia. Some forms of hepatitis are reversible if the offending agent is identified and avoided. Alcoholic and drug-induced hepatitis are examples. Many forms of hepatitis are either not reversible or not detected until serious injury to the liver has already occurred. Long-standing inflammation leads to substantial loss of hepatocytes and severe scarring of the liver, or **cirrhosis**. The most common causes of cirrhosis in the United States are alcohol and hepatitis C virus infection. Cirrhosis is not reversible and will result in liver failure. Also, the most common primary neoplasm of the liver, **hepatocellular carcinoma**, tends to arise in cirrhotic livers. Chronic liver disease is the 12th most common cause of death in the United States, and cirrhosis caused by chronic hepatitis C virus infection is the most common reason for liver transplantation. Livers are the second most commonly transplanted organs, after kidneys.

Hepatocellular carcinoma arising in cirrhotic livers is the most common primary neoplasm of the liver. It is the fifth most common cause of cancer deaths worldwide, but it shows considerable geographic variability: 50% of the world's cases occur in China, but in the United States it causes only 2–4% of cancer deaths. This variability is caused by differences in the distribution of risk factors. In Asia and parts of Africa, hepatocellular carcinoma is linked to chronic hepatitis B virus infection, which is much more prevalent there than in Western countries. In contrast in Western nations, the incidence of hepatocellular carcinoma has nearly doubled in the past 20 years because of a surge in chronic hepatitis C virus infection. In Western nations, the most common neoplasm of the liver is actually metastatic disease. Any cancer can metastasize to the liver, including melanoma, lymphoma, and sarcoma, but the most common liver metastases are from cancers arising in the digestive tract.

The most common problems affecting the pancreas are also inflammation and neoplasia. Inflammation of the pancreas is usually associated with alcohol or with gallstones and ranges in severity from mild and self-limited to severe and fulminant. Carcinoma of the pancreas is the fourth most common cause of cancer deaths in the United States. Although insulin is produced in the pancreas, diabetes mellitus is not usually related to any obvious pancreatic disease.

Symptoms, Signs, and Tests

Jaundice is an obvious sign of liver disease. The first place in which jaundice becomes manifest is usually the scleraes, or the whites of the eyes. Jaundice can be caused by increased hemoglobin breakdown (as occurs, for example, with hemolytic anemias), liver disease, or bile duct obstruction. **Biliary colic** refers to severe right upper quadrant and flank pain caused by obstruction of the biliary ductal system by stones. The pain caused by pancreatitis is usually in the upper abdomen and radiates to the back. Unintentional weight loss may signify serious disease of the pancreas or liver, such as chronic pancreatitis or cancer. **Steatorrhea** is the passage of greasy, smelly stools that often float in toilet water, and is indicative of malabsorption of fats. The size of the liver can be assessed by palpation of the lower edge of the liver in the right upper quadrant just inferior to the rib cage. An increase in the size of the liver, or **hepatomegaly**, is particularly prominent in alcoholic fatty liver and metastatic disease.

Laboratory tests are essential to the analysis of diseases of the liver, pancreas, and gallbladder. A routine battery of tests performed to assess the status of the liver includes bilirubin, total protein, albumin, **aspartate aminotransferase (AST)**, and **alkaline phosphatase**. The causes of elevated bilirubin are the same as the causes of jaundice. The serum bilirubin is at least twice normal when jaundice becomes apparent. Low levels of serum protein, particularly albumin, occur with severe chronic liver disease. AST is elevated with hepatocyte injury, as occurs in hepatitis, and alkaline phosphatase is usually elevated with disorders of bile metabolism and excretion, often even before bilirubin is elevated. Blood coagulation tests assess the liver's ability to make the coagulation factors.

Enzymes produced by the pancreas can be measured in the serum as well. Elevated levels of amylase and lipase are indicative of acute pancreatic injury, because these pancreatic enzymes leak into the blood from destroyed pancreatic tissue.

More specific tests target specific etiologies: unconjugated versus conjugated bilirubin allows assessment of whether elevated bilirubin is the result of increased destruction of red blood cells or inherent liver disease; specific viral proteins are indicative of acute or chronic infection; autoimmune antibodies are present in the various autoimmune forms of hepatitis. The sophistication of these tests makes laboratory analysis the primary tool for diagnosis of liver disease and monitoring of its treatment.

Imaging techniques such as radiography, endoscopy, and ultrasound cannot detect derangements in hepatocellular function, but they are useful in the evaluation of certain structural or mechanical diseases. Twenty percent of gallstones are calcified and can be seen radiographically (**Figure 15–5**), but ultrasound is the preferred method of demonstrating them because ultrasound does not expose the patient to radiation, detects most stones, and can even detect the presence of inflammation if it is severe. Endoscopic retrograde cholangiopancreatography, or **ERCP**, combines direct visualization of the duodenum with radiography. A radiopaque dye is injected into the biliary tree through an endoscope threaded through the upper digestive tract to the ampulla of Vater. Radiographs taken after injection of the dye illustrate strictures or blockages of the extrahepatic biliary tree. This technique also allows tissue samples of strictures or masses to be taken for microscopic assessment. Computed tomography (CT) scans and magnetic resonance imaging (MRI) are the preferred means for evaluating the pancreas and liver for masses. Therapeutic interventions often rely on further evaluation by ultrasound to detect whether the lesion

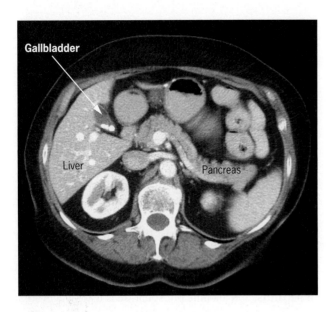

FIGURE 15–5 CT scan demonstrating three round, white stones in the gallbladder. (Courtesy of Dr. Donald Yandow, Department of Radiology, University of Wisconsin School of Medicine and Public Health.)

is primarily cystic or solid, aspiration of cyst fluid for amylase and lipase levels, or tissue biopsy.

Specific Diseases

Genetic/Developmental Diseases

Neonatal Liver Disease

Almost every newborn develops unconjugated hyperbilirubinemia because the hepatic enzyme system necessary for conjugation of bilirubin is not yet fully mature at birth. In addition, there is increased red blood cell breakdown after birth, as fetal red blood cells are cleared and adult red bloods produced, and enzymes in breast milk may interfere with the conjugation of bilirubin. If the hyperbilirubinemia becomes very severe, it can cause permanent brain damage. Usually, however, if it is severe, it is detected very early and can easily be reversed. Most often, it is mild and transient, clearing within a few days to a week. Phototherapy, or exposing the infant to direct sunlight or blue light, is helpful in cases of frank jaundice. The light breaks the bilirubin down into water-soluble substances that can be cleared directly, without need of conjugation.

Not all hyperbilirubinemia in infants is innocuous, however, and neonates should be carefully monitored for persistent hyperbilirubinemia. Hyperbilirubinemia persists if there is excessive red blood cell breakdown, parenchymal liver disease, or atresia of the bile ducts. Hemolysis also occurs with erythroblastosis fetalis as maternal antibodies attack antigens on the neonate's red blood cells. Intrauterine and neonatal infections can produce parenchymal liver injury. Also, in some rare genetic diseases the metabolism of bilirubin is impaired. These diseases result from mutations affecting the enzymes that conjugate bilirubin or transport it into the canalicular system. Most of these genetic conditions are not fatal.

Biliary atresia, or progressive obstruction of the extrahepatic biliary tree in the first 3 months of life, is a serious and often fatal condition. It is the primary reason for liver transplantation in the pediatric age group. Inflammatory conditions, either autoimmune or viral infections, cause progressive narrowing and obliteration of the lumen of the biliary ducts. If the damage is limited to the extrahepatic biliary ducts, a surgical procedure that bypasses these can be performed. However, the inflammation often extends into the intrahepatic bile ducts, causing fibrosis of the portal areas. Cirrhosis develops rapidly in these infants.

Cystic Fibrosis of the Pancreas

Cystic fibrosis is more commonly known as a disease of the lung. It gets its name, however, from its effects on the pancreas: the pancreas is disfigured and destroyed by cystic dilation of ducts and fibrosis of the parenchyma. Blockage of the pancreatic ducts by thick viscid mucus causes cystic dilation of the ducts upstream from the obstruction and impaired delivery of digestive enzymes to the small intestine. The patient therefore suffers repeated bouts of pancreatitis as the pancreatic digestive enzymes escape from the damaged ductal system and destroy the pancreatic tissue, and malabsorption and malnutrition because of the lack of enzymatic activity on nutrients in the bowel. The latter effect can be circumvented by administration of pancreatic enzymes by the oral route, but the damage to the pancreas is not reversible. Patients therefore secondarily develop diabetes mellitus as the pancreatic islets producing insulin are destroyed by the chronic inflammation. It should be remembered that although cystic fibrosis is a genetic disease, its expression can be quite variable. Most patients have predominantly pulmonary complications, but some have predominantly pancreatic insufficiency, and others may have only severe and intractable chronic sinusitis.

Inflammatory/Degenerative Diseases

Viral Hepatitis

Various viruses can affect the liver, including Epstein-Barr virus, cytomegalovirus, the virus causing yellow fever, and the hepatitis viruses A, B, C, D (delta), and E. The latter are called "hepatotropic" because their primary effects are on the liver. Because the hepatotropic viruses are the most prevalent cause of liver failure worldwide, the discussion here focuses on these. They are differentiated in name only by a letter, but they vary considerably in their pathologic effects, epidemiology, and molecular nature (**Table 15–2**). The hepatitis viruses were named sequentially as they were discovered in the laboratory. Hepatitis A virus was the first to be discovered, in 1972,

TABLE 15-2	Comparison of Hepatotropic Viruses				
Virus	**Hepatitis A**	**Hepatitis B**	**Hepatitis C**	**Hepatitis D**	**Hepatitis E**
Type	RNA	DNA	RNA	RNA	RNA
Route of transmission	Fecal–oral	Parenteral, perinatal, sexual contact	Parenteral	Parenteral	Fecal–oral
Chronic liver disease	Never	10%	~80%	5%	Never
Diagnosis	IgM	HBsAg or antibody to HBcAg	Molecular test for HCV RNA	IgM, IgG, or viral-specific antigens	IgM, IgG, or viral-specific antigens
Highest prevalence	Rural areas with poor sanitation and hygiene	Asia	Western nations, United States	Requires HBV for infection	Zoonotic reservoir; India
Fatality	<1%				Highest in pregnant women

and hepatitis G virus was discovered in 1995. Hepatitis G is not purely hepatotropic and is not known to cause disease in humans, so it is not discussed here.

Hepatitis A virus (HAV), an RNA virus, is the most prevalent of the hepatitis viruses and mostly causes a benign illness. It is found all over the world and is particularly prevalent in areas where there is poor hygiene and sanitation. The virus is spread sporadically or in epidemics by fecal contamination of water and food. Close personal contact increases the risk of spread. The incubation period is 2–4 weeks and the virus is shed in the stool during this time and for 1 week after manifestation of symptoms. The onset of symptoms is abrupt, with fever, nausea, vomiting, and loss of appetite. Jaundice may be the first clue to the presence of liver disease, although not all patients become yellow. Physical examination reveals an enlarged, tender liver and the urine appears dark. Serum aspartate aminotransferase (AST) is always strikingly elevated, indicating hepatocyte necrosis. Diagnosis is made by finding elevated immunoglobin M (IgM) anti-hepatitis A antibodies in the serum. Elevated IgG anti-hepatitis A antibodies without IgM antibodies indicates past illness. There is no specific treatment other than rest and a good diet. Most patients recover by 6 weeks after the onset of symptoms, and there are no long-term sequelae: the liver regenerates completely and there is no risk for the development of chronic hepatitis. Because the immune system responds to the virus by producing specific antibodies, subsequent exposures do not result in illness, and vaccination is effective. HAV vaccine is one of the routine childhood vaccines in the United States.

In contrast, **hepatitis B virus** (HBV) can cause chronic liver disease. Like HAV, HBV can cause an acute illness that manifests with fever, malaise and jaundice; however, unlike HAV, HBV can persist in the liver. The infected individual can become a carrier who is asymptomatic but can transfer the virus to others, or may develop chronic hepatitis and eventually cirrhosis. HBV is the main cause of chronic liver disease and hepatocellular carcinoma worldwide. Its prevalence in parts of Asia and

Africa is much higher than in Western nations. In high-prevalence regions, 90% of transmission occurs across the placenta. Transmission also can occur during childhood through minor cuts in skin and mucous membranes. In low-prevalence areas, transmission usually occurs through sharing of needles and unprotected sexual intercourse. Blood transfusions were a source of transmission in the past, but careful screening for hepatitis viral antigens has reduced this risk to virtually zero in the United States.

The incubation period of HBV is long, 1 to 6 months, and the onset of symptoms is gradual. Some patients do not develop any symptoms at all. Diagnosis is made by detecting serum antigens and antibodies (**Figure 15–6**).

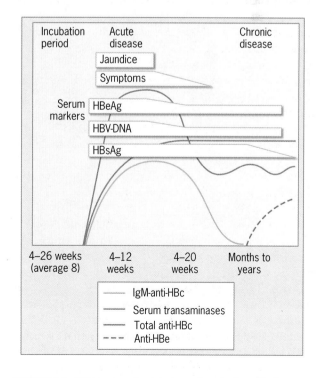

FIGURE 15–6 Sequence of serologic markers for hepatitis B.

The antigen in the surface coat of the virus is called hepatitis B surface antigen (HBsAg), and two antigens in the core of the virus are called core (c) antigen and e antigen (HBcAg and HBeAg, respectively). The surface antigen is shed into the blood for several weeks before the onset of illness, persists into the recovery period, and declines and disappears from the blood approximately 6 months after the acute infection. Antibody to HBsAg rises after recovery; it is actually not detectable until after HBsAg has disappeared from the blood. Anti-HBsAg confers lifetime immunity against reinfection but does not alter the development of chronic hepatitis. Presence of HBeAg parallels disease activity and its persistence suggests chronic disease, including continued viral replication and infectivity. Antibodies to HBcAg and HBeAg indicate recent infection and do not confer immunity. These markers have proved useful in sorting out the various clinical forms of hepatitis B. Liver biopsy is usually not necessary to establish the diagnosis, but if it is performed, the classic finding is of a "ground glass" or finely grainy appearance of the cytoplasm (**Figure 15–7**) that is the result of accumulation of HBsAg in the smooth endoplasmic reticulum of the cells.

Individuals infected with HBV can have very different clinical manifestations. Acute hepatitis, which may or may not be symptomatic, may resolve entirely with complete clearance of the virus. This is actually the outcome in about 90% of infected individuals. Fewer than 1% develop **fulminant hepatitis**, or very severe, life-threatening hepatitis. About 5% develop chronic hepatitis, of whom about 20% develop cirrhosis. These percentages may not appear impressive at first, but by keeping in mind that close to 100% of the population of large areas of the world—about 3 billion people—are infected with HBV during infancy and childhood, you can appreciate how staggering the figures are, and why chronic liver disease is one of the major public health concerns worldwide. A vaccine prepared from HBsAg confers lifelong immunity and is also one of the routine childhood vaccinations in the United States. As usual, the public health problem is getting the vaccine to the populations most in need of it.

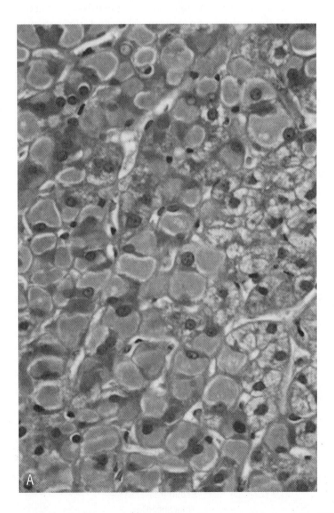 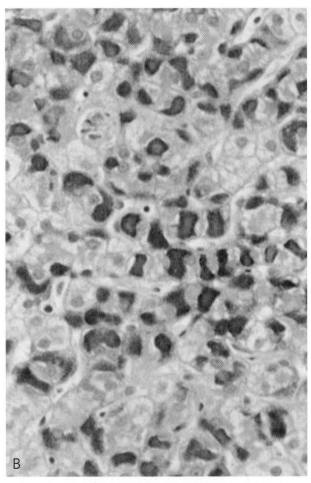

FIGURE 15–7 Hepatitis B virus–infected hepatocytes. **A.** On routine H&E stained sections, the cytoplasm of the hepatocytes has a "ground glass" appearance (compare to those of normal hepatocytes, Figure 15–2). **B.** Immunohistochemistry for hepatitis B antigens shows positivity (brown color) in the cytoplasm of the cells. (Courtesy of Dr. Rashmi Agni, Department of Pathology and Laboratory Medicine, University of Wisconsin School of Medicine and Public Health.)

Hepatitis C virus (HCV) is the major cause of chronic viral hepatitis in the United States. HCV is an RNA virus with an incubation period of 2 weeks to 6 months. It is also spread parenterally—that is, via contaminated blood or bodily secretions. Until HCV was discovered in 1989 and effective screening methods developed, its primary mode of transmission in the United States was via transfused blood products. Nowadays, transmission via transfusions is virtually nil and the primary mode of transmission is via sharing of needles by intravenous drug users. In the United States, about 1.6% of the population is infected.

Acute infection is usually asymptomatic, so it goes undetected. HCV is capable of undergoing antigenic shifts, or changing its protein makeup, once it has infected the liver. This antigenic instability allows it to evade detection by the body's immune system. For the same reason, it has not yet been possible to develop a vaccine against HCV. It is thought that repeated reactivation of the disease by slightly mutated virus causes the prolonged, subclinical, smoldering inflammation that is characteristic of HCV infection.

Unlike with hepatitis B, the majority of patients with hepatitis C lapse into a chronic disease state and 20% progress to cirrhosis in 5–20 years. Laboratory testing reveals episodes of elevation of AST, thought to correspond to flares in disease activity, and nearly persistent circulating HCV RNA. Liver biopsy is performed to monitor the degree of inflammation and the severity of fibrosis (**Figure 15–8**). It is usually not necessary for establishment of the diagnosis. Histologically a chronic inflammatory infiltrate floods the portal triads, and necrotic hepatocytes are present around portal areas and within the hepatocyte lobules. Over time, fibrous bridges develop between portal triads, which become progressively replaced by fibrous tissue, and small bile duct twigs proliferate as they attempt to reestablish a functional bile transport system. Hepatocytes are capable of regenerating to some degree, but as the native hepatic architecture is destroyed, blood from the portal vein cannot get to the hepatocytes and therefore remains largely unfiltered of wastes.

Treatment with pegylated interferon-alpha and ribavirin may clear the infection or delay progression to

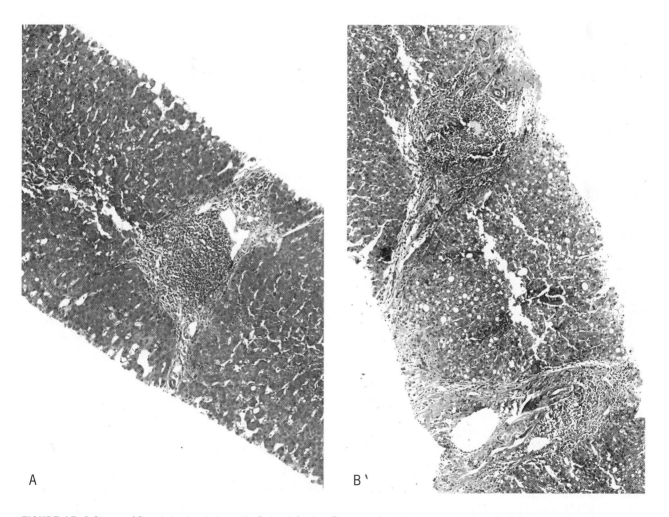

A

B

FIGURE 15–8 Stages of fibrosis in chronic hepatitis C virus infection. These two liver biopsies are stained with trichrome, which colors collagen, a major constituent of fibrous tissue, blue. In **A**, irregular spikes of collagen radiate from a portal triad and extend into the parenchyma for variable distances. This is an example of Stage II fibrosis. In **B**, the collagen is denser and forms a bridge between two portal triads. This is Stage III fibrosis. Figure 15–11 illustrates cirrhosis.

cirrhosis, but it has significant side effects and is not recommended for all patients. Once cirrhosis has developed, the only means for avoiding death as a result of liver failure is liver transplantation. Unfortunately, reinfection of the liver occurs in all cases, and the development of cirrhosis is often accelerated: about 30% of patients develop cirrhosis within 5 years after transplantation.

Delta agent, or hepatitis D virus, is a defective strand of RNA that requires the cellular synthetic machinery of HBV to replicate. In other words, HDV can only infect an individual who is already infected with HBV, and antibody to HBV, either naturally acquired or by vaccine, is protective against the delta agent. Simultaneous infection or infection with HDV after established HBV infection can result in greater severity of acute hepatitis or exacerbation of chronic hepatitis and increased rate of development of cirrhosis.

Hepatitis E virus is another enterally transmitted cause of acute hepatitis. It is a zoonotic disease: the primary reservoir for the virus is in animals, including domestic pigs. It has a greater prevalence than hepatitis A in some areas of Asia. It is usually a self-limited disease, but it can cause severe, fulminant, life-threatening hepatitis in pregnant woman.

BOX 15–1   Viral Hepatitis

Causes

Hepatitis viruses A, B, C, D, E

Lesions

Necrosis of hepatocytes

Inflamed liver

Fibrosis

Manifestations

Anorexia

Malaise

Jaundice

Large tender liver

High AST

Persistent serum antigens, antibodies

Liver failure

Chemical Injuries to the Liver

Virtually every pharmaceutical drug and some herbal preparations have been linked to hepatic injury, though a cause-and-effect relationship cannot always be proven. Toxic injury to the liver can be predictable, occurring in a dose-dependent fashion, or unpredictable, or idiosyncratic. The unpredictable reactions are caused either by individual differences in the metabolism of toxic agents— for example, in the activity of the CYP enzyme— or by individual differences in immune reactions to drugs or their metabolites. Patients with severe acute or chronic liver disease are more susceptible to toxic hepatic injury because their waste-clearing machinery is already compromised. Liver injury is the most common type of acute drug reaction in the United States, and chemical injury accounts for 10% of cases of fulminant hepatitis.

The most common dose-dependent adverse drug reaction (in the United States) occurs in response to acetaminophen. This is the drug of choice for people attempting suicide and is also the most common drug accidentally ingested in large doses by children. If large doses of acetaminophen are taken, its usual clearance mechanism is overwhelmed and cytochrome p450 begins to metabolize the drug. It produces a metabolic by-product that is highly toxic to hepatocytes. If the overdose is detected in time, gastric evacuation and acetylcysteine administration can save the patient's life. Other dramatic presentations occur in patients who receive the commonly used anesthetic agent halothane, especially if they had received it already in the past. A very small percentage of patients anesthetized with halothane develop very severe massive necrosis of hepatocytes much like that occurring in acutely fatal cases of viral hepatitis.

Drugs and toxins can cause damage to any part of the liver: the hepatocytes, the bile ductules, or the enzymatic machinery of hepatocytes. They can cause acute or chronic hepatitis, cholestasis, steatosis, and even fibrosis. Some drugs can induce thrombosis of the hepatic vein, and some may cause a granulomatous inflammation, or even induce the formation of neoplasms. The manifestations of chemical injury to the liver are therefore quite varied and overlap considerably with other diseases. The most important factor in the recognition of drug- or toxin-induced liver injury is a high index of suspicion. There are no specific tests, so all other causes of that pattern of liver injury must be ruled out with serologic tests for viruses, imaging studies for neoplasms, analysis of the pattern of abnormalities in liver function tests, and so forth. Improvement of liver function after discontinuation of the drug is the final "proof" that injury was incurred by toxic damage.

BOX 15–2   Chemical Injuries to the Liver

Causes

Hypersensitivity to drugs

Chemical action of drugs or toxic intermediates of metabolism

Lesions

Damage to hepatocytes

Damage to bile ducts

Manifestations

Jaundice

Abnormal laboratory test values

History of exposure to agent

Fatty Liver Disease

Steatosis refers to the accumulation of fat in hepatocytes. This is also called "fatty change." The most common causes of steatosis in the United States are alcohol and obesity. Some drugs can also induce fat accumulation in the hepatocytes, and fulminant hepatic failure can develop in women who develop pregnancy-associated fatty liver disease.

Alcohol poisons the cellular machinery that is required for the transport of fatty acids out of hepatocytes, so these accumulate. Even social drinking can induce the accumulation of lipids in hepatocytes, and the ability of the liver to metabolize fatty acids even in the presence of high levels of alcohol is quite individual. Not all alcoholics develop steatosis, even after many years of heavy drinking, whereas others may develop cirrhosis from alcohol-induced liver injury even when drinking to a socially accepted degree.

Why fat accumulates in the liver of obese people is not understood, but there appears to be more involved than merely increased levels of lipids in the body, generally. Steatosis is not seen in all obese individuals, and the patient does not have to be morbidly obese to develop it. Obesity is often associated with peripheral insulin resistance, which is another risk factor for the development of steatosis. Accumulation of fat in the liver is more commonly seen in patients who have the **metabolic syndrome**, or the constellation of central (abdominal) obesity, insulin resistance or type 2 diabetes mellitus, hypertension, and dyslipidemia.

Steatosis is reversible in both alcoholic and non-alcoholic fatty liver disease, either with cessation of alcohol ingestion or with a moderate diet and controlled weight loss. (Paradoxically, rapid weight loss and starvation can both induce fatty change.) Steatosis in and of itself does not cause symptoms unless it is very severe and compromises the function of hepatocytes. However, steatosis can be associated with inflammation. This is called **steatohepatitis**. The inflammation causes necrosis of hepatocytes, which are eventually replaced with fibrous tissue. With continuing or repeated bouts of inflammation, steatohepatitis can lead to cirrhosis and its sequelae.

Clinically, steatosis and steatohepatitis are usually asymptomatic. Slight abnormalities in liver function tests may prompt a liver biopsy, which shows the characteristic fat vacuoles, inflammation, and fibrosis, if present. Clinically significant steatosis can sometimes be detected by CT scan. Women with pregnancy-associated fatty liver disease usually present in an emergent fashion with signs and symptoms of massive liver failure.

Autoimmune Diseases of the Liver

Autoimmune diseases of the liver are rare, but they are serious because they result in cirrhosis and hepatic insufficiency secondary to long-standing inflammation. The inflammation in **autoimmune hepatitis** targets

---

BOX 15–3   Steatosis

Causes

Alcohol

Obesity

Rapid weight loss, starvation

Certain drugs

Pregnancy

Lesions

Fatty change

Steatohepatitis

Fibrosis

Finely nodular cirrhosis

Manifestations

Other clinical manifestations of alcohol consumption, obesity

Enlarged liver

Altered liver function tests

Findings of cirrhosis

---

hepatocytes, causing their death and eventual replacement by fibrosis. This disease is more common in women and may be associated with other forms of autoimmune disease, such as systemic lupus erythematosus or celiac disease. It may come to detection in the form of vague symptoms that can be attributed to hepatitis, but it may also go undetected until the liver is completely disfigured by scar tissue. Without appropriate immune suppressant therapy, death can occur within a few months after diagnosis.

Primary biliary cirrhosis is also a disease that primarily affects women. Its pathogenesis is not understood but is attributed to an autoimmune reaction to the bile ductular epithelium. In this case, it is not the hepatocytes that are destroyed, but rather the intrahepatic bile ducts, which become obliterated by fibrous tissue. The disease manifests with symptoms of cholestasis, steatorrhea, and, eventually, jaundice. This disease also results in cirrhosis.

Primary sclerosing cholangitis is a disease that is very strongly associated with ulcerative colitis. The bile ducts are the targets of the inflammation, but the pattern of injury is different from that seen in primary biliary cirrhosis. Both intrahepatic and extrahepatic bile ducts are affected by discontinuous foci of inflammation separated by intervening unaffected areas. The inflammation causes segmental scarring and obliteration of the ducts, so with imaging studies that highlight the biliary tree there is a characteristic "beaded" appearance of the bile ducts, caused by alternating strictured and dilated segments. This disease also presents with nonspecific symptoms of liver injury and cholestasis and results in irreversible scarring of the liver. Patients with primary sclerosing cholangitis have a higher incidence of **cholangiocarcinoma**, or carcinoma of the bile ducts.

Cholelithiasis and Cholecystitis

Bile is rich in cholesterol, which is barely held in solution by bile salts and phospholipids. In the gallbladder, bile is concentrated by absorption of its water content by the absorptive cells of the gallbladder mucosa. If the cholesterol comes out of solution, it forms crystals, which, along with the bilirubin pigment and calcium in the bile, form stones (**Figure 15–9**). The stones vary greatly in number, size, shape, and color. The reason why some people develop cholelithiasis and others do not is not clear, although women are much more prone to develop gallstones than men, and the likelihood of developing gallstones increases with age and in obese persons. Native Americans have a very high rate of development of cholelithiasis.

Cholelithiasis can manifest in several ways. Often, the stones cause no complications at all and the person may not even know s/he has them. The two most common complications are *acute cholecystitis*, which is painful and makes the patient quite ill, and migration of stones down the cystic duct into the common bile duct, obstructing its distal narrow end to produce biliary colic and jaundice.

The stones in the gallbladder can also cause low-grade inflammation, called *chronic cholecystitis*. Uncomplicated chronic cholecystitis is usually asymptomatic but may be associated with symptoms such as pain following meals, especially when fatty or spicy food is ingested. However, the symptoms of chronic cholecystitis are vague and can be mimicked by other things. Other complications of gallstones are acute pancreatitis and, very rarely, carcinoma of the gallbladder or extrahepatic bile ducts.

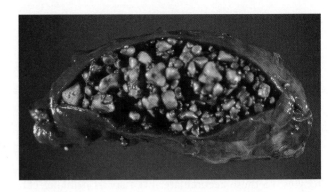

FIGURE 15–9 Cholelithiasis. The gallbladder is opened longitudinally to expose numerous faceted, yellow stones.

Pancreatitis

When the pancreas is inflamed, the powerful digestive enzymes produced by acinar cells escape from the cells or ducts to digest the pancreas itself and surrounding adipose tissue. This is called **enzymatic necrosis**. In pancreatitis, injury to the pancreas is therefore incurred by both inflammation and autodigestion by pancreatic digestive juices. If the inflammation occurs only once and is limited, the pancreatic tissue can regenerate, but if the inflammation is prolonged or repeated and extensive, the pancreas will be replaced by scar tissue, analogous to the development of cirrhosis in the liver.

The most common triggers of **acute pancreatitis** are alcohol and gallstones. It is thought that gallstones, or even thick biliary "sludge," stimulate inflammation by blocking outflow of pancreatic juices from the pancreatic duct. How alcohol causes acute pancreatitis is not understood. Other risk factors or causes of acute pancreatitis include hypertriglyceridemia, infections (e.g., mumps), certain medications, diseases of the arteries supplying the pancreas, surgical trauma, and shock. A familial predisposition is also recognized.

Severe **chronic pancreatitis** is a slowly progressive disease. Patients develop malabsorption as a result of replacement of pancreatic acini by fibrous tissue, and may develop diabetes mellitus as a result of destruction of the islets of Langerhans. End-stage pancreatitis in the alcoholic person is less common than cirrhosis is, and the two conditions may or may not be present together. The most common cause of chronic pancreatitis is repeated episodes of acute pancreatitis, which eventually causes irreversible scarring of the organ. Cystic fibrosis causes chronic injury to the pancreas, as do the familial form of acute pancreatitis, repeated attacks of gallstone pancreatitis, obstruction of the pancreatic ducts by diseases within the pancreas, and autoimmune inflammation of the pancreas that is centered on the ducts and causes their eventual obliteration.

The manifestations of acute pancreatitis usually include pain in the midabdomen that may feel like it is boring through to the back. The pain may be referred

---

BOX 15–4   Cholelithiasis and Cholecystitis

Causes

Precipitation of cholesterol in bile salts

Risk factors:

  Age

  Female

  Obesity

  Native American

Lesions

Gallstones

Mild chronic inflammation

Manifestations

Usually none

Pain after meals

Biliary colic

Pain, fever, and leukocytosis

to the left shoulder. Chronic pancreatitis can also cause severe, crippling abdominal pain. Acute pancreatitis is associated with increased levels of amylase and lipase in the blood and amylase in the urine. In severe chronic pancreatitis, the acini may be destroyed to such an extent that enzyme levels are no longer elevated. Chronic pancreatitis can manifest in the form of malabsorption or diabetes.

The sequelae of acute pancreatitis can be very severe. Autodigestion of the pancreas and the surrounding tissues results in cavitary lesions, called *pseudocysts*, filled with necrotic debris. When these become very large they tend to rupture, spilling the necrotic contents into the abdominal cavity and causing severe peritonitis. Pseudocysts may also become secondarily infected, resulting in an abscess. Bleeding into the pseudocyst or into the damaged pancreatic tissue itself causes *hemorrhagic pancreatitis*, which is a surgical emergency and often fatal. Regional complications include ileus, or paralysis of the small intestine, and gastrointestinal bleeding. One of the pancreatic enzymes, trypsin, can activate the kinin, clotting, and complement systems, which in turn can lead to a generalized systemic inflammatory reaction, shock, and disseminated intravascular coagulation.

BOX 15–5   Pancreatitis

Causes

Alcohol

Gallstones

Hypertriglyceridemia

Other (trauma, shock)

Lesions

Enzymatic necrosis of pancreas and surrounding adipose tissue

Pseudocysts, abscess, GI bleeding (acute)

Fibrosis (chronic)

Manifestations

Abdominal pain

Malabsorption (late)

Diabetes mellitus (late)

Shock (acute)

Hyperplastic/Neoplastic Diseases

In the liver, metastases are much more common than is primary cancer. Hepatocellular carcinoma is the most common primary tumor of the liver, and it most often occurs as a complication of cirrhosis. Gallbladder cancer and cancer of the intrahepatic biliary tree, or cholangiocarcinoma, are rare and usually fatal. Because hepatocellular carcinoma and cholangiocarcinoma are quite rare, they are not discussed in further detail here.

Metastatic Cancer in the Liver

Abdominal cancers, such as carcinoma of the colon, stomach, and pancreas, characteristically metastasize to the liver, but metastases of other neoplasms, such as lymphoma, lung cancer, and breast cancer, are also common. A few patients present with liver metastases without symptoms referable to the primary cancer site. They develop large, nodular livers before the underlying disease manifests. Once a cancer has metastasized to the liver, it is usually no longer curable, but metastases can be removed if the disease is limited to a single site or a few discrete locations and the patient is otherwise in relatively good health. Even removal of an entire lobe or large segment of the liver does not produce liver insufficiency if the remaining hepatic tissue is healthy.

BOX 15–6   Metastatic Cancer of Liver

Causes

Cancer of abdominal organs

Other cancers, including sarcomas

Unknown primaries

Lesions

One or more nodules of cancer in the liver

Manifestations

May be none

Hepatomegaly

Jaundice (late)

Nodular liver

Cancer on biopsy

Carcinoma of the Pancreas

The most common and deadly neoplasm of the pancreas is ductal adenocarcinoma. Most cases of pancreatic adenocarcinoma develop in the head of the pancreas, producing jaundice because of obstruction of the common bile duct and pain because of involvement of nerves in surrounding tissues. As in pancreatitis, pain is often referred to the back. Some patients with pancreatic cancer develop thromboses in multiple body sites, and this may be how they come to medical attention. Pancreatic carcinoma is a very malignant disease with a 5-year survival rate of 5–10%. In the United States, it is the 10th most commonly diagnosed cancer, but because of its high fatality, it is the 4th most common cause of cancer death. Part of the reason it is so deadly is that it is usually not detected until it is already at a late stage, when surgical cure is no longer feasible. There is no screening tool for it, and symptoms usually do not develop until the malignant cells have grown sufficiently to occlude the pancreatic or common bile ducts or invade nerves. The genetic aberrations in the early stages of pancreatic cancer development are only now beginning to be recognized, but what really causes the disease is not known. The strongest known risk factors are smoking and obesity.

Organ Failure

Acute liver failure results from massive death of hepatocytes. Viral hepatitis and drug reactions are the most common causes. Active liver failure can be fatal. Chronic liver failure is associated with cirrhosis, discussed later. Failure of function of the gallbladder is usually the result of obstruction of the cystic or common bile ducts, such as by a stone or inflammatory stricture. The gallbladder can be removed without any deleterious effects to the patient's digestive system. Acute pancreatic failure is not a recognized condition, though acute pancreatitis can be lethal because the tissue destruction causes overwhelming release of cytokines, which induce shock. Chronic pancreatic failure leads to malabsorption if pancreatic acini are extensively destroyed and to diabetes mellitus if islets of Langerhans are extensively destroyed.

Cirrhosis

Cirrhosis is the term used to describe the end stage of most serious chronic types of liver disease. It is characterized by fibrosis and nodular regeneration of hepatocytes. Normally, damaged hepatocytes can be replaced. However, if the delicate connective tissue framework of the liver is destroyed by inflammation and replaced by bands of fibrous tissue, regenerating hepatocytes' connections to the biliary tree and to the venous and arterial networks are defective. Although the hepatocytes have normal enzymatic machinery, the disordered architecture prevents the liver from functioning properly.

Of the many causes of cirrhosis, alcohol consumption and chronic hepatitis account for the largest portion of cases in the United States. Other types of cirrhosis, such as biliary cirrhosis resulting from prolonged bile duct obstruction, pigmentary cirrhosis of hemochromatosis resulting from massive storage of iron, genetic conditions such as biliary atresia or Wilson disease (a genetic defect in copper metabolism), and alpha-1-antitrypsin deficiency are uncommon. In many cases, the exact cause of the cirrhosis cannot be determined.

In cirrhosis, wide bands of fibrosis separate nodules of hepatocytes that lack portal triads and central veins

(**Figures 15–10** and **15–11**). The pattern of injury may be helpful in determining the cause of the cirrhosis. Most instances of alcoholic cirrhosis produce a finely nodular liver. Cirrhosis associated with chronic viral hepatitis generally has larger regenerative nodules and broader and more irregular bands of fibrous tissue.

The development of cirrhosis takes many months to years. It is usually asymptomatic until serious destruction of the architecture of the liver has occurred. Cirrhosis leads to several complications. **Portal hypertension** refers to increased blood pressure in the portal vein resulting from increased resistance to flow through damaged veins in the liver. The increased pressure in the portal venous system causes blood to find alternate pathways to the vena cava, called portosystemic shunts. Common sites for these shunts are the veins at the distal end of the esophagus, hemorrhoidal veins, and the umbilical veins in the skin of the abdomen (**Figure 15–12**). These dilate

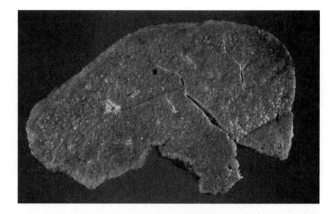

FIGURE 15–10 Cirrhosis. The finely nodular pattern of the cut surface of the liver is suggestive of alcohol-related cirrhosis.

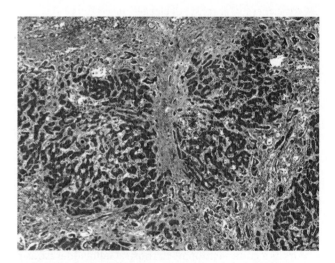

FIGURE 15–11 Cirrhosis. This section of liver is stained with trichrome, which colors collagen blue. Dense bands of fibrosis surround nodules of hepatocytes that do not contain portal triads or central veins.

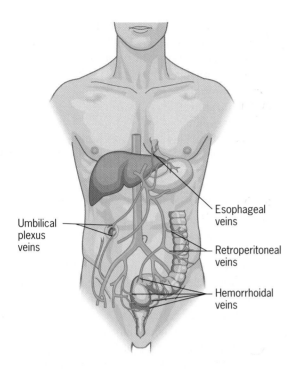

FIGURE 15–12 Common locations of portal-venous shunts in cirrhotic patients.

Labels: Umbilical plexus veins; Esophageal veins; Retroperitoneal veins; Hemorrhoidal veins

as they receive increased blood flow, causing **varices**, and are subsequently prone to rupture. Ruptured esophageal varices are a common cause of death in cirrhotic patients. In addition, portal hypertension can cause passive congestion and enlargement of the spleen. Splenomegaly increases destruction of blood cells by the spleen, leading to anemia, leukopenia, and thrombocytopenia.

Because the hepatocytes are no longer bathed in portal venous blood, they are no longer able to filter it of wastes, such as ammonia. Hyperammonemia is associated with **hepatic encephalopathy** or depression of the central nervous system, resulting in stupor or coma. The shunting of blood away from the hepatocytes also explains why drugs are poorly metabolized in cirrhotic patients, and why cirrhotic patients are more susceptible to infection (the macrophages resident in the liver normally clear bacteria that gain access to the blood stream).

Another complication of cirrhosis is **ascites**, or accumulation of excessive fluid in the abdomen. People can accumulate about 1,500 mL of fluid within the abdomen without it being noticed, but anything more than this will cause the belly to bulge. The etiology of ascites is complicated. Because hepatocyte function is depressed, the circulating blood does not contain enough albumin, produced by the liver, to maintain osmotic pressure. In addition, portal hypertension increases oncotic pressure. Low osmotic and high oncotic pressures induce the movement of fluid out of the circulatory system. Ascitic fluid is susceptible to infection from bacteria in the gut, a condition called **spontaneous bacterial peritonitis**.

Reduced production of plasma proteins results in **coagulopathy**. Altered metabolism of sex hormones by the liver leads to estrogenic effects, including small dilated blood vessels in skin (spider angiomas) and breast enlargement in men (gynecomastia). Also, failure of connections with the biliary tree results in bile backing up in hepatocytes and being passed into the circulation, resulting in jaundice. In the very late stages of chronic liver failure, blood flow is reduced to the kidneys and to the lungs, resulting in the hepatorenal and hepatopulmonary syndromes. These are ominous developments and require intensive medical care.

Chronically inflamed and scarred livers, whatever the cause, are at increased risk for developing hepatocellular carcinoma. As already discussed, this is a major cause of death in regions of the world in which hepatitis B virus is endemic, and its incidence in the United States is increasing as hepatitis C virus–infected individuals are increasingly coming to attention. This cancer is often detected at a late stage, and its treatment is complicated by the generally poor state of health of the patient.

The average cirrhotic patient comes to medical attention because of the development of one or more of the signs or symptoms of cirrhosis: gynecomastia, palmar erythema, spider angiomas, or visible umbilical or hemorrhoidal varices. Often, cirrhosis comes to attention because of derangements in liver function tests performed routinely as part of a screening exam. Ascites and jaundice usually develop more insidiously and in later stages of the disease. Bleeding esophageal varices can have a very dramatic, acute presentation with the loss of a large volume of blood into the gastrointestinal system. Hepatic encephalopathy and hepatorenal and hepatopulmonary syndromes are often end-stage manifestations.

If the cirrhosis is well advanced, the patient dies within a few years from bleeding or infection. If chronic liver disease is discovered at an earlier stage, when fibrosis is not yet advanced, removal of the causative agent can prevent the development of cirrhosis. Unfortunately, some causes cannot be removed, such as hepatitis C virus or autoimmune diseases. They can, however, be carefully managed to at least delay the progression of fibrosis. The aim of therapy for established complications is surgical or medical management: reversal is not an option. For example, esophageal varices, can be embolized or clipped so that they cannot accommodate blood flow, and diuretics can be administered to reduce ascites. Nutritional support, antibiotics, lactulose (which prevents the accumulation of ammonia), and avoidance of toxins that can do further injury to the liver, such as alcohol and pharmaceutical agents, all play a role in the management of the cirrhotic patient. Eventually, however, the patient will die unless s/he is a candidate for transplant surgery. Liver transplantation is the only "cure" for cirrhosis but carries significant risks and toxicities. In addition, the underlying disease, such as hepatitis C virus infection or some of the autoimmune disorders, can recur aggressively in the transplanted liver.

BOX 15–8 Cirrhosis

Causes

Alcohol

Viral hepatitis

Genetic diseases

Bile duct obstruction

Autoimmune diseases

Idiopathic

Lesions

Fibrous bands

Nodules of hepatocytes

Manifestations

Jaundice

Hepatic encephalopathy

Varices

Ascites

Spider angiomas

Gynecomastia

Cirrhosis on tissue biopsy

Splenomegaly

Coagulopathy

Hepatocellular carcinoma

Practice Questions

1. A 12-year-old boy becomes acutely ill with fever, loss of appetite, and jaundice 3 weeks after returning from summer camp. He recovers uneventfully 2 weeks later. His disease is most likely
   A. hepatitis A.
   B. hepatitis B.
   C. hepatitis C.
   D. hepatitis D.
   E. hepatitis E.

2. Severe, acute pancreatitis is most commonly caused by
   A. cholelithiasis.
   B. cystic fibrosis.
   C. trauma.
   D. pancreatic carcinoma.
   E. shock.

3. Accumulation of which of the following substances, usually cleared by the liver, results in hepatic encephalopathy?
   A. Urea nitrogen
   B. Ammonia
   C. Bilirubin
   D. Vitamin K
   E. Triglycerides

4. The biggest risk factor for the development of hepatocellular carcinoma is
   A. smoking.
   B. cirrhosis.
   C. gallstones.
   D. chemicals.
   E. alcohol.

5. A patient complains of foul-smelling, gray, greasy stools that float in the toilet water. Which of the following is the most likely cause of this problem?
   A. Pancreatic carcinoma
   B. Hepatocellular carcinoma
   C. Impaired digestion of fats in the diet
   D. Portal hypertension, resulting in impaired delivery of fatty acids to the liver
   E. Cirrhosis

6. A 68-year-old woman in otherwise good health visits the doctor stating that she can feel masses in her abdomen. Palpation reveals an enlarged, nodular liver. This most likely represents
   A. hepatocellular carcinoma.
   B. cirrhosis.
   C. metastatic colon cancer.
   D. pancreatic pseudocysts.
   E. metastatic thyroid cancer.

CHAPTER 16

Kidney, Lower Urinary Tract, and Male Genital Organs

OUTLINE

OBJECTIVES

1. Review the structure and function of the urinary and male genital tracts.
2. Recognize some of the most common medical diseases, cancers, and surgical interventions of the urological and male genital tracts.
3. Describe the implications of urinary frequency, dysuria, nocturia, urgency, flank pain, hematuria, oliguria, and anuria.
4. Describe the elements of the physical and laboratory examination of the urological and male genital organs, including cystoscopy and visual inspection of the urine.
5. Compare and contrast the nephrotic and nephritic syndromes and give examples of diseases manifesting in these manners.
6. Describe the role of PSA, radiography, and renal biopsy in diagnosing diseases of the urological and male genital tracts.
7. List and describe the most common genetic and congenital conditions of the urological and male genital tracts.
8. Compare and contrast autosomal recessive and autosomal dominant polycystic kidney diseases.
9. Describe the risk factors, causes, and complications of urinary tract infections.
10. Describe the causes, manifestations, and treatments of kidney stones.
11. Describe the role of immune-mediated injury in glomerular diseases, and give specific examples of immune-mediated diseases of the kidneys.
12. Identify the most common causes of chronic glomerular injury in the United States.
13. Describe the most common infectious diseases of the male genital tract.
14. Compare prostatic hyperplasia and prostatic carcinoma in terms of causes, lesions, manifestations, treatment, and possible complications.
15. Compare and contrast carcinomas of the prostate, bladder, kidney, and testes in terms of incidence, age at diagnosis, stage at diagnosis, 5-year survival, treatment, methods of detection, and risk factors.
16. Define Gleason score and describe its importance in estimating prognosis in prostate cancer.
17. Differentiate acute and chronic renal failure in terms of causes, manifestations, and treatments.
18. Describe the modalities with which chronic renal failure can be treated, including the complications that can develop with each.
19. Define and use in proper context all words and terms in headings and bold print in this chapter.

KEY TERMS

acute kidney injury
acute postinfectious
   glomerulonephritis
aldosterone
angiotensin II
antidiuretic hormone
autosomal dominant
   polycystic kidney disease
autosomal recessive
   polycystic kidney disease
azotemia
bacterial prostatitis
benign prostatic hypertrophy
bladder
chlamydia
chronic kidney failure
collecting tubules
creatinine
cryptorchidism
cystoscopy
digital rectal examination
end-stage renal disease
epididymis
focal segmental
   glomerulosclerosis
Gleason score
glomerulonephritis
glomerulosclerosis
glomerulus
gonorrhea
hemodialysis
HLA
hydronephrosis
interstitium
kidney
kidney stone
lithotripsy
membranous nephropathy
mesangium
minimal change disease
mumps orchitis

nephritic syndrome
nephroblastoma
nephron
nephrotic syndrome
penis
podocyte
proliferative
   glomerulonephritis
prostate cancer
prostate gland
prostate-specific antigen
pyelonephritis
renal biopsy
renal cell carcinoma
renal cortex
renal medulla
renal pelvis
renin
resorption
secretion
seminal vesicle
seminiferous tubule
seminoma
syphilis
systemic lupus
   erythematosus
testis
transplant rejection
transplantation
tubular casts
tubule
urea nitrogen
uremia
ureter
urethra
urinalysis
urinary tract infection (UTI)
urolithiasis
urothelial carcinoma
vas deferens
vesicoureteral reflux

Review of Structure and Function

The **kidneys** are bilateral retroperitoneal organs that receive blood from the renal arteries and are drained by the renal veins (**Figure 16–1**). Urine formed by the kidney passes through the **ureters**, which lie in the retroperitoneum, to the **bladder**, a muscular sack that sits in the pelvis. A sphincter at the base of the bladder effectively seals it off until it is induced to relax by a voluntary urge to urinate. Urine is drained from the bladder through the **urethra**. In women, the urethra is only a few centimeters in length, but in men, it first traverses the **prostate gland** and then the length of the **penis**. The secretions of the male genital organs also pass through the urethra. Sperm are produced in the **testes**, bilateral organs sitting in the scrotum slightly outside the body cavity, and stored in the tightly coiled **epididymis** that partially encircles each

testis (**Figure 16–2**). They then pass through the **vas deferens** (pl., vasa deferentia), which courses from the epididymis out of the scrotum and around the bladder to enter the prostate posteriorly. On their way through the urethra, sperm are admixed with fluid from the prostate and from the paired **seminal vesicles** lying behind the prostate.

Because of the close anatomic relationship between the male genital organs and the lower urinary tract, this chapter discusses diseases of the urinary tract and the male genital organs.

The kidneys consist of cortex, medulla, and pelvis (**Figure 16–3**). The **renal cortex** contains the major functional units of the kidney, the **glomeruli** (sing., glomerulus) and most of the **tubules**. The **renal medulla** contains the specialized distal parts of the tubules, also called the loops of Henle, and the **collecting tubules**. The collecting tubules transport urine to the **renal pelvis**, a space lined by urothelium and continuous with the ureters.

The term *upper urinary tract* refers to the kidney and ureters. The kidneys are essential for the control of blood pressure, excretion of waste products of metabolism, and maintenance of acid–base balance. They perform these

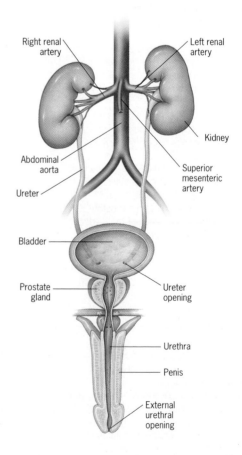

FIGURE 16–1 Schematic diagram of the anatomy of the urogenital system.

FRONT VIEW

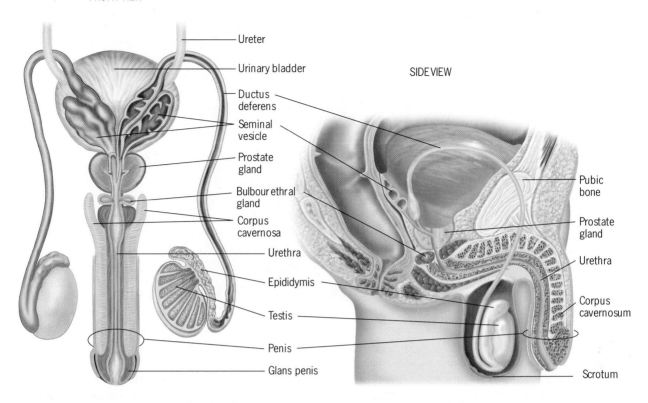

- Ureter
- Urinary bladder
- Ductus deferens
- Seminal vesicle
- Prostate gland
- Bulbourethral gland
- Corpus cavernosa
- Urethra
- Epididymis
- Testis
- Penis
- Glans penis

SIDE VIEW

- Pubic bone
- Prostate gland
- Urethra
- Corpus cavernosum
- Scrotum

FIGURE 16–2 Schematic diagram of male genital organs.

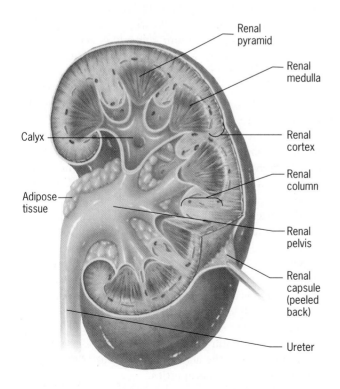

- Renal pyramid
- Renal medulla
- Renal cortex
- Calyx
- Renal column
- Adipose tissue
- Renal pelvis
- Renal capsule (peeled back)
- Ureter

FIGURE 16–3 Schematic diagram of the structure of the kidney.

functions by regulating the concentration of salt, water, and hydrogen ion in the body and filtering the blood of waste substances, including drugs and toxins. The kidneys receive 20% of the cardiac output each minute. The main renal arteries branch several times into smaller arteries and arterioles, which eventually supply the renal glomeruli.

The basic functional unit of the kidney is called the **nephron** and consists of glomerulus, tubules, and associated vessels (**Figure 16–4**). Each glomerulus is a tuft of capillaries covered with a layer of epithelial cells, called **podocytes** (**Figure 16–5**). The capillary tufts are held together by specialized cells that form the **mesangium** of the glomerulus. Between the endothelial cell lining of the capillary and the epithelial cell cytoplasm is a thin basement membrane. Foot processes of the podocytes cover the basement membrane and interconnect extensively, leaving only small slits through which filtration occurs. The endothelial cell, epithelial cell, and basement membrane thereby form a porous filter allowing molecules within the blood to be secreted into Bowman's space around the glomerulus. From there, the filtrate enters tubules lined by epithelial cells and surrounded

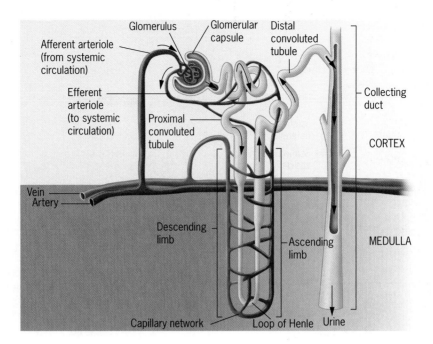

FIGURE 16–4 Components of a nephron.

by a rich plexus of capillaries (**Figure 16–6**). The tubules eventually merge to form the collecting ducts that traverse the medulla to the renal pelvis. All the supporting tissue between the tubules and glomeruli is referred to as the **interstitium** of the kidney.

The tubular epithelial cells are specialized to transport molecules between the tubule lumen and the capillaries around them. This process is highly complex, and it is not within the scope of this text to discuss the intricate physiologic details of fluid and electrolytic exchange in the renal cortex. Suffice it to say that selective activity of the renal tubular epithelial cells maintains blood at a uniform volume and with a stable concentration of sodium, potassium, and hydrogen ions. Throughout the length of the tubules there is constant exchange of fluid, waste molecules, and molecules involved in blood pressure and acid–base balance between the tubules and the capillary networks of the interstitium. Consequently, the urine that emerges from the kidney has a much different chemical composition than the initial filtrate emerging from the glomeruli. Passage of substances from the capillaries to the tubules is termed **secretion**, while the opposite, passage from the tubules to capillaries, is termed **resorption**. The final composition of urine is determined by the collecting tubules, where water is absorbed from urine back into the blood.

Secretion, resorption, and absorption are directed not only by a strong osmotic gradient set up in the renal cortex and medulla, but also by circulating hormones that directly influence the activity of the renal tubular epithelial cells. **Antidiuretic hormone** is released by the posterior pituitary gland in response to reduced plasma volume or increased plasma oncotic pressure. It acts on the epithelial cells of the collecting duct to increase their permeability so that more water is resorbed back into the bloodstream. This increases blood volume and pressure and makes the blood more dilute. In addition, specialized cells in the walls of arterioles supplying the glomerulus are stimulated to release **renin** when there are changes in blood pressure or sodium chloride concentration in the glomerular filtrate. Renin is an enzyme that catalyzes the first step in the formation of **angiotensin II**, a potent vasoconstrictor. Angiotensin II stimulates vasoconstriction of vessels throughout the body, thereby elevating the blood pressure. Renin also stimulates secretion of **aldosterone** from the adrenal gland. Aldosterone increases the resorption of sodium and water by the renal tubules and thereby expands blood volume. These hormonal pathways are important in the pathogenesis of essential hypertension.

The testes basically consist of tightly packed **seminiferous tubules** where sperm are produced (**Figure 16–7**). Testosterone-secreting cells lie in the interstitium between the seminiferous tubules. Sperm production takes place continuously, but sperm are released from the epididymis and propelled through the muscular vasa deferentia only during ejaculation. Prostatic secretions account for the major portion of seminal fluid. Seminal fluid induces maturation of sperm, provides nourishment, neutralizes the acidic environment of the vagina, and has antibacterial properties.

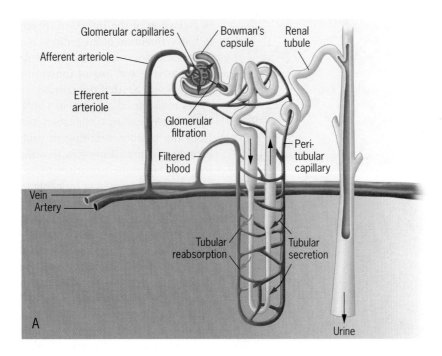

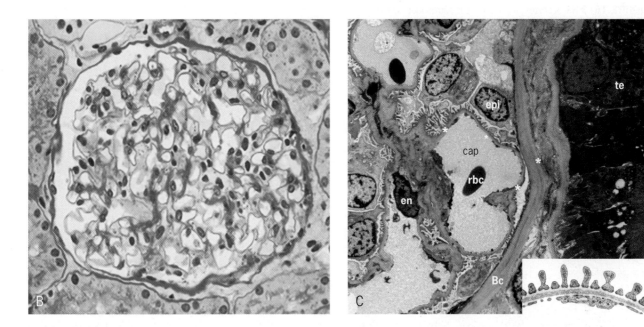

FIGURE 16–5 Components of a glomerulus. **A.** Schematic diagram. **B.** Light microscopy. This glomerulus is stained with PAS, which stains the basement membrane and mesangium dark pink. Notice how very thin the walls of the capillary loops are and how sparse the mesangium is. Bowman's capsule is the thicker pink line around the periphery of the capillary loops. The afferent and efferent arterioles and origin of the proximal convoluted tubule are not captured in this section. (Courtesy of Dr. Jose Torrealba, Department of Pathology, University of Wisconsin School of Medicine and Public Health.) **C.** Electron micrograph. The large, darkly staining cells on the right of the image are tubular epithelial cells (te). Bowman's capsule, which encloses the capillary tuft of the glomerulus, is a wide gray line running down the center of the image (Bc). A red blood cell (rbc) sits in the center of a capillary lumen (cap), which is surrounded by the thin line of the basement membrane (asterisks). Small, filamentous processes adhere at right angles to the outer surface of the basement membrane. These are the podocytes, or foot processes (not labeled), which are highly specialized outpouchings of the epithelial cells. An epithelial cell nucleus is labeled (epi), as is the nucleus of an endothelial cell, which is visible in an adjacent capillary loop (en). The inset shows the relationship of the podocytes and the basement membrane at higher magnification. Podocytes are on top of the basement membrane in this orientation, and the endothelial cell cytoplasm lines the inner (bottom) surface. The gaps in the endothelial cell cytoplasm and the spaces between the podocytes form the slits, or fenestrations, across which filtration occurs. (Courtesy of Dr. Weixiong Zhong, Department of Pathology, University of Wisconsin School of Medicine.)

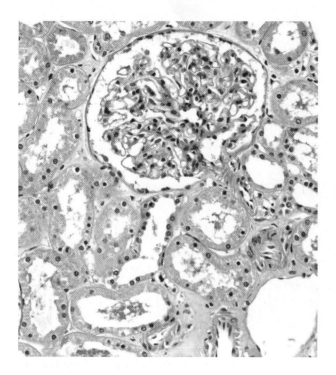

FIGURE 16–6 Renal cortex. A glomerulus is surrounded by tightly packed tubules. There is very little intervening tissue, or interstitium, around the tubules and the glomerulus. The capillary network around the tubules is difficult to appreciate on H&E stained sections. (Courtesy of Dr. Jose Torrealba, Department of Pathology, University of Wisconsin School of Medicine and Public Health.)

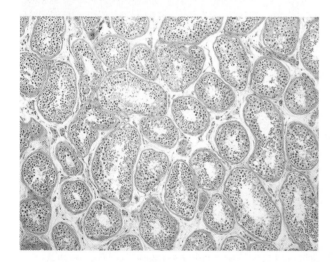

FIGURE 16–7 Testis. Seminiferous tubules are tightly packed with little intervening stroma. Occasional nests of Leydig cells, which produce testosterone, are present between the seminiferous tubules.

Most Frequent and Serious Problems

Urinary tract infections (UTIs) are the second most common infection in the human body, after upper respiratory tract infection. They are more common in women, and it is estimated that about one in five women will have a urinary tract infection in her lifetime. One of the serious complications of lower urinary tract infection is ascension of the infection through the ureters to the kidneys. Infection of the kidneys is called **pyelonephritis**. This is a serious disease, because it can result in permanent scarring and loss of function of the kidney, as well as sepsis and death if not treated.

As men age, their prostates enlarge. **Benign prostatic hypertrophy** causes obstruction of the outflow of urine from the bladder, resulting in problems with urination, including increased urgency to urinate, incontinence, and frequent nighttime urination. More than 4 million office visits are made every year for benign prostatic hypertrophy, about 60% of men older than the age of 60 years have symptoms related to it, and it is the most common diagnosis made by urologists in men between 45 and 75 years of age. Medical therapies for reducing the size of the prostate are available but not always successful. Transurethral resection of the prostate is therefore one of the most common surgical procedures performed on the male urogenital tract.

Kidney stones, or calculi, are exquisitely painful when they lodge in the renal pelvis, ureters, bladder, or urethra and obstruct the flow of urine. They are also very common: about 10% of people will have a symptomatic kidney stone by the age of 70 years, and the incidence of symptomatic kidney stones has been increasing in the past decades. Most kidney stones pass on their own, given time, patience, painkillers, and plenty of fluid. If they are too large to pass through the narrow ureters or urethra, however, they require medical attention. One of the newer methods for removing kidney stones is **lithotripsy**, whereby the stones are shattered by externally applied, high-intensity shock waves. The resulting small fragments of stones are then passed spontaneously. Lithotripsy is more common now than is surgery for removal of stones, and it is one of the most common procedures performed on the urinary tract.

Although everyone has two kidneys and the kidneys have a large reserve of function, **end-stage renal disease**, or irreversible loss of function, is unfortunately all too common. The diseases responsible for most end-stage renal disease in the United States are diabetes mellitus and hypertension. People with end-stage renal disease have two options: kidney transplantation and hemodialysis. Kidney **transplantation** is limited by the supply of donors. In the United States, about 17,000 patients with end-stage kidney disease receive kidney transplants every year. People who are not eligible for organ transplantation because of their age or comorbidities, and those waiting for a donor kidney, have waste products periodically removed from their bloodstream by **hemodialysis** (usually just called dialysis). This is a mechanism by which blood is filtered through an external device and returned to the patient's bloodstream. More than half a million people are on dialysis in the United States.

Malignancies of the urinary tract are primarily diseases of older individuals (see Table 16–5). Testicular cancer, in contrast, is a disease of young men, the median age of diagnosis being 34 years. The most common malignancy of urogenital organs is prostate cancer. More than 2 million men in the United States carry a diagnosis of prostate cancer, 200,000 will be diagnosed with it every year, and prostate cancer is the second most common cause of death in men (after lung cancer). Bladder and kidney cancer are less common, but they are still among the top 10 most common cancer diagnoses. All of these cancers are most commonly found when they are still localized, so 5-year survival is on the order of 90%. These cancers are detected at an early stage either because there is a screening tool available (serum PSA for prostate cancer, manual palpation for testicular cancer) or they produce symptoms (e.g., blood in the urine) early in their natural history.

Symptoms, Signs, and Tests

Most patients with urinary tract infection experience *frequency* of urination, *dysuria* (painful urination), *nocturia* (increased nighttime urination), and *urgency* (almost continuous urge to urinate). In addition, the urine may be clouded by pus. Prostatitis may manifest simply as low back pain. Pyelonephritis classically presents acutely with intense flank pain and systemic signs of infection such as fever and leukocytosis. Diseases of the renal glomeruli present with *hematuria* (blood in the urine) or systemic signs such as edema and hypertension. Renal calculi characteristically cause intense, sharp flank pain that radiates to the groin as the calculi migrate from the renal pelvis to the bladder. Acute necrosis of the renal tubules can result from severe insults to the kidney and manifests as *oliguria* (decreased urine output) or *anuria* (complete absence of urine production).

Physical examination of the urinary tract and genital organs consists of inspection of the penis or vulva for signs of exudation or ulceration from venereal infections, palpation of the abdomen for tumors of the kidney or a distended bladder, and, in the male, palpation of the inguinal ring for hernia or undescended testis and palpation of the testes for tumors. **Digital rectal examination** refers to palpation of the posterior of the prostate by a finger inserted into the rectum. This is performed to assess the size of the prostate and to feel for nodularities that may portend carcinoma.

The urethra and bladder can further be visualized by **cystoscopy**, which entails insertion of tubes fitted with lenses and lights through the urethra. This allows inspection of the mucosal lining of the lower urinary tract, as well as removal of stones and collection of biopsies for microscopic examination. Thinner, longer tubes can even be threaded up the ureters to remove stones and inspect the urothelium higher up in the tract.

Inspection of the urine is also an integral part of the physical exam. Urine can be turned an abnormal color by medications and foods (the antimycobacterial drug rifampin, for example, is notorious for turning urine orange, and vitamin B complex supplements can turn it neon yellow), and some diseases also cause changes in color. Dehydration makes the urine very dark, urinary tract infections can make it cloudy, and blood in the urine, even in very small amounts, can make the urine appear pink or red. In addition, various foods, drugs, and diseases can give urine an unusual odor. The pungent odor imparted by asparagus is probably well known to you. Urinary tract infections can make the urine very foul smelling, and uncontrolled diabetes can make it smell sweet.

Visual inspection of the urine also involves microscopic examination. This can detect the presence of crystals in the blood, which indicates aberrant metabolism and the risk of developing calculi, as well as red blood cells, white blood cells, bacteria, and casts (**Figure 16–8**). **Tubular casts** are tightly packed collections of proteins, lipids, or cellular debris that precipitated in renal tubules or collecting ducts and were washed out by the flow of urine. Various forms of acellular casts signify dehydration or chronic renal failure and compromised flow through the distal tubules. The presence of red blood cell casts is indicative of glomerular injury, while white blood cell casts are formed when there is infection in the kidneys. Epithelial cells can also form casts when there is severe

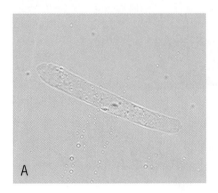
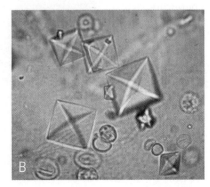
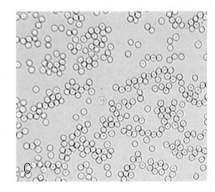

FIGURE 16–8 Microscopic examination of urine. **A.** Hyaline cast. This is the most common form of cast, composed of a tubular epithelial protein that solidifies in the tubule in states of dehydration or low urine flow. **B.** Crystals. These are composed of calcium oxalate, which is the most common constituent of renal stones. **C.** Red blood cells. The presence of red blood cells indicates damage to the urinary system anywhere along its tract, from the renal cortex to the urethra. Inflammatory lesions, cancer, stones, and mechanical trauma can all cause hematuria. (Courtesy of Ms. Stacy Walz, Clinical Laboratory Science Program, University of Wisconsin School of Medicine and Public Health.)

renal tubular injury, such as occurs with acute tubular necrosis.

In the past, doctors would taste the urine for changes in pH and the presence of glucose, but we now, thankfully, have laboratory tests to quantitate such changes. **Urinalysis** can detect the presence of many common urinary tract disorders. A dipstick, a piece of paper with reagents on it that change color in the presence of certain chemicals, can be used to detect specific gravity, pH, and the presence of protein, sugar, nitrite, ketones, or leukocyte esterase. The latter is elevated when there are white blood cells in the urine—for example, when there is a urinary tract infection. A positive leukocyte esterase result can be followed by urine culture and sensitivity tests in the microbiology laboratory. In addition, numerous other chemicals can be detected by more specialized procedures in the laboratory. These include metabolites of drug of abuse, immunoproteins, catecholamines and their metabolites, uric acid, and many others.

Renal function is easily evaluated by measuring levels of two substances in the blood that are excreted by filtration through the glomerulus—namely, **urea nitrogen** and **creatinine**. The blood level of these substances reflects an equilibrium between normal breakdown of nitrogenous compounds (urea nitrogen) and muscle (creatinine) and the activity of the nephron. When the glomeruli are damaged and cannot adequately filter the blood, urea nitrogen and creatinine rise. The level of these substances in the blood gives a clinical estimate of the capability of the glomeruli to adequately clear the blood of waste products.

Two constellations of physical findings and abnormal laboratory tests that are indicative of certain patterns of injury are the nephrotic and nephritic syndromes. The **nephrotic syndrome** results from damage to the glomerular filtering apparatus. Essentially, protein, primarily albumin, is lost through the kidneys, with resultant loss of oncotic pressure in the blood. The patient becomes edematous as fluid escapes the vascular system and displays laboratory evidence of heavy proteinuria (>3 g/24 hr; normal is <150 mg/24 hr) and decreased serum albumin. Hyperlipidemia may also occur with the nephrotic syndrome, and increased lipid may be present in the urine. The most common causes of the nephrotic syndrome are primary glomerular diseases such as minimal change disease and systemic diseases such as diabetes mellitus, amyloidosis, and systemic lupus erythematosus. The **nephritic syndrome** occurs when there is inflammatory damage to the kidneys, usually the glomeruli. The urine contains blood and red blood cell casts, and the patient additionally has signs of decreased renal function such as elevated blood urea nitrogen and creatinine and low urine output.

Laboratory techniques are also available for assessing the function of the male genital organs. Seminal fluid can be analyzed for its composition. Sperm are visualized under the microscope and assessed for shape and motility during infertility workups. One of the most common

tests performed is measurement of **prostate-specific antigen** (PSA) in the blood. This is a protein produced by the prostate in low quantities. It rises a little as men age, but a greater-than-normal rise in PSA is highly suggestive of prostate cancer. It is currently recommended that all men between the ages of 55 and 70 years should have PSA measured annually.

Radiologic techniques can be used to assess the structure of the urinary tract. A *cystogram* is obtained to determine the size and shape of the bladder and the pattern of flow of urine. A contrast agent is instilled through a catheter into the bladder, and radiographic images obtained. Abnormal flow of bladder contents, as for example up into the ureters in cases of urinary reflux, can be detected with this method. The *intravenous pyelogram (IVP)* is used to look for gross structural changes in the kidneys and ureters. Radiopaque contrast material, injected intravenously, is filtered by the glomeruli into the tubules and concentrated in the renal pelvis and ureters. Dilation of the pelvis or ureter indicates obstruction to the flow of urine farther down the tract (**Figure 16–9**). Distortion of the normal pattern of dye in the collecting system suggests a mass or cyst. Calculi in the renal pelvis appear as filling defects. Cystography and intravenous pyelography have largely been replaced with sophisticated computerized tomography (CT) techniques that allow three-dimensional reconstruction of portions of the urinary tract (**Figure 16–10**). Conventional CT images and ultrasound techniques are also useful for diagnosis of renal and testicular masses such as cancer or cystic disease.

Renal biopsies are often performed to evaluate the integrity of the structures of the renal cortex. A thin needle is inserted through the skin of the flank to extract a

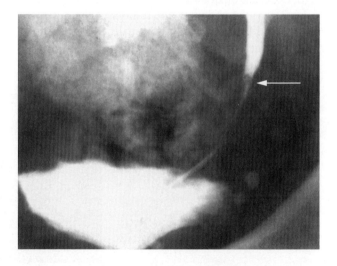

FIGURE 16–9 Intravenous pyelogram. Contrast material fills the bladder at the bottom of the image and the proximal portion of the right ureter. A stone (white arrow) is lodged in the ureter, causing dilation of the ureter above it and preventing urine from filling the distal portion. The dye in the bladder comes from urine passing through the opposite ureter.

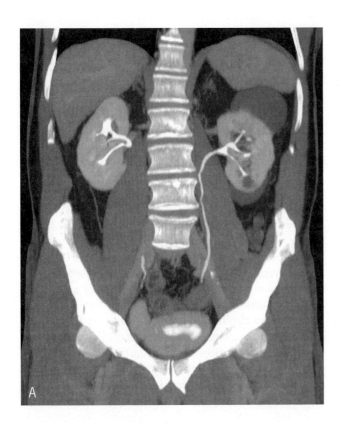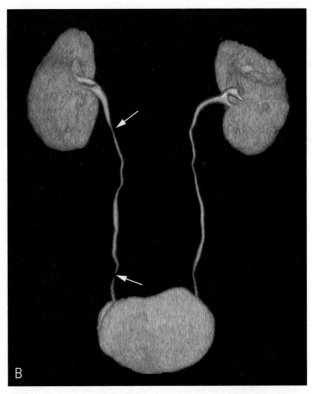

FIGURE 16–10 CT urogram. **A.** In this coronal view, the left ureter can be followed from the kidney to the bladder. The central portion of the right ureter is not filled with contrast. **B.** The relationship of the kidneys, ureters, and bladder is rendered in three dimensions. Even small cysts can be seen on the surface of the kidney. Two strictures are present in the right ureter (arrows), and the segment of ureter above them is slightly dilated in comparison to the left ureter. (Courtesy of Dr. Myron Pozniak, Department of Radiology, University of Wisconsin School of Medicine and Public Health.)

core of tissue. This is then examined by light microscopy, immunofluorescent techniques, and electron microscopy. Examples of these can be seen in the discussion of specific diseases later in this chapter. Biopsies are especially useful in determining the nature of glomerular diseases, and, performed sequentially, they can be used to track the development and document the severity of glomerular injury in chronic diseases such as diabetes mellitus or systemic lupus erythematosus.

Specific Diseases

Genetic/Developmental Diseases

Of all organ systems in the body, the urogenital organs are most commonly affected by congenital anomalies. The kidneys play a crucial role in fetal development, in that they produce the amnionic fluid that surrounds the fetus *in utero*. If the kidneys are not functioning properly and there is insufficient fluid, a characteristic set of anomalies develops, termed the *Potter syndrome*. These include impaired lung development, impaired growth of the fetus, limb deformities, and characteristic facial features. The fetus usually does not survive to birth. In contrast, the conditions and diseases discussed in this section are not incompatible with life, and some are not even detected until adulthood, if at all.

Anomalies of Kidney Number, Size, and Shape

Complete agenesis of the kidney occurs infrequently and is obviously incompatible with life if bilateral. However, agenesis is usually unilateral, and because the other kidney is normal, the patient may not develop renal insufficiency. Hypoplasia, however, even if unilateral, does come to attention. The glomerular filtration rate is decreased because of a decrease in the number of functioning nephrons, and this leads to the release of hormones that cause hypertension, even in childhood. In addition, the intact nephrons are overburdened by the amount of blood they have to filter and rapidly become damaged themselves. This leads to end-stage renal failure. Renal hypoplasia is the most common cause of end-stage renal disease in the pediatric population. Transplant is curative. Rarely, more than two kidneys can develop, and sometimes normally developing kidneys become fused at their lower poles, resulting in a so-called horseshoe kidney (**Figure 16–11**). This does not come to clinical attention because renal function is entirely normal, despite the odd shape of the kidney.

Renal Dysplasia

Malformation of the renal parenchyma during embryonic development can result in disorganized renal cortical tissue, poorly developed glomeruli and tubules, and abnormal differentiation of the mesenchymal component into

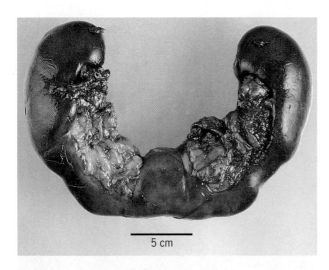

FIGURE 16–11 Horseshoe kidney. The two kidneys fused at their lower pole during fetal development.

cartilage or bone. Dysplastic kidneys are also often disfigured by cysts of varying sizes. If the renal pelvis and ureters are also abnormally developed, stasis or even reflux of urine and repeated urinary tract infections can ensue. If unilateral, and the contralateral kidney is entirely normal, the condition may not cause renal insufficiency. However, if bilateral, symptoms of renal insufficiency can occur. The condition affects about 3 in 1,000 births, and the prognosis depends on whether one or both kidneys are involved.

Congenital Anomalies of the Ureters, Bladder, and Urethra

Hereditary Polycystic Kidney Diseases
Polycystic kidney is a descriptive term that connotes ballooning of the renal tubules. The processes causing multiple cysts to form are usually degenerative: cysts of varying sizes are often seen in end-stage kidneys, regardless of cause. Two genetic diseases that result in polycystic kidneys are described here.

The infantile version, called autosomal recessive polycystic kidney disease, is often present at birth or comes to attention in infancy and early childhood and always has associated liver involvement. The genetic defect involves a large gene called *PKHD1*, which encodes a protein that is normally present in the cells of the collecting ducts and tubules of the kidney and the bile ducts of the liver. Exactly how a derangement in this protein leads to polycystic kidneys and fibrosis of the liver is not known. The condition affects only 1–4:10,000 births. If severe, polycystic kidneys can be seen on prenatal ultrasound and can result in the Potter syndrome. This is rare, however, and children usually survive and develop insidious signs of renal failure, including renal tubular dysfunction and hypertension, as they mature. Hepatic involvement does not manifest clinically until fibrosis is advanced.

The other form of hereditary polycystic kidney disease is called autosomal dominant polycystic kidney disease. In contrast to the infantile recessive form, the dominant form is fairly common, affecting 1:400–1:1,000 live births; it usually does not manifest until adulthood, and liver involvement is less severe. Most autosomal dominant polycystic kidney disease results from mutations in either the *PKD1* or *PKD2* gene, both of which encode a protein that is present in renal tubular cells. As with recessive cystic kidney disease, the pathophysiologic link between this abnormality and dilation of the renal tubules is not known. The cysts develop insidiously, and by the time the patient has full-blown renal failure requiring dialysis, the kidneys are hugely enlarged and disfigured by thin-walled cysts of varying sizes that have entirely replaced the renal parenchyma (**Figure 16–12**). The disease is usually not discovered until adulthood, when hypertension or chronic renal failure occurs. Patients may also develop cysts in other organs, such as the liver and pancreas, and there is a higher incidence of aneurysmal dilation of vessels in the brain, which are prone to rupture. Genetic testing can therefore be useful to guide screening for renal failure and for potentially lethal cerebral vessel aneurysms.

BOX 16–1   Hereditary Polycystic Kidney Diseases

Causes

Autosomal recessive (*PKHD1*)

Autosomal dominant (*PKD1* or *PKD2*)

Lesions

Multiple renal cysts of various sizes, bilateral

Biliary cysts and hepatic fibrosis

Cysts in other organs (pancreas, spleen); cerebral vascular aneurysms (adult form only)

Manifestations

Slowly progressive renal failure, manifesting in infancy or childhood (recessive form) or adulthood (dominant form)

Cryptorchidism

Cryptorchidism means "hidden testis." The testes develop in the abdomen during the fetal period and are pulled down through the pelvis and the inguinal ring into the scrotal sac during the last months of fetal development. They are usually both in the scrotal sac at the time of birth, but in about 1% of male babies one or both of the testes is arrested in its descent. If the testis has not descended by 1 year of age, it is unlikely that it will do so in the future. Instead, it will undergo steady degeneration, with replacement of the seminiferous tubules by scar tissue. If bilateral, testicular degeneration will cause sterility. If the testis is trapped in the inguinal ring, a hernia is also likely to be present. In addition, cryptorchid testes are vulnerable to developing cancer. The risk is greater if both testes are undescended, and the risk for the normally descended testis in cases of unilateral cryptorchidism is also higher than in the general population. It is currently recommended that cryptorchid testes be surgically removed before puberty to reduce the cancer risk.

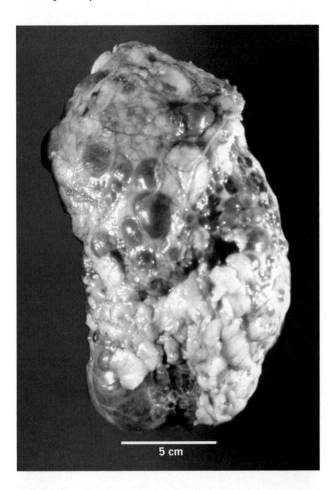

FIGURE 16–12 Adult polycystic kidney. The kidney is much larger than normal and the cortical surface is disfigured by numerous cysts of varying sizes, to which perirenal adipose tissue is densely adherent.

BOX 16–2   Cryptorchidism

Causes

Failure of testes (one or both, usually unilateral) to descend to scrotum

Lesions

Testis present in the abdomen, pelvis, or inguinal canal

May be associated with inguinal hernia

Manifestations

Empty scrotum

Possible sterility if bilateral and uncorrected

Increased risk of testicular cancer

Inflammatory/Degenerative Diseases

Urinary Tract Infection and Pyelonephritis

Infection of the urinary tract is most commonly caused by contamination of the urethra by colonic bacteria and their subsequent spread into the higher reaches of the tract. The bacteria causing most urinary tract infections come from the bowel; of these, *Escherichia coli* is by far the most common. The symptoms of UTI are dysuria, urinary frequency, and urgency. Urinalysis of clean-catch urine can show increased leukocyte esterase, and microscopy can reveal the presence of bacteria and white blood cells. A short course of antibiotics is usually sufficient to treat an uncomplicated UTI.

There are numerous risk factors for UTIs, enumerated in **Table 16–1**. The biggest risk factor is having female anatomy: about half of all women will develop a UTI sometime during their lives. The reason women are more susceptible to UTIs than are men may be because the female urethra is short, so the bacteria have less distance to travel to get to the bladder, and the urethra is close to the anus, so bacterial contamination is more common. Urine is an excellent culture medium, so if urine becomes contaminated and is not flushed from the urinary tract, bacteria can rapidly proliferate. Obstruction to urinary flow is therefore a cause of UTI in patients with kidney stones or prostatic

TABLE 16–1   **Risk Factors for Urinary Tract Infections**

Risk Factor	Reason
Female sex	Short urethra, urethra close to anus; atrophy of urethral/vaginal epithelium after menopause
Sexual activity	Irritation of urethra
Diaphragm for birth control	Unknown
Obstruction: kidney stones, benign prostatic hypertrophy, congenital anomalies	Bacteria grow in stagnant urine
Diabetes, chronic illness	Decreased immunity
Ureteral reflux	Urine is washed back up into the kidney from the bladder
Instrumentation, catheterization	Introduction of bacteria to urinary tract; irritation of urothelium
Infection elsewhere	Hematogenous dissemination of bacteria and infection of kidney

hypertrophy, which cause impaired emptying of the bladder and stagnation of the urine.

Pyelonephritis, or infection of the kidney, is the most serious form of urinary tract infection. It usually develops from infection spreading from the lower urinary tract, but it can also occur if bacteria from some other infection in the body spread through the bloodstream to the kidneys. In children, especially in boys, **vesicoureteral reflux** predisposes them to pyelonephritis. In this condition, the usual anatomic and functional relationship of the ureters to the bladder is disturbed, allowing urine to flow back up from the bladder to the kidneys. The ureter and renal pelvis on the affected side become excessively dilated, and impaired flow of urine potentiates the growth of bacteria. The increased hydrostatic pressure of the urine and repeated episodes of pyelonephritis can completely destroy the kidney if the infections are not rapidly treated. Reflux can be surgically corrected.

The patient with acute pyelonephritis has sudden onset of flank pain, fever, and leukocytosis. Microscopically, the kidney has white cell casts in addition to the other urinalysis findings of UTI. The urine may be so replete with bacteria and white blood cells that effectively it is *pyuria*, or pus-filled urine. The inflammation affects the interstitial tissue and the tubules, with relative sparing of the glomeruli. The renal tissue that is destroyed by the inflammation cannot regenerate, so once the infection has cleared, it is replaced by scar tissue. Deep, wide scars that traverse the cortex and medulla are indicative of prior pyelonephritis. The treatment of pyelonephritis is appropriate antibiotic therapy and alleviation of whatever has predisposed to its development (reflux, obstruction, other infection), if necessary. In some patients, the disease may smolder for a long time despite antibiotic therapy. Chronic pyelonephritis is usually fostered by continued or intermittent obstruction of the urinary tract or vesicoureteral reflux. Another complication of pyelonephritis is sepsis from seeding of the bloodstream by the causative organism. Sepsis can be fatal.

> ### BOX 16–3 Urinary Tract Infection and Pyelonephritis
>
> **Causes**
>
> Bacterial contamination of urethra by colonic bacteria
>
> Ascending infection from urethra to bladder, ureters, and kidney
>
> **Lesions**
>
> Inflammation of urethra, bladder (cystitis) in UTI
>
> Inflammation of renal cortical interstitium and tubules in pyelonephritis
>
> **Manifestations**
>
> Dysuria, urinary urgency and frequency (UTI)
>
> Flank pain, fever, leukocytosis, sepsis (pyelonephritis)
>
> Urinalysis: increased leukocyte esterase; bacteria and white blood cells by microscopy; white blood cell casts in pyelonephritis
>
> Possible renal failure in chronic pyelonephritis

Urolithiasis (Kidney Stones, Renal Calculi)

Kidney stones (**Figure 16–13**) are most often composed of calcium, either calcium oxalate or calcium phosphate. The most important factor in the development of renal calculi is an excess concentration of the stones' chemical constituents so that they precipitate and crystallize in the urine. For this reason, certain hereditary metabolic defects predispose individuals to the formation of stones: these include gout, in which there is hyperuricemia, and cystinuria. In these cases, the stones are formed primarily of uric acid and cystine, respectively. In addition, low urine volume, such as occurs with dehydration or prolonged bed rest, diseases of the parathyroid gland, which stimulate release of calcium from the bones, and some bacterial infection can predispose patients to the formation of renal calculi. By far the majority of stones form for no known predisposing reason, however.

Stones containing calcium are visible on x-ray, but these account for only about 80% of renal calculi. A negative finding therefore does not mean that the patient does not have

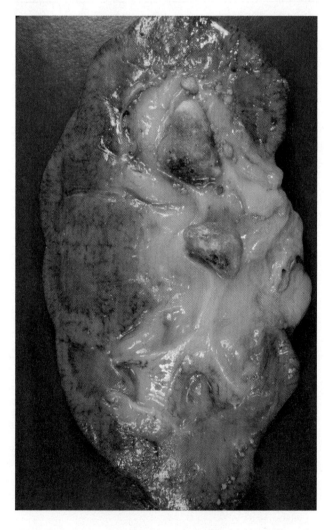

FIGURE 16–13 Kidney stones. The kidney has been opened to expose the collecting system. Gray calculi with rough surfaces lie within the pelvis and extend up into the calyces.

a renal stone. A more sensitive test is ultrasound. Passage of a small stone from the renal pelvis into the ureter produces sudden, severe flank pain, which patients describe as worse than anything they have ever experienced. Immediate treatment consists of pain medications and ingestion of large volumes of water, with the hope that the stone will pass down the urinary tract on its own. The patient may notice blood in the urine. If the stone fails to dislodge from the ureter, a urologist may have to remove the stone using catheters passed through the urethra, bladder, and ureter. Lithotripsy is a noninvasive procedure that breaks kidney stones into small pieces that are then spontaneously cleared.

A stone impacted in the ureter can lead to **hydronephrosis** or massive dilation of the urinary system proximal to the blockage (**Figure 16–14**). It can also lead to urinary tract infection, including pyelonephritis, and thus can incur extensive damage to the urinary tract. Occasionally, large stones fill the renal pelvis. These are referred to as "staghorn" calculi because of their branched appearance. Staghorn calculi are also called struvite or triple-phosphate stones, reflecting their chemical composition, and they form only in the context of infections of the urinary tract by urease-producing bacteria.

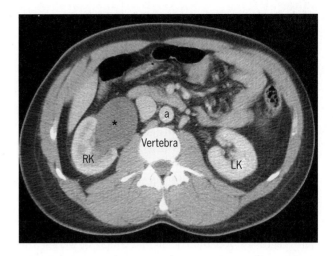

FIGURE 16–14 Hydronephrosis, CT scan. LK = left kidney, RK = right kidney, a = aorta. The asterisk is on the grossly dilated proximal portion of the right ureter. The patient had hydronephrosis from a renal stone that had lodged in the ureter. (Courtesy of Dr. Myron Pozniak, Department of Radiology, University of Wisconsin School of Medicine and Public Health.)

BOX 16–4 Kidney Stones

Causes

Usually no known predisposing condition

Dehydration

Prolonged bed rest

Metabolic disorders, such as gout and cystinuria

Infection by urease-producing organisms

Lesions

Stones form in kidney and pass through ureter, bladder, and urethra

Manifestations

Intense radiating flank or groin pain

Hematuria

Visualization of stone by x-ray or ultrasound

Glomerular Diseases

The clinical hallmarks of glomerular injury are edema, proteinuria, hematuria, increased blood urea nitrogen and creatinine, and decreased protein in blood, in varying combinations. The nephrotic and nephritic syndromes were described in the earlier section on signs, symptoms, and tests. One way of learning about glomerular diseases is to memorize which produce nephrotic syndrome, which nephritic, and which neither, but progress insidiously to end-stage renal disease. Another way of classifying these diseases is to divide them into those that cause inflammation and those that cause sclerosis, or scarring, of the glomeruli. The former pattern of injury is called **glomerulonephritis**, reflecting inflammatory damage to the glomeruli, while scarring of the glomeruli is called **glomerulosclerosis**. These can further be defined by chronicity (acute versus chronic), by whether the injury involves the majority of the glomeruli or some of the glomeruli, by whether the entire glomerulus or only parts of it are involved, and by what anatomic part of the glomerulus is affected. Glomerular diseases can also be considered in terms of whether they are primary to the kidney or secondary to some other, systemic disease such as diabetes mellitus or systemic lupus erythematosus. The classification and nomenclature of these diseases can be overwhelming to students first exposed to them, so in this discussion, the pathogenesis of glomerular diseases is discussed in general terms, and then examples are provided to illustrate how disease processes cause damage to the glomeruli and manifest clinically.

Most diseases of glomeruli are caused by immune-mediated injury. This can be of two types. In one, antigen–antibody complexes form in the blood in response to a non-kidney-related disease and are deposited on the basement membrane of the glomerulus as the blood filters through it. The second type of injury occurs when antibodies are formed against the basement membrane of the glomerulus. The antibodies in this type of nephritis may be generated against a foreign, possibly viral, protein that shares common antigenic properties with the glomerular basement membrane. The antibodies are therefore said to cross-react with basement membrane antigens. Both types of immune-mediated injury cause damage to the basement membrane and impair its ability to retain protein as the blood filters through it. If the immune complexes subsequently stimulate an inflammatory reaction, red blood cells may also leak into the urine.

A prototypical immune complex disease is **acute postinfectious glomerulonephritis**. This follows an infection with certain strains of group A streptococci, usually causing pharyngitis. One to 3 weeks after the initial infection, antibodies are formed against streptococcus antigens, and the resultant antigen–antibody complexes get stuck on the glomerular basement membrane and incite an acute inflammatory response (**Figure 16–15**). Inflammation of the basement membrane leads to nephritic manifestations: hematuria, edema, hypertension, and decreased urine output. There usually also is protein in the urine. Antibiotics are not effective in treating acute poststreptococcal glomerulonephritis because the initial bacterial infection has already cleared by the time this complication develops. Instead, treatment is supportive: managing fluid overload and hypertension while the disease spontaneously regresses over the course of a couple of weeks. The recovery rate is approximately 95% in children and slightly lower in adults; the remainder in both groups develop progressive renal failure. Acute poststreptococcal glomerulonephritis is the most common cause of acute nephritis globally, but it is quite uncommon in developed countries, affecting fewer than 1 in 100,000 people annually. It is most common in children between the ages of 5 and 12 years.

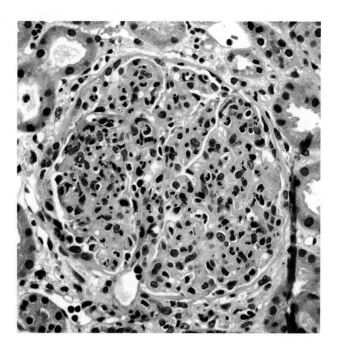

FIGURE 16–15 Acute postinfectious glomerulonephritis. There are numerous polymorphonuclear leukocytes (neutrophils) in this glomerulus. The capillary lumens are inconspicuous due to the inflammation. (Courtesy of Dr. Weixiong Zhong, Department of Pathology, University of Wisconsin School of Medicine and Public Health.)

BOX 16–5 Acute Postinfectious Glomerulonephritis

Causes

Antigen–antibody complexes lodge in glomerular basement membrane

Prior streptococcal infection

Lesions

Acute inflammation of glomeruli

Manifestations

Hematuria, edema, hypertension, proteinuria

Very rare progression to chronic renal failure

Not all immune complex–mediated injury of the glomeruli results in inflammation and the nephritic syndrome. Injury to the filtering capability of the glomerulus in the absence of inflammation results in the nephrotic syndrome. In adults, one of the most common causes of the nephrotic syndrome is **membranous nephropathy**. In this condition, immune complexes are deposited along the basement membrane of the glomerulus (**Figure 16–16**) without inciting an inflammatory reaction. In most cases, the underlying condition giving rise to the immune complexes is not known. In the remainder, antibodies are generated against a wide variety of exogenous or endogenous antigens (**Table 16–2**). Deposition of the immune complexes results in thickening of the basement membrane. In addition, the immune complexes activate the complement pathway, with subsequent generation of the membrane attack complex. It is thought that it is the activity of the membrane attack complex that makes the basement membrane leaky. Membranous nephropathy usually presents with the insidious onset of

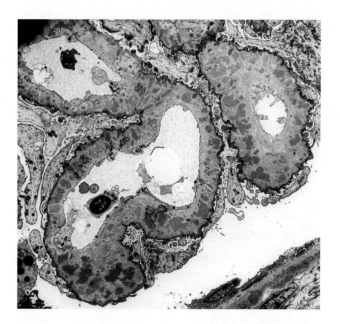

FIGURE 16–16 Membranous glomerulopathy. The basement membranes of these capillaries are very thick (compare to the basement membrane in Figure 16–5C) and contain irregular, electron-dense deposits. Podocytes are present, but they are fused, thickened, and irregular. This is a secondary change in membranous glomerulopathy. (Courtesy of Dr. Jose Torrealba, Department of Pathology, University of Wisconsin School of Medicine and Public Health.)

the nephrotic syndrome. The disease does not respond to corticosteroids, and its course is highly variable: some patients go into spontaneous remission, some progress slowly, and about 40% progress to renal failure.

TABLE 16–2	Causes of Membranous Nephropathy
Cause	**Examples**
Idiopathic	
Drugs	Penicillamine, captopril, gold, NSAIDs
Malignancy	Lung cancer, colon cancer, melanoma
Infections	Hepatitis B, hepatitis C, syphilis, malaria
Autoimmune diseases	Systemic lupus erythematosus, thyroiditis

BOX 16–6   Membranous Nephropathy

Causes
Idiopathic
Drugs
Malignancy
Infections
Autoimmune diseases
Lesions
Immune complex deposition in basement membrane
Thickening of basement membrane
Manifestations
Nephrotic syndrome
End-stage renal disease (over time)

BOX 16–7   Minimal Change Disease

Causes
Usually idiopathic
Infection
Drugs
Neoplasia
Allergy
Other kidney diseases
Lesions
Effacement of podocyte foot processes
Manifestations
Usually in children
Sudden onset nephrotic syndrome

In children, the most common cause of the nephrotic syndrome is **minimal change disease**. It accounts for 80% of cases of nephrotic syndrome in children and 15% in adults. Unlike the other diseases discussed here, it is not caused by deposition of immune complexes. Instead, the foot processes of podocytes that cover the basement membrane are damaged (**Figure 16–17**). A wide variety of clinical and research observations suggest that the cause of minimal change disease is aberrant T-lymphocyte function, which results in the elaboration of cytokines that increase the permeability of the basement membrane. The altered architecture of the foot processes appears to be a secondary phenomenon and not related directly to the altered immune regulation itself. Minimal change disease is so called because there is no alteration to the appearance of the glomerulus by light microscopy or by immunofluorescence. The only change that is seen is effacement of the podocyte foot processes on electron microscopy. As with membranous nephropathy, most cases of minimal change disease are idiopathic. **Table 16–3** lists some of the conditions known to be associated with minimal change disease. The nephrotic syndrome caused by this condition is of sudden and acute onset. Glomerular function and urine output are usually not disturbed.

Minimal change disease typically resolves with steroid therapy, leaving no residual decrease in glomerular function or morphologic evidence of glomerular injury. In another pattern of glomerular disease, which appears to be pathogenetically related to and possibly even a variant of minimal change disease, chronic glomerular injury does take place. This disease is called **focal segmental glomerulosclerosis**. *Focal* refers to the observation that

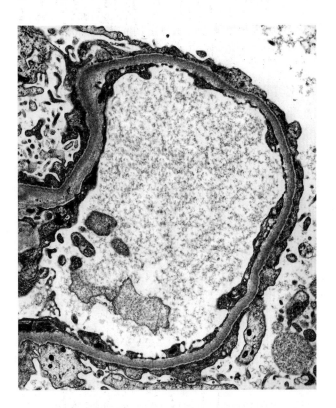

FIGURE 16–17 Minimal change disease. The foot processes are fused and form a continuous line along the epithelial side of the basement membrane. The basement membrane itself is of the usual thickness. Compare to Figure 16–5C. (Courtesy of Dr. Jose Torrealba, Department of Pathology, University of Wisconsin School of Medicine and Public Health.)

TABLE 16–3	Clinical Associations of Minimal Change Disease
Cause	**Comments or Examples**
Idiopathic	By far the majority of cases in children and adults
Infection	Often precedes onset of minimal change disease in children
Drugs	NSAIDs, antibiotics, immunizations, lithium, others
Neoplasia	Hematologic malignancies may precede or be preceded by minimal change disease
Allergy	Poison ivy, fungi, ragweed, house dust, grass pollen, bee stings, cat fur
Other kidney diseases	Systemic lupus erythematosus, type 1 diabetes, polycystic kidney disease, HIV nephropathy

not all glomeruli are affected, and *segmental* means that only parts of the affected glomeruli are sclerotic, or scarred (**Figure 16–18**). As in minimal change disease, the epithelial cell foot processes are disrupted. Over time, proteins that are filtered through the hyperpermeable areas of the basement membrane get trapped within the membrane. These deposits can become so large that they occlude the capillary. They can also be admixed with lipid droplets. The glomeruli become progressively sclerotic, and if the condition cannot be reversed with corticosteroid therapy, progression to end-stage renal disease occurs and renal replacement therapy (dialysis or transplantation) is necessary. Unfortunately, focal segmental glomerulosclerosis recurs in 25–50% of patients receiving a renal transplant, possibly because of a circulating immune factor that is not replaced with the renal transplant procedure and that causes the same kind of injury to the new kidney. Focal segmental glomerulosclerosis is the second most common cause of nephrotic syndrome in children and adults.

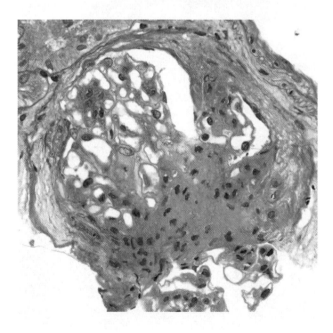

FIGURE 16–18 Focal segmental glomerulosclerosis. In the upper part of the glomerulus there are thin capillary loops, but in the lower portion, the glomerulus is disfigured by a solid growth of cells. The sclerosing, or fibrosing, process affects only a portion of the glomerulus at first. Over time, the entire glomerulus will become sclerotic. (Courtesy of Dr. Jose Torrealba, Department of Pathology, University of Wisconsin School of Medicine and Public Health.)

> **BOX 16–8   Focal Segmental Glomerulosclerosis**
>
> **Causes**
> Unknown
> Genetic
> Infections (e.g., HIV)
> Toxins (e.g., heroin)
> Secondary to damage to nephron in other disease states (diabetes, hypertension, obesity, sickle cell disease)
>
> **Lesions**
> Thickening of basement membrane due to trapped immune complexes
> Progressive scarring of glomeruli
>
> **Manifestations**
> Nephrotic syndrome
> Gradual development of end-stage renal disease

Other patterns of glomerular injury can occur: HIV induces a characteristic nephropathy; some patterns of immune complex disease present with clinical abnormalities that are neither nephritic nor nephrotic, such as isolated hematuria (IgA nephropathy); and some diseases cause increased cellularity of glomeruli because of inflammation or proliferation of the glomerular connective tissue (proliferative glomerulonephritis). Usually, diseases affecting glomeruli cause one or another pattern of injury, but **systemic lupus erythematosus** can cause a variety of different types of injury.

Systemic lupus erythematosus (SLE, or simply lupus) is an autoimmune disease that can affect a large number of organ systems, from the skin to the nervous system, hematologic system, joints, kidneys, and serosal surfaces. In fact, by definition, four different recognized manifestations of SLE have to be present before a patient is diagnosed with this disease. Renal involvement occurs in

50–70% of patients. It presents with persistent proteinuria and casts in the urine. If severe, symptoms can include weight gain, swelling, foamy urine, and hypertension. Histologically, lupus nephritis is classified based on the pattern of injury. Immune complexes consisting of DNA and anti-DNA antibodies are deposited in the connective tissue of the glomerulus (the mesangium) or in the basement membrane of the glomerular tufts. The latter is a form of membranous nephropathy. The most common finding is inflammation of portions of the glomeruli, with resultant necrosis and eventually scarring of the glomeruli. This kind of injury is called **proliferative glomerulonephritis** because the glomeruli are infiltrated by leukocytes that make it look hypercellular, or proliferative (**Figure 16–19**). By immunofluorescence, complement proteins are present within the glomerulus (**Figure 16–20**), and immune complex deposits can be seen by electron microscopy. In addition, immune complexes can deposit on the basement membrane of tubules and capillaries in the kidney, impairing the function of these structures as well. With appropriate therapy, most patients survive beyond 10 years, but renal failure does occur eventually as the glomeruli become irreversibly scarred.

Except for lupus, the diseases we have discussed so far are primary diseases of the glomerulus, meaning the disease process begins here and all its manifestations are attributed to inhibition of glomerular function. The two

diseases that account for, by far, the majority of cases of chronic renal failure as a result of glomerular injury are systemic diseases, however: hypertension and diabetes mellitus. Hypertension causes thickening of the walls of small arterioles that supply the cortical tissues. Not enough blood can get through these narrowed arterioles to meet the metabolic needs of the tissues, so they undergo ischemic injury. Glomeruli eventually scar down, tubules become atrophic, and the interstitium is infiltrated by chronic inflammatory cells and replaced by fibrous tissue (**Figure 16–21**). In diabetes,

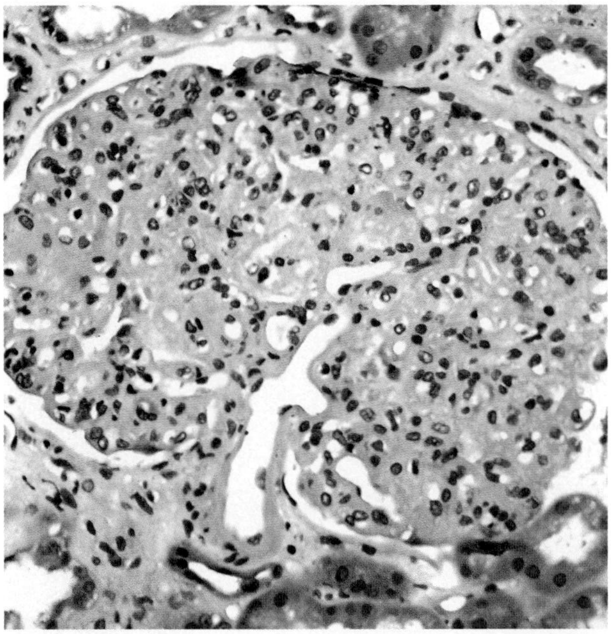

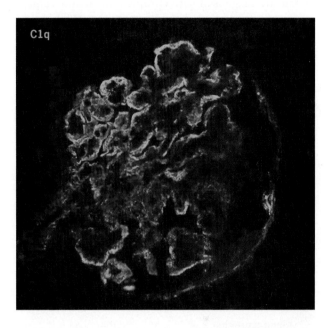

FIGURE 16–20 Immunofluorescence with C1q, lupus. C1q is one of the complement proteins. In lupus, this complement protein is deposited along the basement membrane of the capillary loops. (Courtesy of Dr. Jose Torrealba, Department of Pathology, University of Wisconsin School of Medicine and Public Health.)

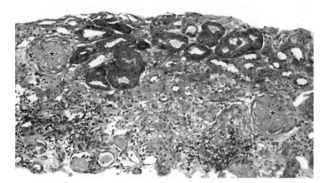

FIGURE 16–21 Renal sclerosis. This renal biopsy has been stained with trichrome, which makes fibrous tissue appear blue and the renal tubules dark pink. Two glomeruli are entirely sclerotic, or replaced by fibrous tissue (asterisks), and the interstitium, which is normally inconspicuous (see Figure 16–6), is expanded by fibrosis. There are large areas in which the tubules are atrophic or have entirely disappeared. (Courtesy of Dr. Jose Torrealba, Department of Pathology, University of Wisconsin School of Medicine and Public Health.)

FIGURE 16–19 Proliferative glomerulonephritis, lupus. There are many more nuclei in this glomerulus than normal (compare to Figure 16–5B), giving the glomerulus a "proliferative" appearance. The small, darkly staining nuclei are those of lymphocytes. The basement membranes are thickened, and the capillary lumens are inconspicuous. (Courtesy of Dr. Weixiong Zhong, Department of Pathology, University of Wisconsin School of Medicine and Public Health.)

metabolic and hemodynamic defects result in altered glomerular filtration. Glucose intolerance appears to disturb the biochemical makeup of the basement membrane so that it becomes leaky. In early diabetes, there are also, for reasons that are not entirely clear, increased glomerular filtration and increased capillary pressure, which result first in hypertrophy of the glomerulus and eventually damage to the capillary loops. Over many years, the glomeruli undergo irreversible injury and become scarred. Both these diseases take a long time to develop, but because of their prevalence, they constitute a considerable health burden. More than 100,000 people are diagnosed with chronic renal failure requiring renal replacement therapy every year: 44% because of diabetes, 27% because of hypertension. By contrast, the primary glomerular diseases discussed in this section account for fewer than 10% of the cases of chronic renal failure.

BOX 16–9 End-Stage Glomerulosclerosis

Causes

Diabetes

Hypertension

Chronic immune complex deposition in glomeruli

Other systemic diseases (lupus, amyloidosis)

Lesions

Glomerular injury depending on underlying disease: membranous, membranoproliferative, mesangial, inflammatory

Glomerulosclerosis

Manifestations

None (early)

Weight gain, edema, foamy urine, fatigue

Proteinuria, hematuria, casts

Hypertension

Uremia (late)

Inflammation of the Male Genital Organs

Sexually transmitted diseases account for by far the majority of inflammatory conditions of the male genital organs. The most common of these diseases is **chlamydia**, which causes urethritis, manifesting as a thin, watery discharge from the urethra and dysuria. Not all chlamydial infections come to clinical attention, however, and it is thought that the prevalence of the disease is much higher than clinically documented. **Gonorrhea** can also manifest in men with urethritis, but it can also infect other organs, including the epididymis, seminal vesicles, and prostate. Gonorrhea can cause abscesses in these organs and can disseminate to other tissues, primarily the joints. In addition, transmission via the oral route can result in gonococcal pharyngitis. The shallow,

painless ulcer of **syphilis** is more easily detected on the surface of the penis (**Figure 16–22**) than in the vagina. Nevertheless, most cases of syphilis are detected in the secondary stage, in both men and women. Genital herpes and genital warts also occur in men.

Although the sexually transmitted diseases affect both men and women, serious consequences are much less common in men: the diseases rarely impair men's fertility and will not be passed on to their offspring. Nevertheless, it is imperative that men be screened for these diseases at routine physical checkups, and treated, even in the absence of symptoms, because the consequences of the transmission of these diseases to sexual partners can be devastating.

The testes are relatively impervious to infection. The common sexually transmitted diseases may affect the epididymis but usually do not involve the testes. One of the infectious agents that can infect testicular tissue is the mumps virus. In up to 40% of postpubertal males, mumps can involve the testes and epididymis, often bilaterally. This presents as acute, severe scrotal pain and swelling and fever. Usually, **mumps orchitis** clears without any residual damage, but it can cause testicular atrophy or impaired

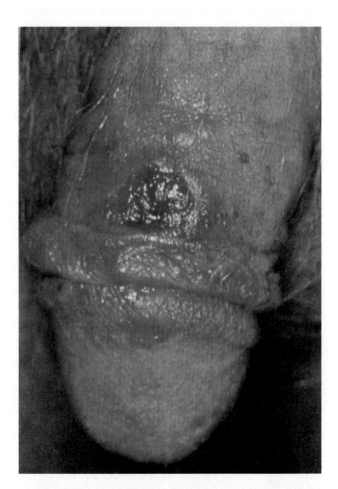

FIGURE 16–22 Syphilis. Primary chancre.

fertility. Widespread vaccination against mumps virus has decreased the incidence of this disease.

Inflammation of the prostate is a poorly understood and vexatious condition for patients and doctors. Unfortunately, it is also quite common, accounting for about 2 million office visits every year in the United States alone. Acute or chronic **bacterial prostatitis** accounts for some of these. Bacterial prostatitis is caused by the same organisms that cause urinary tract infections and manifests with urgency, frequency, and perineal pain. Acute infection can cause tenderness of the prostate upon palpation during the digital rectal exam. The patient may also have fever and other symptoms of an acute inflammatory reaction (fatigue, malaise). The urine can be cloudy and contains white blood cells and bacteria. In cases of chronic prostatitis, the white blood cells and bacteria may have to be encouraged to appear in the urine by gently massaging the prostate before urine is collected for laboratory studies. Sometimes, more serious complications occur, including prostatic or seminal vesicle abscesses or, in very severe cases, sepsis. Antibiotics are curative. In contrast, *chronic pelvic pain syndrome* presents with symptoms of frequency, urgency, and perineal pain, but no infectious organisms can be cultured. Most cases of "prostatitis" unfortunately fall into this category. The symptoms are extremely aggravating, the diagnosis is one of exclusion, the cause is not known, and there is no treatment for it other than warm sitzbaths and nonsteroidal anti-inflammatory drugs (NSAIDs).

Hyperplastic/Neoplastic Diseases

Benign Prostatic Hypertrophy

Enlargement of the prostate is caused by hyperplasia of the prostatic tissue in the periurethral area. Both glandular and stromal cells proliferate, but stromal cells much more so. In addition, the peripheral zones of the prostate undergo atrophy, and the hyperplastic process does not take place evenly throughout the tissue but induces the development of multiple nodules (**Figure 16–23**). As the central tissue enlarges, it impinges on the outflow of the urinary bladder. The symptoms of benign prostatic hypertrophy (BPH) include frequency, urgency, nocturia, hesitancy, incomplete bladder emptying, and weak urinary stream. If the obstruction is severe, it can predispose to the development of urinary tract infections.

The frequency of benign prostatic hypertrophy increases with age. Only about 8% of men ages 31–40 years have BPH, while 80% of men older than the age of 80 years have it. In addition, there is great racial variation in the prevalence of BPH: it is more common and develops at a younger age in black men than in white men or Asians. The cause of prostatic hyperplasia is not known. Both androgens and estrogens are implicated in its development, but excesses or imbalances of these hormones are not sufficient to cause the disease.

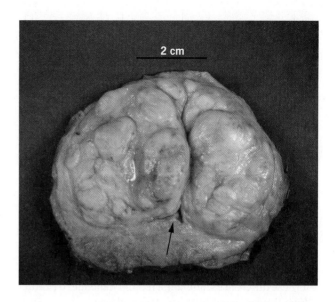

FIGURE 16–23 Benign prostatic hypertrophy. This prostate gland is cut transversely. The gland is large, and multiple nodules bulge from the cut surface. They also impinge on the ureter, which is compressed to a narrow slit (arrow).

The decision to treat BPH is based on the severity of symptoms. Medical therapy includes drugs that act on the muscular component of the prostatic stroma to induce it to contract (alpha-1-adrenergic antagonists) or that inhibit the action of testosterone and thereby cause a decrease in the proliferation of the prostatic tissue (5-alpha-reductase inhibitors). Both these drugs have side effects that can be intolerable to patients. Numerous surgical techniques have recently been developed to minimize the trauma and potential irreversible loss of sexual function that accompanies complete excision of the prostate. Transurethral resection involves cutting away the hypertrophic tissue from inside the urethra. Similar effects can be achieved with laser surgery and electrical energy. If the prostate is only slightly enlarged, incisions made through the prostate but without removal of prostatic tissue can provide symptomatic relief.

BOX 16–10   Benign Prostatic Hypertrophy

Causes

Unknown

Excess androgens and estrogens potentiate hyperplasia

Lesions

Multinodular growth with excessive stromal and glandular tissue

Periurethral tissue most involved

Manifestations

Frequency, urgency, hesitant stream, nocturia

Incomplete bladder emptying, urinary retention

Urinary tract infection

Adenocarcinoma of the Prostate

Cancer of the prostate is generally a disease of the older adult: it is very rare in men younger than the age of 50 years, and some experts claim that every man will develop it if he lives long enough. One in six men will develop prostate cancer in the United States. It is the most commonly diagnosed cancer in men, but lung cancer causes more mortality. The natural history of prostatic adenocarcinoma is variable. Some incidentally found cancers are indolent and patients survive a decade or more even without treatment. Others are very aggressive, growing and metastasizing despite therapy. There is also considerable racial variation in the incidence of prostate cancer: the incidence among white men is two-thirds that among black men, and among Asian men it is half that of white men. There is currently no explanation for these differences, and it is a major challenge to predict which cancers need to be treated, and how.

In addition to race and age, other risk factors for prostate cancer include family history, genetic mutations (such as *BRCA2*, better known for its role in breast cancer in women), elevated androgen levels, and as yet unknown but presumably dietary environmental factors. It is unlikely that androgens drive prostatic epithelial cells to become malignant. Rather, testosterone is a potent growth factor for prostatic epithelial cells, which retain their responsiveness to testosterone even after they have transformed to a malignant genotype. This responsiveness is targeted by one of the treatments for prostatic cancer, medical or surgical inhibition of androgen production. Medically, this can be achieved by administering estrogen, which blocks androgen receptors. Surgically, this is achieved by removing the bulk of testosterone-producing tissue, the testes. Although antiandrogen therapy is useful for slowing the progression of prostate cancer, it is not curative, and eventually the cells lose their dependence on the growth-promoting effect of androgen and grow even in its absence. This portends a turn for the worse in the natural history of the cancer.

Most prostate cancer is detected at an early stage because the level of prostate-specific antigen (PSA), a protein produced only by prostatic epithelial cells, including malignant ones, can easily be measured in the serum. PSA levels tend to trend upward slightly as men age and their prostates enlarge, but excessive elevations are concerning for prostate cancer and should be followed by biopsy. Most cancers grow in the periphery of the prostate—in other words, that part of the tissue that abuts the rectum—so if they form a discrete nodule, they can be detected by a palpating finger during the rectal digital examination or by transrectal ultrasound. Unfortunately, many men escape detection by screening and physical examination: these are usually men without health insurance or men with poor health education. They tend to present with symptoms of advanced prostate cancer: weight loss and low back pain caused by bony metastases. Prostate cancer tends to metastasize to bone, especially the lower vertebrae and pelvis.

Screening for prostate cancer with the PSA test has been invaluable for detecting cancers whose progression can be significantly delayed with appropriate therapy, but it also detects a lot of cancers that would never have become symptomatic. Separating the cancers that need treatment from those that do not, or at least not yet, is a clinical challenge. There is no ideal modality for the treatment of prostate cancer. Most chemotherapeutic drugs work on actively and rapidly dividing cells by inhibiting successful cell division. In slowly growing cancers, such as most cases of prostate cancer, chemotherapy is not effective because the percentage of cells undergoing active replication is so low. The same is true of radiation therapy, although radiation is more effective than chemotherapy in reducing the bulk of malignant cells. Surgery to remove the entire prostate is also not necessarily curative, because there is no clearly defined capsule around the prostate and glandular epithelium can be located in the periprostatic connective tissue, so cancer can recur even if the prostate is apparently entirely excised. Antiandrogen therapy has already been discussed. Men who have newly diagnosed, early-stage cancer may decide to postpone therapy until the cancer begins to show signs of increased rate of growth. This option is called *active surveillance*. Postponement of therapy in select cases does not seem to cause a worse outcome.

The timing and sequence of therapies used to reduce the progression of prostate cancer are dependent on numerous factors. Physicians use complex *nomograms* or algorithms to tailor treatment strategies for each patient. These algorithms include the PSA level, the age of the patient, the clinical stage of the tumor (**Table 16–4**), the number of biopsy cores that contain cancer and the extent of involvement of each core by cancer (this predicts how much of the prostate is actually involved by the cancer), the patient's preferences for surgical, hormonal, or radiation treatment, as well as the **Gleason score** of the cancer. The Gleason score is the grade of the cancer—that is how aggressive it appears under the microscope. There are five grades of cancer, scored from 1 to 5. Grades 1 and 2 are the best differentiated, least aggressive appearing. These are extremely rare, whereas grade 3 is the most common (**Figure 16–24**). Grades 4 and 5 are the highest grades and are associated with a worse prognosis. Usually prostate cancer displays a variety of growth patterns. The two most abundant patterns constitute the Gleason score. For example, a cancer displaying grade 3 and 4 patterns would be reported as Gleason score 3 + 4 = 7. Gleason scores are highly predictive of clinical outcome: cancers with scores of 6 or 7 are moderately growing, while cancers with scores of 8–10 are aggressive.

The outcome of prostate cancer is highly variable. Some patients die "with" prostate cancer; in other words, they have it and may even have been treated for it but die of unrelated diseases such as coronary vascular disease or chronic obstructive pulmonary disease (COPD).

Others are afflicted with it at a young age and experience rapid progression and death. In general, cure rates are very low: treatment modalities are temporizing measures and not curative. Most prostate cancers grow relatively slowly: 5-year survival is close to 100%, and 10-year survival is 91%. However, prostatic cancer is so prevalent that despite the impressive survival statistics, it still kills about 27,000 men every year in the United States.

Urothelial Carcinoma of the Bladder

Carcinoma of the urinary bladder (**Table 16–5**) is the fifth most common cancer in the United States, much more common in men than in women, and typically diagnosed in the seventh decade. Cigarette smoking is the strongest known risk factor: about half the cases occur in smokers. There is also a strong association with exposure to chemicals, such as aniline dyes (used primarily in leather and woodworking industries). It is thought that concentration of toxic chemicals in the urine causes damage to the epithelial lining of the bladder, and this predisposes individuals to the development of cancer.

The lining of the bladder used to be called transitional epithelium, but this term has now given way to the more appropriate *urothelium*; hence, cancer of the mucosal lining of the bladder is called **urothelial carcinoma**. The urothelium is a multilayered epithelium supported by a submucosa of loose connective tissue and blood vessels. Urothelial carcinomas are characterized by proliferation

---

BOX 16–11 Adenocarcinoma of Prostate

Causes

Unknown

Risk factors: African American men, increasing age, family history, dietary factors

Lesions

Adenocarcinoma

Metastases to bone, other organs if advanced

Manifestations

Elevated PSA

Nodule on digital rectal exam or by ultrasound

Tissue biopsy with adenocarcinoma

If metastatic: weight loss, bone pain

TABLE 16–4 Prostate Cancer Staging

Stage	Description
Stage I	Cancer involves less than half of one lobe of the prostate and is confined to the prostate, and Gleason score no more than 6, and PSA < 10
Stage IIA	Cancer involves no more than one lobe of the prostate and is confined to the prostate, and Gleason score no more than 7, and PSA < 20
Stage IIB	Cancer involves both sides of the prostate and is confined to the prostate, or Gleason score 8 or higher, or PSA ≥ 20
Stage III	Cancer has spread to periprostatic tissue or the seminal vesicle
Stage IV	Cancer has spread to bladder, rectum, or pelvic wall, or to lymph nodes, or has metastasized

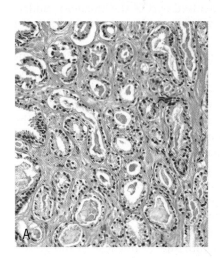
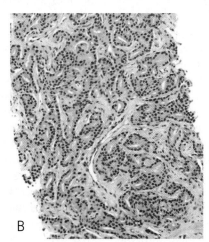
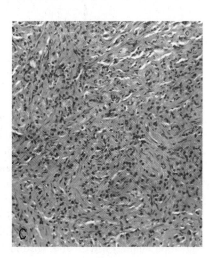

FIGURE 16–24 Gleason grade. **A.** Grade 3. The malignant cells are growing in tightly packed but still recognizable glands. **B.** Grade 4. The glands are no longer small and discrete but arrayed in branching networks. **C.** Grade 5. Glands are not identifiable at all. Instead, individual malignant cells are diffusely infiltrating the stroma.

TABLE 16–5 Comparison of Age of Occurrence, Risk Factors, Stage at Which Most Commonly Diagnosed, and 5-Year Survival for Cancers of the Kidney, Lower Urinary Tract, and Male Genital System

	Incidence	Median Age at Diagnosis	Stage at Which Most Commonly Diagnosed	5-Year Survival	Risk Factors
Kidney (renal cell carcinoma)	14:100,000	64 years	Stage I	68%	Smoking, increasing age, male sex
Bladder (urothelial carcinoma)	21:100,000	73 years	Carcinoma *in situ* and Stage I	80%	Smoking, chemicals (e.g., aniline dyes), male sex
Prostate (prostatic adenocarcinoma)	159:100,000	68 years	Stage I	99%	Increasing age, African American race
Testis (germ cell tumors)	5:100,000	34 years	Stage I	95%	Unknown

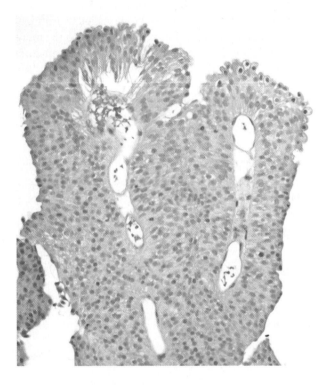

FIGURE 16–25 Papillary urothelial carcinoma, low grade. The malignant cells are growing in a fairly orderly arrangement around a papillary stalk that contains capillaries and connective tissue. This kind of lesion would be growing out into the lumen of the bladder.

of the urothelial cells along fibrovascular cores, a so-called *papillary* pattern of growth (**Figure 16–25**). Papillary urothelial neoplasms can be low grade or high grade: the distinction is made by how differentiated the cells appear under the microscope and predicts how aggressively the cancer will behave. There is also a urothelial carcinoma *in situ* (CIS), characterized by malignant-appearing cells spreading along the surface of the bladder without inducing a papillary growth and without invading into the submucosa.

Most papillary urothelial carcinomas of the bladder are noninvasive, meaning they proliferate on their fibrovascular stalks but do not break through the basement membrane to grow into the submucosa or deeper. When they do invade, they are usually high grade. Papillary carcinomas are readily seen on cystoscopy and can be removed by a device inserted through the cystoscope that snares the growth and burns it off. Generally, low-grade carcinomas tend to recur, often frequently and sometimes extensively. It is important to remove these papillary growths to prevent them from becoming high grade or invasive. Carcinoma *in situ* spreads extensively over the surface of the bladder and can give rise to high-grade, invasive carcinomas without warning. CIS appears as irregular red spots on cystoscopic examination of the bladder lining. Fulguration, or burning, of the red spots keeps the CIS in check to some extent. CIS and low-grade papillary urothelial neoplasms are sometimes also treated with a type of immune therapy involving bacillus Calmette-Guérin (BCG). BCG was initially developed as a vaccine against tuberculosis. When instilled into the bladder, it incites a low-grade inflammation that inhibits malignant growth. With recurrent CIS or invasive urothelial carcinoma, surgical resection of all or only the involved part of the bladder is undertaken. Some surgeons can create a new bladder out of a loop of intestine.

Bladder carcinomas usually present with painless hematuria. Diagnosis is made by cystoscopy and biopsy. Prognosis depends on the grade of the tumor and the stage. Most urothelial carcinomas are detected at an early stage, before they have invaded into the bladder muscle, and when they are still amenable to treatment by transurethral resection, fulguration, or intravesical immune therapy. These treatments are only temporizing measures, however: up to 80% of tumors recur despite treatment. Patients must be followed after therapy with frequent cytologic examination of the urine, which detects atypical urothelial cells that are sloughed into the urine. Five-year survival for early-stage urothelial carcinoma is close to 100%, but for muscle-invasive carcinoma, 5-year survival drops to 60%.

Cancer of the Kidney

One of the more common solid tumors occurring in children is **nephroblastoma**, or *Wilms' tumor*, a malignancy derived from primitive cells in the renal cortex. Only about 500 cases of nephroblastoma are diagnosed in the United States annually, and the prognosis is excellent because the tumor tends to respond very well to chemotherapy. In adults, a large variety of benign and malignant tumors can afflict the kidney. **Renal cell carcinoma** (Table 16–5) is the most common malignant one. It counts among the top 15 cancers in the United States in terms of both incidence and mortality, but its position on that list is quite low: it is the 8th most common cancer diagnosis and 13th most common cause of cancer-related deaths. About 58,000 people are diagnosed with it annually in the United States.

Risk factors for renal cell carcinoma are common to many other cancers: smoking, age, and male sex. Some pharmaceutical drugs, chronic kidney disease, dialysis, and family history are also predisposing factors. Renal cell carcinoma can also occur in cancer syndromes, such as von Hippel–Lindau disease, in which patients develop cysts and neoplasms in various tissues in the body, including the eyes, brain, adrenal gland, spinal cord, pancreas, and kidney. Classically, renal cell carcinoma presents with the triad of flank pain, hematuria, and a palpable flank mass; however, it is rare that a patient has all three manifestations, and most cases come to attention for investigation of painless hematuria or are incidental findings on radiographic procedures done for other reasons.

Renal cell carcinoma grows as a spherical, usually well-circumscribed, bright yellow mass in the cortex of the kidney (**Figure 16–26**). It has the tendency to grow into the renal vein and from there can rapidly grow into the inferior vena cava and even fill and occlude the right side of the heart. The cancer arises from the epithelial lining of the proximal tubules. Renal cell carcinoma can grow in a variety of patterns, some of which have prognostic implications. For example, tumors that are growing in a papillary pattern (malignant cells growing along fibrovascular cores) tend to have a better prognosis than the conventional clear cell carcinoma (cells have abundant,

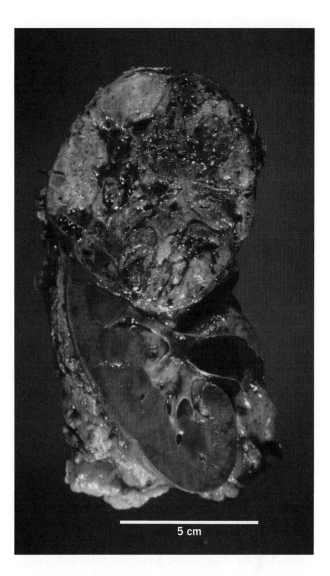

FIGURE 16–26 Renal cell carcinoma. A neoplasm has taken over the upper pole of this kidney. The renal tissue in this area is entirely destroyed, and the tumor is causing the capsule of the kidney to bulge outward. The cut surface of the neoplasm reveals soft, partially hemorrhagic and partially necrotic tissue.

optically clear cytoplasm). In addition, grade as determined by nuclear features has a bearing on prognosis.

The first line of treatment is surgical eradication, either by resection or, if the tumor is small, by ablating it with cryotherapy (cold) or high-frequency radio waves. Embolization of the arteries that supply it to deprive it of its oxygen supply may also be attempted if the tumor is so large that it is not amenable to surgical resection. Chemotherapy and radiotherapy are usually not effective. Therapy targeted against certain receptors that are known to drive cancer growth or drugs that enhance the body's own immune system to eliminate the cancer cells are under clinical investigation. As with any other cancer, prognosis depends on the stage of the tumor. Overall, the 5-year survival is about 70%, but survival varies from more than 90% for small, localized tumors to 10% for tumors that have already metastasized.

BOX 16–13   Kidney Cancer

Causes

Cigarette smoke

Increasing age

Male sex

Family cancer syndromes (e.g., von Hippel–Lindau)

Lesions

Yellow, spherical mass in cortex of kidney

Growth into renal vein, inferior vena cava

Manifestations

Classic triad of flank pain, hematuria, and palpable renal mass is rare

Radiography

Cancers of the Testis

Testicular germ cell neoplasms (Table 16–5) are unusual in that they occur in men at a much younger age than cancers occur generally: the median age at diagnosis is 34 years. They form a discrete, palpable lump in the testis and therefore are usually detected when they are still localized. Germ cell neoplasms can have a variety of morphologic appearances, and each of the histologic types responds to treatment slightly differently. The most common and most easily cured type is **seminoma**. Most of the testicular cancers are very responsive to chemotherapy and radiation therapy, and cures have been achieved even after the cancer has metastasized. The 5-year survival is close to 100% and even 10-year survival is not much lower. Testicular germ cell cancers are uncommon: the lifetime risk of developing testicular cancer is only 0.4% (as compared to 16% for prostate cancer), and testicular cancer represents less than 1% of malignant tumors in men. These cancers are more common in white than in African American men, and the strongest risk factor is cryptorchidism. Prior infections, trauma, or tight-fitting clothes have not been statistically linked to testicular cancer.

Organ Failure

Many of the organs of the urinary and male genital tracts are paired and have a large reserve of function. For example, removal of one testis for cryptorchidism, cancer, or testicular torsion does not cause infertility as long as the other testis is intact. However, diseases that destroy both organs cause morbidity. Failure of the testes results in decreased or no sperm production and subsequent infertility. In up to 30% of couples seeking treatment for infertility, the cause of the infertility is attributable to the male. This is not always because of primary destruction of the testis: causes of male infertility range from genetic diseases that impair testicular development

(e.g., Klinefelter syndrome), to abnormal hormonal control of sperm production, to impaired motility of sperm, to sexual dysfunction.

Failure of the kidneys occurs in two distinct forms. One, caused by toxic or ischemic insults, is called **acute kidney injury**, and the other, caused by smoldering diseases that slowly scar the kidneys, is **chronic kidney failure**. These two forms of kidney injury have different clinical presentations, different etiologies, different consequences and sequelae, and different treatments.

When the renal tubular epithelial cells sustain a sudden, severe injury they are liable to undergo necrosis. The two most common causes of acute tubular necrosis (ATN) are ischemia, or low blood flow secondary to volume loss or shock, and toxins (certain antibiotics, contrast agents used in radiography, as well as some common poisons such as ethylene glycol [antifreeze], toxic mushrooms, and heavy metals such as mercury) that cause direct injury to the epithelial cells. Obstruction of the outflow of urine secondary to renal stones or prostatic hypertrophy can also result in ATN, presumably because the backpressure of urine damages the epithelial cells. Some intrinsic renal diseases such as glomerulonephritis or lupus nephritis can also result in ATN. Whatever the reason for the injury, the dead renal tubular epithelial cells slough into the proximal or distal tubules, where they accumulate and block the flow of urine. This results in oliguria and even anuria if the injury is very severe. Consequent water retention and electrolyte imbalances can be life-threatening even before metabolic toxins rise to dangerous levels. Patients with ATN have to be closely monitored and treated for fluid and electrolyte imbalances. Drugs that enhance the filtering capacity of nondamaged nephrons are given, and in severe cases patients need dialysis to remove accumulating waste products. If the underlying cause of the injury is removed, the tubular epithelium can usually regenerate. Immature renal tubular epithelial cells cannot efficiently resorb water, so in the healing phase, patients may have excessive urine output and run the risk of dehydration. It is therefore important to monitor patients closely during the recovery phase.

In contrast to acute renal injury, chronic renal failure develops insidiously. The earliest signs of it are laboratory evidence of rising blood urea nitrogen and creatinine levels. In most cases, the patient has an underlying condition known to cause slow destruction of the kidneys, such as lupus nephritis or diabetes, and so kidney function is frequently monitored. Certain drugs that alter the flow and pressures in the glomerular capillaries, such as angiotensin-converting enzyme (ACE) inhibitors, can slow the progression of the disease. Progressive renal failure results not only in the retention of nitrogenous wastes in the blood, called **azotemia**, but also in retention of fluid and imbalances of acids, electrolytes, and hormones. When these abnormalities come to clinical attention, the condition is called **uremia**. Signs and symptoms of uremia include fatigue, coagulopathy, anorexia, muscle weakness, pericarditis and pericardial effusions, mental status changes, and eventually coma.

Patients with chronic renal failure require dialysis to prevent azotemia and uremia. Exactly when in the course of the disease dialysis is initiated depends on a variety of factors. Fluid overload, metabolic acidosis, severe electrolyte abnormalities, and signs or symptoms of uremia are all indications for dialysis, but in many cases, dialysis is initiated before these complications develop, when there is laboratory evidence of markedly increased creatinine and the calculated glomerular filtration rate is low.

There are two main types of dialysis: hemodialysis and peritoneal dialysis. With hemodialysis, blood passes through a series of thin tubes made of permeable membranes bathed in dialysis solution. The substances in the blood and dialysis solution readily pass through the walls of the tubes. With peritoneal dialysis, a dialysis solution is instilled into the peritoneal cavity. The peritoneum is richly vascularized and thin, so wastes in the capillaries of the peritoneum accumulate in the dialysis solution. After several hours, the fluid is drained off the peritoneal cavity again. The more common form of dialysis is hemodialysis. Usually, a fistula that connects a vein to an artery is surgically created in the arm to provide convenient access to the blood. Each hemodialysis session is several hours long, and patients require at least three of them every week. Peritoneal dialysis is not as efficient as hemodialysis and needs to be performed four to five times a day. It is also very uncomfortable because of the large volumes of fluid that are introduced into the peritoneal cavity with each cycle. Both hemodialysis and peritoneal dialysis can be performed at home with specialized equipment, but even so, dialysis is cumbersome, and neither technique is free from the risk of infection.

The alternative to dialysis is transplantation. Kidneys are the most common solid organs transplanted. In the United States, close to 17,000 kidney transplants are performed annually. Both living related and deceased donor kidneys can be used. Not everyone on dialysis is eligible for a renal transplant: the major limiting factors are age and comorbid conditions such as heart or liver failure. Usually only one kidney is needed for the patient to gain independence from dialysis machines. Kidney transplants can tremendously improve a patient's quality of life, but patients still need frequent monitoring of their new kidney's function. For one, the old disease can recur in the new kidney. More important, the patient's immune system recognizes the new kidney as "foreign" and attempts to get rid of it. The patient therefore must be on chronic immunosuppressive therapy to prevent rejection, and the immunosuppressive drugs can themselves be toxic to the kidney and to other organ systems.

Rejection of the transplanted kidney occurs in three forms. *Hyperacute* rejection occurs when there is a major mismatch, usually of blood group antigens, between the donor and the recipient so that the recipient already has circulating antibodies against donor antigens that cause immediate—in other words, within milliseconds of establishment of vascular connections, right under the surgeon's eyes—immune attack of the donor kidney. With appropriate screening, this type of rejection is virtually unheard of nowadays. *Acute rejection* begins about 1 to 6 weeks after transplantation. This depends on the match between the donor's and recipient's human leukocyte antigens (HLA). Because complete HLA matching occurs only in identical twins, some degree of acute rejection can be expected in virtually every kidney transplant. This form of rejection needs to be controlled with chronic immunosuppressive therapy. *Chronic rejection* occurs years after the transplant. The mechanism by which it occurs is not known: it appears to be a mixture of smoldering acute rejection and additional immune injury. Most transplanted kidneys survive for 1 year, but about 30% of patients experience graft failure by 5 years. Even so, many donor kidneys can function adequately for decades.

Although patients experience morbidity from chronic immunosuppressive therapy and need frequent monitoring of their kidney function, kidney transplantation is a very attractive alternative to dialysis for most patients. However, donor shortages make the median wait time for a kidney about 44 months in the United States. Many people argue that healthy people should be encouraged to donate one of their organs in return for money. Sale of organs for transplantation is legalized in only one country, Iran, but all over the world poor and vulnerable people are illegally preyed upon by rapacious middlemen to sell a kidney. Medical tourism—traveling to another country for medical care, usually to receive an illegally acquired organ—is a multi-billion dollar industry. Not only are the organs derived from people, including minors, who have little to no understanding of what risks they are incurring, but the organs are not necessarily well matched or prepared and the recipients have a much greater rate of complications. Ethical and humanitarian appeals to the general United States population to donate their organs have not resulted in a yield to meet the needs of patients with chronic renal failure. How to increase organ donation is therefore a hotly debated topic in the medical, bioethical, and legal fields.

Practice Questions

1. The part of the kidney in which blood is filtered is called the
   A. medulla.
   B. glomerulus.
   C. nephron.
   D. mesangium.
   E. podocyte.

2. A 42-year-old woman is seen in the emergency room because of a high fever of acute onset and

severe flank pain. A urinalysis shows white blood cells and casts. The most likely diagnosis is

A. acute glomerulonephritis.
B. kidney stones.
C. pyelonephritis.
D. cystitis.
E. kidney cancer.

3. A 6-year-old girl is seen by her pediatrician because her parents notice edema of her ankles. Subsequent laboratory testing reveals proteinuria, hypoproteinemia, and hyperlipidemia. She most likely has

A. acute glomerulonephritis.
B. pyelonephritis.
C. nephrotic syndrome.
D. interstitial nephritis.
E. nephritic syndrome.

4. Most diseases of the glomeruli are caused by

A. infection of the kidney.
B. immune-mediated injury.
C. cross-reacting antibodies.
D. altered blood flow through the glomerulus.
E. glycosylation of the glomerular basement membrane.

5. Which of the following patients is most likely to require long-term renal replacement therapy (dialysis)?

A. A 21-year-old man who had a kidney removed for recurrent pyelonephritis caused by unilateral vesicoureteral reflux
B. A 68-year-old man with kidney cancer
C. A 72-year-old woman with diabetes and poorly controlled hypertension
D. A 7-year-old with minimal change disease
E. A 52-year-old who experienced acute tubular necrosis after severe blood loss in a motor vehicle accident

6. Gleason score is an important prognostic factor in prostate adenocarcinoma. Gleason score

A. describes how aggressive the tumor looks under the microscope.
B. is the sum of the patient's age and percentage of the prostate involved.

C. predicts response to chemotherapy.
D. is not as important as stage in prognosis.
E. cannot be determined on biopsy specimens.

7. Cryptorchidism should be surgically treated because undescended testicles

A. have a high risk for developing testicular cancer.
B. can predispose men to incarceration of an inguinal hernia.
C. cause infertility.
D. overproduce testosterone.
E. are physically uncomfortable.

8. Differences between acute and chronic renal failure include all of the following except which one?

A. Acute renal failure is usually reversible, but chronic renal failure is not.
B. The cause of acute renal failure can be determined by renal biopsy, but the cause of chronic renal failure cannot.
C. Chronic renal failure eventually requires renal replacement therapy, but most cases of acute renal failure do not.
D. Chronic renal failure results from injury to the nephron, whereas acute renal failure results from damage to renal tubular epithelial cells.
E. Chronic renal failure results in elevated blood urea nitrogen and creatinine levels, whereas acute renal failure results in diminished urine production.

REFERENCES

1. Altekruse SF, Kosary CL, Krapcho M, Neyman N, Aminov R, Waldron W, et al. *SEER Cancer Statistics Review, 1975–2007.* Bethesda, MD: National Cancer Institute.
2. American Cancer Society. *Cancer Facts and Figures 2010.* Atlanta, GA: American Cancer Society, 2010.

Female Genital Organs

OUTLINE

OBJECTIVES

1. Review the anatomy of the female genital tract and hormonal regulation of menstruation.
2. List the most frequent conditions of the genital system for which women seek medical attention.
3. Describe the signs and symptoms by which disorders of the female genital tract come to attention, and define the words by which menstrual irregularities are described.
4. Describe the components of a gynecologic history and physical examination.
5. Describe the role of Pap smear, colposcopy, cone biopsy, dilation and curettage, ultrasound, and laparoscopy in evaluation of female genital diseases.
6. List the common sexually transmitted diseases and the complications they cause in the female genital tract.
7. List common causes of vaginal or vulvar itching and describe their cause, predisposing conditions, and treatments.
8. Define endometriosis, describe how it arises, and identify the symptoms and complications it causes.
9. Describe the cause and treatment of dysfunctional uterine bleeding, and recognize how this is differentiated from normal menstruation.
10. Describe how obesity contributes to the pathogenesis of diseases in the female genital tract.
11. Describe the causes, lesions, and manifestations of polycystic ovary disease.
12. Define menopause and list its short-term and long-term effects on the health of women.
13. List the most common benign neoplasms of the uterus and ovary and describe how they come to medical attention.
14. Compare the risk factors, relative incidence, and mortality of cancers of the uterus, ovary, and cervix.
15. Describe the role of high-risk HPV in the pathogenesis of cervical cancer and describe how Pap tests are used to recognize HPV infection and preinvasive squamous lesions of the cervix.
16. Discuss how ectopic pregnancy arises and why it is life threatening.
17. Define placental abruption and describe why it can be life threatening to the fetus and the mother.
18. Define preeclampsia and eclampsia and describe the current understanding of how these conditions arise and how to definitively treat them.
19. Describe what is meant by a "molar pregnancy" and describe how it arises.

20. Understand that infertility can be caused by a variety of anatomic, psychologic, and physiologic derangements, and recognize how much infertility results from "male" versus "female" factors.

21. Define and use in proper context the words and terms in bold print throughout the chapter.

KEY TERMS

abortion	human chorionic
acute salpingitis	gonadotropin (hCG)
amenorrhea	human papillomavirus (HPV)
ASCUS	hydatidiform mole
blastocyst	hysterectomy
candidiasis	infertility
cervical canal	leiomyoma
cervical intraepithelial	lichen sclerosus
neoplasia (CIN)	lichen simplex chronicus
cervical os	luteinizing hormone
cervix	menarche
chlamydia	menopause
choriocarcinoma	menorrhagia
condyloma acuminatum	menses
conization	menstrual cycle
corpus luteum	menstrual history
dilation and curettage	menstruation
disorders of placentation	metrorrhagia
dysfunctional uterine	molar pregnancy
bleeding	obstetrics
dysmenorrhea	ovarian cancer
dysplasia (LGSIL, HGSIL)	ovary
eclampsia	polycystic ovarian disease
ectopic pregnancy	ovulation
endometrial	ovum
adenocarcinoma	Pap smear
endometriosis	pelvic inflammatory disease
endometrium	placental abruption
estrogen	preeclampsia
fallopian (uterine) tubes	progesterone
fertilization	pseudomyxoma peritonei
fibrothecoma	syphilis
follicle	teratoma
follicle-stimulating	trichomoniasis
hormone	tubal ligation
fundus of uterus	uterus
gonorrhea	vagina
gynecology	venereal disease
herpes simplex virus (HSV)	vulva

Review of Structure and Function

Female genital organs include the vulva (labia majora, labia minora, clitoris), vagina, uterus (cervix, body), fallopian (or uterine) tubes, and ovaries (Figure 17–1). Each of these organs has a very different role to play in achieving, maintaining, and terminating pregnancy.

The vulva, vagina, and outer aspects of the cervix are lined by a protective stratified nonkeratinized squamous epithelium. Bartholin's glands at the outlet of the vagina produce a mucoid secretion that lubricates the vagina during sexual intercourse. The uterine cervix is the distal, narrow portion of the uterus that projects into the vagina. The cervical canal is continuous with the uterine cavity. At the cervical os, or opening of the cervical canal into the vagina, there is a transition from stratified squamous to columnar mucus-secreting epithelium. The thick mucus produced by these columnar cells makes the cervical canal and endometrial cavity virtually impervious to bacteria—and to sperm. At around the time of ovulation, or release of an egg from the ovary, the mucus changes in consistency to allow sperm to get through and access the uterine cavity. The glandular mucosa lining the uterine cavity is called the endometrium. This is the site of implantation of a fertilized ovum (pl., ova; egg). The body or fundus of the uterus is a very muscular organ. The muscular wall stretches and hypertrophies during pregnancy, as the fetus grows, and its contraction is important in accomplishing childbirth.

The ova rest in the ovarian cortex in specialized structures called follicles. Once a month, one of the eggs is stimulated by hormones produced in the pituitary to finish the first part of meiotic reduction—that is, to "mature." (The first part of meiotic reduction began during the fetal period, and the eggs are in a state of arrested reduction until stimulated by pituitary hormones.) Once mature, the ovum is released from its follicle and expelled from the surface of the ovary. This process is called ovulation. The egg is then quickly scooped up by the frondlike end of the uterine tube and propelled into the lumen of the tube. Fertilization, or fusion of sperm and egg, occurs in the uterine tube. The ovum, fertilized or not, travels along the uterine tube and then drops into the uterine cavity. If the egg is fertilized, it immediately finishes meiosis and then begins to undergo mitotic divisions to form the blastocyst, which implants in the endometrial lining of the uterine cavity. If it is not fertilized, it is expelled with the menstrual purge, and a new egg is stimulated to mature in the ovary one month later.

The ovaries and endometrium function synchronously to provide a suitable environment for pregnancy to occur and progress. In repeated menstrual cycles (Figure 17–2), the endometrium is stimulated to proliferate, or develop a rich blood supply and produce secretions that provide nourishment for the growing blastocyst. It is sloughed during menstruation if pregnancy does not occur, and then immediately begins to proliferate again. Menarche is the first menstrual period of a pubertal girl. The menstrual cycle is timed each month from the onset of bleeding because this date is easily determined. However, the critical events are more accurately timed from the day of ovulation. This event can be determined by a rise in a woman's basal body temperature. Ovulation occurs about 2 weeks after menstruation begins. In the 2 weeks before ovulation, the endometrium is in the proliferative, or actively and rapidly growing, phase. In the 2 weeks following ovulation, the endometrium undergoes secretory changes to prepare for possible pregnancy.

Endocrine control of the menstrual cycle and pregnancy involves hormones from the pituitary glands, adrenal glands, ovaries, and placenta (Figure 17–2). Follicle-stimulating hormone, produced by the pituitary

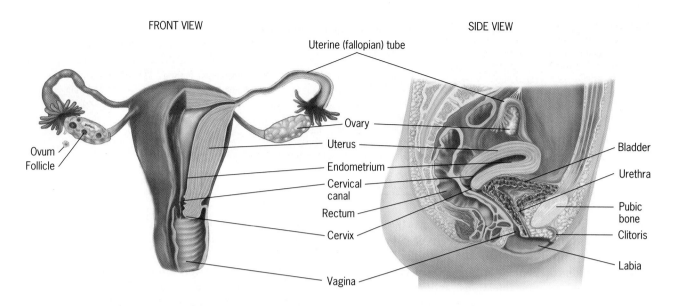

FRONT VIEW

SIDE VIEW

FIGURE 17–1 Anatomy of the female genital organs.

gland, stimulates maturation of a follicle in the ovary. The maturing follicle produces estrogen, which stimulates the endometrial glands to proliferate. When the level of **estrogen** reaches a critical threshold, the pituitary gland releases **luteinizing hormone**, which stimulates the release of the ovum from the follicle. The empty follicle continues to grow into a large mass of lipid-rich cells, called the **corpus luteum** (pl., corpora lutea). These cells produce **progesterone**, which encourages the endometrium to undergo secretory changes that make it hospitable to the blastocyst. If pregnancy occurs, the developing embryo produces **human chorionic gonadotropin (hCG)**, which maintains the corpus luteum; if pregnancy does not occur, the corpus luteum slowly involutes, and the withdrawal of progestogens causes the endometrium to degenerate and menstruation to occur. As progesterone and estrogen both fall, the pituitary is again stimulated to produce follicle-stimulating hormone, and the cycle starts again.

Most Frequent and Serious Problems

The field of obstetrics and gynecology (OB/Gyn) is one of the largest and most diverse in medicine. **Obstetrics** refers to childbirth, while **gynecology** refers to treatment of conditions specific to women—in other words, of diseases of the female organs of reproduction. The practice of OB/Gyn encompasses a wide spectrum of activities, from primary care (e.g., Pap smears for cervical cancer and prenatal assessments of pregnant women) to surgery (e.g., cesarean section and removal of tumors), from endocrinology (e.g., management of dysfunctional uterine bleeding) to dermatology (e.g., treating diseases of the vulva), from radiology (e.g., imaging of fetuses with

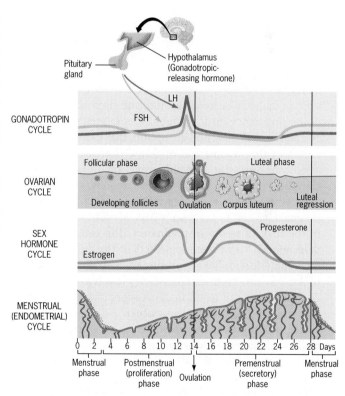

FIGURE 17–2 The menstrual cycle. Temporal relationship of changes in the endometrium, maturation of an ovum, and levels of hormones through one cycle.

ultrasound) to midwifery (assisting uncomplicated vaginal births). In addition, infertility treatment and management of high-risk pregnancies are ever more in demand as older women and women with complicated medical conditions seek to achieve pregnancy.

The conditions for which women seek help from an OB/Gyn change as a woman grows older (**Table 17–1**).

TABLE 17–1   Most Common Complaints of the Female Genital System, by Age

Puberty and Adolescence	Reproductive Age	45–55 Years	55 Years+
• Amenorrhea • Dysmenorrhea • HPV vaccination	• Birth control • Pap smears • Pregnancy • Infertility • Sexually transmitted diseases • Pelvic inflammatory diseases • Dysfunctional uterine bleeding • Endometriosis • Polycystic ovary syndrome	• Dysfunctional uterine bleeding • Menopause	• Cancer • Uterine prolapse

Overall, the most frequent problems relating to the female genital system that require medical care or counseling include birth control and its opposite, infertility. Prenatal care and childbirth, control of menopausal symptoms, diagnosing and treating infections, and screening for cervical cancer are some of the more "routine" activities in OB/Gyn practice.

By far the majority of pregnancies are not complicated, meaning they do not require any kind of medical intervention. Prenatal monitoring of the health of the fetus and mother and help during childbirth are sufficient to ensure a good pregnancy outcome. However, serious complications can occur with pregnancy. Some maternal conditions have an adverse effect on the fetus, such as diabetes or hypertension, and there are diseases of the pregnancy itself, such as ectopic pregnancy, preeclampsia, and placental abruption, that can impair the health of the mother and/or fetus. Complications can also occur during and after delivery. The most common complication of pregnancy is spontaneous abortion, or "miscarriage." It is estimated that up to a quarter of all pregnancies end in pregnancy loss. Most of these occur in the first 12 weeks of pregnancy. The cause is rarely determined. Major genetic defects of the fetus that are incompatible with life are presumed to account for most of these losses. Recurrent pregnancy loss is a devastating condition that can result in depression, marital conflict, and loss of self-esteem in the mother.

The most contentious issue surrounding pregnancy is elective abortion. This procedure has been legal in the United States since the 1973 Supreme Court ruling, in *Roe v. Wade*, that women had a right to abortion in the first two trimesters of pregnancy. Although abortion remains technically legal, many federal and state initiatives have curtailed women's access to surgical abortion. The synthetic progesterone antagonist RU-486, or mifepristone, was approved for termination of pregnancy in the United States by the Food and Drug Administration (FDA) in 2000. Surgical and medical abortions are fraught with moral and ethical dilemmas, which pull the right of women to control the productivity of their own bodies into political and religious disputes. It is not within the scope of this text to elaborate on these arguments.

Sexually transmitted diseases (STDs), also called **venereal diseases**, produce both acute and long-term problems in women. Gonorrhea is the most commonly reported communicable disease, but infections caused by chlamydia, which are often not reported because they are not detected, are even more common. Gonorrhea and chlamydia infections, when they spread to the fallopian tubes, cause **pelvic inflammatory disease**. Pelvic inflammatory disease not only causes pain and discomfort, but, more seriously, can cause infertility and ectopic pregnancy. Herpes simplex virus commonly affects the cervix, vagina, and vulva. It causes repeated outbreaks of small but exquisitely painful vesicles that rupture, crust over, and heal over the course of a couple of weeks.

Human papillomavirus (HPV) infections cause genital warts and carcinoma of the cervix. The malignant changes HPV causes in cervical squamous cells can be detected by microscopic examination of squamous cells scraped with a small, stiff brush during a gynecologic exam. This is the **Pap smear**. Before the 1950s, when the Pap smear first began to be popularized, cervical cancer was one of the most common cancers in women. Today, preinvasive lesions can easily be detected and treated, and the incidence rates are steadily dropping. The incidence of cervical cancer is now less than that of uterine cancer. Ovarian cancer is less common than uterine cancer, but more likely to be fatal. This is because it is usually not detected until it has already reached a high stage. The pelvic and abdominal cavities are rather roomy and can accommodate a lot of ovarian tumor before its presence is detected. Endometrial cancer usually makes its presence known before it has spread extensively, by causing abnormal vaginal bleeding.

The most common tumors of the female genital tract are not cancers. A **leiomyoma** (pl., leiomyomata) is a nodular overgrowth of smooth muscle cells in the uterus. This is commonly referred to as a "fibroid." Fibroids can cause abnormally heavy or irregular menstrual cycles, and they can cause problems with the attachment of the placenta to the uterine wall. Leiomyomata causing menstrual irregularities are one of the most common reasons for **hysterectomy**, or surgical removal of the uterus, which in turn is one of the most common invasive operations on the female genital system. **Tubal ligation**, or surgical interruption of the uterine tubes, is another common surgical procedure, performed for birth control.

Irregularities in menstruation are common as well. **Amenorrhea** is the absence of menstruation. Menses can also be irregular and/or excessive. These abnormalities can be caused by structural defects (e.g., a leiomyoma causing excessive bleeding during menstruation), but more often they are the result of an underlying hormonal derangement. Excessive bleeding caused by an imbalance of hormones is called **dysfunctional uterine bleeding** and affects most women at least once during their reproductive years. The most common times are in the first few years after menarche and in the years preceding menopause. All women eventually go through **menopause**, the permanent cessation of menstruation. In the United States, this time of life is generally accompanied with nuisance symptoms, such as "hot flashes." More importantly, decreased estrogen levels can have adverse effects on other organs, such as the heart and bone, in the postmenopausal years.

Symptoms, Signs, and Tests

Major symptoms referable to the female genital tract involve bleeding, pain, vaginal discharge, and endocrine effects. Normal menstrual bleeding, or **menses**, must be distinguished from abnormal uterine bleeding. Bleeding may be abnormal in amount, timing, or character. Hormonal changes are the most common cause of abnormal bleeding, but bleeding is also one of the principal symptoms of endometrial cancer. Several names differentiate various patterns of bleeding: **menorrhagia** refers to excessive menstrual bleeding, **metrorrhagia** refers to irregular bleeding from the uterus between menses, vaginal spotting refers to small amounts of bleeding not associated with menses, and dysfunctional uterine bleeding refers to abnormal bleeding caused by derangements in the usual flux of hormones during the menstrual cycle.

Dysmenorrhea is cramping pain during menstruation. Many women experience sharp, one-sided abdominal pain at midcycle because of peritoneal irritation caused by rupture of an ovarian follicle at the time of ovulation. This is called "Mittelschmerz" (German *mittel* = mid, *schmerz* = pain). Causes of severe pain include ruptured ectopic pregnancy, acute pelvic inflammatory disease, and twisted or ruptured ovarian cysts. Itching of the vulva is commonly associated with atrophic changes in the vulvar skin in postmenopausal women and infections of the vulva and vagina in younger women.

Nonbloody vaginal discharge is associated with mild superficial infections, such as trichomonas and *Candida* vaginitis. Symptoms related to endocrine changes are common prior to onset of menstruation (often called "premenstrual syndrome") and at the time of menopause, when the monthly hormonal cycles slowly cease. Although all women undergo monthly hormonal fluxes and, eventually, menopause, there is considerable variation between cultures and between individuals in the degree to which premenstrual and menstrual symptoms

are perceived. These variations should be acknowledged and not labeled "abnormal" at either end of the spectrum.

The **menstrual history** is an important part of the gynecologic examination. Information on the length of the menstrual cycle (the time between menses), the duration of menses, the amount of menstrual blood flow, and the regularity of the cycles gives an indication of the integrity of the hormonal axis. Other signs of endocrine abnormalities include hirsutism, or the growth of male-pattern facial hair, atrophy of the breasts, changes in voice as a result of excess androgens, and itching of the vulva and pain with sexual intercourse because of decreased estrogen.

The pelvic examination involves direct inspection of the vulva; examination of the vagina and cervix with the aid of a speculum, a device that spreads the walls of the vagina apart so that the inner vagina and cervix can be seen; and bimanual palpation of the uterus, fallopian tubes, and ovaries. Carcinoma of the vulva is visible by inspection. The vulva can additionally be involved by many of the known skin diseases and condylomata acuminata, or genital warts, can also be seen by direct visual inspection. During the speculum examination, the vaginal wall and outer portion of the cervix are examined for signs of inflammation or neoplasia, and cells are gently scraped from the cervical os for cytologic examination (the Pap smear).

Bimanual examination is so named because one of the examiner's hands is placed on the abdomen while the fingers of the other hand are inserted into the vagina, and the internal organs are palpated between the two hands (**Figure 17–3**). Bimanual rectal examination allows palpation of posterior uterine lesions. The most common pelvic mass is, of course, a growing fetus, but that is usually detected by other means. Leiomyomata of the uterus and the various ovarian tumors are often

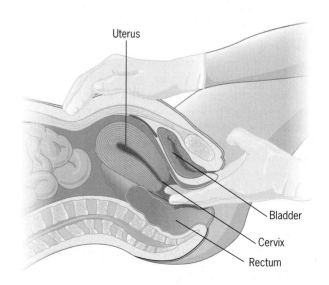

FIGURE 17–3 Bimanual palpation.

discovered by palpation of a mass. Usually, the ovaries are not felt at all, or at the most as a thin little nubbin that barely tickles the examining finger. Any enlargement in the size of the ovaries should be followed up by other imaging procedures.

The most common test is the Papanicolaou (Pap) test of the uterine cervix. Pap tests at regular intervals allow detection of human papillomavirus infection and the neoplastic lesions it causes. Smears of abnormal vaginal secretions can be used for visual detection of some infectious diseases. Blood counts are important for detection of iron-deficiency anemia, a common condition in women because of loss of iron in menstrual blood and transfer of iron to the fetus during pregnancy. Pregnancy tests involve the measurement of hCG, a hormone made first in the developing embryo and then in the placenta, in maternal urine or blood. Other hormones that may be responsible for infertility or abnormal symptoms can also be measured in the blood.

Biopsy is commonly used to determine the nature of lesions in the female genital tract. Vulvar lesions are especially common in postmenopausal women and have malignant potential. The cervix is biopsied whenever there is a visible lesion or suggestive Pap test. Staining of the cervix with agents that highlight premalignant lesions and examination at high magnification with a colposcope (*colpo-*, vagina) aid in selecting the most appropriate biopsy sites. Cone biopsy refers to the removal of a cone of tissue, including the cervical os and endocervical lining, for systematic histologic evaluation. Endometrial biopsy is essential for evaluation of endometrial lesions and abnormal uterine bleeding. It is always necessary to exclude endometrial carcinoma in these settings. One procedure for endometrial biopsy is called **dilation and curettage** (D&C) and involves dilating the cervical os and scraping out tissue from the uterus with a curette. Small samples of endometrium can be obtained without dilating the cervix, with a much thinner biopsy curette.

The fallopian tubes and ovaries cannot directly be visualized and are not easily accessible for biopsy. Diseases of these organs can be evaluated by ultrasound, a noninvasive procedure that is used primarily to assess for masses. Ultrasound is also used to look for placental diseases or structural abnormalities of the fetus during pregnancy (**Figure 17–4**). Radiographic procedures such as computed tomography (CT) scans also are helpful in delineating the anatomy and pathologic processes in the pelvis. Injection of radiopaque material into the uterus can help determine whether the uterine tubes are patent. Laparoscopy or insertion of an endoscope into the peritoneal cavity through an incision at the umbilicus is often necessary for direct inspection of the abdominal and pelvic contents. This procedure is particularly useful in diagnosis of ectopic pregnancy, endometriosis, and pelvic inflammatory disease and may also be used to assess the stage of a carcinoma before definitive treatment is planned.

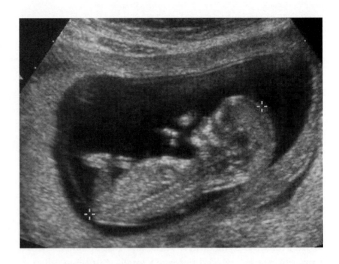

FIGURE 17–4 Ultrasound image of a fetus *in utero*. (Courtesy of Dr. Myron Pozniak, Department of Radiology, University of Wisconsin School of Medicine and Public Health.)

Specific Diseases
Genetic/Developmental Diseases

Compared to other organ systems, congenital anomalies of the female genital organs are relatively uncommon. Various degrees of uterine duplication can occur. A uterine septum that divides the endometrial cavity into two compartments is a congenital anomaly that sometimes prevents a pregnancy from developing normally. Resection of the septum improves the chances of a successful pregnancy. Cysts formed from embryonic remnants occur adjacent to the fallopian tubes and in the lateral wall of the cervix and vagina. These rarely come to clinical attention.

Inflammatory/Degenerative Diseases

Those aspects of the infections that pertain directly to the female genital system are discussed. Many of the other infectious diseases affecting this area of the body are also sexually transmitted (**Table 17–2**). Inflammatory conditions of the vulva occur predominantly in postmenopausal women and may evolve into carcinoma. Hormonal problems are discussed in this section for lack of a better place to put them.

Gonorrhea, Chlamydia, and Syphilis

The bacteria responsible for **gonorrhea**, **chlamydia**, and **syphilis** infect millions of people in the United States each year. These are usually sexually active teenagers and young adults, but any person practicing unprotected sex with multiple sex partners is at risk. In women, these infections often are silent, meaning they cause no symptoms. Chlamydial and gonorrheal infection may go completely unnoticed by the woman, even though the bacteria set up a smoldering infection in the uterine tubes that can cause irreversible scarring and infertility. If the organisms do cause symptoms, they are usually

TABLE 17-2 Comparison of Sexually Transmitted Diseases in Women			
Disease	**Organism**	**Effect on Female Genital Tract**	**Effect on Fetus or Neonate**
Gonorrhea	*Neisseria gonorrhoeae*	Pelvic inflammatory disease	Blindness, arthritis, sepsis
Chlamydia	*Chlamydia trachomatis*	Pelvic inflammatory disease	Prematurity, "pink eye," pneumonia
Syphilis	*Treponema pallidum*	Not specific	Intrauterine death, congenital syphilis
Herpes	Herpes simplex virus-2	Blisters on external genitalia	Disseminated infection, death
HPV (low risk)	Human papillomavirus	Condylomata acuminata	Laryngeal papillomatosis (very rare)
HPV (high risk)	Human papillomavirus 16, 18	Cervical cancer	None known
Trichomoniasis	*Trichomonas vaginalis*	Itching, odor, vaginal discharge	Low birth weight (rare)

mild urethritis (pain and urgency with urination) or vaginal discharge. Rarely, acute salpingitis resulting in pain, fever, and nausea may occur, or nonspecific pelvic pain. The latter is usually vague and intermittent, and thereby defies diagnosis unless the physician has a high index of suspicion for chlamydial or gonorrheal infection.

Pelvic inflammatory disease (PID) refers to the complications of infection by chlamydia or gonorrhea in the uterus, uterine tubes, and tissues around the tubes. This is a very common disease, diagnosed in more than 1 million women in the United States every year. The resulting scar tissue can seriously distort the uterine tubes so that ova can no longer pass through them into the uterine cavity. This results in two serious complications: ectopic pregnancy, or implantation of a fertilized egg in the fallopian tube, and infertility. Ectopic pregnancy is life threatening, for the tube cannot accommodate a growing embryo and will therefore rupture, causing excruciating pain and potentially fatal bleeding in the mother. Infertility can be psychologically devastating and, in the case of PID, usually cannot be reversed because it is not possible to make the tubes patent by surgical means. *In vitro* fertilization is the only means by which pregnancy can be achieved, because this does not require patency of the uterine tubes.

The primary lesion of syphilis, a painless ulcer called a *chancre*, usually develops in the vaginal canal, where it is not seen or felt by the infected woman. The woman may not know she is infected until the typical symptoms of secondary syphilis (a rash on the palms, soles, and mucous membranes accompanied by nonspecific symptoms such as headache, fatigue, and lymphoglandular swelling) occur.

All three of these organisms can be transmitted to a developing fetus. Chlamydia can cause pneumonia and "pink eye" in an infant that has passed through an infected birth canal. More serious disease, including infection of joints and sepsis, can occur when the fetus picks up gonorrheal organisms from the birth canal. The bacteria causing syphilis can be transmitted across the placenta. About 40% of syphilis-infected fetuses will die *in utero*, and about 10% of those who survive have or

will develop abnormalities after birth. These can involve virtually any organ, from the nervous tissue (seizures, deafness) to bones, spleen, liver, skin, and lymph nodes. Developmental delays and skeletal deformities are the most common complications in infants and children with *congenital syphilis*.

Poor pregnancy outcomes are especially unfortunate if the woman does not even know that she is infected. For these reasons, all pregnant women with access to health care are tested for gonorrhea, chlamydia, and syphilis as soon as pregnancy is established. Treatment of these infections is very simple: nonteratogenic antibiotics rapidly eradicate the infection. Treatment for the complications of these diseases is much more difficult, and it is therefore necessary to have a high index of suspicion for these diseases in young, sexually active women who present with vague and nonspecific symptoms.

Herpes Infection

Herpes simplex virus (HSV) causes blistering lesions of the squamous epithelium of the vulva and cervix (**Figure 17-5**). This is also a sexually transmitted infection. HSV-1 is the virus that causes "cold sores" on the lips and oral mucous membranes. If it infects the genital tract, transmission most likely occurred via oral–genital contact, and the blisters are less severe and less predictable than those caused by HSV-2.

HSV-2 causes only genital herpes. Transmission can occur when a person has blisters, but the virus can also be shed from normal-appearing skin. About 2 weeks after transmission, the patient develops a "crop" of blisters in the outer genital tract. These are exquisitely painful and persist for about 2 weeks. The virus takes up residence in nervous tissue and periodically reactivates, causing recurrent lesions. In addition to the pain and discomfort this condition causes, the patient feels stigmatized and inhibited in sexual encounters. Active genital herpes at the time of delivery can cause serious, disseminated infection in a newborn if it is delivered vaginally. Babies are delivered via cesarean section in women with active lesions.

Typically, an infected woman will have about five genital herpes outbreaks a year, but their frequency and

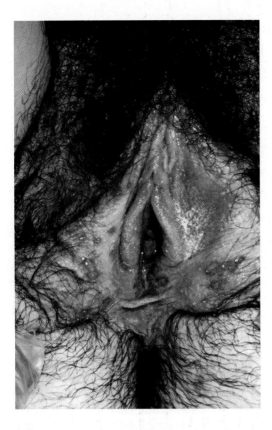

FIGURE 17–5 Genital herpes. (© Wellcome Trust Library/Custom Medical Stock Photo.)

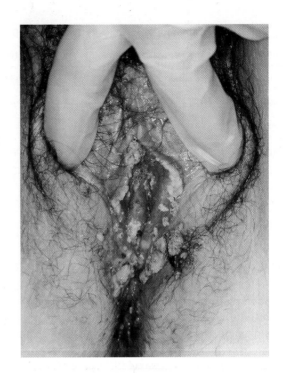

FIGURE 17–6 Condyloma acuminatum. (Courtesy of Joe Millar/CDC.)

intensity tend to diminish over time. There is no known agent that will eradicate the virus for good, but some antiviral medications can decrease the intensity and duration of the periodic recurrences.

BOX 17–1 Infections of the Female Genital Tract

Causes

Sexually transmitted bacteria, viruses, or parasites

Overgrowth of yeast

Lesions

Infection of the uterine tubes, paratubal tissue, cervix, vagina, and vulvar skin

Manifestations

Often, none

Pelvic inflammatory disease

Poor pregnancy outcomes

Infertility

Pain, itching, vaginal discharge

Discomfort with sexual intercourse

Condyloma Acuminatum

Several serotypes of **human papillomavirus (HPV)** are known to cause diseases in humans. Some of these cause cervical cancer, others cause squamous papillomas of the vulva, anus, and vagina, called **condylomata acuminata** (sing., condyloma acuminatum), and commonly known as genital warts (**Figure 17–6**). These lesions are similar to the common skin wart (verruca vulgaris), except that they are transmitted venereally and they tend to occur on moist mucous membranes. Condylomata do not herald an increased risk for cervical cancer because the HPV viruses causing these conditions are different. However, the HPV virus does appear to be transmitted by oral–genital contact as well as by genital–genital contact. Recurrent squamous papillomas of the larynx are thought to be caused by HPV, and HPV is also increasingly becoming linked to laryngeal squamous carcinoma.

Condylomata are easily seen during the gynecologic examination. They are usually small bumps on the genital skin and mucous membranes, though occasionally they can be quite large. Often, they go away on their own. If they are bothersome they can be treated with liquid nitrogen, or, if they are very large, they can be removed surgically.

Superficial Vaginal Infections

Trichomonas vaginalis (**Figure 17–7A**) is a protozoan parasite that is also sexually transmitted, so **trichomoniasis**, the disease it causes, is most common in the same demographic set as the other sexually transmitted diseases discussed previously. *Trichomonas* causes a green-yellow, frothy, foul-smelling discharge from the vagina, itching of the vagina and vulva, discomfort with sexual intercourse, and sometimes urethritis. Because it does not infect the upper reproductive tract, it does not

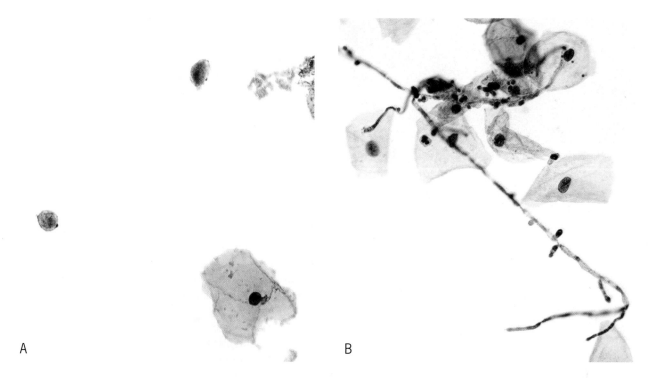

FIGURE 17–7 A. *Trichomonas vaginalis*. The large blue cell with tissue-paper–like cytoplasm on the bottom right is a normal squamous cell. The two small round structures are *Trichomonas* organisms. **B.** *Candida.* Normal squamous cells and acute inflammatory cells are clustered around a long, filamentous hyphal form of *Candida*. (Courtesy of Dr. Josephine Harter, Department of Pathology and Laboratory Medicine, University of Wisconsin School of Medicine and Public Health.)

interfere with ovulation or implantation, and it does not interfere with pregnancy. The vaginitis is very uncomfortable, however. Diagnosis is by inspection of the vaginal discharge for the organism, which is readily seen, and treatment is by antibiotics.

Candida (**Figure 17–7B**) are fungi that are normally present in the vagina. Under certain conditions, they can grow in excessive numbers and produce a superficial vaginitis or vulvovaginitis. This is commonly called a "yeast infection". Symptoms of **candidiasis** include itching, pain, discomfort with intercourse, and a thick, white discharge that resembles cottage cheese. The overgrowth of *Candida* is prevented by the presence of other bacteria that normally reside in the vagina and do not cause any symptoms or abnormalities. If these bacteria are diminished, for example, with antibiotic use, then *Candida* can proliferate. Other conditions that facilitate candidal overgrowth include immune suppression, chemotherapy, pregnancy, diabetes mellitus, and the use of oral contraceptives. Candidiasis can be diagnosed by smear or culture of vaginal discharge. Treatment consists of antifungal agents that are topically applied or taken by mouth and control of any underlying condition that may have contributed to its development.

Endometriosis

Endometriosis is the occurrence of endometrial tissue outside the uterus, usually in the ovary, but also on the peritoneal surface of adjacent organs (uterus, bladder, rectum). The origin of this tissue is unclear. The "metastatic" hypothesis is based on the observation that in up to 90% of women, little bits of endometrium that are shed during menstruation travel backward, up the fallopian tube and into the abdominal cavity. These little bits of endometrium can implant on the pelvic organs or the peritoneal lining. The other, "metaplastic" hypothesis suggests that the mesothelial lining of the peritoneal cavity and pelvic organs can itself give rise to endometrial-type glands and stroma.

However it got there, the endometrial tissue in these ectopic locations is responsive to estrogen, and therefore undergoes cycles of proliferation and degeneration just as the endometrial glands in the uterus do. Bleeding from these little foci of endometriosis causes severe pain: pain with menstruation, pain with intercourse, pain with defection, pain with urination, and generalized, nonspecific pelvic pain. The pain can be caused by the endometriotic foci themselves or from adhesions that eventually form. Endometriosis affects about 15% of women in the United States, primarily in the 25- to 35-year age group, and is the most common cause of pelvic pain: about 80% of women with pelvic pain have endometriosis. Endometriosis is one of the most common reasons for laparoscopic surgery, which is undertaken to ablate endometriotic foci and to lyse adhesions.

Other complications occur as well. Scarring of the uterine tube can cause infertility. Large *endometriomas* or hemorrhagic cavities on the surface of the ovary

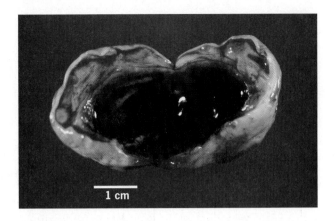

FIGURE 17–8 Endometrioma. The cystic ovary has been opened to reveal hemorrhagic contents.

(Figure 17–8) can result in torsion of the ovary, or twisting of the ovary around its vascular stalk, with resultant ischemic injury. This causes severe, acute pain and is a surgical emergency. Finally, endometriosis is commonly associated with certain carcinomas of the ovary, and molecular studies have demonstrated common genetic changes in these two conditions, suggesting that endometriosis may be a precursor for cancer.

BOX 17–2   Endometriosis

Causes

Endometrial tissue outside uterine cavity is responsive to monthly flux of hormones

Lesions

Foci of endometrial glands and stroma outside uterus (ovary, peritoneum most common)

Endometrioma

Manifestations

Pain

Ovarian torsion

Infertility

Dysfunctional Uterine Bleeding

Dysfunctional uterine bleeding (DUB) is the most common cause of abnormal vaginal bleeding in the United States. It is defined as abnormal uterine bleeding that is not caused by a structural defect, such as endometrial cancer or complications during pregnancy. More specifically, DUB results from derangements in hormonal control of the ovulatory cycle. Failure to ovulate may result in amenorrhea, but it can also cause the opposite, excessive bleeding (menorrhagia and/or metrorrhagia). If ovulation does not occur, the corpus luteum fails to develop, and progesterone is not produced. Estrogen stimulates the growth of the endometrium, so when the endometrium is exposed to continuous estrogen unopposed by progesterone, it grows throughout the cycle, without

undergoing secretory changes. The endometrium eventually becomes so thick that it outgrows its blood supply. Menstrual flow then occurs because the endometrium is necrotic, and because there is so much of it, the flow is much more abundant than usual. It should be recognized that there are many hormones that coordinate ovulation, and disturbances anywhere along the pathway can result in menstrual abnormalities. For example, the production of luteinizing hormone is inhibited by extreme athletic activity, resulting in anovulatory cycles and amenorrhea.

There are many other diseases that can result in amenorrhea or excessive uterine bleeding, so women who present with these symptoms should be thoroughly worked up for nutritional, endocrine, structural, and neoplastic diseases before this diagnosis is rendered. Pregnancy can also cause abnormal bleeding, especially in the early weeks, when a woman may not yet recognize that she is pregnant. Various pharmaceutical contraceptives can cause hormonal imbalances that result in abnormal bleeding. DUB is therefore a diagnosis of exclusion, and it is less a diagnosis than a descriptor, for often the exact hormonal excess or deficiency is simply surmised on the basis of the timing of the bleeding and its relationship to the woman's menstrual cycles rather than determined by clinical or laboratory investigations.

DUB can be associated with infertility because ovulatory cycles are unpredictable. It often occurs at the end of a woman's childbearing age, when the hormonal cycles become disregulated in a prelude to menopause. Premenopausal women often have severe, protracted bleeding that can result in iron-deficiency anemia. In rare cases, the bleeding is so severe that it results in hemorrhagic shock. DUB is usually treated with pharmaceutical control of the hormonal cycle—in other words, with birth control pills that equilibrate the endometrial environment. Progesterone may be given to stabilize the endometrium so that it can mature and slough normally. Hormonal manipulation is preferred if the woman is of reproductive age and wants to maintain her fertility. If the bleeding is very severe or the hormones provided by birth control pills cannot control it, hysterectomy puts a permanent end to the bleeding.

BOX 17–3   Dysfunctional Uterine Bleeding

Causes

Hormonal imbalance resulting in anovulation

Lesions

Excess endometrial tissue

Manifestations

Menorrhagia

Metrorrhagia

Iron-deficiency anemia

Hemorrhagic shock if severe

Obesity

Obesity is obviously not only a female problem, but many of the adverse effects of excessive adipose tissue in women involve the female organs. Adipose tissue contains the enzyme *aromatase*, which converts circulating androgens, such as androstenedione and testosterone, to estrogenic hormones. The androgenic hormones are normally produced in the adrenal gland and in the ovaries in women, albeit in much lower quantities than in men. Fat cells convert these androgenic compounds to estrogenic ones, so the levels of circulating estrogens in obese women are elevated. Excessive estrogen interferes with the release of the pituitary hormones that stimulate follicles to mature and be released from the ovary. Obese women therefore often have anovulatory cycles. Excessive estrogen also stimulates the proliferation of the endometrium, causing dysfunctional uterine bleeding. Obese women therefore can suffer irregular menstrual cycles, amenorrhea, DUB, and infertility. In addition, prolonged estrogenic stimulation is the biggest known risk factor for the development of endometrial carcinoma and breast carcinoma.

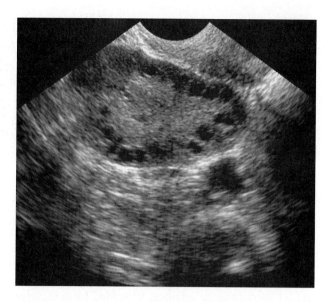

FIGURE 17-9 Polycystic ovaries. This is an ultrasound showing multiple cysts around the periphery of an ovary. (Courtesy of Dr. Myron Pozniak, Department of Radiology, University of Wisconsin School of Medicine and Public Health.)

BOX 17-4   Estrogen Excess due to Obesity

Causes:

Caloric consumption greater than expenditure

Adipose tissue converts circulating androgens to estrogenic compounds

Lesions:

Obesity

Endometrial proliferation

Manifestations:

Irregular menstrual cycles

Amenorrhea

Dysfunctional uterine bleeding

Infertility

Uterine (possibly also breast) cancer

Polycystic Ovarian Disease

Polycystic ovarian disease is another condition that is associated with derangements in the control of ovulation. This is a fairly common condition, affecting about 5% of women and resulting in irregular menstrual cycles and infertility. The condition gets its name from the numerous large cystic follicles protruding from the surface of the affected ovary (**Figure 17-9**). These are the remains of follicles that were stimulated to grow but did not release their ova. The exact hormonal derangement underlying this disease has not been thoroughly worked out. Women with polycystic ovary disease often also have signs of androgen excess, such as profuse male-pattern hair growth, insulin resistance (if not frank diabetes

mellitus type 2), and obesity. Excess androgens, excess estrogens (from excess adipose tissue), and insulin resistance are all known to inhibit the proper maturation of follicles. Treatment of this condition usually revolves around controlling insulin resistance/diabetes and obesity, primarily by diet and exercise, and birth control pills to reestablish regular endometrial shedding.

BOX 17-5   Polycystic Ovary Disease

Causes

Unknown

Lesions

Polycystic ovaries

Manifestations

Irregular menstrual cycles

Infertility

Associated with symptoms of androgen excess, insulin resistance, obesity

---

Menopause

The ovulatory cycle becomes increasingly irregular and eventually ceases in women around the age of 50 years. Menopause is defined as permanent cessation of menstruation. While a woman is pregnant and lactating, she will most likely not have a menstrual cycle, but this state of physiologic suppression of ovulation is reversible and ovulatory cycles eventually recommence once the baby relies more on solid foods than on mother's milk. Obviously, if a woman undergoes bilateral oophorectomy, or surgical removal of the gonads, menopause will occur earlier, and there are various medical conditions that cause premature ovarian failure and early menopause, but in general, the natural cessation of menstruation occurs about 40 years after menarche.

Cessation of menstruation is caused by the cessation of estrogen and progesterone production in the ovary. As estrogen levels decline, the remainder of the ova in the ovaries undergo atresia, or wither away, and the endometrium ceases to proliferate. Estrogen has wide-ranging effects in other organs, so decreased estrogen levels can manifest in many different ways. The symptoms most frequently reported in the United States include hot flashes, mood changes, problems with memory, depression, anxiety, insomnia, pain with sexual intercourse, and itching and dryness of the vagina. Some of these symptoms go away on their own; for example, hot flashes eventually become less common and then cease entirely. Other problems, such as vaginal dryness and itching, will not go away because estrogen is needed to moisturize this area. The most serious effects will not be felt for several years, however. These are impaired mineralization of bone, causing osteoporosis, and accelerated atherosclerosis, which leads to heart disease and stroke.

Vaginal dryness and itching can be treated with the topical application of estrogen-containing creams. The role of oral hormone replacement therapy to counteract the symptoms of menopause and the long-term effects of low levels of estrogen is, however, controversial. Well-designed studies have demonstrated that estrogen supplementation is quite effective at controlling menopausal symptoms, and that women who take estrogen replacement therapy suffer less morbidity from osteoporotic bone fractures, but the incidence of atherosclerotic cardiovascular disease and stroke is actually increased. In addition, women who take hormone replacement therapy are at greater risk of developing hormone-dependent cancers such as endometrial and breast cancers. The role of hormone replacement therapy in treating menopausal symptoms and the long-term effects of decreased estrogen are still not clearly defined. Its use should be tailored to each individual woman depending on the severity of symptoms and other risk factors she might have. Both osteoporosis and heart disease can be prevented by other means, including lifestyle adjustments (exercise, diet) and use of drugs that provide increased calcium, improve mineralization in bone, control hypertension, and decrease hyperlipidemia.

Finally, not every woman will experience menopause in the same way. There is considerable variation among women in the same socioeconomic class, and there is even more variation between women of different cultures. In the United States, menopause has always been defined as the time when women lose their fertility, a definition that by itself can engender anxiety in a culture in which youth and productivity are valued over age and knowledge. In contrast, in Asian countries, menopause is viewed as a time of liberation: liberation from childbearing and virtual enslavement by the husband's family. In Japan, for example, there is no word for menopause and women report none of the nuisance symptoms that plague women in the United States, such as hot flashes. This is not to say that menopausal symptoms are "all in the head," but to underscore that societal norms and cultural factors have a profound, though poorly understood, impact on how diseases are perceived. It is necessary to recognize this wide variation so as not to label a particular woman's complaints, or lack thereof, as abnormal.

BOX 17–6   Menopause

Causes

Decreased hormone production by the ovary

Lesions

None

Manifestations

Menopausal symptoms (hot flashes, anxiety, insomnia, memory problems)

Vaginal dryness, itching, pruritus

Accelerated osteoporosis

Accelerated cardiovascular disease and stroke

Lichen Sclerosus and Lichen Simplex Chronicus

Virtually all of the diseases that can affect the skin can also arise in the vulvar region, including melanoma, nonmelanoma skin cancers, blistering disorders, warts and herpes infections, psoriasis, and eczema. Two diseases that are common in the vulvar region are lichen sclerosus and lichen simplex chronicus. Both present as white plaques on the vulvar skin. There are many other conditions that cause leukoplakia, including malignant ones, so these lesions should always be biopsied and examined by a pathologist for a specific diagnosis. The term *lichen* in the names of these two diseases refers to their resemblance to the lichen that grows on rocks: flat, thin, rough, and with irregular contours.

Both of these diseases tend to occur in postmenopausal women, and they are both inflammatory. In **lichen sclerosus**, the epidermis becomes very thin, almost parchment paperlike, while the underlying dermis becomes thickened with fibrosis. This disease can spread to involve the entire vulva, and in so doing constricts the vaginal opening. A sparse inflammatory infiltrate consisting almost entirely of T cells is usually present underneath the epidermis, suggesting that autoimmune dysregulation plays a role in its pathogenesis. Women with this disease are at increased risk for developing squamous cell carcinoma of the vulva.

Lichen simplex chronicus is related to extreme vulvar pruritus that often occurs with decreased levels of estrogen after menopause. In this condition, the epidermis becomes hyperplastic, or thickened, because of rubbing or scratching of the vulvar skin. This condition is best treated with topical estrogen creams. It is not a risk factor for squamous cell carcinoma.

Hyperplastic/Neoplastic Diseases

All of the organs of the female genital tract can be affected by hyperplastic and/or neoplastic diseases. The list of such diseases fills heavy volumes of textbooks, but many of these are quite rare. Leiomyomata, common benign tumors of the ovaries, and the most common carcinomas of the uterus, ovaries, and cervix (**Table 17–3**) are the focus of the discussion here.

Leiomyoma of the Uterus

A leiomyoma (pl., leiomyomata) is a benign tumor that arises from the smooth muscle of the uterus (**Figure 17–10**). Leiomyomata are commonly known as fibroids. These tumors are clonal, meaning that the cells share a common genetic makeup that is presumably derived from a single progenitor cell and that gives them a growth advantage. The cells require estrogen to grow. Leiomyomata will not develop before puberty, and they regress after menopause. They most commonly occur in women between 25 and 35 years of age, and they are very common. Sensitive imaging studies that can detect

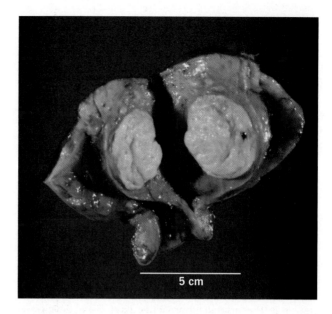

FIGURE 17–10 Leiomyoma. The uterus has been opened, and the cut surface reveals a well-circumscribed, solid white nodule.

very small leiomyomata demonstrate these neoplasms in up to 75% of women of childbearing age. Most of these tumors are entirely asymptomatic. They produce problems that require medical or surgical intervention in less than 25% of women.

Symptoms of leiomyomata relate to their size and location. If they block the opening of the uterine tube into the uterus, or if they are so large that they entirely fill the uterine cavity, they can result in infertility. If they are located immediately underneath the endometrium, they can interfere with implantation of a fertilized egg or proper development of the placenta. Usually, if pregnancy is established, they do not interfere with the growth of the fetus or of the placenta, though they themselves can continue to increase in size because of the increased circulating estrogen during pregnancy. If the leiomyoma is

TABLE 17–3   Comparison of Malignancies of the Female Genital Tract

Cancer	Incidence	Mortality	Age at Diagnosis	Stage at Which Most Frequently Detected	Risk Factors	Most Common Histologic Type
Endometrial	23:100,000 women	4:100,000 women	Postmenopausal (median = 62 yrs)	I	Unopposed estrogen	Endometrioid
Ovarian	13:100,000 women	9:100,000 women	Postmenopausal (median = 63 yrs)	IV	Genetic (family history)	Serous
Cervical	8:100,000 women	2.5:100,000 women	Premenopausal (median = 48 yrs)	I	Sexually transmitted disease: HPV	Squamous cell
Vulvar	2:100,000 women	0.5:100,000 women	Postmenopausal (median = 68 yrs)	I	HPV, lichen sclerosus	Squamous cell
Choriocarcinoma	25:100,000 pregnancies	0.25:100,000 pregnancies	Following pregnancy	IV	Pregnancy	Choriocarcinoma

growing on the serosal surface of the uterus on a stalk, the stalk can twist and compromise the tumor's vascular supply, resulting in acute and severe abdominal pain. And if the tumor is very large, it can cause symptoms of pelvic pressure, or compress the bladder, resulting in urinary stress incontinence.

In addition, leiomyomata can cause excessive menstrual bleeding, often leading to fatigue and anemia. Excessive menstrual bleeding as a result of leiomyomata is the most common reason for hysterectomy in the United States. Hysterectomy is a major, invasive surgery that has to be performed under full anesthesia and requires a considerable recovery period. The expense involved, as well as the psychological anguish that can accompany this surgery, are not to be taken lightly. Various alternatives to surgery do exist. Hormonal therapies—specifically, administration of drugs that counteract the effect of estrogen on the uterus—can shrink the tumors. In the past few decades, newer interventional approaches have been developed that are less invasive, require much shorter recovery periods, and can preserve the uterus. These include enucleation, or shelling out of the tumor from the surrounding smooth muscle, ablation of the tumor by focused ultrasound, and uterine fibroid embolization, where the main artery that supplies the tumor is identified and a synthetic material injected to occlude it so that the cells downstream lose their blood supply and die.

BOX 17–8   Leiomyoma of the Uterus

Causes

Clonal

Dependent on estrogen for growth

Lesions

Benign neoplasm of smooth muscle

Often multiple

Manifestations

Excessive bleeding

Abdominal fullness or pain

Infertility

Benign Ovarian Neoplasms

The ovary has the potential to produce a greater variety of tumors than any other organ. The tumors can be cystic or solid. The most common cysts are not neoplasms at all, but cystically dilated follicles or corpora lutea that have become hemorrhagic. Foci of endometriosis may also undergo excessive bleeding, resulting in endometriomas (Figure 17–8). Polycystic ovaries, in which follicles have been arrested in their development before ovulation occurs (Figure 17–9), have already been discussed. Cysts come to attention either when they become so large that the ovary "loses its balance," so to speak, and twists around its vascular pedicle, causing excruciating pain, or when they rupture and spill their contents

into the abdominal cavity, which also causes severe pain. Sometimes they are detected incidentally on bimanual examination. Commonly, they are detected on imaging studies performed for other reasons.

Benign tumors of the ovary are much more common than malignant ones. In general, tumors that arise in young women tend to be benign, while those arising in older (peri- or postmenopausal) women tend to be malignant. There are three "compartments" in the ovary, each of which can give rise to benign and malignant tumors. These are the surface epithelium, the germ cells, and the stroma. Surface epithelial tumors are by far the most common tumors, benign or malignant. These are further classified histologically by the type of epithelium the tumor is composed of. The surface epithelium of the ovary can differentiate into any type of epithelium in the female genital tract: glandular epithelium resembling that in the cervix, endometrioid glands, or columnar cells resembling those in the fallopian tubes. The latter is called "serous" epithelium, because the columnar cells produce a clear, watery ("serous") liquid. Most benign surface epithelial tumors are serous cysts and mucinous cysts (**Figure 17–11**). These tumors may also have varying degrees of fibrous tissue and are accordingly called serous cystadenoma or mucinous cystadenoma.

Ovarian tumors derived from ovarian germ cells or stroma tend to be benign. The most common germ cell tumor is a **teratoma**, commonly called a dermoid cyst because it contains mature tissue resembling skin and skin appendages. The pathogenesis of this tumor is not understood. It is thought to arise from an ovum in which the cells derived from the first meiotic division autonomously divide and differentiate into mature tissue. Teratomas rarely contain only one kind of tissue. Usually they comprise a variety of tissues including skin, gastrointestinal epithelium, cartilage, brain, and even teeth (**Figure 17–12**). They are usually cystic, and the cysts contain various substances including hair, sebum (oil generated by sweat glands), and keratinous debris. In women, malignant teratomas are very rare.

The most common benign stromal tumors are **fibrothecomas**. The fibrous component arises from the fibrous tissue in the ovary; thecoma cells are lipid containing and hormonally active stromal cells that normally form a dense coat around a follicle. Fibrothecomas account for about 4% of all ovarian neoplasms and usually go undetected. There is a curious syndrome associated with them—the so-called Meigs syndrome, which is the occurrence of ascites and usually only right-sided hydrothorax in association with a fibrothecoma. Pure thecomas and many other stromal tumors can come to attention when they secrete female or male hormones, thus causing cessation of menstruation, irregular menstrual cycles, the development of androgenic features such as facial hair, atrophy of the breasts, and changes in voice.

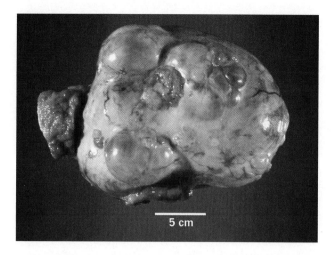

FIGURE 17–11 Serous cysts of the ovary. The ovary is very large and the external surface is distorted by numerous thin-walled cysts.

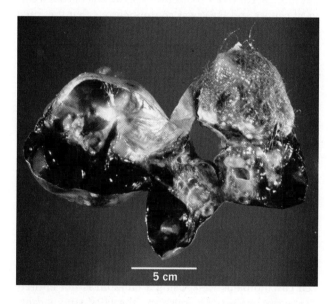

FIGURE 17–12 Teratoma. The ovary has been opened to reveal cystic spaces of various sizes, some filled with blood, interspersed with solid areas that represent nodules of ectopic tissue. In the upper right corner of the teratoma is a compact mass of hair and oily sebum.

The diagnosis of ovarian tumors is based on pathologic examination after their removal. Because most ovarian tumors are small and benign, professional judgment is required to decide which ones should be removed. Thorough familiarity with the age range in which specific tumors tend to occur, their natural history, and their association with known syndromes, body habitus, menstrual histories and fertility is necessary to make an informed judgment on how best to manage them. Obviously, an acute abdomen from ovarian torsion or hemorrhage is a surgical emergency, but every operation should be undertaken with an understanding of the woman's wishes pertaining to her fertility.

Carcinoma of the Endometrium

Endometrial adenocarcinoma is the most common female genital tract cancer in the United States, and the fourth most common cancer (excluding nonmelanoma skin cancers) detected in women overall (Table 17–3). Most cases occur in postmenopausal women and are associated with prolonged, unopposed estrogen stimulation, as occurs, for example, in obese women, women who take unopposed estrogens to counteract the effects of menopause, and women who were infertile because of anovulatory cycles. Other conditions associated with endometrial cancer include diabetes and hypertension.

Because most endometrial cancers arise after menopause, the bleeding they cause is recognized by the patient as abnormal, so the cancers are usually detected before they have spread beyond the uterine cavity. About 70% of endometrial cancers are detected while they are still confined to the uterine cavity, with a corresponding 5-year survival over 90% after hysterectomy. If the tumor has grown deeply into the wall of the uterus or spread beyond the uterus, some combination of radiotherapy and chemotherapy is necessary for control, and survival is no longer so high.

Histologically, endometrial adenocarcinomas can have a variety of appearances. The most common type resembles benign endometrial glands, and is therefore called *endometrioid* adenocarcinoma. Endometrium that is exposed to continuous, excess estrogen becomes hyperplastic and is vulnerable to acquire additional mutations that render it frankly neoplastic. These changes can be detected in endometrial biopsies and appear to form a continuum from simple hyperplasia, to hyperplasia with cytologic atypia, to adenocarcinoma. Hyperplasia of the endometrium and hyperplasia with atypia should be treated to prevent the development of cancer.

> **BOX 17–9 Carcinoma of the Endometrium**
>
> **Risk Factors**
> Unopposed estrogen
> Obesity
> Hypertension
> **Lesions**
> Adenocarcinoma
> **Manifestations**
> Abnormal uterine bleeding
> Usually detected in Stage 1

Carcinoma of the Ovary

Malignant ovarian neoplasms are much less common than benign ones, but they still represent the eighth most common cancer type in women and the fifth most common cause of cancer death in women (Table 17–3). Like benign neoplasms, they are classified as to whether they are of surface epithelial, germ cell, or sex cord-stromal origin, and surface epithelial cancers (serous, endometrioid, and, very rarely, mucinous) account for by far the majority of malignant neoplasms. The cause of **ovarian cancer** is not known. One strong association is having a first-degree relative with ovarian or breast cancer. Obesity, nulliparity (not ever having been pregnant), prolonged estrogen supplementation, and postmenopausal age all seem to confer additional risk for the development of ovarian cancer.

Ovarian cancers are usually detected late in the disease process, when they have already spread beyond the ovary to involve other organs in the pelvis, lymph nodes, or distant sites. This is because there is usually no specific symptom to herald their growth. Women may complain of pelvic pressure, abdominal fullness, bloating, urinary symptoms, or constipation. They are often diagnosed with irritable bowel syndrome, depression, or stress before worsening of their symptoms prompts diagnostic imaging. Only about 15% of cancers are detected in Stage I (limited to the ovaries), compared to 60% diagnosed in Stage IV. Surgical removal of the involved ovary or ovaries and their tubes in Stage I disease achieves a cure more than 90% of the time. Advanced disease requires a combination of chemotherapy and radiotherapy for additional control after surgical removal of both ovaries, the uterus, and pelvic lymph nodes. The overall (all stages combined) 5-year survival rate for ovarian cancer is around 50%, and more women die of it every year than of endometrial cancer, even though the incidence of endometrial cancer is higher.

Aside from stage, the histologic grade of the tumor is also of prognostic value. There is a form of serous tumor that is not clearly benign and not really malignant when examined microscopically. This is called a serous tumor of borderline malignant potential. Some of the patients with this kind of tumor are entirely free of the disease for the rest of their life, while in others, the tumor can recur and behave in a malignant fashion. At the other end of the spectrum, clear cell carcinoma of the ovary is a particularly aggressive neoplasm with a very low survival rate.

The ovary is an infrequent site of metastasis from cancers in other organs. The most common cancers to metastasize to the ovaries are from the colon, breast, stomach, and pancreas. Because the appearance of ovarian cancers can be quite variable under the microscope and can mimic cancers from any of these other sites, it is necessary to have a high index of suspicion that a cancer may be metastatic to the ovary rather than primary. A particularly striking phenomenon is the co-occurrence of mucinous tumors in the ovaries with an appendiceal mucinous tumor. Often, the mucinous component of these tumors spreads to fill the entire abdominal cavity, a condition termed **pseudomyxoma peritonei**. It is increasingly becoming recognized that the primary tumor is actually the appendiceal one, and that ovarian and peritoneal involvement are secondary features.

BOX 17–10   Carcinoma of the Ovary

Risk Factors

Genetic (family history)

Prolonged estrogen exposure (obesity, nulliparity, estrogen supplementation)

Postmenopausal

Lesions

Adenocarcinoma

Manifestations

Abdominal fullness, pelvic pressure

Bloating, nausea, urinary frequency, constipation

Carcinoma of the Cervix

Squamous cell carcinoma of the cervix, the most common type of cervical cancer, is caused by the human papillomavirus (HPV). Discovery of the link between cervical cancer and HPV was so momentous that it earned the Nobel Prize in Medicine and Physiology in 2008. The following year, the FDA approved a vaccine against the HPV strains causing cervical cancer for use in all women between the ages of 9 and 26 years. Though cervical cancer was once the leading cause of cancer death in women, the means of controlling and preventing this disease are now readily and cheaply available.

Cervical carcinoma is a sexually transmitted disease. HPV is passed between sexual partners. Women at risk of contracting this virus are those who have sex with multiple (male) partners, or with male partners who themselves have multiple sexual partners, and women who begin to have sex at a young age. The virus is also transmitted between male sexual partners, causing anal squamous cell carcinoma, and can apparently be transmitted via oral sex, as it is associated with oral squamous cell carcinoma as well. Using a condom is not entirely protective against transmission. The HPV strains causing cervical cancer do not cause visible lesions in men, so the male carrier of the virus does not even know he is infected. The fact that men can develop HPV-related anal and oral squamous cell carcinoma, and transmit the virus to their sexual partners when infected, makes a cogent argument for vaccination of boys and young men (not only women) against HPV

HPV infects immature cells at the site of the transition zone in the cervix, where the glandular lining of the cervical canal transforms to squamous epithelium lining the outside of the cervix and vagina (**Figure 17–13**). Here, the immature cells are close to the surface and therefore exposed to the virus. As the cells mature, genes carried by the virus induce longevity in the squamous cells, as well as genetic instability, or the propensity to acquire mutations that give them additional growth advantage. The presence of the virus in the cell can be seen histologically by morphologic alterations of the nuclei of the squamous cells. The nuclei become large and swollen,

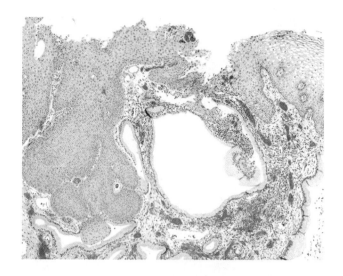

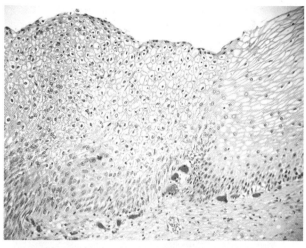

FIGURE 17–13 Squamous metaplasia at the transition zone. Normal stratified squamous mucosa is present on the right side of the image. Underlying the mucosa are mucinous glands lined by a single layer of columnar cells. On the left side of the image, the contour of the glands is still visible, but they are filled with squamous cells. These cells have not assumed the orderly, stratified arrangement of the squamous lining to the right. They are still immature. A small cluster of squamous cells is growing into a gland in the bottom left of the field. This is the usual appearance of the junction of the glandular and squamous mucosae of the cervix. (Courtesy of Dr. Josephine Harter, Department of Pathology and Laboratory Medicine, University of Wisconsin School of Medicine and Public Health.)

FIGURE 17–14 Dysplasia. On the right side of the image, the squamous mucosa has its usual stratified appearance, with an orderly maturation from small, linearly arranged basal cells at the base of the mucosa to plump, polygonal cells that gradually lose their nuclei as they move up to the surface. On the left side, the cells appear crowded and jumbled and have irregular nuclear sizes and shapes. Disordered maturation is the hallmark of dysplasia in the squamous mucosa of the cervix. (Courtesy of Dr. Josephine Harter, Department of Pathology and Laboratory Medicine, University of Wisconsin School of Medicine and Public Health.)

or contracted and wrinkled, and are often surrounded by a "halo" of cytoplasmic clearing. These changes are called *koilocytosis*. Altered maturation of the cells is also seen microscopically, (**Figure 17–14**) and is the basis of identification of cervical **dysplasia**. Actually, because we know that dysplasia is already the precursor to invasive carcinoma in the cervix, dysplastic lesions seen on biopsy samples are called **cervical intraepithelial neoplasia (CIN)** and graded according to severity into CIN-1, CIN-2, and CIN-3, with the last also called squamous cell carcinoma *in situ*.

More than 100 HPV types are known, but only a few of these cause cervical cancer. Some of them cause condylomata, or genital warts, which are not precursors to cancer. The HPV strains that cause the majority of cervical cancers in the United States are HPV 16 and 18. These are called high-risk HPV. Moreover, not all cases of demonstrated HPV infection progress to cancer. In fact, most HPV infections go away on their own. This is why a genetic test for the presence of HPV is currently not recommended as a screening tool: many women would be identified as having the virus, but we would not be able to predict which need intervention. The Pap smear is still the primary screening test for cervical cancer, followed by a test for high-risk HPV only if the results are equivocal.

Koilocytosis and degrees of dysplasia are easily seen on the Pap smear. Cells from the cervical transition zone, which is usually identified at the cervical os during the speculum examination, are collected with a little brush and, after fixation and staining, examined through the microscope. **Figure 17–15** illustrates the morphologic changes in the squamous cells with increasing dysplasia. Pap smears are read as low-grade squamous intraepithelial lesion or high-grade squamous intraepithelial lesion (abbreviated to **LGSIL** and **HGSIL**, respectively), or frank squamous cell carcinoma. Sometimes, inflammation at the transition zone obscures the characteristic morphology of HPV infection, and the Pap smear is read as **ASCUS**, or "atypical squamous cells of uncertain significance." ASCUS smears are then further tested for the presence of HPV by genetic tests.

Screening and treatment recommendations for cervical lesions are continually changing. In general, every sexually active woman should be screened by Pap smear every year. Abnormal test results should be followed with more frequent screening. A diagnosis of LGSIL or HGSIL should be followed with colposcopy. Visible lesions are biopsied, and further treatment designed according to the biopsy results. CIN-2 and CIN-3 lesions are treated with **conization**, which involves removing the end of the cervix including the area of squamous metaplasia. This procedure physically removes the area of virally infected mucosa, preventing the spread of the infection and the development of carcinoma. Conization does not impair the ability of the woman to bear children in the future. Invasive carcinoma requires more extensive treatment, including radiation therapy.

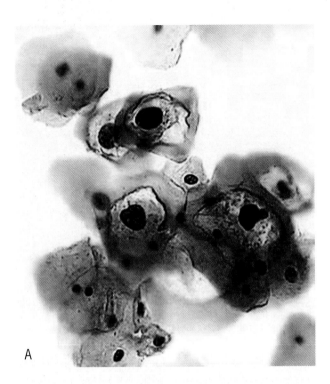

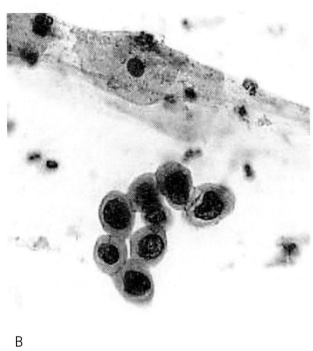

A

B

FIGURE 17–15 A. Low-grade squamous intraepithelial lesion (LGSIL), Pap smear. A few normal squamous cells with small nuclei are present at the periphery of the field. In the center of the field are cells with larger and somewhat irregular nuclei. These are cells of low-grade dysplasia. **B.** High-grade squamous intraepithelial lesion (HGSIL). A normal squamous epithelial cell is present at the top of the field. The small cells with large nuclei and scant cytoplasm are cells of high-grade squamous dysplasia. (Courtesy of Dr. Josephine Harter, Department of Pathology and Laboratory Medicine, University of Wisconsin School of Medicine and Public Health.)

BOX 17–11 Carcinoma of the Cervix

Causes

HPV, sexually transmitted

Lesions

Squamous cell carcinoma

Adenocarcinoma (rare)

Premalignant changes: LGSIL, HGSIL

Manifestations

Abnormal cells on Pap test

Abnormal vaginal bleeding

Cervical mass

Diseases of Pregnancy

The number of problems that can complicate pregnancy is so large that they are separately dealt with in the sub-specialty of obstetrics. We discuss only a few of the more common problems, both degenerative and neoplastic, that might arise during or after pregnancy.

Spontaneous Abortion

At least one out of five pregnancies terminates spontaneously during the first third of pregnancy. These abortions result from a major defect in embryonic development due to abnormal chromosomes. The chromosome abnormality is usually confined to the individual sperm or ovum involved, so the next pregnancy is likely to be normal. The patient presents with cramps and bleeding, and the placental tissue either passes spontaneously or is found in the cervical os or vagina. Dilation and curettage may be needed to remove remaining placental tissue to prevent infection. The pathologist frequently finds only placental tissue without evidence of the embryo.

Ectopic Pregnancy

Ectopic means out of place, and an **ectopic pregnancy** is one in which the fertilized ovum implants outside the uterine cavity, usually in the fallopian tube (**Figure 17–16**).

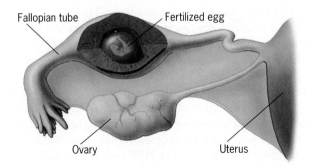

Fallopian tube

Fertilized egg

Ovary

Uterus

FIGURE 17–16 Ectopic pregnancy.

The embryo and placenta can develop in this abnormal location, but the tube is not plastic enough to accommodate the growing embryo and is not vascular enough to supply sufficient blood to the growing placenta. The embryo is destined to die, in any case, but the mother also faces life-threatening complications if the fallopian tube or the blood vessels supplying the placenta rupture. This is a surgical emergency and is usually heralded by increasing abdominal pain, vaginal bleeding, or light-headedness from internal bleeding. The diagnosis is often complicated by the fact that the woman may not know that she is pregnant, so her pain is confused with acute appendicitis or ovarian torsion.

Diagnosis of ectopic pregnancy involves demonstrating elevated levels of hCG, which will usually not be as high as in an intrauterine pregnancy of the same age, and demonstration of a mass by pelvic exam and ultrasound. If complications have not yet occurred, methotrexate, a teratogenic agent, is given at doses that are lethal to the developing embryo. The aborted pregnancy will then pass or regress on its own. Close follow-up, meaning frequent monitoring of hCG levels, is necessary to ensure that the pregnancy has indeed been terminated.

Ectopic pregnancies occur in about 2% of pregnancies; however, previous scarring of the fallopian tube makes it much more likely for a blastocyst to implant in the tubes. Pelvic inflammatory disease or, less commonly, endometriosis or prior surgical interventions are the strongest risk factors for the development of this condition. Smoking is another very strong risk factor for ectopic pregnancies, because some chemicals in cigarettes appear to inhibit the normal movement of an egg down the fallopian tube. Having had one ectopic pregnancy puts a woman at risk for having another one, but achieving an intrauterine pregnancy is still possible in many cases.

BOX 17–12   Ectopic Pregnancy

Causes

Implantation of fertilized ovum in fallopian tube or abdominal cavity

Risk factors: pelvic inflammatory disease, endometriosis, prior abdominal surgery, smoking

Lesions

Fetus and placenta in fallopian tubes or abdominal cavity

Internal hemorrhage

Manifestations

Pain

Vaginal hemorrhage

Ectopic pregnancy detected by ultrasound

Hemorrhage, mass seen by laparoscopy

Septic Abortion

Septic abortion refers to infection of the uterus after an abortion. It more commonly occurs when abortions are carried out by untrained persons using nonsterile technique. The infection may spread to the peritoneal cavity and cause death. Treatment consists of removal of the infected tissue and administration of antibiotics.

Placental Disorders

Intrauterine infections are common causes of pregnancy loss and perinatal/neonatal complications.

Development of the placenta occurs about 7–8 days after fertilization, after the embryo has implanted into the lining of the uterine cavity. Implantation of the placenta is called *placentation*. Usually, the placenta develops within the endometrium in the fundus of the uterus (**Figure 17–17a**). Complications can occur if it develops

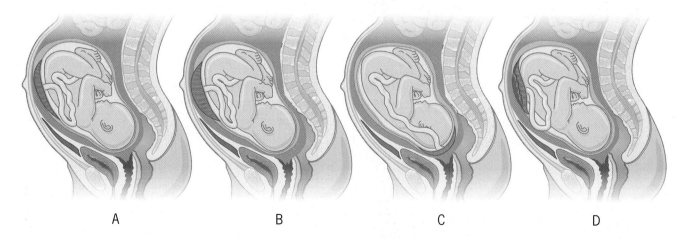

FIGURE 17–17 Disorders of placental position. **A.** Placenta in normal position. **B.** Placenta accreta. **C.** Placenta previa. **D.** Placental abruption.

at an abnormal location. If the placental nidus burrows deeply through the endometrium, it may develop within the myometrium, a condition called *placenta accreta* (**Figure 17–17b**). This does not necessarily interfere with the development of the fetus, but it can lead to life-threatening hemorrhage of the mother during and after birth. If the placenta implants low in the uterine cavity, it can partially or completely cover the cervical os, a condition called *placenta previa* (**Figure 17–17c**). This is an indication for cesarean section, because the placenta blocks the fetus's exit from the uterus and life-threatening bleeding can occur as the cervical os expands and tears the placenta during labor.

Another **disorder of placentation** is **placental abruption** (**Figure 17–17d**). *Abruption* refers to separation of the placenta from its attachment to the uterus. The uterine vessels nourishing the placenta remain wide open and bleed extensively into the space between the placenta and the uterine wall. This has adverse effects on the mother and the fetus. The mother can lose large volumes of blood and go into hemorrhagic shock, while the fetus is deprived of its oxygen supply.

Placental abruption complicates about 1% of pregnancies, usually after the first 20 weeks. It is most common in cases where the mother is hypertensive or uses drugs that induce hypertension, such as cocaine, or in cases of trauma (motor vehicle accidents, falls). It is also more common at the extremes of maternal age. Treatment involves emergent delivery of the fetus by cesarean section and hemodynamic support of the mother (transfusion of blood products, blood volume expanders, and prevention of disseminated intravascular coagulation [DIC]). If the fetus has not died *in utero*, it will suffer the complications of prematurity and, possibly, anoxic brain injury. About 10% of babies born in settings of abruption die.

> ### BOX 17–13   Placental Abruption
>
> **Causes**
> Maternal hypertension
> Cocaine
> Trauma
>
> **Lesions**
> Hematoma formation between placenta and uterine wall
>
> **Manifestations**
> Maternal: severe pain and massive vaginal blood loss, leading to hemorrhagic shock
>
> Fetal: Prematurity, anoxic brain injury, death

Preeclampsia and Eclampsia

Preeclampsia is a life-threatening disease characterized by hypertension and maternal endothelial dysfunction. It occurs in about 5% of pregnancies and accounts for about 20% of deaths resulting from complications during pregnancy and childbirth, and 15% of premature births in the United States. **Preeclampsia** is defined by maternal hypertension, proteinuria, and edema. If the woman additionally develops signs of central nervous system involvement, such as seizures or coma, the condition is called **eclampsia**. The goal of therapy is to stabilize the mother long enough to bring the fetus to maturity and to deliver it as quickly as possible because delivery of the fetus—more specifically, of the placenta—reverses the derangements in the mother. Preeclampsia is more common in the last third of pregnancy but tends to be more severe if it develops earlier. It does not develop before 20 weeks of pregnancy.

The pathogenesis of preeclampsia and eclampsia is not entirely clear. It is thought that these disorders begin with faulty maturation of the endometrial arteries that nourish the placenta. As the placenta perceives low oxygenation, it releases factors that result in systemic endothelial dysfunction in the mother. Endothelial dysfunction manifests as hypertension, increased permeability of vessels resulting in edema and proteinuria, and in some cases hypercoagulability. The latter manifests as fibrin thrombi forming in small vessels throughout the body, or disseminated intravascular coagulation. This impairs perfusion of maternal tissues, leading to ischemic damage of the kidneys, lungs, liver, brain, and other organs.

Preeclampsia is most common in first pregnancies and in pregnancies with multiple fetuses. The mother usually feels completely fine until she suddenly notices swelling, headache, or visual disturbances or, much more commonly, she notices no symptoms at all and the condition is detected at one of her regularly scheduled prenatal exams.

> ### BOX 17–14   Preeclampsia and Eclampsia
>
> **Causes**
> Impaired placental perfusion results in release of a placental factor that causes maternal endothelial dysfunction
>
> **Lesions**
> Vasoconstriction
> Increased permeability of vessels
> Hypercoagulability
>
> **Manifestations**
> Hypertension
> Edema, proteinuria
> Convulsions, coma
> DIC

Gestational Trophoblastic Neoplasms

Placental tissue can develop and grow independent of growth signals from a fetus. Neoplastic placental tissue is related to pregnancy in some way, developing either during pregnancy or thereafter. The malignant cells are derived from the trophoblast, or the layer of cells that immediately surrounds an embryo and develops into the villi of the placenta.

Most gestational trophoblastic neoplasms are benign. These are called **hydatidiform mole**, and the condition that ensues is called a **molar pregnancy**. Hydatidiform moles are derived from duplication of spermatic chromosomes. Either the sperm undergoes duplication after it has fertilized an egg, or two sperm fertilize a single egg. If the egg itself does not contain any genetic material, the result is a "complete" hydatidiform mole, and a fetus is entirely absent. If the egg does contain genetic material, an "incomplete" hydatidiform mole forms, and a fetus may develop, but it is incompatible with life. In either case, placental tissue forms, but the individual villi are grossly swollen, resembling a bunch of grapes (**Figure 17–18**). In some hydatidiform moles, the abnormal chorionic villi invade deeply into the myometrium. **Choriocarcinoma** is an invasive and metastatic malignancy that grows rapidly and spreads widely. It can arise from a preexisting hydatidiform mole or from a completely normal placenta.

Gestational trophoblastic neoplasms secrete hCG that can be measured in blood or urine. In fact, in many molar pregnancies, the woman may believe she is having a normal pregnancy until she develops vaginal bleeding or uterine growth inappropriate with gestational age, or a prenatal ultrasound detects the abnormal placental tissue and absence of a fetus. Treatment of benign molar pregnancies involves surgery to remove all the neoplastic tissue, followed by sequential hCG measurements to make sure it does not regrow. Choriocarcinoma grows very quickly, and because it is so mitotically active it is quite sensitive to chemotherapeutic agents, even when it has already metastasized widely.

Molar pregnancies are rare in the United States. Hydatidiform moles occur in only 1 in 1,000–2,000 pregnancies, invasive moles develop from only a fraction of molar pregnancies, and choriocarcinoma develops in about 1 of 40,000 pregnancies. In other areas of the world, such as Africa and Asia, the rates of these diseases are much higher, for unexplained reasons. In general, gestational trophoblastic diseases account for about 1% of gynecologic cancers in the United States.

> ### BOX 17–15 Gestational Trophoblastic Disease
>
> **Causes**
>
> Duplication of paternal chromosomes
>
> Malignant transformation of prior molar or nonmolar pregnancy
>
> **Lesions**
>
> Hydatidiform mole
>
> Choriocarcinoma
>
> **Manifestations**
>
> Vaginal bleeding
>
> Uterine size inappropriately large for gestational age
>
> hCG inappropriately high for gestational age
>
> Ultrasound reveals "mole" and (usually) absence of fetus

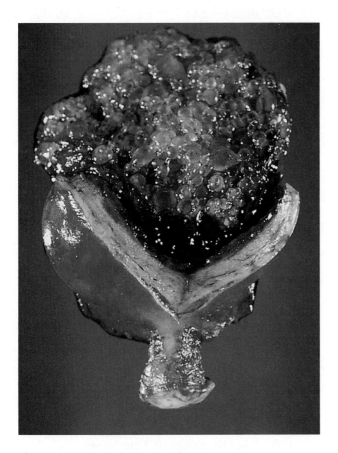

FIGURE 17–18 Hydatidiform mole. The uterus has been opened (the cervix is the conical structure at the bottom of the uterus). Clusters of translucent blisters extrude from the lumen of the uterus.

Organ Failure

Fertility and infertility are both major healthcare problems. The majority of women desire temporary or permanent infertility at some time during their childbearing years. Temporary infertility, or birth control, can be achieved by mechanical blockage of the cervix (diaphragm), spermicidal chemicals, mechanical prevention of implantation (intrauterine device), hormonal prevention of ovulation (oral contraceptives), and hormonal prevention of implantation (the morning-after pill). Permanent infertility can be accomplished by clamping or resecting a portion of the fallopian tubes. Obviously, removal of the uterus and/or ovaries can also achieve infertility, but these surgeries are not performed for that purpose. The condom is another very effective way to prevent pregnancy. It not only prevents transmission of sperm but also prevents transmission of most sexually transmitted diseases, including the HIV virus that causes AIDS. Vasectomy, or severing the vasa deferentia that carry sperm from the testes to the penis, causes permanent infertility in the man. All of these techniques have desirable and undesirable features. Medical expertise and counseling are often necessary to help a woman or couples determine which type of birth control is most suitable to her/them, taking into consideration their current and future desires for pregnancy.

Undesirable, involuntary infertility is also a common problem. **Infertility** is defined as the inability to achieve pregnancy after 1 year of unprotected sex. About 10% of couples of childbearing age seek medical help to establish pregnancy. Reproductive endocrinology and infertility, which addresses the concerns of infertile couples, is a subspecialty within the field of obstetrics and gynecology, requiring additional training of doctors who are already certified in OB/Gyn. Twenty percent of cases of infertility are caused by problems with the production or delivery of sperm, 50% are caused by problems of the female genital organs, and the remaining 30% are caused by problems in both the man and woman. Many factors can impair fertility in men and women, including lifestyle (smoking, marijuana use, extreme athletics in women, stress), increasing age, problems with the physical act of sex (e.g., inability to achieve erection, retrograde ejaculation), problems with sperm production or ovulation, and underlying medical conditions ranging from hormonal imbalance to autoimmune diseases. Evaluation of a couple's infertility requires a holistic approach to both the male and female partners, and complete evaluation of the endocrine, metabolic, medical, psychological, and anatomic parameters systems discussed earlier in the chapter. It involves hormones produced by the pituitary, ovary, adrenal gland, thyroid, and adipose tissue. Excesses and deficiencies of these hormones can lead to anovulatory cycles. Pelvic inflammatory disease causes blockage of the lumen of the uterine tube by scar tissue, preventing an egg from traveling through it to the uterus. The patency of the tube can rarely be reestablished by surgical means.

Numerous other causes of female infertility range from low-grade endometritis that impairs implantation to antisperm antibodies present in the cervical mucus, from advanced maternal age to congenital anomalies of uterine structure, from leiomyomata blocking the opening of the uterine tube to polycystic ovarian syndrome, from smoking to obesity. Infertility may also be the result of inhospitable uterine environments and systemic diseases, such as hypertension or lupus erythematosus, that impair perfusion of the placenta.

The treatments for infertility are as numerous as the causes. These range from surgery to sexual counseling, hormonal induction of ovulation, psychological counseling, and *in vitro* fertilization. The latter can be accomplished with donor sperm or egg, followed by implantation into the natural or a surrogate mother. Some of these techniques take the definition of parenthood into morally, legally, or ethically fraught domains. Even without such complications, infertility is a cause of severe stress and anxiety to the mother and her partner. Marital discord, sexual dysfunction, depression, anxiety, and actual or perceived social stigmatization are common sequelae of infertility.

Practice Questions

1. Which of the following tests or procedures can confirm the presence of an ovarian cyst?
   A. Chorionic gonadotropin levels
   B. Speculum examination
   C. Pap test
   D. Ultrasound
   E. Bimanual examination

2. The term for painful menstruation is
   A. menorrhagia.
   B. dysmenorrhea.
   C. menarche.
   D. metrorrhagia.
   E. menopause.

3. Which of the following diseases is not associated with a venereally transmitted infection?
   A. Cervical cancer
   B. Pelvic inflammatory disease
   C. Candidiasis
   D. Trichomoniasis
   E. Secondary syphilis

4. Permanent cessation of menstruation
   A. occurs around the age of 60 years.
   B. is best treated with oral estrogen supplementation.
   C. rarely causes symptoms in women in the United States.
   D. is associated with accelerated osteoporosis and cardiovascular disease.
   E. does not cause symptoms outside the female genital tract.

5. A 71-year-old woman who has never been pregnant and always had normal Pap tests notices spotty vaginal bleeding. A workup is performed and a biopsy reveals cancer. Which is she most likely to have?
   A. Stage I endometrial carcinoma
   B. Stage IV cervical carcinoma
   C. Stage I ovarian cancer
   D. Stage III endometrial carcinoma
   E. Stage I vulvar carcinoma

6. A 35-year-old woman attends a routine prenatal exam in her 32nd week of pregnancy complaining of recent severe headaches and swelling of her feet. Her blood pressure is 160/90 mm Hg and urinalysis shows markedly elevated protein. What is her diagnosis?
   A. These changes are normal for pregnancy
   B. Preeclampsia
   C. Gestational hypertension
   D. Eclampsia
   E. Gestational diabetes

7. *Molar pregnancy* refers to
   A. a teratoma in which teeth have formed.
   B. growth of a placenta derived only from paternal chromosomes.
   C. a rapidly fatal malignancy of the placenta.
   D. growth of a fetus with an abnormal placenta derived only from paternal chromosomes.
   E. a pregnancy developing outside the uterus.

Breast

OUTLINE

OBJECTIVES

1. Review the structure and function of mammary tissue.
2. Recognize the magnitude of the problem of breast cancer in the United States, and be able to cite key statistics relating to lifetime risk, prevalence, mortality, and median age at diagnosis of breast cancer.
3. Name the most common surgical procedures performed on the breast.
4. List the components of the physical examination of the breast.
5. Name the lesions that can mimic breast cancer by forming a palpable lump.
6. Describe the role of mammography and ultrasound in evaluating mammary tissue, and cite the screening recommendations for breast cancer.
7. Describe acute mastitis, under what conditions it occurs, and how it is treated.
8. Describe the lesions encompassed by the term *fibrocystic change*, and list those lesions that impart a higher risk for the subsequent development of breast cancer.
9. Name and describe the benign and malignant stromal tumors of the breast.
10. List the risk factors for breast cancer.
11. List the prognostic factors for breast cancer.
12. Describe the difference between *in situ* and invasive carcinoma.
13. Describe the most common lesions of the male breast.
14. Be able to define and use in context all terms and phrases in bold print in this chapter.

KEY TERMS

acinus	invasive mammary carcinoma
acute mastitis	(ductal, lobular)
areola	lactation
atypical ductal	lactiferous duct
hyperplasia	lobule
BRCA	lumpectomy
carcinoma *in situ* (CIS)	lymphedema
duct ectasia	mammography
ductal hyperplasia	mastectomy
ER/PR positive	nipple
fibroadenoma	oxytocin
fibrocystic change	phyllodes tumor
galactorrhea	prolactin
gynecomastia	sentinel lymph node
Her2/neu	stroma
intraductal papilloma	supernumerary nipple

Review of Structure and Function

The mature female breast is composed of 10–20 separate lobes made up of glandular units that empty to the **nipple** by means of an excretory duct, the **lactiferous duct** (**Figure 18–1**). The glandular units, called **lobules** (**Figure 18–2**), overlap one another in three-dimensional space. The small glands of the lobules, also called **acini**, are the milk-producing units of the breast. The ducts and acini are lined by two layers of cells: an inner epithelial

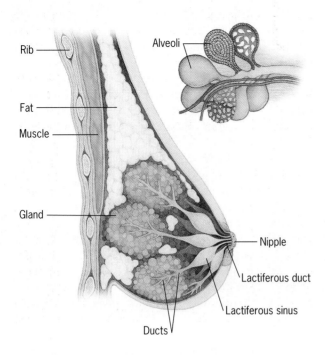

Rib
Fat
Muscle
Gland
Alveoli
Nipple
Lactiferous duct
Lactiferous sinus
Ducts

FIGURE 18–1 Anatomy of the breast ducts and lobules.

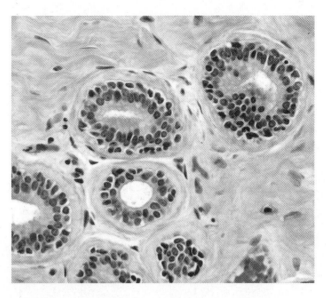

FIGURE 18–3 Breast glands. Each gland is lined by two layers of cells: an inner epithelial layer and an outer layer of myoepithelial cells.

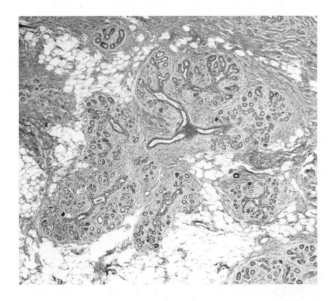

FIGURE 18–2 Breast lobule. The tissue surrounding the lobule is fibrous (top) and adipose (bottom) tissue. A large duct in the center of the lobule branches extensively to end in tightly clustered, small glands, or acini.

layer and an outer myoepithelial layer that can contract and thereby facilitates the transport of milk to the nipple (**Figure 18–3**). Between the lobules is a variable amount of fibrous and adipose tissue.

At birth, male and female breasts consist only of ducts. The ducts may be hypertrophied, giving the impression of slight breast prominence, as a result of the influence of maternal hormones *in utero*. Otherwise, the breasts remain quiescent until puberty, when both male and female breasts undergo ductal hyperplasia. This is minimal in the male and usually regresses. Proliferation of ducts, glandular buds within lobules, and connective tissue accounts for enlargement of the female breast at puberty. Estrogen and progesterone produced during the menstrual cycle cause mild hyperplasia of the breast ducts and lobules. In some women, this results in a feeling of fullness and tenderness of the breasts just before menstruation. After menopause, there is gradual atrophy of glands so that in older women the breasts consist mainly of ducts, adipose tissue, and some dense connective tissue.

High levels of the hormones estrogen, progesterone, and **prolactin** produced during pregnancy cause a striking change in the structure of the breast. The glands proliferate so that the entire breast appears to be composed of lobules. Milk production by the epithelial cells of the glands does not occur until after birth, when the level of progesterone suddenly drops. The hormone **oxytocin** stimulates contraction of the myoepithelial cells so that milk is expressed into the ducts and transported to the nipple. **Lactation** refers to the secretion of milk and to the period of time that a mother produces milk. Following lactation, the physiologic glandular hyperplasia gradually regresses, although glands remain somewhat more abundant than before the first pregnancy.

The prefixes *mammo-* and *mast-* both refer to the breast. *Mammo-* is used in reference to breast tissue, while *mast-* refers to the breast itself. Thus, a *mammography* is a radiographic examination of the breast, while *mastectomy* is surgical removal of a breast.

Most Frequent and Serious Problems

Carcinoma of the breast is by far the most serious disease of the breast. In the United States, approximately 1 in every 8 women will develop breast cancer and about 40,000 die from it each year. Other lesions of the breast are important because they may be causally related to breast cancer (e.g., epithelial hyperplasia) or mimic it on physical exams and imaging studies (e.g., fibroadenoma). The relative frequency of lesions of the breast that are biopsied out of concern for cancer is shown in **Figure 18–4**. As you can see, benign lesions far outweigh malignant ones, but because breast cancer is such a common and deadly disease, care must be taken not to miss it. The age range at which hyperplastic and neoplastic breast lesions are most commonly diagnosed is shown in **Figure 18–5**.

The most common inflammatory condition of the breast is **acute mastitis**, or bacterial infection of the breast tissue. This usually occurs when a woman is breastfeeding. Lactation itself may be difficult to establish and maintain by first-time mothers, but usually not because of any underlying medical condition. Lactation specialists help teach the baby how to latch on to the nipple properly and advise the mother on other aspects related to breastfeeding that may be causing her anxiety or discomfort.

Breasts vary greatly in size, and surgeries to both increase and decrease the size of breasts are some of the most common elective procedures performed in the United States. Women with excessively large breasts often develop neck, shoulder, and back pain from the weight of the breasts and they may even develop problems with breathing because the weight of the breasts restricts the movement of the thorax. To put the magnitude of breast weight in perspective, about twice as many women have breast reduction surgery as die of breast cancer every year. Even this figure pales in comparison to the women who are dissatisfied with the small size of their breasts and undergo breast augmentation—almost 300,000 every year, according to the American Society of Plastic Surgeons (2009 data). Men are not spared worries about breast size. **Gynecomastia**, or enlargement of the breasts, is a source of discomfort and embarrassment to many men. As in women, breast size increases in men secondary to increased circulating estrogens. Obesity is the most common cause of gynecomastia in men.

Symptoms, Signs, and Tests

Diffuse tenderness of the breasts often occurs in the latter part of the menstrual cycle. Acute mastitis is accompanied by localized pain, redness, and swelling. Neoplastic lesions of the breast usually do not cause pain. They come to attention by producing a palpable lump. This may be discovered accidentally but hopefully is detected during the monthly breast self-exam that women are encouraged to perform on themselves. Not all lumps are cancer: fibrocystic changes and benign fibroadenomas can also present as lumps. The breast can also produce abnormal secretions. **Galactorrhea** is production of milk unassociated with pregnancy. Milk production in these cases is usually driven by a prolactin-producing tumor in the pituitary gland. Bloody, watery, or cloudy discharges are usually associated with a papilloma, a benign growth within a duct, or with fibrocystic changes. Cancer rarely causes a discharge.

Physical examination of the breasts begins with visual assessment. Asymmetry of the breasts, inversion of the nipple, and focal changes in skin color or texture may all be indicative of underlying breast pathology. Visual inspection is followed by breast palpation. The breasts usually feel "lumpy" because of variation in the consistency of the adipose and fibrous tissues that make up the bulk of normal breast tissue. Fibrocystic changes can also cause lumpy-feeling breasts. Mammary tissue is located not just over the pectoralis muscle, but also extends high up to the clavicle and laterally into the armpit, or axilla. It is therefore important to palpate all the way up to the

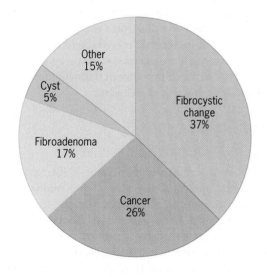

FIGURE 18–4 Relative frequency of lesions of the breast that are biopsied out of concern for cancer.

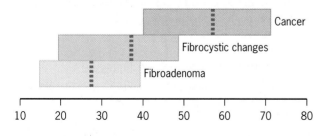

FIGURE 18–5 Age range at which hyperplastic and neoplastic lesions are commonly diagnosed. The dashed red lines indicate the mean.

clavicle and into the axilla for lumps. An experienced professional can usually tell the difference between "lumpy-bumpy" breasts caused by fibrocystic changes and lumps that are due to a neoplastic process or enlarged lymph nodes.

Mammography and ultrasound are used to further investigate lumps detected during the physical examination, and as screening techniques for breast cancer. Ultrasound can help differentiate whether a lump is composed of solid tissue, which is concerning for cancer, or is a fluid-filled, benign cyst. Mammography is a radiographic procedure that "sees through" the adipose tissue of the breast to highlight areas of solid growth as well as clusters of dystrophic calcifications. Abnormal calcifications can be as concerning for breast cancer as dense areas with irregular outlines (**Figure 18–6**). The main role of mammography is not to evaluate palpable lumps, however, but to serve as a screening procedure. The goal of breast cancer screening is to detect growths at a very early stage, before they have become palpable lumps. Breasts that are very dense are not amenable to mammographic examination because the fibrous tissue of the breast can obscure abnormal, solid growths. This is why mammography is not used to screen women less than 40 years old.

The current screening recommendation set forth by the American Cancer Society is that all women should have annual screening mammograms beginning at the age of 40 years. Women who are at higher-than-average risk of developing breast cancer, for example, because of a family history of breast cancer, should begin screening earlier. Ultrasound, which is much more time consuming, may be the screening modality of choice for young women because the density of their breasts inhibits adequate visualization of the mammary tissue by mammography. At the time this chapter is being written, these recommendations are being hotly contested and may have been revised by the print date. There does not seem to be a benefit from screening all women between 40 and 50 years on an annual basis. In addition, newer magnetic resonance imaging (MRI) modalities appear to be much more sensitive in picking up breast cancer in young and at-risk women than mammogram and ultrasound.

Regardless of which radiographic modality is used, radiographic techniques do not make a diagnosis of breast cancer. They highlight suspicious masses and areas of calcification, but diagnosis is made by tissue biopsy. Biopsies are performed under radiographic guidance: the suspicious area is first visualized, and then a fine, hollow needle is inserted into it to extract tissue. The tissue is examined microscopically. If cancer is present, it can be graded (an assessment made of how aggressive it appears), and various cell surface receptors detected by ancillary laboratory techniques. Grade of the tumor and the presence or absence of cell surface receptors are used to choose the particular treatment that will most likely be effective for each particular cancer.

Specific Diseases

Genetic/Developmental Diseases

Primates are unusual among mammals for having only two breasts, one on either side of the midline. These develop from paired milk lines or ridges that form on the ventral surface of the embryo at about 4 weeks' gestation. The milk lines extend from the clavicle to the groin. In other mammals, paired lactiferous units and nipples develop all along this line, and occasionally, in humans, **supernumerary nipples** develop along this line, as well. During puberty, under the influence of estrogens and androgens, the breast tissue underlying the nipples begins to grow, causing considerable discomfort and embarrassment. Supernumerary nipples are easily surgically removed.

Inflammatory/Degenerative Diseases

Acute mastitis develops in lactating women. When a baby is first born and begins to suckle, the nipples and surrounding pigmented skin, or **areolae**, become very dry and chapped. Bacteria can enter cracks in the skin and set up infections and even abscesses. Acute mastitis is terribly painful and associated with redness and swelling of the breast and fever. It is important that the mother

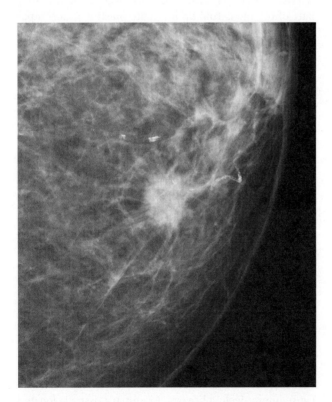

FIGURE 18–6 Mammogram. A dense, stellate lesion in the center of the breast turned out to be infiltrating carcinoma when it was biopsied. (Courtesy of Dr. Lonie Salkowski, Department of Radiology, University of Wisconsin School of Medicine and Public Health.)

be encouraged to continue to breastfeed despite the pain because the infection can be eradicated with appropriate antibiotics and the originally painful and uncomfortable cracks and fissures in the skin soon heal.

There is a form of chronic inflammation of unknown cause called **duct ectasia** that affects one or more of the major ducts and occurs near the time of menopause. The ducts become filled with necrotic and inflammatory debris that can be extruded through the nipple. Duct ectasia is primarily of importance because it can produce a lump or cause scar formation that retracts the overlying skin and thereby mimics cancer. Likewise, trauma to the breast can produce localized fat necrosis, which becomes scarred and produces a hard lump mimicking carcinoma on breast examination.

BOX 18–1   Acute Mastitis

Causes

Cracks in nipple and areola when a newborn first begins to suckle

Bacteria, primarily *Staphylococcus aureus*

Lesions

Acute inflammation

Abscess

Manifestations

Pain, redness, heat, swelling

Drainage of pus

Hyperplastic/Neoplastic Diseases

Fibrocystic Changes (Fibrocystic Disease)

Fibrocystic change is a term used to encompass a variety of alterations that occur in the epithelial and stromal compartments of the breast. The reason some experts refer to it as fibrocystic "disease" is that some of the changes are associated with an increased risk of breast cancer. Fibrocystic changes are extremely common: it is estimated that 60% of women have some degree of fibrocystic change. This is usually bilateral. The most innocuous of these changes, meaning they are not associated with an increased risk of breast cancer, are cysts and fibrosis. These manifest as "lumpy bumpy" tissue on physical exam and may cause tenderness or fluctuant palpable masses that grow and regress with changing levels of circulating hormones.

The fibrocystic changes that are associated with an increased risk of breast cancer are proliferative lesions, in which the epithelial component of the breast grows abnormally. A localized growth of epithelial cells around slender fibrovascular cores within a large duct is called an **intraductal papilloma** (**Figure 18–7**). This often comes to attention by causing a serous or bloody nipple discharge or a small mass. Surgical removal is indicated because a papilloma cannot be distinguished clinically

or radiographically from carcinoma. The most common proliferative lesion is **ductal hyperplasia**, or an increase in the number of layers of epithelial cells lining ducts (**Figure 18–8**). Ductal hyperplasia may come to attention by mammography because, especially if it is "florid," or widespread, it can be associated with dystrophic calcifications that mimic those seen in cancer. It usually does not form a mass lesion or result in a discharge. Intraductal papilloma and ductal hyperplasia double the lifetime risk of developing cancer. It is not necessarily the case that, if left in place, the lesion itself will develop into cancer.

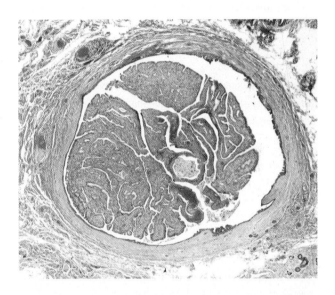

FIGURE 18–7 Intraductal papilloma. This photomicrograph shows a cross section of a breast duct that is filled and expanded by a growth with tightly compressed, finger-like processes, or papillae. An intraductal papilloma can occlude the duct it is growing in, resulting in obstruction, discharge, or a palpable mass.

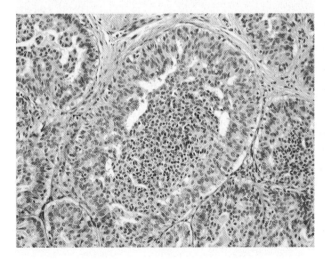

FIGURE 18–8 Ductal hyperplasia. Rather than having a lining composed of only two layers of cells, the lining of these ducts is multilayered. Epithelial cells are growing into and virtually occluding the lumens of the ducts.

Cancer can develop in the same breast far away from the lesion or in the opposite breast. Ductal hyperplasia may also be associated with cytologic atypia, meaning the cells resemble those seen in ductal carcinoma *in situ* (noninvasive cancer, described later). This is called **atypical ductal hyperplasia** and is associated with a four- to five-fold risk of developing cancer.

> **BOX 18–2   Fibrocystic Changes**
>
> **Causes**
> Unknown
> Fluctuating levels of hormones
> **Lesions**
> Fibrosis, cysts
> Proliferative epithelial lesions
> **Manifestations**
> Mass, nipple discharge on physical examination
> Mass, cyst, dystrophic calcifications on radiography
> Often bilateral
> Biopsy necessary for definitive diagnosis

Stromal Tumors

Overgrowth of the **stroma**, or fibrous connective tissue component, of lobules results in firm mass lesions. Stromal tumors can be benign or malignant. In a benign **fibroadenoma**, the stroma of a lobule expands and compresses the epithelial ducts and glands (**Figure 18–9**). It manifests as a painless, movable lump, most commonly in women 15 to 35 years of age. Fibroadenomas do not need to be removed because they do not impart an increased risk for the development of cancer. However, any change that affects the ductal epithelium—fibrocystic changes, atypical ductal hyperplasia, and cancer—can develop in the epithelium of a fibroadenoma. Such complications are very rare.

The malignant version of a stromal tumor is called a **phyllodes tumor**. The word *phyllodes* refers to the characteristic "leaflike" proliferation of malignant stroma, with individual bulbous processes surrounded by a benign epithelium (**Figure 18–10**). Like fibroadenoma, this tumor comes to attention by producing a mass lesion. It grows very quickly, can be very large when it is detected, and often recurs despite wide surgical excision. Phyllodes tumor usually occurs in women 40–50 years of age, or about 10 years older than those with fibroadenoma, and it is quite rare, representing only about 1% of all breast cancer.

> **BOX 18–3   Fibroadenoma**
>
> **Causes**
> Unknown
> **Lesions**
> Benign neoplasm of glandular and fibrous tissue
> **Manifestations**
> Discrete, movable mass
> Occurs in young women
> Biopsy for diagnosis

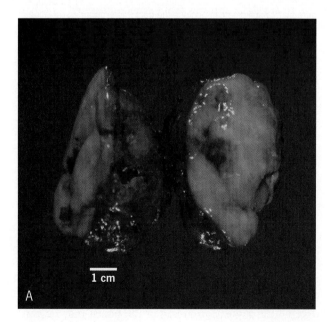

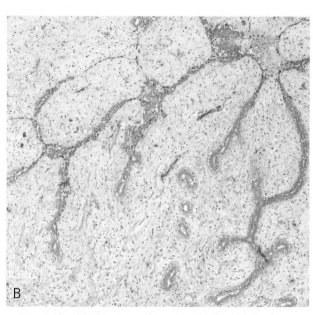

FIGURE 18–9 Fibroadenoma. **A.** Gross appearance. Notice how sharply circumscribed the lesion is and how solid it looks. You can imagine being able to feel this as a discrete lump in an otherwise soft breast. **B.** Microscopic appearance. Very dense, fibrous stroma is compressing the glands into long, narrow slits.

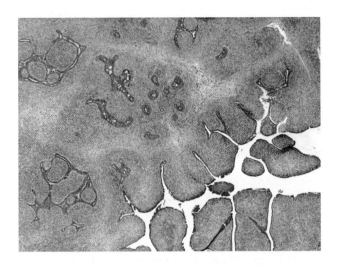

FIGURE 18–10 Phyllodes tumor. As in fibroadenoma, the stroma compresses the breast glands into narrow slits; however, the stroma is much more cellular than in fibroadenoma, and forms large bulbous processes (lower right).

Carcinoma of the Breast

Breast cancer is the cancer most frequently diagnosed in women in the United States and is the second leading cause of cancer-related deaths in women (lung cancer, though of lower incidence, causes more deaths). In terms of numbers, about 2.5 million women alive in the United States have a personal history of breast cancer, and about 40,000 women die each year of breast cancer. The lifetime risk of developing breast cancer is 12%. The median age at which breast cancer is diagnosed is 61 years, though the age range at which it affects women is very wide. Breast cancers are very rare before 30 years, but there is no upper limit to the age at which they can occur. The overall 5-year survival rate (all stages) is 90%, but 5-year survival varies tremendously by age, stage, and race. There is wide geographic variation in the occurrence of breast cancer. Breast cancer death rates are highest in industrialized Western nations and lowest in China, Japan, and Central American states (compare 26 deaths per 100,000 women in Denmark to 6 deaths per 100,000 women in China). The reasons for these wide discrepancies are the topic of much research in breast cancer epidemiology.

The strongest risk factor for development of breast cancer is a mutation in one of the **BRCA** genes (*BRCA-1* or *BRCA-2*); however, *BRCA* gene mutations account for only about 1–5% of breast cancers. The *BRCA* genes are tumor suppressor genes. They repair damaged DNA and prevent cell division in case the DNA damage cannot be repaired. Inheriting a mutation in one of these genes makes women five times more likely to develop breast cancer (in other words, the risk goes from 12% prevailing in the general population to 60%). Women with this mutation are also more susceptible to developing cancer in other organs, including the ovaries. Men who inherit abnormal *BRCA* genes are also at risk for developing male breast, pancreatic, testicular, and prostate cancer.

In addition to *BRCA*, many other genes have been linked to breast cancers arising in familial cancer syndromes such as Li-Fraumeni, Peutz-Jeghers, and Cowden syndromes. Genetic testing for specific mutations in these genes is available for individuals with a strong family history of cancer. Although there is a proven strong link between certain defective genes and breast cancer, altogether, inherited predispositions account for only about 10% of all breast cancers.

By far the majority of breast cancer is sporadic, meaning it does not occur in familial clusters. Sporadic breast cancers are genetically very heterogeneous, and the exact molecular pathways involved in their pathogenesis are not worked out. It is thought that they involve the same genes that are implicated in familial forms of breast cancer, but there are no firm data to support this speculation. Likewise, although we can say in general terms what the risk factors are for the development of sporadic breast cancer, we cannot say in any particular instance what precipitated its development. The pathogenesis of breast cancer appears to involve a complex interplay among genes, hormones, and possibly environmental, even dietary, factors.

Generally speaking, the biggest risk factor for the development of breast cancer is female sex, including both having breast tissue and being exposed to high levels of circulating estrogens during the reproductive years. **Mastectomy**, or surgical removal of all breast tissue, is protective against the development of breast cancer. Prophylactic mastectomy is advised for women with inherited breast cancer genes when they are done with childbearing and nursing. However, having breast tissue alone is not what puts women at risk because men also have breast tissue, but male breast cancer accounts for only 1% of breast cancer. Lifetime exposure of breast tissue to estrogen appears to be crucial. Women who had early menarche, late menopause, no or few children, did not breastfeed their infants (breastfeeding usually delays the onset of menstruation after childbirth by several months), are obese, and/or received exogenous estrogen therapy are more likely to develop breast cancer. Long-time exposure to estrogen somehow appears to drive the growth of malignant cells, though we do not know by what mechanism. Increasing age, white race, higher socioeconomic status, prior radiation exposure, alcohol consumption, and lack of physical activity also confer a higher risk of breast cancer.

Carcinoma of the breast can arise from the ductal or the lobular epithelium and is called *ductal carcinoma* or *lobular carcinoma*, accordingly. These look different under the microscope, and there are some differences in their behavior (e.g., lobular carcinoma tends to be low grade but does not always form a mass lesion, so it may not be detected until it is large), but clinically they are treated the same. Carcinoma of the breast may be confined to ducts or lobules, in which case it is called **carcinoma *in situ* (CIS)**, or it can infiltrate the surrounding tissue, in which case it is called **invasive**. **Figure 18–11**

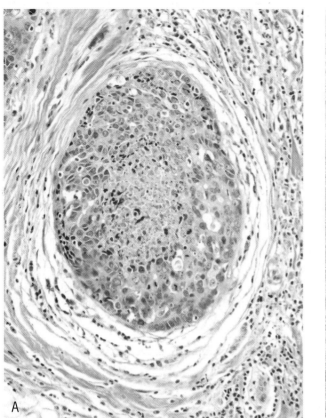 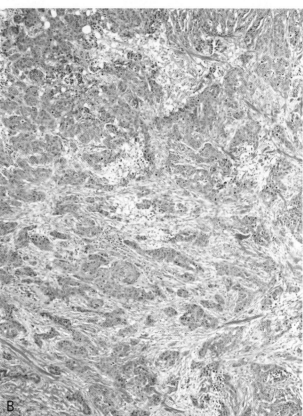

FIGURE 18–11 Ductal carcinoma of the breast. **A.** *In situ* ductal carcinoma (DCIS). The malignant cells fill and expand a duct lumen, but do not extend beyond the wall of the duct. **B.** Invasive ductal carcinoma. Malignant cells infiltrate extensively through the tissue, without regard to the preexisting structures of the breast.

illustrates the different histologic appearances of *in situ* and invasive ductal carcinoma. Ductal carcinoma *in situ* (DCIS) and lobular carcinoma *in situ* (LCIS) increase a woman's risk of developing invasive carcinoma by about 10 times. DCIS may itself progress to carcinoma, and surgical excision with wide margins is usually curative. LCIS, in contrast, is a marker for a generally increased risk of breast cancer in either breast. It is therefore usually not excised, but when it is found, usually incidentally on biopsy performed for some other reason, the woman is followed more closely by mammography or other radiographic technique.

The first modality for treatment of breast cancer is surgical excision. If the cancer is small, surgery may simply entail the removal of the cancer and a rim of benign mammary tissue around it. This is called **lumpectomy**. Lumpectomy is just as good as mastectomy for treatment of cancers that are less than 2 cm in diameter and have not spread to lymph nodes (see **Table 18–1** for stage groupings and 5-year survival for breast cancer). If cancers are more extensive than this, then some combination of radiation and chemotherapy is added to the treatment protocol.

Hormone therapy and targeted therapy are also treatment options. Their use depends on whether the malignant cells are expressing certain receptors on their cell surfaces. If the cells express estrogen receptor or progesterone receptor (in medical lingo this is called **ER positive**

or **PR positive**), they are responsive to and grow under the influence of estrogen. Antiestrogenic agents such as tamoxifen block estrogen signaling, which slows the growth of the malignant cells. Likewise, **Her2/neu** is a growth factor receptor that can be blocked with the agent trastuzumab. Cancers that express Her2/neu are generally very aggressive, but trastuzumab is effective in reducing their growth and preventing recurrence after surgery and chemotherapy.

In planning treatment, it is crucial to know the status of the lymph nodes. This is initially assessed by histologic examination of the **sentinel lymph node** (**Figure 18–12**). This is the first lymph node that receives lymph drainage from the area of the cancer. The sentinel lymph node is discovered by injecting a radioactive dye into the area of the cancer, and then massaging the tissue and waiting for the dye to be taken into the lymphatic spaces. Within a few minutes, the radioactive dye will have traveled to a lymph node, usually in the axilla but sometimes, especially if the cancer is more medially located, in the thoracic cavity. A probe can detect the radioactive substance emitted by the lymph node, effectively locating it for the surgeon to dissect. The node is then examined histologically. If there is cancer in the node, the likelihood is very high that there will be cancer in other lymph nodes as well, and the surgeon will then proceed to remove the additional nodal tissue. If the sentinel lymph node does

TABLE 18-1	Breast Cancer Stage Groupings and Corresponding Survival	
Stage	**Simplified Description**	**5-Year Survival**
Stage 0	Carcinoma *in situ*	100%
Stage IA	Tumor less than 2 cm	100%
Stage IB	Tumor less than 2 cm, with microscopic foci* of cancer in lymph nodes	
Stage IIA	Tumor less than 2 cm with spread to 1–3 axillary lymph nodes** OR Tumor between 2 and 5 cm without spread to lymph nodes	86%
Stage IIB	Tumor between 2 and 5 cm with spread to 1–3 axillary lymph nodes OR Tumor larger than 5 cm without extension to lymph nodes	
Stage IIIA	Tumor no more than 5 cm, with spread to 4–9 axillary lymph nodes or enlarged internal thoracic lymph nodes, OR Tumor larger than 5 cm with spread to up to 9 axillary lymph nodes	57%
Stage IIIB	Tumor of any size that has grown into chest wall or skin, with or without nodal spread	
Stage IIIC	Tumor of any size that has spread to 10 or more axillary lymph nodes, to axillary and internal thoracic lymph nodes, or to infra- or supraclavicular lymph nodes	
Stage IV	Cancer of any size with any degree of lymph node involvement, with spread to distant sites	20%

*Microscopic foci are tumor deposits less than 2 mm in diameter.
**Regional lymph nodes include both axillary and internal thoracic lymph nodes. Axillary lymph nodes are easily accessible to the surgeon, but internal thoracic (mammary) ones are usually sampled only when they are highlighted by the sentinel lymph node procedure. Involvement of internal thoracic lymph nodes imparts a slightly worse prognosis than involvement of axillary lymph nodes.

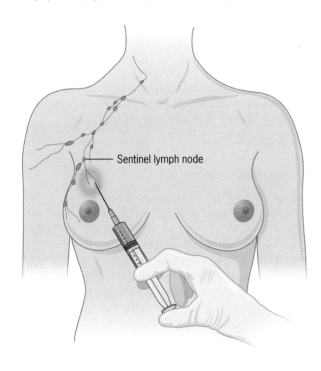

Sentinel lymph node

FIGURE 18-12 Schematic diagram of sentinel lymph node biopsy.

not contain cancer, the likelihood is very slim that there is cancer in the other lymph nodes, and they can be left in place. Preservation of the axillary lymph nodes prevents the morbidity associated with axillary lymph node dissection. Because these nodes also drain lymph from the arm, their removal causes obstruction to lymphatic flow and subsequent development of **lymphedema**, or extensive, unsightly, and uncomfortable swelling of the arm.

The most important prognostic factors for breast cancer are the size of the tumor, the status of the lymph nodes, ER/PR and Her2/neu status, and the grade of the tumor. The size of the tumor and the status of lymph nodes are incorporated into the stage grouping (Table 18–1), and ER/PR and Her2/neu expression are used to tailor therapy. The grade of the tumor is assessed microscopically, by determining how much of the tumor is composed of recognizable glands, how variable the nuclear morphology is, and how mitotically active the tumor is (**Figure 18–13**). Also, certain patterns of growth have been associated with clinical behavior. These correlations are not entirely predictive of behavior, however, and recently the traditional classification of breast cancer on the basis of morphology has been challenged by a molecular approach that classifies tumors by ER/PR and Her2/neu expression. Cancers that do not express any of these markers are called "triple negative" and have a poor prognosis because they are not responsive to hormonal or targeted therapy.

With the advent of widespread mammography as a screening tool, breast cancers are mostly detected in Stage I—in other words, when they are still small lesions confined to the breast. Also, many cancers are found when they are still in the *in situ* stage, and surgical excision prevents the progression of these lesions to invasive carcinoma. The 5-year survival for Stage I breast cancers after surgical excision with wide margins is 100%. These reassuring statistics should not lull us into thinking that we have a good handle on breast cancer, however. The death rate has not decreased significantly in the past few years. Hormonal and targeted therapy have had limited success in preventing death, and breast cancer is still the second leading cause of cancer-related deaths in women.

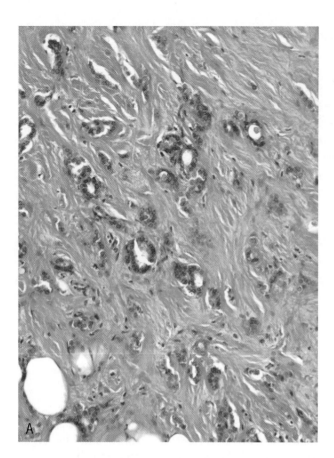
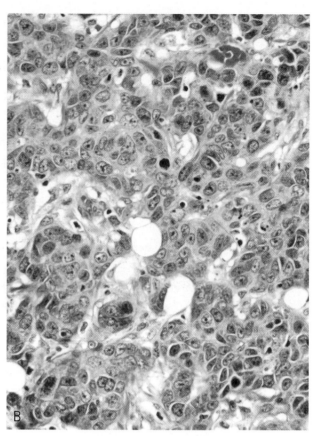

FIGURE 18–13 Grade of mammary carcinoma. **A.** Low-grade invasive ductal carcinoma. The malignancy consists of small, irregular but recognizable glands infiltrating through a fibrous stroma. The cells have nuclei of fairly uniform size. **B.** High-grade invasive ductal carcinoma. The cells are not forming glands, but are clustered together haphazardly. The nuclei are large and of irregular sizes and shapes.

When advanced, breast cancer can metastasize widely, primarily to the lungs, liver, bone, or brain.

BOX 18–4   Carcinoma of the Breast

Causes

Proliferative fibrocystic changes

Genetic predisposition (*BRCA* genes, *p53, PTEN*)

Female sex

Lifetime estrogen exposure

Age, radiation, alcohol

Geographic variation

Lesions

Ductal or lobular adenocarcinoma

Metastases to regional lymph nodes and other organs

Manifestations

Mass detected on mammography or physical examination

Clusters of abnormal calcifications on mammography

Rarely, secondary changes in breast (nipple retraction, skin ulcer), palpable lymph nodes or distant metastasis

Diagnosis by biopsy and microscopic examination

Lesions of the Male Breast

Enlargement of the male breast tissue caused by proliferation of ducts and connective tissues is called gynecomastia. Male breast tissue does not contain terminal lobular units, only ducts, and, as in women, the ducts and their surrounding stroma proliferate under the influence of circulating estrogens. Estrogen can be increased in men secondary to estrogen-secreting neoplasms, estrogenic drugs such as digitalis and marijuana, cirrhosis of the liver with decreased metabolism of the normally small amounts of estrogen produced by males, Klinefelter syndrome, obesity, and aging with decreased countereffects of androgens. Gynecomastia presents as subareolar swelling, which can be mistaken for cancer. Surgical excision is curative, but the underlying cause of hyperestrinism should be determined and treated.

Carcinoma of the male breast accounts for 1% of all breast cancers, and the lifetime risk of developing it is 0.11%. It can occur in familial settings. The *BRCA*-2 gene is the one most strongly linked to male breast cancer. In sporadic cases, male breast cancer is a disease of the older adult with a somewhat worse prognosis than cancer of the female breast because it is usually detected at a higher stage.

Practice Questions

1. Which of the following statements about breast cancer is correct?
   A. Breast cancer is the leading cause of cancer-related deaths in women in the United States.
   B. Breast cancer usually occurs in the setting of familial (inherited) cancer syndromes.
   C. The incidence of breast cancer is about the same all over the world.
   D. In the United States, breast cancer is usually detected at an early stage.
   E. Breast cancer is usually diagnosed in premenopausal women.

2. The milk-producing part of the breast is called the
   A. nipple.
   B. lactiferous duct.
   C. lobule.
   D. adipose tissue.
   E. areola.

3. A 25-year-old woman notes a round, movable, painless lump in her breast. A biopsy would most likely show
   A. lobular carcinoma.
   B. duct ectasia.
   C. intraductal papilloma.
   D. fibroadenoma.
   E. phyllodes tumor.

4. Which of the following statements about mammography is correct?
   A. Mammography cannot be used reliably in older women because fibrous tissue increases with age.
   B. Dense areas with irregular outlines and clusters of calcifications are concerning for breast cancer.
   C. Mammography cannot detect lumps that are not palpable.
   D. Mammography can be used to differentiate between solid lesions and fluid-filled cysts.
   E. Mammography is no better than ultrasound in detecting cancer.

5. A positive sentinel lymph node
   A. means the cancer is widely metastatic.
   B. means the patient has to have a mastectomy rather than lumpectomy.
   C. is usually detected by palpation of a lump in the axilla.
   D. means the patient will require hormone therapy.
   E. needs to be followed with dissection of the remaining axillary lymph nodes.

Skin

OUTLINE

OBJECTIVES

1. Review the structure and function of the skin.
2. Name the most common life-threatening conditions and malignant neoplasms of the skin.
3. Recognize that some skin lesions are manifestations of systemic disease, and name some of the systemic diseases that can manifest on the skin.
4. Be able to define the terms used to describe skin lesions (*macule, patch, papule, plaque, nodule, pustule, vesicle, bulla, wheal, scale, crust*).
5. Identify the role of biopsy and microscopic examination in the diagnosis of skin diseases, including melanoma.
6. Compare and contrast albinism and xeroderma pigmentosum.
7. Define *dermatitis*, and name some of the more common causes of dermatitis.
8. Identify the causative agent of verrucae, name the locations at which verrucae are likely to occur, and list the names given to verrucae at different locations.
9. Describe the etiology of acne and define *comedone* and *pustule*.
10. Name the various types of skin abscesses.
11. Name and describe the superficial fungal infestations (what they are caused by and where they occur).
12. Compare and contrast atopic and contact dermatitis, and give examples of each.
13. Describe the clinical manifestation of impetigo, urticaria, seborrheic dermatitis, and psoriasis.
14. Differentiate between melanoma and nonmelanoma skin cancers in terms of cell of origin, risk factors, age of occurrence, treatment, and prognosis.
15. Name and describe the benign and malignant conditions of the skin that are related to sun exposure.

[handwritten notes at top of page: "4 levels D: Basal layer B: Granular Layer C: Spinous layer A: Cornified Layer"]

16. Describe how to clinically differentiate benign from malignant melanocytic proliferations.
17. Describe the life-threatening complications that occur with extensive denudation of the skin, and explain how these need to be managed.
18. Define and be able to use in context all the words in bold print and in headings throughout the chapter.

KEY TERMS

acral lentiginous melanoma	lentigo
actinic	lentigo maligna melanoma
actinic keratosis	macule
albinism	marsupialization
alopecia	melanin
apocrine gland	melanocyte
atopic dermatitis	melanocytic nevus
basal cell carcinoma	melanoma
basal layer	melanoma *in situ*
biopsy	melasma
boil	mole
burn unit	nevocellular nevus
candidiasis	nodular melanoma
carbuncle	nonmelanoma skin cancer
chancre	papule
comedone	paronychia
compound nevus	pilonidal cyst
condyloma	port wine stain
acuminatum	pruritus
congenital nevus	rash
cornified layer	ringworm
cradle cap	sebaceous gland
dermatitis	seborrheic keratosis
dermis	shingles
dysplastic nevus	solar elastosis
eccrine gland	solar keratosis
eczema	solar lentigo
ephelides	spinous layer
epidermis	squamous cell carcinoma
eruptive xanthoma	subcutis
exfoliative	superficial spreading
flare	melanoma
furuncle	telangiectasia
granular layer	tinea (various types)
hirsutism	toxic epidermal necrolysis
intradermal nevus	verruca plana
junctional nevus	verruca vulgaris
keratinocyte	wheal
keratosis	xeroderma pigmentosum

Review of Structure and Function

The skin functions as a barrier between the body and its external environment, protecting the body from injury by external forces and preventing excessive loss of body fluids. The skin also constitutes a major sense organ; cutaneous sensations of touch, temperature, pressure, and pain are essential to maintain orientation in the environment. In addition, the skin plays a vital role in regulation of body temperature, both by controlling the amount of blood brought near the surface for heat exchange and through the process of sweating, which lowers skin temperature through vaporization.

Histologically, as depicted in **Figure 19–1**, the skin consists of an outer covering of stratified squamous epithelium (**epidermis**); an underlying layer of fibrous connective tissue (**dermis**), which contains the hair follicles, sebaceous and sweat glands, blood vessels, and sensory nerves; and a deep layer of adipose tissue (**subcutis** or subcutaneous tissue).

The epidermis is a stratified squamous epithelium composed of cells called **keratinoyctes**. It has four major morphologic divisions (**Figure 19–2**). The deepest, the **basal layer**, is a single layer of predominantly cuboidal germinative cells that gives rise to all other epidermal cells by mitotic division. The broad middle zone known as the **spinous layer** consists of several layers of keratinocytes undergoing progressive maturation while producing keratin fibrils. In the **granular layer**, the keratinocytes acquire keratohyaline granules and form rows parallel to the skin surface. These cells eventually die and shed their nucleus to form the outermost layer known as the **cornified layer**. The thickness of this layer varies greatly in different body sites; for example, it is very thick over the palm and fingers and very thin on the eyelid. Scattered throughout the basal layer are larger, pale cells that may contain brown granules. These cells, called **melanocytes**, are embryologically derived from the neural crest and produce brown **melanin** pigment, which helps protect the skin from sunlight damage and contributes to skin color. The concentration of melanocytes varies widely, with melanocytes being almost twice as numerous in the genital area as on the back. Melanin production is increased when the skin is exposed to sunlight. This is why fair-skinned individuals tan when exposed to sun.

The dermis consists of fibrous tissue intermixed with elastin fibers. The high collagen concentration provides great skin resistance to mechanical force and the elastin allows the skin to return to its normal form after mechanical deformation. When elastin fibers are destroyed with aging or disease, the skin becomes loose and wrinkled. A gel-like ground substance holds the dermal fibers together. **Eccrine glands** (Figure 19–1) are present in the deep dermis over nearly the entire surface of the body and are responsible for the production of sweat in response to heat stress. **Apocrine glands** occur in a restricted distribution (axillae, pubis, perineum, periumbilical region, nipples, ear canal, margin of the lips) and produce a sticky proteinaceous and lipid-rich fluid in response to hormonal stimuli. Apocrine glands are largely dormant until puberty. With the exception of palms, soles, and portions of the genitalia, the entire body surface is covered by hair. Individual hairs are produced by division of cells lining the hair follicle. Each hair follicle, or bulb, undergoes recurring cycles of hair growth, regression, and rest. Attached to each hair follicle is a **sebaceous gland** (Figure 19–1), which secretes lipid-rich sebum. Sebum waterproofs skin and hair and protects them from dehydration.

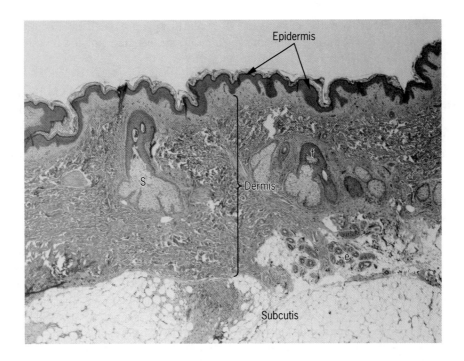

FIGURE 19–1 Histologic components of the skin. The fairly thin epidermis lies over a much thicker, collagenous dermis, which contains skin appendages such as the eccrine glands (e) and sebaceous glands (s). Sebaceous glands empty sebum, or oil, into hair follicles (f), which extend from the dermis to the surface of the epidermis and are composed of the same cell layers as the epidermis.

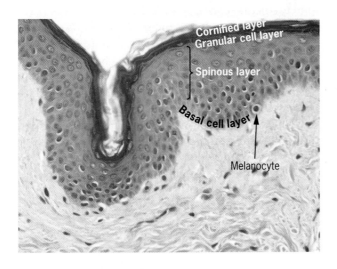

FIGURE 19–2 Layers of the epidermis.

Most Frequent and Serious Problems

Among the most common dermatologic problems that may prompt a person to seek medical attention are cuts, abscesses, acne, nevi (moles), warts (verrucae), eczematous dermatitis, seborrheic dermatitis (dandruff), and rashes of various types. Brown-black, stuck-on-appearing, warty lesions called **seborrheic keratoses** commonly occur on the face, trunk, and extremities of persons past middle age and are usually multiple. Older persons who have been exposed to sunlight for many years frequently have small precancerous lesions, so-called **actinic** or **solar keratoses**, or early skin cancers on exposed surfaces.

Life-threatening skin conditions include extensive burns and severe drug reactions with sloughing of portions of the epidermis, a condition called **toxic epidermal necrolysis.** Loss or destruction of large areas of epidermis is always potentially lethal because of the resulting loss of body fluids and because of the high risk of secondary infection by organisms such as *Staphylococcus aureus* and *Pseudomonas aeruginosa.* There are about 700,000 visits to emergency departments in the United States every year for burn injuries. At greatest risk of sustaining burns are young children, who are at risk for scalding accidents; young men who engage in risky activities involving fires; and older patients whose skin receptors for heat are compromised and who are thus likely to sustain injury from hot surfaces such as electric heating pads. People who have lost more than 20% of their body surface area because of burns or **exfoliative** conditions such as toxic epidermal necrolysis must be treated in specialized intensive care units called **burn units**. The serious sequelae of burn injuries emphasize the critical importance of skin in thermoregulation, preservation of fluid, and protecting the internal environment from bacteria and toxins.

Skin lesions may be important indicators of systemic disease. Cutaneous eruptions, most commonly a red rash over both cheeks and the bridge of the nose, occur in many patients with systemic lupus erythematosus and often constitute an early sign of this disease. Deposits of urate crystals frequently occur in patients with gout. These chalky deposits most commonly occur in the subcutis of the helix of the ear and over the elbows and digits of hands and feet. Well-circumscribed areas of brown, slightly atrophic skin are common on the lower extremities of diabetics. An eruption of small yellow papules on the extensor surfaces of the extremities and buttocks, called **eruptive xanthoma**, is indicative of a significant elevation in plasma triglyceride levels as can be seen in hereditary disorders of lipid metabolism or uncontrolled diabetes. Some degree of hyperpigmentation of skin occurs in 90% of pregnant women, with the most striking manifestation being mask-like pigmentation of the face known as **melasma**. Freckles and nevi may appear darker during pregnancy.

Skin cancers are the most common malignancy overall. In fact, basal cell carcinoma and squamous cell carcinoma, so-called **nonmelanoma skin cancers**, are so common that they are by convention left out of cancer statistics. When we say, for example, that lung cancer is the number one cancer in the United States, this is bending the facts: about 219,000 people are diagnosed with lung cancer in the United States every year, but about 3.5 million people are diagnosed annually with nonmelanoma skin cancer. The reason this type of cancer is left out of the statistics is that, in contrast to all other cancers, nonmelanoma skin cancer very rarely metastasizes and even more rarely causes death. **Melanoma**, however, is included in the cancer statistics for exactly those reasons: it is a malignant neoplasm of melanocytes that can be deadly. Melanoma is the eighth most commonly diagnosed cancer in the United States; about 69,000 people will develop it every year; and the overall 5-year survival is about 90%. Melanoma has a propensity to gain access to the lymphovascular system and metastasize even if it has not invaded very deeply at its site of origin. Although melanoma and nonmelanoma skin cancers are quite different in pathology, natural history, and prognosis, they share a common risk factor: sun exposure. Premalignant and early neoplastic lesions, including squamous cell carcinoma *in situ*, actinic keratosis, melanoma *in situ*, and dysplastic nevi, are much more commonly removed than are the frankly malignant and invasive counterparts.

Symptoms, Signs, and Tests

Most skin diseases are not life threatening, but many are distressing to patients because of unsightly appearance, itching (**pruritus**), or pain. Unlike diseases of other body systems, skin diseases are readily visible—if they are looked for. Lesions on the face, arms, legs, hands and feet, and abdomen are readily seen by the patient himself/herself. Those on the back, neck, axillae, and posterior surface of the legs or ears may be seen by a concerned friend or family member. Other areas require a little more diligence to inspect—the perineal region, the skin in the gluteal fold, the skin of the scalp, behind the ears, between the toes, and other nooks and crannies of the body. Distress over the appearance of skin lesions and fear of cancer are perhaps the most common concerns of patients with skin disease, but it cannot be stressed enough how important it is to visually examine every square centimeter of a patient's body for potential lesions.

Often, the gross appearance of the lesions and the history of their development are sufficient to make a diagnosis. The gross appearance is described in terms of size, location on the body, multiplicity, color, shape, and texture. Lesions that are flat are termed **macular** and those that are raised are called **papular**. **Rashes** are temporary eruptions on the skin that can have a multitude of causes, including systemic infections (measles, rubella, chickenpox, scarlet fever, secondary syphilis), hypersensitivity reactions to food or drugs, and local reactions to surface contact with topical drugs and allergenic or irritating substances. The following terms are commonly used to describe the gross appearance of skin lesions. Their appearance is depicted in **Figure 19–3**.

- *Macule*: Change in skin color; not raised or depressed, <10 mm
- *Patch*: Change in skin color; not raised or depressed, 10 mm or larger

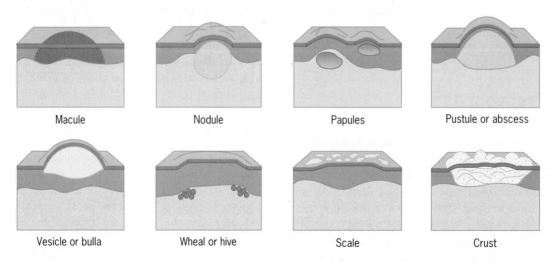

| Macule | Nodule | Papules | Pustule or abscess |
| Vesicle or bulla | Wheal or hive | Scale | Crust |

FIGURE 19–3 The appearance of various types of skin lesions.

- *Papule*: Raised lesion, <10 mm
- *Plaque*: Elevated lesion, 10 mm or larger
- *Nodule*: Knot or lump, typically a thick (and/or deep), solid lesion
- *Pustule or abscess*: Elevated skin lesion containing pus
- *Vesicle or bulla (blister)*: Bubble-like swelling containing air or fluid
- *Wheal or hive*: Ridge-like reddened elevation caused by edema
- *Scale*: Flaky superficial material (keratin) that easily separates from the skin
- *Crust*: Hardened, adherent serum on skin surface over a lesion

Visual examination of the skin, sometimes with the help of a magnifying glass, is extended to microscopic examination of **biopsies** taken from lesions. This allows differentiation of inflammatory eruptions and neoplastic lesions. Excisional biopsy may be used in the evaluation of cutaneous malignancies and often constitutes the sole treatment. Laboratory tests are indicated under selected circumstances, including culturing a purulent lesion for bacteria, preparing a smear when fungal infection is suspected, or ordering blood tests when there is a concern for systemic disease.

Specific Diseases

Genetic/Developmental Diseases

Hemangiomas and neurofibromatosis are mentioned elsewhere in this text. Major inherited disorders of hair distribution and pigmentation are included in this category because they can be considered specific diseases. Acquired problems of hair distribution and pigmentation are possible manifestations of a wide variety of diseases and are not specifically discussed.

Vascular Lesions (Hemangiomas and Capillary Malformations)

Infantile hemangiomas arise in the neonatal period. They are proliferations of small blood vessels in the dermis that present as elevated red or blue-purple lesions. They have an early rapid growth phase followed by slower spontaneous involution. **Port wine stains** (capillary malformations) appear faint pink in early infancy and become progressively darker and thicker with age. Port wine stains that involve one segment of the forehead may be associated with vascular lesions in the brain, seizure disorders, and developmental delay.

Hair Disorders

The distribution, color, and texture of scalp and body hair are genetically determined and influenced by hormones. Excessive body hair is called **hirsutism** and may be particularly distressing to female patients. Early onset

of baldness, or **alopecia,** in men is determined by polygenic inheritance and environmental factors. Though by far less common, it can also occur in women.

Disorders of Pigmentation

Albinism is an uncommon autosomal recessive hereditary condition in which melanocytes are unable to produce normal amounts of melanin pigment. Patients lack normal pigmentation in skin, hair, and irises. The absence of normal cutaneous melanin renders the patient markedly sensitive to sunlight and predisposes him or her to increased incidence of basal and squamous cell cancers. **Xeroderma pigmentosum** is a rare autosomal recessive condition characterized by intolerance of skin and eyes to sunlight, with development of skin cancers in childhood or early adult life. Affected patients lack enzymes necessary to repair damage to DNA caused by sunlight.

BOX 19–1   Disorders of Pigmentation

Causes

Autosomal recessive inheritance

Lesions

Diminished skin pigmentation (albinism)

Impaired DNA repair mechanisms (xeroderma pigmentosum)

Manifestations

Pale skin, hair, irises (albinism)

Dyspigmentation with multiple skin cancers (xeroderma pigmentosum)

Infectious and Inflammatory Diseases

The first part of this section deals with the various types of skin infections and the situations in which they occur. This is followed by a discussion of the various forms of dermatitis. Although **dermatitis** literally means inflammation of the skin, the term is usually used in a narrower sense to describe patchy noninfectious inflammations that may be chronic or allergic in nature. Finally, acute edema (urticaria) and chronic scaling skin diseases are discussed.

Viral Exanthems

Rashes of various viral diseases are most often seen in children, and their clinical appearance and distribution are the basis for diagnosis of measles, rubella, and chickenpox. Varicella zoster virus, the causative agent of chickenpox, can lie dormant in nerve cell bodies for decades after the childhood infection and flare suddenly to cause **shingles**. This is an exquisitely painful rash that is usually limited to a specific region of the body and does not cross the midline. It resolves within a few weeks, but patients may have residual nerve pain for months or years afterward. Shingles usually occurs in older patients or in patients who are immunosuppressed.

Verrucae (Warts)

Human papillomaviruses of several strains cause neoplastic proliferations of stratified squamous epithelium. Most of these are benign, but some carry a risk of malignant transformation. Three different patterns of disease, caused by different strains of papillomavirus, are **verruca vulgaris** (common wart), **verruca plana** (flat wart), and **condyloma acuminatum** (genital wart).

Verruca vulgaris (**Figure 19–4**) occurs on exposed body parts, particularly the fingers and back of the hand, and is a raised, papillated, dry lesion. Warts on the palms and soles (Figure 19–4A) are flat or elevated lesions that may be painful, especially when pressure is applied on them. Warts on the face and neck may form tiny finger-like projections. Verrucae vulgares are common in children but may occur at any age. Although warts eventually regress spontaneously, they may cause considerable pain and discomfort, especially when frequently traumatized. Verrucae planae, or flat warts, are small smooth-topped, skin-toned papules that can present in a linear array if inoculated via trauma. Condylomata acuminata occur on oral (Figure 19–4B) and anogenital mucous membranes and can be spread by venereal contact, particularly in young adults.

Various techniques are used to destroy verrucae, including freezing them with liquid nitrogen and burning them with electrocautery, but eradication is difficult because of persistence of the virus in the basal keratinocytes, which are not always destroyed by these methods. Also, the skin adjacent to lesions may already be infected by virus by autoinoculation, but not yet demonstrate a verrucous growth, so it would be spared destruction. If very large and uncomfortable, the lesions can be removed by surgery.

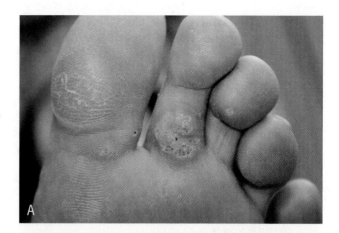

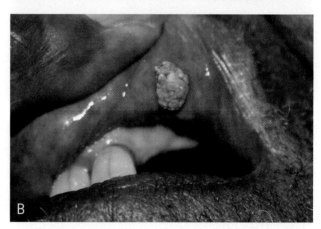

FIGURE 19–4 Verrucae. **A.** Verruca vulgaris on the plantar aspect of a foot. **B.** Condyloma acuminatum on the mucous membrane of the lip. (Courtesy of Yale Residents' Slide Collection, Dermatology Department, Yale University School of Medicine.)

BOX 19–2   Verrucae (Warts)

Causes

Human papillomavirus

Lesions

Discrete raised proliferation of squamous epithelium, often with a rough surface

Manifestations

Verrucous papule on exposed parts of body (verruca vulgaris, verruca plana)

Papule on mucous membranes (condyloma acuminatum)

Acne

The presence of **comedones** (blackheads and whiteheads) and multiple recurrent crops of pustules on the face, neck, and upper back during puberty and early adulthood are characteristic of acne (**Figure 19–5**). The comedone is the basic lesion of acne. It is caused by plugging of hair follicles and associated sebaceous gland ducts with lipid and keratin, producing a slightly raised lesion

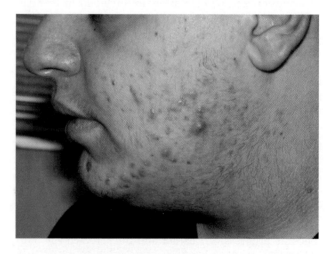

FIGURE 19–5 Acne on the face of an adolescent. (Courtesy of Dr. Richard Antaya, Department of Dermatology, Yale School of Medicine.)

that can be closed (whitehead) or open (blackhead). Comedones can subsequently become colonized by the bacteria *Propionibacterium acnes*. The accumulating keratin, oil, and bacterial colonies eventually cause the blocked duct to rupture, spilling debris into the dermis and precipitating a brisk acute inflammatory reaction. Other, more virulent organisms may infect the lesions secondarily, producing tiny abscesses.

The severity of acne varies greatly among individuals, suggesting hereditary and hormonal influences on sebaceous glands. Acne may be aggravated by emotional stress and administration of corticosteroids. Severe cases lead to scarring, which may be disfiguring. Treatment is directed toward reduction of follicular plugging by gentle washing of the face, reduction of bacterial burden with topical or oral antibiotics, regulation of the development of the squamous lining of the hair follicle and sebum production with topical or oral retinoid drugs, and, in very severe cases, reduction of inflammation with steroids.

BOX 19–3   Acne

Causes

Plugs of keratin and sebum in hair follicles

Propionibacterium acnes

Chemical irritation

Secondary infection

Endocrine factors (androgen release during puberty)

Hereditary factors

Lesions

Comedone

Inflammatory papules and pustules

Manifestations

Open and closed comedones and pustules

Occurs in adolescents and young adults

Facial scarring (late)

Abscess

Skin abscesses are localized skin infections forming walled-off collections of pus. *S. aureus* is the most common infectious organism. Skin abscesses can occur at sites of skin trauma, around hair follicles, and around embedded foreign material, such as splinters. **Paronychia** is the occurrence of abscesses in the folds around the nails (**Figure 19–6**). A **pilonidal cyst** is an abscess occurring around ingrown hair in the skin just above the gluteal fold. Other common sites of abscess formation are around the anus and on the back of the neck. Small abscesses centered about a hair follicle are known as **furuncles** or **boils.** These begin as painful, elevated, red areas, and then develop a white, soft center that represents liquefaction necrosis of tissue with accumulation of purulent exudate. If uncomplicated, the furuncle is gradually walled-off, ruptures to release the exudate, and then collapses to heal with a small scar. Healing of an abscess is accelerated by incision and drainage. Recurrent abscesses, such as pilonidal cysts, may require excision of the sinus tract or **marsupialization** (incising the cyst

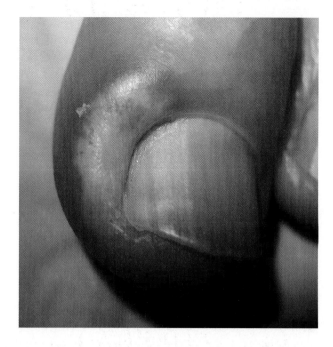

FIGURE 19–6 Paronychia, with swelling due to collection of purulent exudate around the nail. (Courtesy of Yale Residents' Slide Collection, Dermatology Department, Yale University School of Medicine.)

and suturing the exposed flap to adjacent tissue) so that the cyst is open and can drain to the surface. Splinters and other foreign materials should be removed, preferably before an abscess develops. A **carbuncle** is a group of furuncles with associated connecting sinus tracts and multiple openings on the skin. This uncommon lesion usually occurs on the back of the neck. Diabetics are especially prone to develop carbuncles because of their reduced resistance to infection.

BOX 19–4   Abscess

Causes

Trauma

Foreign bodies

Lesions

Abscess in dermis or subcutis

Furuncle carbuncle

Paronychia

Pilonidal cyst

Manifestations

Pain, swelling, heat, redness

Purulent discharge

Impetigo

Impetigo is a superficial bacterial skin infection that occurs predominantly in children and is characterized by flaccid bullae that easily rupture to form crusted erosions (**Figure 19–7**). The face is a common site of involvement. *S. aureus* is most commonly the causative organism. Impetigo is contagious and may spread rapidly in crowded conditions.

> ### BOX 19–5   Impetigo
>
> **Causes**
>
> Unknown factors
>
> *Staphylococcus aureus*
>
> **Lesions**
>
> Multiple superficial facial inflammatory foci developing into pustules
>
> Flaccid vesicles and bullae, erosions with honey-colored crusting
>
> **Manifestations**
>
> Occurs in children
>
> Facial lesions in varying stages from mild inflammation to blisters to pustules

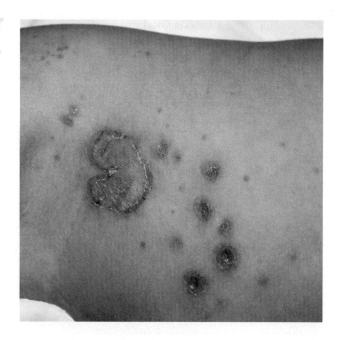

FIGURE 19–7 Bullous impetigo. (Courtesy of Yale Residents' Slide Collection, Dermatology Department, Yale University School of Medicine.)

Syphilis

The primary lesion of syphilis, known as a **chancre**, occurs at the site of entry of the causative organism, *Treponema pallidum*, and takes about 3 weeks to develop. Common sites of chancres include the mucous membranes of the penis, vagina, cervix, anus, and mouth. The chancre is usually a single, painless ulcer that heals spontaneously in 4 to 12 weeks. It contains many spirochetes and is highly contagious even though serologic tests for syphilis may be negative at this stage. The secondary stage of syphilis may be associated with a variety of cutaneous manifestations, most commonly a maculopapular eruption on the trunk or extremities (**Figure 19–8**), often with involvement of the palms and soles.

Superficial Fungal Infections

In superficial fungal infections, the fungi are located in the cornified layers of the skin, nail, or hair and can often be demonstrated in a smear prepared from skin scrapings. The dermis is not infected. The two main types of superficial fungal infection of the skin are **ringworm** (**tinea**) and **candidiasis**. Ringworm is not caused by a worm but by various fungi. Regardless of the site affected, the lesions are typically pink or red scaly patches; blisters, pustules, or fissures may also occur. The lesions may itch. Different forms of tinea are transmitted from person to person, from animal to person, or from soil/environmental sources to humans. The most common form of superficial fungal infection is **tinea pedis** (athlete's foot), which affects the soles and interdigital spaces of the feet. Hereditary and immunologic factors, sweating, and type of foot covering all appear to play a part in the etiology of this infection. **Tinea cruris** (jock itch) is a superficial fungal infection involving the perineum, buttocks, and/or inner thighs. Infection of the scalp

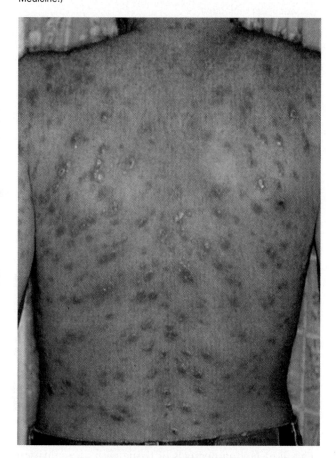

FIGURE 19–8 Secondary rash of syphilis.

(**tinea capitis**) and beard (**tinea barbae**) cause breaking of hairs and focal hair loss. Fungal infections of the nails produce opaque, discolored painless patches within the nail. In late stages of infection, the nail is deformed and

TABLE 19–1	Classification and Characteristics of Dermatitis			
Type	**Morphologic Pattern**	**Location**	**Frequency**	**Severity**
Contact	Eczema	Site of allergen contact	Most common	Distressing, recurrent
Atopic	Eczema	Begins on face, extremities late	Common	Disfiguring, impaired function
Seborrheic	Greasy, scaling	Scalp, face, trunk	Common	Widely variable
Light-induced	Eczema or rash	Exposed skin	Common	Usually mild
Exfoliative	Sloughing of superficial epidermis	Total body	Uncommon	May be fatal

eventually destroyed. Most cutaneous superficial fungal infections are eradicated by treatment with topical agents. Nail fungus is particularly difficult to eradicate.

Superficial infections with *Candida albicans* (cutaneous candidiasis) may be focal or widespread and produce moist red plaques, characteristically with pustules at the margin. Factors that predispose to superficial *Candida* infection include diabetes mellitus, leukemia, lymphoma, treatment with antibacterial or immunosuppressive drugs, and chronic exposure to moisture. Involvement of folds of skin or skin between the digits is frequent in diabetics. Candidiasis of the perioral skin (perleche) produces red cracks (fissures) at the corners of the mouth. People who chronically have their hands in water, such as bartenders and dishwashers, may develop chronic paronychia and candidiasis of the fingernails manifested as painless, red swelling of the skin around the nail, loss of the cuticle, and yellow discoloration of the nail. Chronic paronychia associated with candidal infection can be difficult to eradicate.

BOX 19–6   Superficial Fungal Infections

Causes

Tinea

Candida

Lesions

Fungi in cornified layer

Moist red patches or thin plaques with satellite pustules

Manifestations

Scaling skin lesions in characteristic areas

Dermatitis in General

Dermatitis is a generic, clinical term used to describe a wide variety of skin conditions, all characterized by inflammation of the skin. Dermatitis occurs in response to a wide variety of stimuli, including drugs, chemical allergens, ultraviolet radiation, local trauma, and various metabolic and immunologic disorders. **Eczema** is a term often used as a synonym for **atopic dermatitis**, a chronic, relapsing form of dermatitis with a genetic basis.

Dermatitis accounts for about one-third of patients who consult a dermatologist. Acute dermatitis is red and exudative, with many minute erosions and crusts. In later stages, the skin becomes scaly and thickened, with accentuation of normal skin lines (lichenification). Severe pruritus may accompany any stage of disease. Thickening of the lesion is largely a reaction to prolonged scratching.

Histologic features in dermatitis are usually nonspecific, and diagnosis of the specific type of dermatitis depends primarily on the clinical evolution and distribution of the lesions. Ideally, classification of dermatitis is based on etiology. In many patients, however, a cause cannot be determined. The types described in **Table 19–1** represent a mixed classification based on cause and morphology.

Contact Dermatitis

This is a type of eczematous dermatitis that occurs as a delayed-type hypersensitivity reaction to chemical allergens in items such as clothes, cosmetics, jewelry, and various metals. Because skin changes occur at the site of allergen contact, the location and configuration of the skin eruption often provides an important clue as to the causative agent (**Figure 19–9**). A suspected substance can be placed on a patch on the patient's back to test for reactivity (patch test). A local reaction to the offending substance will manifest under the patch after 48 to 72 hours. Avoidance of the causative allergen is imperative for resolution of the eruption and often entails a change in work or personal activities. Contact dermatitis may be subclassified by the causative agents.

Poison ivy is a common example of contact dermatitis (**Figure 19–10**). Vesicles, often linear, develop at the site of contact with the oil of poison ivy leaves. This reaction occurs in previously sensitized persons within 1–2 days

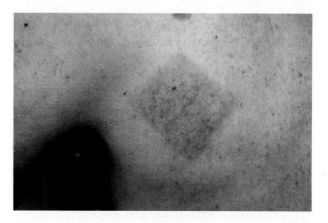

FIGURE 19–9 Allergic dermatitis resulting from reaction to nicotine patch. (Courtesy of Yale Residents' Slide Collection, Dermatology Department, Yale University School of Medicine.)

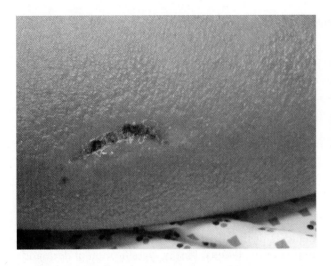

FIGURE 19–10 Poison ivy. The skin is red and swollen, and there are numerous tiny fluid-filled vesicles all over the skin surface. (Courtesy of Dr. Richard Antaya, Department of Dermatology, Yale School of Medicine.)

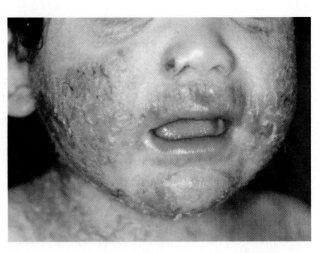

FIGURE 19–11 Atopic dermatitis (eczema) on the face of a small child. (Courtesy of Dr. Richard Antaya, Department of Dermatology, Yale School of Medicine.)

of contact. Spread of the plant oils to other body parts may extend the eruption beyond the initial site of contact. When poison ivy is severe, it may be advisable to treat the patient with systemic corticosteroids to reduce the inflammatory reaction. In sensitized individuals, poison oak plants and sumac bushes can also produce allergic contact dermatitis.

BOX 19-7   Contact Dermatitis

Causes

Environmental allergens, such as can be found in clothes, cosmetics, metals, plants, chemicals

Specific example: poison ivy

Lesions

Inflammation of skin

Blister formation in epidermis

Manifestations

Erythematous, eczematous pruritic patch or plaque corresponding to area of contact

Blisters in region of contact with poison ivy oil

Appearance of rash within hours of contact in previously sensitized individual

---

Atopic Dermatitis

Atopic dermatitis is a multifactorial disease with a genetic basis that is influenced by environmental factors. Atopic dermatitis, also called eczema, most commonly occurs in individuals having other manifestations of atopy (allergy), such as asthma and allergic rhinitis (hay fever). It usually begins in infancy with eczema of the face (**Figure 19–11**), scalp, and extensor surfaces such as knees, and then transitions in children and adults to characteristic involvement of the neck and inner (flexor) surfaces of the elbows

and knees. This condition is characterized by severe itching. Edematous papules and exudative plaques, often with crusting, predominate in infants, while children and adults develop scaling erythematous papules and plaques and chronic, thickened plaques. Exacerbations of this disease have been related to substances in the environment, such as wool clothing, temperature variations, sweating, and emotional stress. Patch testing is not relevant as a means of diagnosing atopic dermatitis.

BOX 19-8   Atopic Dermatitis

Causes

Hereditary predisposition

Lesions

Eczematous dermatitis, early

Skin thickening (lichenification), chronic

Manifestations

Multiple patchy skin lesions varying from moist to dry, with or without erosions

Pruritus

Other atopic diseases (asthma, allergic rhinitis)

Seborrheic Dermatitis

This common form of dermatitis occurs in sites of greatest concentration of sebaceous glands: the scalp, central face, ears, chest, and areas where different skin surfaces touch, such as the groin. Seborrheic dermatitis usually begins in childhood as fine scaling of the scalp (**cradle cap**) and may continue throughout life with variable extension to other areas. The pink-red patches usually have a greasy, yellow scale. The specific cause is unknown, but aberrant sebum production and the yeast *Malassezia furfur* are thought to play roles.

BOX 19–9 **Seborrheic Dermatitis**

Causes

Unknown

Lesions

Increased production and sloughing of keratin layer of epidermis

Manifestations

Scaling of scalp and other areas

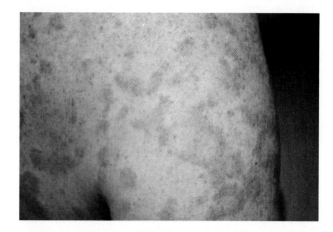

FIGURE 19–12 The characteristic "wheal and flare" of urticaria. (Courtesy of Yale Residents' Slide Collection, Dermatology Department, Yale University School of Medicine.)

Urticaria (Hives)

Urticaria is an acute patchy eruption with raised edematous areas (**wheal**) surrounded by erythema (**flare**) (**Figure 19–12**). The lesions itch. They seldom persist for more than 48 hours but may recur in successive episodes. Urticaria results from local release of histamine in the skin and is frequently the result of an allergic reaction, which can be caused by an allergen in a medication (such as penicillin) or a food (such as shellfish). It can also be caused by infections and autoimmunity.

BOX 19–10 **Urticaria**

Causes

Histamine release resulting from allergens such as foods or drugs

Infection, autoimmunity

Lesions

Edema of skin with vascular congestion at margin

Manifestations

Large patchy areas of wheal and flare

Pruritus

Psoriasis

Psoriasis is a chronic inflammatory disease of skin with a polygenic basis that is influenced by environmental factors. It is characterized classically by thickened areas of skin with silver-colored scales (**Figure 19–13**). Lesions are most common on the extensor surfaces of the knees and elbows. Disease severity can vary widely among patients. Proliferation of the epidermis is a prominent feature of this disease. A variety of anti-inflammatory ointments and a special ultraviolet (UVB) light are commonly used to control psoriasis; systemic immunosuppressants are used in severe cases. Psoriasis may be quite distressing to the patient but is usually not life threatening.

Benign and Malignant Neoplasms

The skin is fertile ground for various benign, premalignant, and malignant growths. Long exposure to sunlight in association with aging is important in the vast majority of these lesions. Neoplasms derived from the epidermis primarily involve two separate cell lines: the

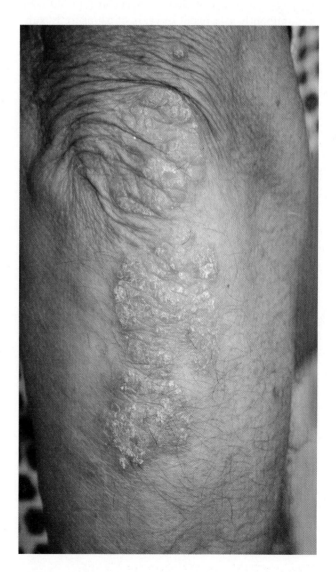

FIGURE 19–13 Psoriasis. Well-demarcated, raised, red, scaly plaques are on the extensor surface of an elbow. (Courtesy of Yale Residents' Slide Collection, Dermatology Department, Yale University School of Medicine.)

keratinocytes and the melanocytes of the epidermis.
The relative frequency of the three major types of cancer
of the skin is shown in **Figure 19–14**.

Solar Degeneration and Actinic Keratosis

With age, a number of changes occur in exposed skin,
predominantly as a result of years of exposure to sunlight. The degree of skin change is directly related to
the duration and intensity of solar exposure. The most
characteristic change is degeneration of dermal collagen and elastic fibers that results in excessive wrinkling of the skin (**Figure 19–15**). This degeneration is
called **solar elastosis**. Other skin changes attributed to
solar, or **actinic**, damage include skin atrophy, areas of
increased pigmentation (**lentigo**), collections of small
blood vessels (**telangiectasia**), and patches of thickened skin (**keratoses**). Thus, the face of an older farmer
or seaman is likely to have areas of dyspigmentation as
well as a ruddy complexion caused by telangiectasia and
keratoses.

Actinic keratoses (also called senile or solar keratoses) occur as multiple, scaly lesions on sun-exposed skin
of persons with extensive sun exposure. They are more

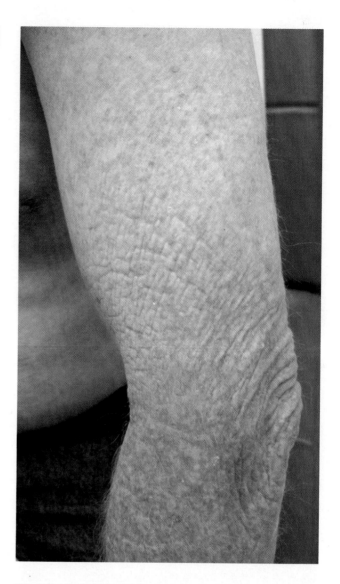

FIGURE 19–15 Solar elastosis. The skin around the elbow of this
elderly individual is wrinkled and sagging due to degeneration of
dermal connective tissue by many years of exposure to sunlight.
(Courtesy of Yale Residents' Slide Collection, Dermatology
Department, Yale University School of Medicine.)

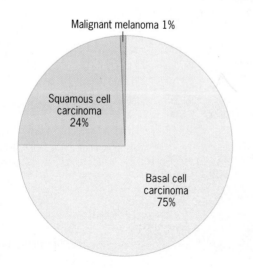

FIGURE 19–14 Relative frequency of skin cancers derived from
squamous cells (basal and squamous cell carcinomas) and from
melanocytes (malignant melanoma).

common in fair-skinned persons. The lesion consists of an
area of atypical epidermal proliferation frequently accompanied by thickening of the keratin layer. Actinic keratosis
is considered to be a precancerous lesion because progression to squamous cell carcinoma can occur in a minority
of lesions. Actinic keratoses are therefore important to
identify so as to recognize patients at risk for developing
subsequent squamous cell carcinomas.

Seborrheic Keratosis

Seborrheic keratoses are benign neoplastic proliferations
of keratinocytes that occur most commonly on the trunk,
face, and arms of persons in middle life and beyond. The
seborrheic keratosis is a warty, brown, greasy lesion that

Causes

Long exposure to sunlight

Aging

Lesions

Degeneration of collagen and elastin fibers (solar elastosis)

Telangiectasia

Increased or decreased pigmentation

Actinic keratoses

Manifestations

Wrinkling of skin of face and hands

Pigmented macules on exposed areas

Ruddy complexion

Small areas of thickened skin

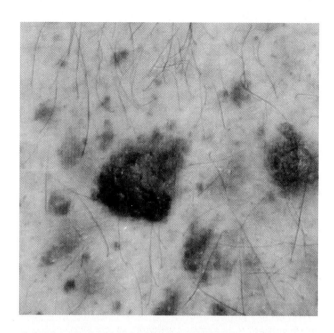

FIGURE 19–16 Seborrheic keratosis. Irregular brown plaques are composed of a thickened cornified layer that has a characteristic waxy and "stuck on" appearance. (Courtesy of Yale Residents' Slide Collection, Dermatology Department, Yale University School of Medicine.)

appears to be tacked on to the skin and can often be easily scraped off (**Figure 19–16**). The etiology underlying their development is not known. Seborrheic keratoses are not premalignant.

BOX 19–13   Seborrheic Keratosis

Causes

Unknown

Lesions

Benign neoplasm of keratinocytes

Manifestations

Brown-black, stuck-on-appearing papules and plaques

Middle age or older

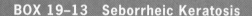

Melanocytic Nevus

The common nevus (**melanocytic nevus, nevocellular nevus, mole**) results from a benign proliferation of melanocytes of the epidermis. At first, the melanocytes or nevus cells proliferate at the junction of the epidermis and dermis (**junctional nevus**); later the cells migrate into the dermis and form clumps of nevus cells (**intradermal nevus**). When clusters of melanocytes are present at the junction as well as in the dermis, the nevus is called a **compound nevus**. Melanocytic nevi develop in most light-skinned individuals any time from childhood to early adulthood and evolve from junctional to intradermal nevi over a number of years. They may eventually involute. They may be brown to black or even skin-toned, depending on the amount of melanin pigment produced. They vary from flat to pedunculated depending on the number of nevus cells present (**Figure 19–17**).

The vast majority of melanocytic nevi are harmless. Though controversial, it is estimated that about 30% of

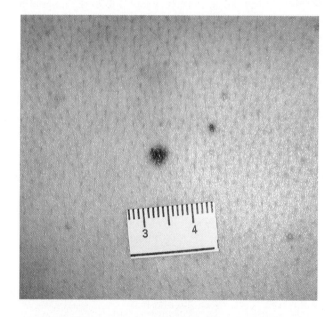

FIGURE 19–17 Melanocytic nevi. Numerous small, circumscribed brown spots are present on this fair skin. (Courtesy of Dr. Richard Antaya, Department of Dermatology, Yale School of Medicine.)

malignant melanomas arise from melanocytic nevi, but the chance of any one nevus becoming malignant is extremely small. The risk is considerably greater in large or giant **congenital nevi**—nevi that cover a large amount of the body surface area in neonates. Clinically, atypical nevi with irregular pigmentation or ill-defined borders can show histologic evidence of architectural and cytologic atypia and are thought to be markers of patients at moderately increased risk for developing melanoma. These kinds of nevi are called **dysplastic nevi**.

Clinical features that suggest a nevus may be dysplastic or frankly malignant can be remembered with the ABCDE criteria (compare Figures 19–17 and **19–18**):

A—Asymmetry: Benign nevi are usually symmetrical. One can draw a line at any angle through the nevus and divide it into two halves that are mirror images of one another. This is not true of melanoma, which usually grows as irregular nests, producing an asymmetrical lesion.

B—Border irregularity: Benign nevi usually have smooth, linear edges, while dysplastic nevi and melanoma grow with irregular, jagged edges.

C—Color: Benign nevi have a uniform color. It can be the same as surrounding skin or any variation of brown from light tan to almost black. There are even blue and pink nevi. Dysplastic nevi and melanoma are more likely to be variegated in color. All the colors that normally occur in nevi can be present in a single dysplastic nevus or melanoma.

D—Diameter: Benign nevi are usually less than 6 mm in greatest dimension, while dysplastic and malignant melanocytic proliferations are larger than 6 mm. This is not to say that any lesion larger than 6 mm is automatically malignant; some large nevi can be benign. However, large size in conjunction with other features listed here is highly suggestive of dysplasia or malignancy.

E—Evolution: A mole that is changing in size, shape, or color is worrisome.

It is imperative that any pigmented lesion removed from the skin, even if only for cosmetic purposes, be examined by a pathologist. It is unfortunately not uncommon for a patient to present with metastatic melanoma, which is invariably lethal, without having an identifiable primary lesion, but recalling a history of having had a spot removed from the skin a few years prior to this and the physician throwing it away rather than sending it to the laboratory because it "looked benign." Even the most experienced dermatologist can be misled by the gross appearance of a pigmented lesion and should refrain from calling something benign on clinical grounds alone. Accurate diagnosis of a melanocytic lesion requires microscopic evaluation, and it is the microscopic, not clinical, characteristics that provide prognostic estimates and guide therapy.

BOX 19–14   Melanocytic Nevus

Causes

Proliferation of melanocytes

Hereditary

Lesions

Clusters of melanocytes at dermal/epidermal junction and/or in dermis

Manifestations

Small macules or papules; may be varying shades of brown or skin-toned

Malignant Melanoma

Malignant melanoma is a malignant neoplasm of melanocytes. It is one of the top 10 cancers diagnosed in the United States, and although the overall 5-year survival is around 90%, about 20% of patients with melanoma die from metastases. This number would be much greater if lesions were not detected and removed at an early stage. Malignant melanoma has a tendency to spread widely to

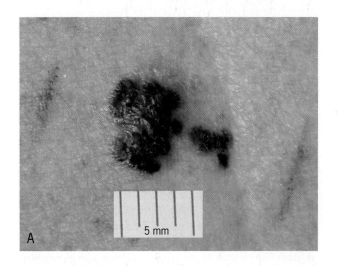

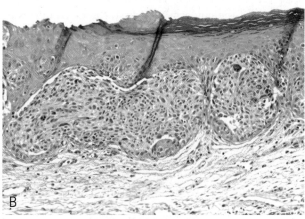

FIGURE 19–18 Malignant melanoma. **A.** Gross appearance. Compare this to the nevi in Figure 19–17 according to the ABCDE criteria. (Courtesy of Yale Residents' Slide Collection, Dermatology Department, Yale University School of Medicine.) **B.** Nests of malignant melanocytes are growing in the epidermis in this melanoma *in situ*.

many organs in the body even before it has spread very widely at the site of origin, and, even more ominously, malignant cells can lie dormant for several years before producing obvious metastases.

Various forms of melanoma are recognized based on clinical and histologic appearance and behavior of the lesions. Melanoma *in situ* is confined to the epidermis, and therefore has a better prognosis as compared to invasive lesions. Lentigo maligna melanoma is a clinical variant of melanoma *in situ* that classically develops as a slowly expanding tan-brown patch with pigmentary variations on the face of an older individual. Superficial spreading melanoma is the most common type of melanoma and is characterized by spreading growth of malignant cells within the epidermis and superficial dermis, producing a flat to slightly raised lesion with often a variegated color pattern. Nodular melanoma grows primarily downward, into the dermis rather than along the epidermis, and expands outward to form a nodule. Acral lentiginous melanoma occurs on the palms, soles, and in or around the nail unit. Nodular and acral lentiginous melanomas are more likely to be diagnosed at a later and more advanced stage than the superficial spreading form is.

Table 19–2 gives the criteria for assigning stage in melanoma. The most important parameters for prognosis are tumor thickness, which measures the "vertical growth phase" of the melanoma, and depth of invasion, measured in fractions of a millimeter under the microscope. Additional prognostic factors include whether the lesion is ulcerated and whether it has spread locally within the skin, as so-called satellite lesions. As with all other cancers, spread to lymph nodes and spread to distant organs are ominous signs. Sentinel lymph node biopsy, analogous to that performed in the breast, is now feasible and standard in all new diagnoses of melanoma. The most common sites of metastasis are the lungs, liver, and brain, but melanoma has the propensity to spread to tissues that do not usually harbor metastases, such as the mucosa of the gastrointestinal tract and spleen.

The most important risk factor for the development of melanoma is sun exposure, particularly blistering sunburns in childhood. This is in contrast to nonmelanoma skin cancers, which appear to arise as a result of cumulative exposure to sun. It is not surprising, given this correlation, that the highest incidence of melanoma occurs in fair-skinned populations living in areas of intense sun exposure—Florida and Australia, for example. Melanoma can occur in black people, but this is quite unusual. Also, melanoma can occur in young individuals. Although the median age of diagnosis is 60 years, many cases are diagnosed in people in their 30s and 40s, and ever more commonly, even in the teenage years. It is the most common form of cancer in young adults (25–29 years old). The incidence of melanoma has been increasing over the past 30 years and will continue to do so until people become more cautious about enjoying sunlight. Protection against the harmful effects of ultraviolet (solar) radiation by sunscreen creams and clothing is effective in inhibiting the development of melanoma as well as actinic degeneration and nonmelanoma skin cancers.

The first line of treatment of melanoma is surgical excision with wide margins, so as to be sure to capture any "in-transit" melanocytes that might later set up satellite lesions. Chemotherapy may be added if the tumor is of high stage or has metastasized. Radiotherapy is used as a palliative measure to reduce the effects of metastatic cancer. Immune therapy has grown out of the observation that there is often a very pronounced inflammatory cell infiltrate in melanomas that appears to delay its growth. Various modalities to boost this natural immune response against the cancer are now being tested.

BOX 19–15   Malignant Melanoma

Causes

Unknown

History of intense sun exposure (blistering sunburns) in childhood

Lesions

Proliferation of malignant melanocytes

Manifestations

Enlarging pigmented skin lesion, either superficial or nodular

Lymph node metastasis

Widespread metastasis

TABLE 19–2   Stage Groupings and 5-Year Survival for Melanoma

Stage	Characteristics	5-Year Survival
Melanoma *in situ*	Melanoma confined to the epidermis; no invasion	~100%
Stage I	Melanoma that has invaded 2 mm or less into the dermis and is not ulcerated, OR Melanoma that has invaded 1 mm or less and is ulcerated	99%
Stage II	Melanoma that has invaded more than 2 mm into the dermis and is not ulcerated, OR Melanoma that has invaded more than 1 mm into the dermis and is ulcerated	~80%
Stage III	Melanoma that has metastasized locally in the skin ("satellite lesions"), OR Melanoma that has spread to distant sites	65%
Stage IV	Melanoma that has spread to lymph nodes	15%

Other Pigmented Lesions

Ephelides (freckles) are focal areas of hyperpigmentation that occur in response to sunlight. Freckles occur only on sun-exposed skin and darken with repeated exposure to sunlight. They begin in childhood but decrease in number with maturity. By comparison, **solar lentigines** (singular, *lentigo*) are lesions of adults and are typically darker brown. They also represent localized areas of increased keratinocytic pigmentation in response to sun exposure. Actinic keratoses, seborrheic keratoses, and basal cell carcinomas may also be dark colored when they contain increased amounts of melanin.

Basal Cell and Squamous Cell Carcinomas

The term *nonmelanoma skin cancers* refers to basal cell and squamous cell carcinomas. Cancers can also arise from the skin appendages, blood vessels, immune cells, and connective tissue in the skin, but these neoplasms are very rare and not included in the general category of nonmelanoma skin cancer.

Squamous and basal cell carcinomas occur most frequently on the face and hands of older adults. They are often multiple, either discovered at the same time or developing in different places on the skin over many years. The biggest risk factor for the development of these lesions is also sun exposure, but in contrast to melanoma, it appears that cumulative sun exposure over many years appears to be the predisposing factor.

Basal cell carcinoma is more common (Figure 19–14) and is made up of cells that resemble those of the basal cell layer of the epidermis (**Figure 19–19B**). Basal cell carcinoma classically presents as a slowly enlarging, pearly papule with prominent telangiectasia and a rolled border. Ulceration can occur with continued growth (**Figure 19–19A**). Untreated, it can become locally destructive, impinging on neighboring tissues, but only in the rarest of cases has basal cell carcinoma been reported to metastasize. Surgical excision, sometimes followed by localized radiation therapy if the lesion is large or deeply invasive, is therefore curative.

Squamous cell carcinoma is composed of a proliferation of cells that resemble those in the spinous layer of the epidermis (**Figure 19–20B**). It has a greater potential for spread and metastasis than basal cell carcinoma does. Squamous cell carcinomas may arise in preexisting skin lesions, such as actinic keratoses, burn scars, or chronic ulcers, and typically present as enlarging, keratotic or ulcerated lesions (**Figure 19–20A**). Untreated, some squamous cell carcinomas may metastasize. The risk

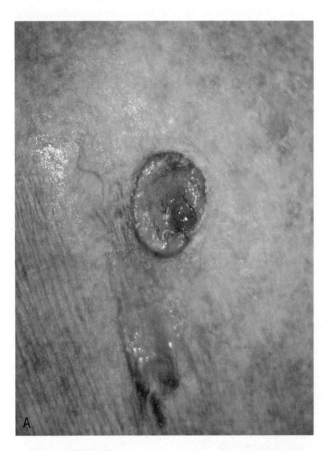
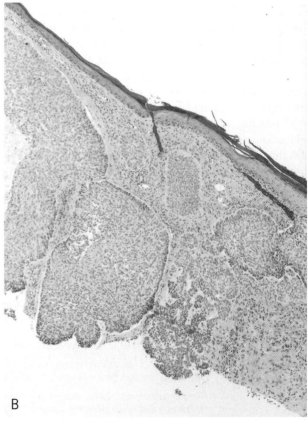

FIGURE 19–19 Basal cell carcinoma. **A.** A pearly lesion with rolled borders and central ulceration. (Courtesy of Yale Residents' Slide Collection, Dermatology Department, Yale University School of Medicine.) **B.** Microscopically, nests of small blue cells are invading the dermis.

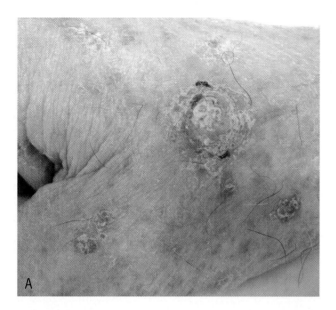 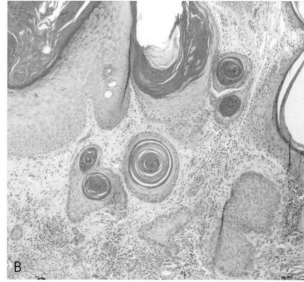

FIGURE 19–20 Squamous cell carcinoma. **A.** A mounded-up, hyperkeratotic, scaly lesion on the hand of an elderly person. (Courtesy of Yale Residents' Slide Collection, Dermatology Department, Yale University School of Medicine.) **B.** Microscopically, this consists of islands of squamous cells within the dermis that are even producing little "pearls" of keratin. This is a very well-differentiated carcinoma.

for metastasis increases with tumor size and underlying immunosuppression.

BOX 19–16   Basal Cell and Squamous Cell Carcinomas

Causes

Cumulative (lifetime) exposure to sunlight

Squamous cell carcinoma can also arise in preexisting scars and chronic ulcers

Lesions

Nodular lesions on skin, sometimes ulcerated and/or keratotic

Manifestations

Enlarging papule or nodule in sun-damaged skin

Organ Failure

Lethal failure of skin function occurs with extensive, severe burns and rare cases of diffuse blistering diseases such as drug-induced toxic epidermal necrolysis. In these conditions, fluid loss and infection become life-threatening emergencies. Patients with extensive skin loss require immediate admission to a burn unit, a specialty department in large referral hospitals that is specially equipped to handle the complex medical issues that occur when the barrier function of the skin is compromised.

Practice Questions

1. Skin adnexal glands that are present all over the body are
   A. apocrine glands.
   B. eccrine glands.
   C. sebaceous glands.
   D. follicular glands.

2. Verrucae and condylomata acuminata are caused by
   A. papilloma virus.
   B. excessive skin moisture.
   C. *Staphylococcus aureus*.
   D. genetic defects.

3. Superficial fungal infections of the skin are caused by which of the following organisms?
   A. *Candida*
   B. *Tinea*
   C. Both
   D. Neither

4. A 19-year-old woman is seen by a dermatologist for red, crusty lesions on her neck, wrists, and the backs of her knees. Other members of her family have a similar affliction. Which of the following is the most likely diagnosis?
   A. Impetigo
   B. Acne
   C. Contact dermatitis
   D. Eczema

5. Which of the following is an example of an immune-mediated skin lesion?
   A. Poison ivy
   B. Atopic dermatitis
   C. Impetigo
   D. Seborrheic dermatitis

6. Which of the following is a precancerous lesion?
   A. Ephelides
   B. Telangiectasia
   C. Seborrheic keratosis
   D. Actinic keratosis

7. A 35-year-old man is treated by ultraviolet light for a chronic skin rash characterized by patches of thickened skin with silver scales on the knees and elbows. This condition most likely is
   A. urticaria.
   B. seborrheic keratosis.
   C. psoriasis.
   D. atopic dermatitis.

Eye

OUTLINE

OBJECTIVES

1. State which symptom is common to most people wearing eyeglasses regardless of their underlying eye disorder.
2. Describe how each of the following instruments or procedures is helpful in evaluation of eye problems: visual acuity tests, visual field tests, funduscopic examination, tonometer, slit-lamp.
3. List the causes, lesions, and major manifestations of each of the specific diseases or disorders discussed in this chapter.
4. Describe how abnormalities in the cornea, lens, or retina lead to strabismus.
5. Describe the pathogenesis of visual loss in glaucoma.
6. Compare the manifestations of diabetic retinopathy with hypertensive retinopathy.
7. Compare the pathogenesis of decreased visual acuity in myopia, hyperopia, presbyopia, and astigmatism.
8. List the leading causes of blindness.
9. Define and use in proper context all the words and phrases in this chapter in bold print.

KEY TERMS

accommodation
amblyopia
aqueous humor
astigmatism
capillary aneurysm
cataract
closed-angle glaucoma
conjunctiva
conjunctivitis
cornea
cyclopia
diabetic retinopathy
enucleation
fovea
funduscopic examination
glaucoma
hyperopia
hypertensive retinopathy
keratitis
legal blindness
lens
macula
macular degeneration
malignant melanoma
microhemorrhages
myopia
nystagmus
open-angle glaucoma
ophthalmoscope
papilledema
photophobia
presbyopia
pupil
refractive error
retinal layer
retinoblastoma
sclera
senile macular degeneration
slit-lamp
strabismus (heterotropia)
tonometer
trachoma
uvea
visual acuity
visual field test
vitreous humor

Review of Structure and Function

The globe of the eye (eyeball) sits inside the bony orbit and is protected anteriorly by the eyelid. The extraocular muscles attach to its outer surface. The optic nerve together with blood vessels enter the globe posteriorly. The globe is composed of three layers (**Figure 20–1**): the outer **scleral** layer, a tough fibrous coating; the **uveal** layer (iris, ciliary body, and choroid), a pigmented layer of connective tissue through which nerves and blood vessels course; and the inner, **retinal layer**.

Anteriorly, the scleral layer is continuous with the **cornea**, the transparent structure through which light first passes into the globe. The cornea is the initial refracting (light-bending) surface of the eye. The exterior of the sclera is covered by the **conjunctiva**, a tissue that reflects onto the inner surface of the eyelids at approximately 1 cm posterior to its origin at the corneoscleral junction. The **lens**, the suspending ligaments of the lens, the iris, and the muscular ciliary body are all located in the anterior portion of the eye. Contraction of the ciliary body controls the focal length of the lens. The iris controls the amount of light reaching the lens by varying the size of its aperture (**pupil**). Decrease in pupil size (miosis) is achieved by contraction of the circular smooth muscles in the iris, which are stimulated by autonomic nerve fibers from the third cranial nerve, the oculomotor.

Posteriorly, the retina is the site of the light- and color-sensing rod and cone neurons. Impulses generated in these cells by light are transmitted by a chain of neurons back through the optic nerve to the visual cortex of the brain. The **macula** is the spot on the retina of greatest visual acuity. The **fovea** is the central portion of the macula. The ciliary body and the lens and its ligaments mark the boundary between the anterior and posterior segments of the globe. Within the anterior segment is the anterior chamber, which is filled with a watery fluid, **aqueous humor**. Aqueous humor is secreted by the ciliary body and diffuses forward, through the pupil, from the posterior to the anterior chamber and serves to nourish and cleanse the avascular lens and retina. It drains out of the anterior chamber slowly through a series of tissue spaces at the periphery of the chamber. The space behind the lens is filled with a clear gelatinous substance, the **vitreous humor**.

Most Frequent and Serious Problems

The most common overall problems affecting the eyes are decrease in visual acuity (indistinct focusing of the visual image on the retina) from refractive error and inflammation. Age-related macular degeneration is the most common cause of legal blindness in persons older than 65 years. Approximately one-third of the population wears eyeglasses for correction of the main types of refractive error, which include myopia, hyperopia, presbyopia, and astigmatism. Trauma to various parts of the eye, especially to the cornea, is a very common problem and can lead to significant pain and disability. Acute conjunctivitis, colloquially called pinkeye, may occur by itself or be associated with another bacterial or viral infection such as an upper respiratory infection. Infections in the adjacent sinuses can spread to the orbit, resulting in serious complications. Strabismus is deviation of one or both eyes that cannot be overcome by the patient. Strabismus is relatively common and is due to several causes. Cataract is an opacity of the lens leading to decreased visual acuity. Cataracts may be the result of birth defect, infection, or trauma, but most commonly they arise *de novo* in older persons. Glaucoma is a disease

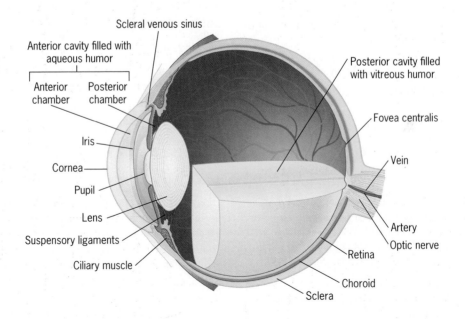

FIGURE 20–1 Schematic drawing of the anatomy of the eye.

caused by an increase in intraocular pressure, with resultant damage to the optic nerve and its fibers inside the eye. Afflictions of the small retinal vessels occur commonly in individuals with hypertension and diabetes. Tumors of the eye, although uncommon, can cause blindness as well as death.

Symptoms, Signs, and Tests

The most common manifestation of eye disease is decreased visual acuity. Decreased visual acuity may be a symptom when experienced by a person or a sign when manifested as a result of a visual acuity test. Decreased visual acuity may result from macular degeneration, cataracts, and vascular diseases, as well as from myopia or hyperopia. Visual field defects (focal areas of blindness) also may be signs or symptoms and result from diseases affecting the optic pathways of the central nervous system or from diseases of the retina. Pain is often a manifestation of trauma, infection, or acutely increased intraocular pressure from closed-angle glaucoma. Blurring of vision accompanies various systemic diseases, especially those of toxic and metabolic origin. **Papilledema** (swelling of the head of the optic nerve as seen through the ophthalmoscope) may reflect an increase in intracranial pressure, usually resulting from an expanding intracranial mass. **Photophobia** (uncomfortable sensitivity to light) is commonly seen with inflammation inside and outside the eyeball. **Nystagmus** (flickering eye movements) may be caused by a variety of central nervous system lesions.

Clinical tests for eye disease include the utilization of eye charts for testing **visual acuity**. The person being examined reads letters or numbers from a chart at a distance of 20 feet. Normal visual acuity (20/20) means that the person can accurately read with either eye the smallest figures that are readable to a normal control population. A visual acuity of 20/40 means that the affected eye can accurately read at 20 feet what a normal eye can read at 40 feet. These charts are widely used as screening devices for school children and for persons applying for driver's licenses.

Tests for mapping visual field defects are employed to detect area(s) of the retina or optic pathways affected by a particular disease process (**Figure 20–2**). In administering **visual field tests**, the person being examined is asked to focus on a small stationary spot while a test spot is moved to different points of a circular map. In those areas where the person cannot see the test spot, he or she has a visual field defect.

The **ophthalmoscope** is a hand-held, light-projecting instrument used to examine the retina by utilizing lenses of various refractive powers to focus the image for the examiner. Visualization of the retina with the ophthalmoscope is referred to as a **funduscopic examination** (**Figure 20–3**). A **tonometer** is a small instrument that

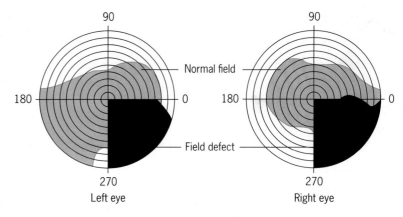

FIGURE 20–2 Visual field chart with visual field defects marked in black.

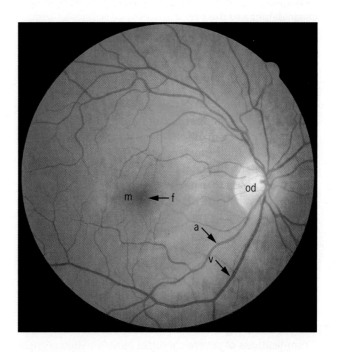

FIGURE 20–3 Normal retina, showing optic disk (od), macula (m) with fovea in center (f), artery (a), and vein (v). (Courtesy of Dr. Daniel Albert, Department of Ophthalmology, University of Wisconsin School of Medicine and Public Health.)

is placed directly on the eyeball to measure the intraocular pressure, which may be elevated in glaucoma. A **slit-lamp** is a binocular magnifying instrument that projects a focused beam of light into the eye and is used for detailed examination of the cornea, anterior chamber, iris, and lens and is useful in the evaluation of glaucoma, trauma, inflammation, and other conditions. Various types of lenses are utilized in the evaluation of myopia and hyperopia to determine the **refractive error** (degree by which the cornea, lens, and humor fail to focus light rays on the retina). Ultrasound is used to evaluate masses in the orbit.

Specific Diseases

Genetic/Developmental Diseases

Serious isolated congenital eye defects are uncommon, but genetic factors appear to predispose individuals to certain eye disorders such as myopia, glaucoma, strabismus, cataracts, and retinoblastoma (a malignant neoplasm). **Cyclopia**, a very rare condition in which a single, malformed eye is centrally situated, occurs in conjunction with severe brain malformation.

lazy eye

Inflammatory/Degenerative Diseases

Except for injuries and infections, the diseases discussed here represent a heterogeneous group of developmental and acquired conditions. Although not discussed further, it should be noted that infections of the maxillary, ethmoid, and frontal sinuses can extend into the orbit and cause damage to the eye.

Trauma and Chemical Injury

The eye is susceptible to many different types of injuries, which include penetrating injuries, blunt injuries, chemical injuries, and commonly, corneal abrasions. The most common penetrating injury occurs when metal strikes metal. The manifestations of penetrating injuries are usually readily apparent and receive the immediate attention of an ophthalmic surgeon. The manifestations of blunt injuries are usually less apparent, but may be no less severe. When the eye is hit directly by a blunt object (e.g., golf ball, hockey puck, or paddle ball), compression/decompression occurs, which can produce damage to several intraocular structures. Such damage can, in time, result in retinal detachment, intraocular hemorrhage, dislocation of the lens, and/or glaucoma. Of the different types of chemicals that can damage the eye, concentrated alkali solutions, such as ammonia, produce the most damage to the cornea and adjacent tissues. Complications of severe chemical burns include corneal ulcer and corneal perforation.

Corneal abrasions occur when the cornea is scratched with an object such as a fingernail, a piece of paper, or a contact lens. Symptoms are severe pain and photophobia. Treatment consists of antibiotic ointment and a pressure bandage over the eye to prevent movement of the eyelid over the cornea.

In older persons, the vitreous humor may become desiccated and retract from the retina at points of attachment. This can lead to progressive retinal detachment. Retinal detachment is treated by laser beam surgery that thermally "glues" the retina to the uvea.

Conjunctivitis and Dry Eyes

Inflammation of the conjunctiva with vascular congestion producing a red or pink eye (**Figure 20–4**) is the most common eye disease; it may be secondary to viral, chlamydial, bacterial, and fungal infections or allergy.

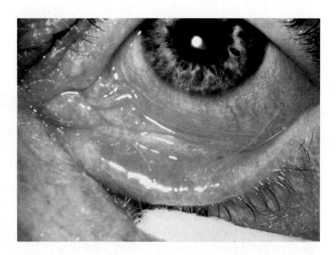

FIGURE 20–4 Conjunctivitis with congested conjunctival vessels and edema. (Courtesy of Dr. Daniel Albert, Department of Ophthalmology, University of Wisconsin School of Medicine and Public Health.)

Symptoms include irritation, blurred vision, and photophobia. **Conjunctivitis** most often occurs in association with an upper respiratory infection but may occur by itself. Measles often presents with conjunctivitis. Conjunctivitis associated with hay fever may be very troublesome because of photophobia and itching. Viral and allergic types of conjunctivitis are prone to secondary bacterial infections; hence, the treatment of conjunctivitis often consists of administration of eyedrops that contain antibiotics and topical antihistamines. Conjunctivitis caused by **trachoma** (a chlamydial disease) is one of the most common causes of blindness in many parts of the world because it results in corneal scarring. Inflammation of other parts of the eye is less common, but **keratitis** (corneal inflammation), uveitis, and retinitis can be devastating to sight.

BOX 20–1   Conjunctivitis

Causes

Bacteria

Viruses

Chlamydia

Fungi

Allergy

Drugs

Lesions

Inflamed conjunctiva

Manifestations

Red eye

Irritation

Blurred vision

Photophobia

Dry eyes are a common similar problem occasionally associated with systemic immune disorders such as rheumatoid arthritis, but more often secondary to systemic drugs such as antihypertensive, antidepressant, and antihistamine medications. Dry eye symptoms include itching, burning, photophobia, "sandy" sensation, blurred vision, and vascular congestion. Dry eyes occur most often in older adults and in women. Treatment consists of eyedrops plus alleviation of the primary condition.

Strabismus (Heterotropia) *Lazy Eye*

Strabismus (heterotropia) is an improper alignment of the visual axis (the line of vision), with one or both eyes at fault. The result is that each eye points in a different direction and the eyes cannot fixate on the same visual object simultaneously (**Figure 20–5**). Strabismus is a common condition, most often manifest in childhood and often referred to as crossed eyes in lay terms. Normally, children attain alignment by 3 to 4 months of age. A variety of factors may cause strabismus—paralysis of an extraocular muscle, refractive errors, opacities of the cornea or lens, diseases of the retina, and diseases of the optic nerve or brain. Some types of strabismus may be corrected with lenses; others are corrected surgically by altering the insertions of extraocular muscles to realign the eyes. If not discovered and treated early, strabismus can cause irreversible loss of vision in one eye called **amblyopia** (lazy eye).

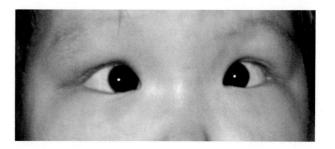

FIGURE 20–5 Strabismus. (Courtesy of Dr. Daniel Albert, Department of Ophthalmology, University of Wisconsin School of Medicine and Public Health.)

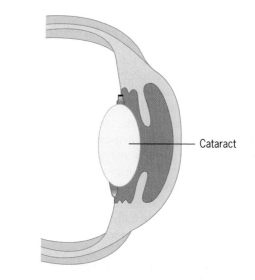

Cataract

FIGURE 20–6 Schematic drawing of cataract.

BOX 20–2   Strabismus

Causes

Extraocular muscle defects

Refractive errors

Corneal opacities

Retinal disease

Nerve or brain disease

Lesions

Varies with cause

Manifestations

Deviation of eyes

Cataract

Cataract is an opacification of the lens (**Figure 20–6**) that most commonly occurs in older individuals (senile cataract). Less commonly, cataracts may be secondary to trauma or may be accelerated by poorly controlled diabetes mellitus. Congenital cataracts are rare, and some types have a familial tendency. Most cataracts develop slowly, resulting in progressive diminution of vision. In most cases, treatment of cataracts consists of surgical extraction of the opacified portion of the lens followed

by insertion of a prosthetic intraocular lens inside the preserved outside capsule of the natural lens.

BOX 20–3   Cataract

Causes

Age-related

Trauma

Diabetes

Congenital diseases

Lesions

Total or partial opacification of the lens

Manifestations

Diminution of vision; may be progressive

Glaucoma

Glaucoma is a condition characterized by a rise in intraocular pressure sufficient to damage optic nerve fibers. The increase in intraocular pressure is almost always caused by obstruction of the normal exit of anterior chamber fluid (aqueous humor) in the angle where the iris meets the corneal–scleral junction. Glaucoma is divided into open-angle, closed-angle, and rare congenital forms. In **open-angle glaucoma**, there are gross or microscopic abnormalities of the angle tissues (**Figure 20–7B**). Open-angle glaucoma is the much more common type and is chronic and insidious in onset. The patient is unaware of slowly progressive damage to the optic nerve with consequent peripheral visual loss until the condition is far advanced.

In **closed-angle glaucoma**, there is obstruction of the angle by the iris (**Figure 20–7A**). The adhesion of the iris to the angle structures may be reversible or, if inflammation and scarring have occurred, permanent. The symptoms of closed-angle glaucoma are usually acute, with pain, nausea, vomiting, and a sudden decrease in vision.

Glaucoma can also be separated into primary and secondary causes. Primary glaucoma is caused by closure of a preexisting narrow anterior chamber angle, found in older persons. Secondary glaucoma is usually associated with uveitis or dislocation of the lens.

Glaucoma is diagnosed by demonstration of increased intraocular pressure as measured with a tonometer and by documented defects in peripheral visual fields. It is treated by various adrenergic and anticholinergic drugs, newer beta-blockers, prostaglandins, and carbonic anhydrase inhibitors, which partially inhibit the formation and secretion of aqueous humor and, to some degree, increase outflow.

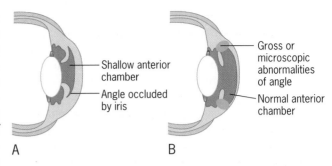

FIGURE 20–7 **A.** Closed-angle glaucoma. **B.** Open-angle glaucoma.

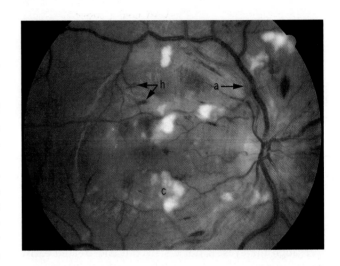

FIGURE 20–8 Hypertensive retinopathy, with flame-shaped hemorrhages (h), narrow, tortuous arteries (a), and cotton wool patches (c) caused by focal ischemia. (Courtesy of Dr. Daniel Albert, Department of Ophthalmology, University of Wisconsin School of Medicine and Public Health.)

BOX 20–4   Glaucoma

Causes
Obstruction of exit flow of aqueous humor

Lesions
Abnormal structure of angle (open angle)

Obstruction of angle by iris inflammation and scarring (closed angle)

Manifestations
Increased intraocular pressure (open and closed angle)

Pain

Nausea and vomiting (closed angle)

Progressive loss of vision

BOX 20–5   Hypertensive Retinopathy

Causes
Hypertension

Lesions
Narrowing of retinal vessels

Microhemorrhages

Exudates from serum

Manifestations
Progressive loss of vision

Hypertensive Retinopathy

Hypertension causes progressive arteriolosclerosis of the retinal vessels, eventually resulting in loss of vision because of compromised oxygen delivery to the retinal neurons. **Hypertensive retinopathy** is diagnosed by funduscopic examination because the sclerosis of the retinal arteries is seen as characteristic alterations in the light reflection from these vessels, along with "flame" hemorrhages and "cotton wool" spots when severe (**Figure 20–8**). Control of the hypertension usually results in some visual improvement.

Macular Degeneration

Macular degeneration is a disease of the older adult and is an important cause of blindness. The degeneration occurs in the retinal pigment epithelium in the macula, the area of the retina with greatest visual acuity. The cause is not known, but the incidence is slightly higher in women and in cigarette smokers, and it is familial in some instances. In the more common form of macular degeneration, called "dry" macular degeneration, the retina becomes thin and small white spots, or "drusen," develop within the retina (**Figure 20–9**). This initially causes blurriness of the central portion of the visual field and can progress to blindness.

Diabetic Retinopathy

Long-standing diabetes mellitus leads to retinal vessel disease manifested by progressive arteriosclerosis similar to that which occurs with hypertension. In addition, diabetes is associated with the development of vascular abnormalities. Early vascular lesions consist of **capillary aneurysms** and **microhemorrhages**, the latter eventually resulting in visual loss. The most advanced vascular lesions consist of proliferation of newly formed abnormal vessels (**Figure 20–10**), which can cause retinal detachment and

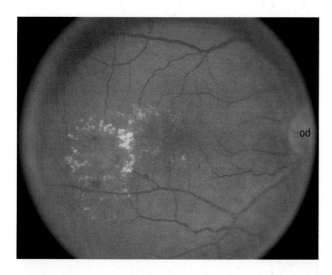

FIGURE 20–9 Macular degeneration. The optic disc is labeled (od). Vessels arch out from the optic disc toward the macula (not labeled), which is covered with small white spots, or "drusen." (Courtesy of Dr. Daniel Albert, Department of Ophthalmology, University of Wisconsin School of Medicine and Public Health.)

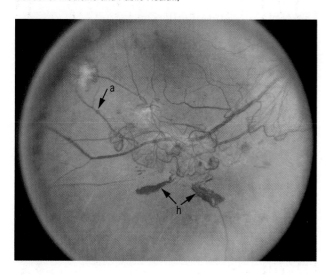

FIGURE 20–10 Diabetic retinopathy, with focal hemorrhages (h), aneurysms (a), and tangles of new vessels proliferating particularly profusely around the optic disc. (Courtesy of Dr. Daniel Albert, Department of Ophthalmology, University of Wisconsin School of Medicine and Public Health.)

vitreous hemorrhage. Treatment of abnormal retinal vessels may be effectively accomplished using a laser beam to coagulate many areas of the retina by thermal energy; this devitalizes large areas of retina and halts the progression of neovascularization. Successful treatment of the underlying diabetes is paramount for prevention of blindness.

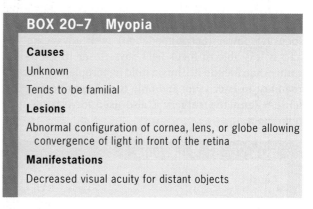

BOX 20–6 Diabetic Retinopathy

Causes

Diabetes mellitus

Lesions

Narrowing of retinal vessels

Capillary aneurysms

Vitreous microhemorrhages from new blood vessels

Manifestations

Progressive loss of vision

Myopia (Nearsightedness)

Myopia is a condition of refractive error in which light entering the eye is focused at a point anterior to the retina (**Figure 20–11**). This may be the result either of abnormal curvature and refractive power of the cornea and lens, or it may be because of relative elongation of the eyeball. Myopia often develops in childhood for poorly understood reasons and progresses until early adulthood, when the condition stabilizes because of normal loss of elasticity of the eye structures. Myopia tends to be familial; it is usually treated successfully with corrective lenses, but refractive surgery is becoming increasingly more common. Severe myopia may be associated with multiple defects in intraocular structures, including the angle and retina.

BOX 20–7 Myopia

Causes

Unknown

Tends to be familial

Lesions

Abnormal configuration of cornea, lens, or globe allowing convergence of light in front of the retina

Manifestations

Decreased visual acuity for distant objects

Hyperopia (Farsightedness)

Hyperopia is different from myopia in that light entering the eye tends to focus at a point posterior to the retina, with resultant poor vision for near objects and better vision for far objects (**Figure 20–12**). Hyperopia is the result of a relatively short eyeball or reduced refractive power of the cornea or lens. Children can often overcome

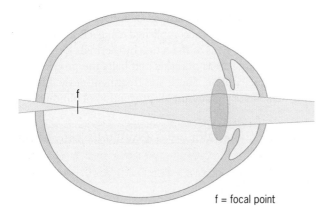

f

f = focal point

FIGURE 20-11 Schematic drawing of myopic eye.

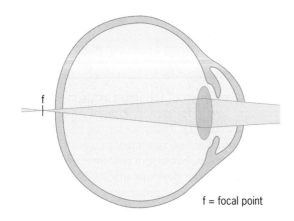

f

f = focal point

FIGURE 20-12 Schematic drawing of hyperopic eye.

an underlying mild hyperopic refractive error because of lens elasticity but often lose this ability as they grow older. The lens loses its elasticity and ability to adjust its focusing power (**accommodation**) with advancing age and is less able to focus light rays closer to the retina rather than behind it. Thus, a mild hyperopia can become manifest in later years and only then require corrective lenses. Refractive surgery is also used for treatment of hyperopia.

BOX 20-8   Hyperopia
Causes
Unknown
Tends to be accentuated with advancing age
Lesions
Abnormal configuration of the eye allowing convergence of light posterior to the retina
Manifestations
Decreased visual acuity, especially for near objects

Presbyopia

Presbyopia is a refractive error produced by loss of elasticity of the lens and/or atrophy of the ciliary muscle, and it starts in the 40s for most persons. It represents an inability to accommodate. Accommodation means the ability of the lens to change its shape to focus light rays from nearby objects onto the retina. Although the optical defect of presbyopia is similar to that of hyperopia inasmuch as light rays are focused behind the retina, the pathogenesis of the two conditions is different. Hyperopia is the result of the relatively short length of the eyeball, whereas presbyopia results from the degenerative effects of aging on the lens. Presbyopia is corrected by reading glasses or bifocals.

Astigmatism

Astigmatism is uneven focusing of light entering the eye because of unequal curvature of the cornea or acquired irregularities in the corneal surface or lens. Astigmatism may occur by itself or may accompany myopia or hyperopia. Unless unusually severe, astigmatism is correctable with appropriate lenses.

Refractive surgery is being used increasingly for treatment of astigmatism as well as myopia and hyperopia.

BOX 20-9   Astigmatism
Causes
Unknown
Tends to be familial
Lesions
Irregularities in cornea or lens
Manifestations
Uneven focusing of light, with decreased visual acuity

Hyperplastic/Neoplastic Diseases

Retinoblastomas and melanomas account for more than 90% of all primary intraocular eye tumors. With rare exceptions, retinoblastoma occurs in children, while melanoma occurs in adults.

Retinoblastoma

Retinoblastoma is a rare malignant tumor of primitive neurons, which are the precursors of the retinal ganglion cells. Retinoblastomas occur in children; they tend to be familial and have an autosomal dominant inheritance pattern with incomplete penetrance. Retinoblastomas are bilateral about 30% of the time. Treatment is removal of the eye (**enucleation**), often combined with chemotherapy or radiation.

Malignant Melanoma

Malignant melanoma is a malignant tumor arising from the choroid pigment-containing cells and is primarily a tumor of adults. Most ocular melanomas arise from the

BOX 20–10	Retinoblastoma

Causes

Unknown

Autosomal dominant inheritance

Lesions

Malignant neoplasm of retinal neurons

Manifestations

Occurs in children

Decreased vision

Mass arising from retina

30% bilateral

choroid layer, although they can arise from the iris or ciliary body. They usually carry a worse prognosis than do melanomas of the skin.

Organ Failure

Approximately 4 of every 1,000 persons in the United States are legally blind. **Legal blindness** is defined as visual acuity of 20/200 or less in the better eye with best correction. Blindness may be caused by lesions of the cornea, lens, vitreous humor, retina, and optic nerve. Congenital blindness or blindness developing in infancy can be caused by a wide variety of developmental, inflammatory, or traumatic conditions. Oxygen toxicity causes fibrosis of the retina, a condition called retinopathy of prematurity. Attention to the amount of oxygen given to newborns with respiratory distress syndrome has greatly reduced the incidence of this condition. The most common of the many causes of blindness in adults are glaucoma, diabetic retinopathy, trachoma, uveitis, macular degeneration, senile cataract, optic nerve atrophy, and retinitis pigmentosa. Degeneration of the macula with resultant loss of central vision may be the result of several causes, the most common of which is an idiopathic condition called **senile macular degeneration** characterized by damage to retinal pigment epithelium with underlying vascular proliferation. Optic atrophy may be caused by occlusion of the small vessels supplying the optic nerve, by optic neuritis such as occurs in multiple sclerosis, and by masses that press on the optic nerve. Retinitis pigmentosa, usually a recessively inherited condition, results in progressive destruction of rods and cones beginning in childhood and leading to blindness.

Practice Questions

1. Legal blindness is defined as diminished visual acuity of at least
   A. 20/40.
   B. 20/100.
   C. 20/200.
   D. 20/400.

2. A 72-year-old woman complains of decreased visual acuity over a period of 18 months. Her physician notes opacification of both of her lenses. The most likely diagnosis is
   A. cataract.
   B. glaucoma.
   C. conjunctivitis.
   D. presbyopia.

3. The most important and effective treatment of diabetic retinopathy is
   A. laser surgery.
   B. treatment of the diabetes.
   C. injection of insulin into the eye.
   D. appropriate corrective lenses.

4. A 76-year-old man complains of progressive loss of peripheral vision that is confirmed by his ophthalmologist by visual field testing. He has no other symptoms and his central visual acuity is good. His most likely problem is
   A. presbyopia.
   B. astigmatism.
   C. cataract.
   D. glaucoma.

5. Presbyopia results from
   A. light rays focusing behind the retina.
   B. light rays focusing in front of the retina.
   C. retinal hemorrhage.
   D. degeneration of the lens.

6. Which of the following conditions results from uneven focusing of light on the retina because of irregularities of the cornea or lens?
   A. Astigmatism
   B. Myopia
   C. Hyperopia
   D. Strabismus

7. Both hyperopia and presbyopia result in
   A. retinal detachment.
   B. decreased accommodation.
   C. decreased visual acuity for distant objects.
   D. opacification of the lens.

Bones and Joints

OUTLINE

OBJECTIVES

1. Review the structure and function of bones and joints.
2. Compare the relative frequency of joint disease and bone disease, and state how they are likely to differ in their consequences.
3. Identify the most common and most serious problems affecting bones and joints.
4. State the common manifestations (symptoms and signs) of bone and joint diseases.
5. Describe the common laboratory, radiographic, and clinical procedures used to diagnosis diseases of the bones and joints.
6. Describe how localized developmental abnormalities differ from generalized genetic abnormalities of the skeletal system in terms of frequency and likely outcome, and give examples of each.
7. Describe the genetic abnormalities in achondroplasia, osteogenesis imperfecta, and Marfan syndrome, and describe the appearance of individuals affected by these diseases.
8. Compare and contrast sprain, strain, and subluxation.
9. List the most common causes of low back pain and describe how a herniated disc develops.
10. Describe the various kinds of fracture and understand how fractures heal and which factors impair healing.
11. Define septic arthritis and describe how it arises and is treated.
12. Compare hematogenous osteomyelitis with secondary osteomyelitis in terms of cause, affected population, and outcome.
13. Define osteopenia and osteoporosis, and describe how bone loss is detected.

14. List some of the causes and complications of osteoporosis and describe who is most likely to have it.
15. Compare osteoporosis and osteomalacia in terms of cause, affected population, and laboratory findings.
16. Understand how degenerative and rheumatoid arthritis differ in frequency, cause, morphology, and location.
17. Describe how primary and metastatic cancers of bone and osteosarcoma differ in frequency, age of occurrence, and outcome.
18. Describe the most common primary malignant neoplasm of bone.
19. Be able to define and use in proper context the words and terms in bold print throughout the chapter.

KEY TERMS

acetabulum	metaphysis
achondroplasia	metaplastic bone formation
alkaline phosphatase	multiple myeloma
ankylosing spondylitis	nucleus pulposus
ankylosis	open fracture
arthritis	ossification
arthroscopy	osteitis deformans
calcitonin	osteoarthritis
chondrocytes	osteoblast
closed fracture	osteoclast
clubfoot	osteogenesis imperfecta
comminuted fracture	osteoid
complete fracture	osteomyelitis
compression fracture	osteopenia
degenerative joint disease	osteophyte
developmental dyplasia of	osteoporosis
the hip	osteosarcoma
diaphysis	pannus
dual-energy x-ray	parathormone
absorptiometry	periosteum
epiphyseal plate	radiculopathy
epiphysis	rheumatoid arthritis
erythrocyte sedimentation	rheumatoid factor
rate	rickets
Ewing sarcoma	sciatica
fibrillin	scoliosis
flat bone	septic arthritis
fracture	sex hormones
ganglion	sprain
gout	strain
hematopoiesis	subluxation
herniated disc	synostosis
hyaline cartilage	synovial fluid
hydroxyapatite crystals	synovial joint
incomplete fracture	tophus
juvenile arthritis	torticollis
kyphosis	T-score
low back pain	uric acid
lumbar spine	vertebral body
Marfan syndrome	vitamin D
meniscus	whiplash injury

Review of Structure and Function

The human body contains 206 bones, most of which have joints at their ends to connect them to adjacent bones. Bone provides a framework for the attachment of muscles, supports weight bearing, and protects internal organs from injury. It also plays a major role in calcium and phosphorus metabolism. Bone marrow may be considered part of bone. Joints allow movement of body parts and control the extent of movement. They can be very tight, such as the fusions between cranial bones after they have stopped growing in childhood. A tight joint is called a **synostosis**. The majority of joints are between bones that move. In this type of joint, ends of the two bones that articulate with one another are covered by **hyaline cartilage**, which has a very smooth surface and allows the two bones to move smoothly against each other. Fibrous bands connect the two bones together and form a tight capsule lined by a serous membrane and filled with lubricating fluid called **synovial fluid**. These types of joints are called **synovial joints**. The major bones and joints are labeled in **Figure 21–1**.

The parts of a typical long bone are shown in **Figure 21–2**. The long, tubular shaft of bone is called the **diaphysis**, the end that articulates with another bone is the **epiphysis**, and the part that flares out between the diaphysis and epiphysis is the **metaphysis**. In children, there is a cartilaginous **epiphyseal plate** between the epiphysis and metaphysis. **Ossification**, or bone formation, occurs on either side of this plate during childhood. The epiphyseal plate is essential for a bone to reach its mature length. Fusion of the plate results in cessation of growth and is a normal part of maturation. Damage to the epiphyseal plate by trauma, cancer, or infection results in permanently impaired growth, short limb length, and asymmetry of the limb (or digit).

The knee joint (**Figure 21–3**) is a particularly frequent site of injury and disease. It is structurally more complex than most other synovial joints. It contains fibrocartilaginous pads called **menisci** and is supported anteriorly by an extra bone, the patella. Numerous tendons and ligaments connect the femur, tibia, and patella to one another. The spinal column (**Figure 21–4**) has discs between vertebral bodies that consist of **nucleus pulposus** surrounded by fibrocartilage. The spinal canal, which houses the delicate spinal cord and emerging spinal nerves, lies posterior to the **vertebral bodies** and anterior to the more complex posterior elements of the spine. Like the knee, the spine is particularly vulnerable to the effects of weight bearing. The **flat bones** such as ribs, sternum, pelvis, and cranium serve to protect the thorax, abdomen, and brain. They also, along with the vertebrae (especially in older individuals), are major sites of **hematopoiesis**, or blood cell formation.

Bone, in spite of its solid consistency, is an active tissue that responds to physical stress, metabolic conditions, injury, and disease, and it continues to remodel throughout life. It is covered on its outer surface by a tough, fibrous membrane, the **periosteum**, from which it receives its blood supply. Bone is formed by **osteoblasts**,

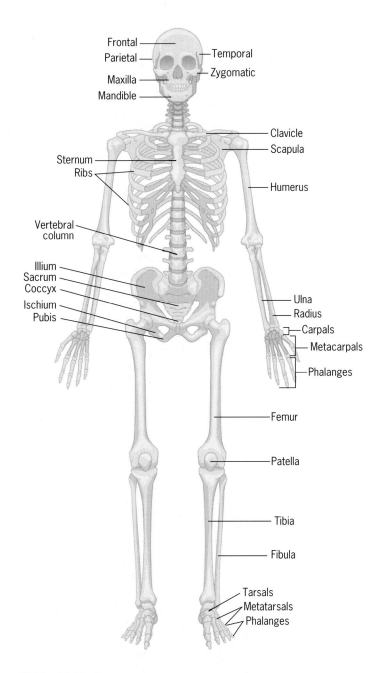

FIGURE 21–1 Major bones and joints of the body.

cells that lay down a collagenous matrix called **oste-oid** and promote deposition of **hydroxyapatite crystals** within this collagenous matrix. **Osteoclasts** are multinucleated cells that dissolve the mineral matrix of bone in response to hormonal signals. Hormones that exert effects on bone are **parathormone**, which stimulates release of calcium by bone; **calcitonin**, which antagonizes the effect of parathormone by stimulating calcium uptake by bone; **sex hormones**, primarily estrogen, which help maintain bone mineral density; and **vitamin D**, which also

promotes bone mineralization. In addition to responding to hormones, bone remodels rapidly in response to changes in load. Bone resorption accelerates after just 24 hours of bed rest, and bone density can be increased with weight-bearing exercises. When injured, such as by fracture, osteoblasts and **chondrocytes** proliferate to form new bone by enchondral ossification. Rarely, osteoblasts are seen at sites far away from bone, such as in severely stenotic aortic valves or at sites of soft-tissue injury. This is called **metaplastic bone formation**.

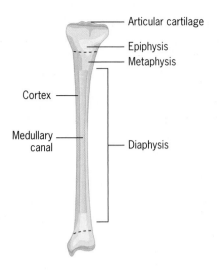

FIGURE 21–2 Structure of a long bone. The tibia is illustrated here.

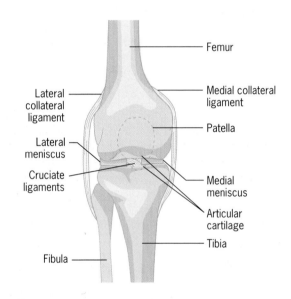

FIGURE 21–3 Anatomy of the knee joint.

Most Frequent and Serious Problems

Inflammation of the joints, or **arthritis**, is the most common disease affecting the bones and joints. There are more than 100 different types of arthritis, with **osteoarthritis**, or "degenerative joint disease," being the most common. The prevalence of arthritis increases with age so that 70% of people older than age 65 years have some degree of arthritis. Even so, more than half the people with arthritis are younger than the age of 65, and this includes nearly 250,000 children. More than $50 billion is spent each year for medical and surgical treatment of the condition.

By far the most frequent affliction of bone is **fracture**. Fractures can be caused by trauma alone or can be pathologic, meaning that the bone was already weakened by other disease such as metastatic cancer or **osteoporosis** and fractured because of a stress that would not have injured a healthy bone. Sites commonly involved with fractures vary with age and sex. For example, traumatic fractures of the extremities are most common in 20- to 40-year-old males. In children, the most common fractures are of the clavicle and the humerus. The risk of pathologic fractures as a result of osteoporosis increases with age. The bones most likely to fracture from osteoporosis are the proximal end of the femur, at the "hip," and the vertebrae. Traumatic injuries to the joints, **strains** and **sprains**, are more common than fractures of bone. They are among the most common reasons for patients' seeking health care for acute disease, while low back problems and degenerative arthritis are among the top reasons for patients seeking health care for chronic disease.

Generalized loss of bone, called **osteopenia**, may be the result of a wide variety of causes such as osteoporosis, osteomalacia, rickets, hyperparathyroidism, and metastatic cancer. Osteoporosis in postmenopausal women is the most common of these conditions and the hip, vertebral column, and forearm are the most common sites of fracture. Osteoporosis increases with age, so as the population of the United States ages, osteoporosis will become even more of a significant problem. Currently, it is estimated that about 12 million people in

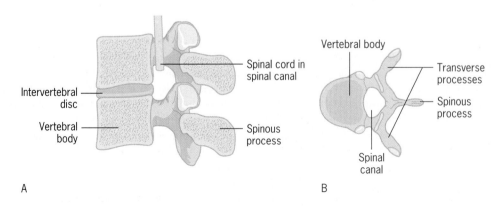

FIGURE 21–4 Anatomy of the spinal column. **A.** Sagittal plane. **B.** Transverse plane.

the United States have osteoporosis; by 2020 this number is expected to increase to 14 million. Every year about 2 million people suffer osteoporotic fractures. Older adults do not heal as easily as young people do, and many of these patients require care in long-term nursing facilities after the fracture. To the financial burden of care, then, is added the emotional and psychological burden of dependency.

Metastatic cancer is the most common malignancy of bone and often requires considerable health care because of associated pain and pathologic fracture. Of the several types of nonmetastatic cancers, **multiple myeloma** is the most common in adults and **osteosarcoma** and **Ewing sarcoma** are the most common in children and adolescents.

Symptoms, Signs, and Tests

The most common symptoms of bone and joint diseases are pain, decreased mobility, and deformity. Almost all fractures of bone are associated with pain resulting from disruption of sensory nerves. Usually, the fracture is obvious because of the attendant deformity, although in some fractures the bone is not displaced. The muscles surrounding a fracture site undergo intense sustained contraction, or spasm, in an attempt to protect the fractured area, and this spasm often causes additional pain. Joint stiffness, decreased mobility, and varying degrees of pain are associated with chronic forms of arthritis such as osteoarthritis and rheumatoid arthritis, whereas the cardinal signs of inflammation (redness, heat, swelling, and pain) are present with acute arthritis.

Physical examination of patients with bone and joint disease involves careful attention to evaluation of joint mobility, gait, and neurologic examination, as well as looking for deformity or masses.

Radiography is the primary diagnostic modality used to evaluate most bone and joint diseases. Plain films allow visualization of fractures and bony abnormalities, for example, at joint surfaces in the various forms of arthritis. Computed tomography (CT) scans are useful in the evaluation of masses. Magnetic resonance imaging (MRI) is helpful to assess problems with soft tissues such as ligaments and disk herniation. The joint space can further be visualized by **arthroscopy**, which involves inserting a fiber-optic scope into the joint cavity so as to see the joint structures, perform repairs of ligaments, remove loose cartilaginous fragments, or take biopsies. Larger joints, such as the knees, shoulders, hips, ankles, and elbows, can be directly examined with this technique.

The metabolic activity of bone is evaluated by a battery of serum tests, including calcium, phosphorus, and alkaline phosphatase. Calcium and phosphorus are principal constituents of bone, and **alkaline phosphatase** is an enzyme produced by osteoblasts that is elevated in many bone diseases that involve proliferation of osteoblasts. The **erythrocyte sedimentation rate** may be used as an indicator of inflammation and is useful in following

patients with rheumatoid arthritis. Tests for **rheumatoid factor** and serum **uric acid** levels may be useful aids in the diagnosis of rheumatoid arthritis and gout, respectively. Cultures are important in the diagnosis of acute arthritis and osteomyelitis. Rarely, a biopsy is necessary to confirm infection or to identify the nature of a bone tumor that has been demonstrated radiographically.

Specific Diseases
Genetic/Developmental Diseases

Developmental abnormalities fall into two broad groups. Selected structural defects include embryonic anomalies and localized deformities that arise during fetal development and childbirth. The most common types, many of which need early diagnosis and treatment to prevent permanent deformity, are discussed here. These include clubfoot, congenital dislocation of the hip, and torticollis. The wide variety of other types include conditions such as missing limbs and extra digits. The second major group of developmental abnormalities is generalized genetic disorders. These are much less common than are the localized types, and their treatment is symptomatic rather than curative. Three types are discussed briefly—achondroplasia, osteogenesis imperfecta, and Marfan syndrome.

Clubfoot (Talipes Equinovarus)

Clubfoot occurs in approximately 1 of every 1,000 births. It consists of a complex structural defect in which there is downward (equino) and inward (varus) turning of the foot, inward turning of the toes (metatarsus adductus), and an elevated arch (cavus deformity) caused by fixed flexion of the foot (**Figure 21–5**). Clubfoot can occur

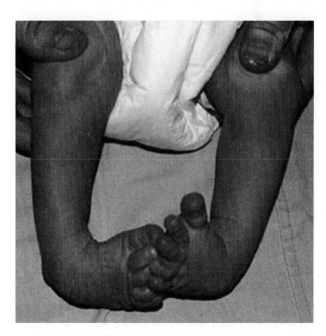

FIGURE 21–5 Clubfoot. (Courtesy of Dr. Kenneth Noonan, Department of Pediatric Orthopedics, University of Wisconsin School of Medicine and Public Health.)

bilaterally and is more frequent in males. Although the precise cause of clubfoot is not known, there is evidence that a genetic factor is involved. The deformity is evident at birth and can usually be corrected by placing the foot in casts for 2 to 6 months.

> ### BOX 21–1   Clubfoot
>
> **Causes**
> Genetic influence
> Other factors unknown
> **Lesions**
> Foot turned down and in (talipes equinovarus)
> **Manifestations**
> Deformity present at birth
> Permanent deformity if untreated

Developmental Dysplasia (Congenital Dislocation) of the Hip

Developmental dysplasia of the hip may be detected during infancy or childhood. It consists of displacement of the head of the femur from the hip socket, or **ace-tabulum**, with resultant deformation of the acetabulum (**Figure 21–6**). The occurrence is influenced by heredity and much more frequently involves girls than boys. Other risk factors are first-born girls and breech position. The most common clinical sign in infants is joint instability. As the child grows, the leg on the affected side shows limited abduction, or movement away from the body. If the condition is not corrected with splinting, the involved

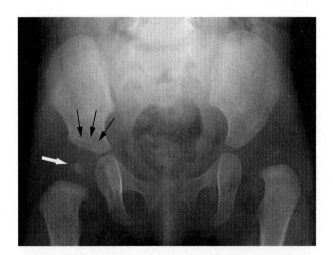

FIGURE 21–6 Developmental dysplasia of the hip, radiograph. The left hip is dislocated. Compare the orientation of the two hip sockets, or acetabula. On the right (normal) side, the acetabulum (thin black arrows) is facing downward, while on the opposite side, the hip socket is shallow, steep, and oriented outward. Also, the ossification center of the femoral head is much smaller on the left than on the right (white arrow). (Courtesy of Dr. Bradley Maxfield, Department of Radiology, University of Wisconsin School of Medicine and Public Health.)

joint may be permanently misshapen with resultant gait abnormalities and shortening of the involved leg. Treatment with appropriate splinting, if done in time, prevents permanent deformity and crippling.

> ### BOX 21–2   Developmental Dysplasia of the Hip
>
> **Causes**
> Genetic influence
> Risk factors: first-born girl, breech presentation
> **Lesions**
> Head of femur not in acetabulum
> Malformed acetabulum
> **Manifestations**
> Joint instability, limited abduction in infancy
> If untreated, gait abnormalities, short leg

Torticollis (Wry Neck)

Torticollis means "turned neck" and presents within the first 3 months of infancy as a neck pulled to one side. Although the cause is usually not clinically evident, it is believed to be due to injury to the sternocleidomastoid muscle during the fetal period by abnormal intrauterine positioning or injury at birth. Scarring and contraction of the muscle lead to pulling of the neck to one side. Treatment consists of manipulative stretching or surgical cutting of the muscle to prevent permanent facial deformity.

> ### BOX 21–3   Torticollis
>
> **Causes**
> Presumed injury to sternocleidomastoid muscle
> **Lesions**
> Scarring of sternocleidomastoid muscle
> **Manifestations**
> Neck turned and fixed to one side
> Onset in early infancy

Achondroplasia

Achondroplasia is a rare autosomal dominant disorder in which there is a mutation in fibroblast growth factor receptor gene 3 (*FGFR3*). This gene is necessary for cartilage formation and inhibits bone growth. In achondroplasia, the gene is constitutively activated. This results in a poorly organized epiphyseal plate so that ossification and subsequent growth of long bones is impaired (**Figure 21–7**). Usually, intramembranous ossification is not affected so that the cranium, for example, is of normal size, and affected individuals have normal intelligence. Homozygosity is lethal, but patients with one copy of the defective gene live a normal life span. The primary

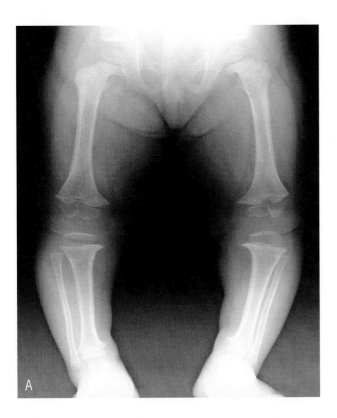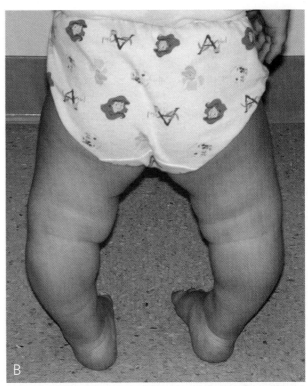

FIGURE 21–7 Achondroplasia. **A.** This is a skeletally immature, or still growing, individual, as can be seen by the presence of a translucent epiphyseal plate between the metaphyses and the epiphyses. **B.** Note the outward bowing of the legs and the disproportionately short long bones. (Courtesy of Dr. Kenneth Noonan, Department of Pediatric Orthopedics, University of Wisconsin School of Medicine and Public Health.)

defect is that they are short: their average height is just over 4 feet.

BOX 21-4   Achondroplasia

Causes

Autosomal dominant

Mutation of fibroblast growth factor receptor 3 gene (*FGFR3*)

Lesions

Failure of growth of long bones resulting from defective epiphyseal cartilage

Manifestations

Short stature (average height 4 feet)

Osteogenesis Imperfecta

Osteogenesis imperfecta is a genetic condition caused by abnormal collagen formation that usually follows an autosomal dominant inheritance pattern. There are several different types of osteogenesis imperfecta, affecting different genes and presenting with different degrees of severity. Very severe disease can cause death *in utero* or soon after birth. Thin bones that fracture with minimal trauma characterize the more common delayed form. The abnormal collagen production results in thin blue sclerae of the eye, fractures of the bony ossicles of the ear leading to deafness, and deformed, hypoplastic teeth.

BOX 21-5   Osteogenesis Imperfecta

Causes

Genetic defect in genes involved with synthesis of collagen

Autosomal dominant

Lesions

Fragile bone

Manifestations

Multiple fractures with slight trauma

Blue sclerae, hypoplastic teeth

Marfan Syndrome

Marfan syndrome is also an autosomal dominant disorder. The gene affected codes for a glycoprotein present in the extracellular matrix, called **fibrillin**. Fibrillin is necessary for the proper modeling of the connective tissue and for maintenance of its elastic properties. The affected tissues include the skeletal system, eyes, aorta and aortic valve, lungs, and dural membrane surrounding the spinal cord. The manifestations of the disease range from very severe to hardly noticeable. Classically, patients have disproportionately long arms and legs, and long, thin fingers (**Figure 21–8**). Other skeletal abnormalities can include **scoliosis**, or curvature of the spine, crowded teeth due to a narrow palate, and abnormalities of the sternum. Astigmatism, nearsightedness, spontaneous

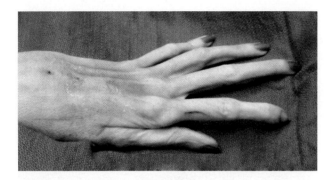

FIGURE 21–8 Marfan syndrome. One can appreciate why this disorder used to be called arachnodactyly, literally "spider fingers."

pneumothorax, and back pain caused by ballooning of the dural membrane can also occur. The potentially lethal complication of this disorder results from structural abnormality of the aorta. The root of the aorta, where it originates from the heart, can become excessively dilated, and the wall weak. This can result in rupture of the aorta and aortic dissection. Aortic rupture can occur in young people and may be precipitated by exercise.

BOX 21–6   Marfan Syndrome

Causes

Autosomal dominant

Mutation in fibrillin gene

Lesions

Weakened connective tissue, loss of elasticity

Manifestations

Tall, thin stature with long, slim limbs and fingers

Dislocation of lens, nearsightedness, astigmatism

Rupture and/or dissection of aorta

Inflammatory/Degenerative Diseases

In this category are discussed the effects of trauma (strains, sprains, fractures), infection (acute arthritis, osteomyelitis), and chronic disorders of varied etiology. Low back pain and curvatures of the spine (scoliosis and kyphosis) are clinical syndromes with multiple causes. Many other inflammatory and degenerative conditions of bones and joints, often made specific by their location and symptomatology, are beyond the scope of this text.

Injuries to Joints and Muscles

An acute injury to a joint with tearing of the joint capsule and ligaments around the joint is called a sprain. Hemorrhage around or into the joint may also be present. Twisting of the ankle is a common cause of a sprain and usually involves rupture of a ligament on the lateral side of the foot. **Whiplash injury**, caused by sudden extension of the neck, is a sprain in which ligaments and other tissues supporting the cervical spine are torn.

Tearing of a muscle and/or its tendon as the result of excessive use and stretching is called a strain. Muscle strains, commonly called "pulled" muscles, are usually accompanied by some degree of hemorrhage and mild inflammation. Athletes use conditioning and warmup exercises to prevent strains. Bones may be traumatically dislocated from their joint sockets. A partial dislocation is called a **subluxation**.

BOX 21–7   Sprains and Strains

Causes

Trauma

Twisting

Excessive exercise

Lesions

Tearing of joint capsule (sprain)

Tearing of muscle or tendon (strain)

Dislocation of bone from its socket (subluxation)

Manifestations

Swollen, tender, nonfunctional joint

Low Back Pain

Owing to their upright posture, humans are uniquely susceptible to **low back pain**. The **lumbar**, or lower part of the spine, essentially carries the entire weight of the torso and buffers it from rattles and jolts with every step we take. The problem of weight bearing is accentuated by obesity, weak abdominal muscles, poor posture, and sudden physical stresses. These factors are more likely to cause problems when there is underlying disease of the spine. The evaluation of persistent low back pain, an extremely common problem, involves evaluation of not just the spine but the entire patient for any signs of underlying disease that might affect bone health.

Back pain is most commonly caused by injury to nerves, muscles, or ligaments. If the back is exposed to a sudden, unaccustomed activity, such as lifting a heavy load, the muscles may undergo a strain, resulting in painful muscle spasms. The disc between the vertebrae is composed of a soft, gelatinous material that usually dries out a little with age and is prone to bulge outward, or **herniate** (**Figure 21–9**). When it does so, it is likely to pinch one of the dozens of nerves that branch off the spinal cord and pass between the vertebrae on their way to innervate peripheral tissues. In addition to causing low back pain, pressure on the nerves can cause **radiculopathy**, or pain in the tissues serviced by that nerve. For example, shooting pain in the leg, which may extend all the way down to the foot, is caused by a particular type of radiculopathy called **sciatica**, because the sciatic nerve is the one that is pinched. Bone spurs developing from osteoarthritis can also cause radiculopathy.

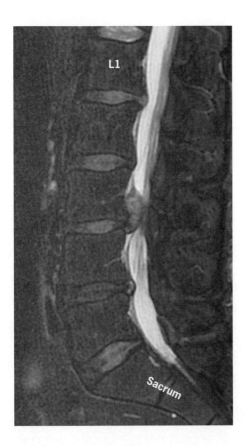

FIGURE 21–9 Herniated intervertebral disc. MRI scan of the lumbar (lower) spine. The vertebral bodies are separated by gray intervertebral discs. The spinal cord lying in the spinal canal is bright white. L1 = first lumbar vertebra. The vertebrae are numbered sequentially moving toward the sacrum. The disc between the third and fourth lumbar vertebrae has herniated. (Courtesy of Dr. Kirkland W. Davis, MD, Department of Radiology, University of Wisconsin School of Medicine and Public Health.)

Generalized diseases that can cause or accentuate low back pain include degenerative arthritis, rheumatoid arthritis, ankylosing spondylitis, osteoporosis, and metastatic cancer. Neurologic examination to evaluate for nerve compression and radiographic exams of the lower spine can reveal most of these conditions. Exercises to improve posture, strengthen muscles, including abdominal muscles, and weight loss are essential for controlling most low back pain. Muscle relaxants can be given if the pain is caused by muscle spasm. Spine surgery is sometimes necessary to remove degenerated discs or bone spurs or to permanently fix vertebrae to one another so as to prevent further degeneration.

Scoliosis and Kyphosis

Scoliosis is abnormal lateral and rotational curvature of the spine (**Figure 21–10**), and **kyphosis** is an abnormal forward bending of the upper spine producing a hunched back (**Figure 21–11**). By the age of 14 years, approximately 2% of people have some degree of scoliosis. Most of the time the cause is unknown. Known causes include

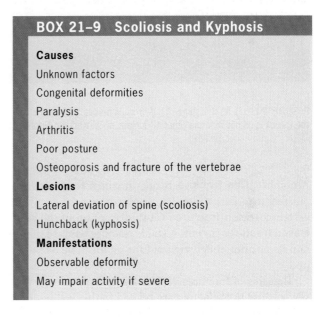

BOX 21–8   Low Back Pain

Causes
Strains
Herniated intervertebral disc
Various forms of arthritis
Metastatic cancer
Lesions
Depends on cause
Manifestations
Low back pain
Radiculopathy

congenital deformity, paralysis, and diseases involving the vertebrae. Kyphosis in young people is often postural, while in older adults it is the result of osteoporosis causing fractures of the vertebrae with resultant forward bowing of the spine.

BOX 21–9   Scoliosis and Kyphosis

Causes
Unknown factors
Congenital deformities
Paralysis
Arthritis
Poor posture
Osteoporosis and fracture of the vertebrae
Lesions
Lateral deviation of spine (scoliosis)
Hunchback (kyphosis)
Manifestations
Observable deformity
May impair activity if severe

Fractures

A fracture is any disruption of the continuity of bone. Most fractures are caused by trauma. Spontaneous fractures or fractures resulting from slight trauma suggest the possibility that the fracture was caused by underlying disease of bone. This is called a pathologic fracture. The pain associated with a fracture results from tearing of the periosteum, which contains sensory nerve endings.

Many terms are used to describe the nature of a fracture (**Figure 21–12**). **Incomplete fractures** produce cracks without separation of the ends of the bone; with **complete fractures**, the bone is separated into two or more parts (**Figure 21–13**). **Comminuted fractures** are ones in which more than two fragments are produced.

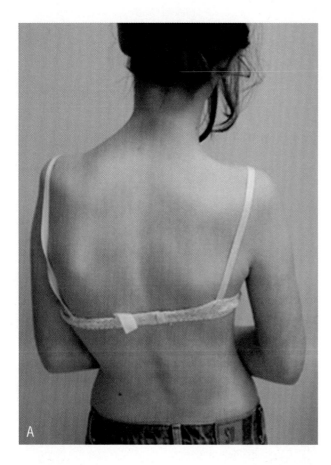
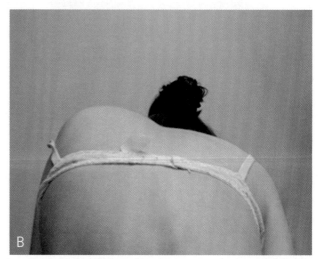

FIGURE 21–10 A. The spine of this woman makes a marked curve to the left when she stands upright. **B.** When she bends over, one side of the thorax is higher than the other. (Courtesy of Dr. Kenneth Noonan, Department of Pediatric Orthopedics, University of Wisconsin School of Medicine and Public Health.)

A **compression fracture** is one in which the bones are pushed together; these fractures commonly occur in vertebrae. **Open fractures** cause disruption of the skin; **closed fractures** do not. A stable fracture tends to maintain its position following fracture, an unstable one does not.

The sites of fractures vary in frequency with age and sex because these factors are related to the likelihood of various types of injury and the possibility of underlying disease. For example, arm fractures are common in children as a result of pulling or falling; spine and hip fractures are common in older women because these weight-bearing bones are affected by osteoporosis. Bone has great power to heal so that continuity can be accomplished in a few weeks and bone can return to normal strength in a few months. Fracture healing is much more rapid in the young than in older adults.

The process of fracture healing involves the proliferation of osteoblasts from the fracture margins to form new cartilage and bone, along with proliferation of vascular channels from the periosteum. The immature bone and cartilage are gradually remodeled into mature bone. Bone is usually produced in excess, but eventually, through the process of remodeling, the bone returns to normal structure.

Several important factors can prevent this normal healing sequence from occurring. The broken fragments must be close to each other or the ends will fail to unite. The fracture must be stabilized using splints, casts, traction (steady pulling by means of weights), or operatively inserted metal pins, screws, or plates. With fractures of the neck of the femur, the head of the femur is sometimes removed and replaced with a prosthesis. Nonstabilized fractures cannot heal. One of the worst complications of fracture is infection. Open fractures, particularly those in which the trauma drives dirt into the wound, and fractures that are artificially opened in the operative room to accomplish immobilization are subject to the possibility of infection. Cleaning of the wound, removal of dead tissue, and antibiotics are used to prevent infection. The consequences of an infected fracture are chronic osteomyelitis, nonunion, and eventual deformity.

Other factors affecting healing are the extent and location of the fracture. Comminuted fractures heal well unless they are displaced, involve joints, or cannot be stabilized. Fractures in the middle of long and flat bones generally heal well, whereas fractures involving joints are likely to produce problems with joint mobility. Fractures that disrupt the blood supply to the bone do not heal

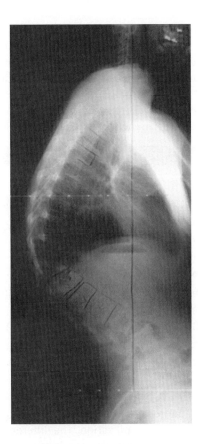

FIGURE 21–11 Kyphosis. This vertebral column has a marked convex deformity on lateral x–ray. (Courtesy of Dr. Kenneth Noonan, Department of Pediatric Orthopedics, University of Wisconsin School of Medicine and Public Health.)

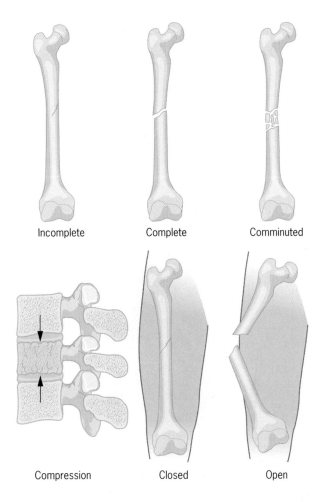

Incomplete   Complete   Comminuted

Compression   Closed   Open

FIGURE 21–12 Types of fractures.

well. Finally, pathologic fractures may not heal unless the underlying cause, such as a bone tumor, is addressed.

BOX 21–10   Fractures

Causes
Trauma
Primary diseases of bone (osteoporosis)
Diseases secondarily affecting bone (metastatic cancer)
Lesions
Break in continuity of bone
Manifestations
Pain
Deformity
Radiographic techniques for diagnosis

Septic Arthritis

Septic arthritis is caused by pyogenic bacteria. Staphylococci and streptococci are the most common bacteria to infect joints. The joint itself is usually sterile, meaning no bacteria grow there. Organisms get to the joint via the bloodstream, from an infection elsewhere, or are introduced directly into the joint via trauma. Infection of

the synovial lining causes painful, red, and swollen joints. Usually only one joint is affected; however, polyarthritis is common in disseminated infection by *Neisseria gonorrhea*. Septic arthritis can produce rapid destruction of the joint lining and is likely to lead to permanent destruction and bony **ankylosis** (stiffening caused by fusion of bones) of the joint.

BOX 21–11   Septic Arthritis

Causes
Infection by pyogenic bacteria (*Staphylococcus*, *Streptococcus* most common)
Lesions
Acutely inflamed joint space
Manifestations
Pain, heat, swelling, redness, leukocytosis, fever
Nonfunction of joint
Destruction of joint and ankylosis

Osteomyelitis

Although **osteomyelitis** literally means inflammation of bone, the term is usually used in a more restricted sense to mean infection of bone. The route of infection is the

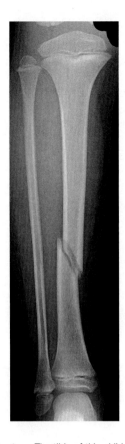

FIGURE 21–13 Fracture. The tibia of this child has sustained a complete fracture. Notice that the epiphyseal plates are still open: the ossification centers at each of the ends of the long bones, or epiphyses, have not yet fused on to the metaphyses. This indicates the patient is "skeletally immature," or a child. The fracture in the diaphysis has broken the bone completely in two. (Courtesy of Dr. Kirkland W. Davis, MD, Department of Radiology, University of Wisconsin School of Medicine and Public Health.)

basis of classification of the two major types of osteomyelitis. Hematogenous osteomyelitis involves spread of the causative organism through the blood to localize in one bone and set up a focus of infection. The site of entry of the organism is often a skin infection, which may go unnoticed. The organism is usually *Staphylococcus aureus*, and the site of the osteomyelitis is usually the metaphysis of a long bone, near but not involving the epiphysis. Children are most commonly affected. If untreated, the infection spreads, producing necrosis of the bone. The purulent infection may produce draining sinuses, and the necrotic bone must be removed because antibiotics will not be effective against bacteria lurking in dead bone. The clinical findings are pain and other local and systemic signs of inflammation. By the time x-ray changes occur, the bone is necrotic. The outcome in advanced cases includes recurrence of the infection and bone deformity with crippling.

The other form of osteomyelitis, which is much more common, is called secondary osteomyelitis because the infection spreads to bone secondarily from an adjacent site of infection or open wound. The most common causes are infected operative sites, soft-tissue infections

adjacent to bone, and gangrene of the toes with ulceration and infection. Treatment consists of removal of dead tissue and bone, open drainage of the infected area, and antibiotics. Treatment with antibiotics must be prolonged because usually the infected sites are poorly vascularized, so drug delivery via the bloodstream is compromised. Permanent damage is likely.

BOX 21–12   Osteomyelitis

Causes

Bacterial infection, *Staphylococcus* most common

Lesions

Acutely inflamed marrow cavity and bone

Necrosis of bone

Manifestations

Manifestations of acute and/or chronic inflammation

Sinuses draining pus

Necrotic bone by x-ray

Recurrence common

Osteoporosis

Osteopenia and osteoporosis both refer to quantitative decrease in bone mineralization. The difference between the two terms is that osteoporosis is more severe and is more likely to result in pathologic fracture. Osteopenia can be demonstrated by a special type of radiographic procedure called **dual-energy x-ray absorptiometry**, which measures how much of each of two x-ray beams with different amounts of energy are absorbed by bone. The result of this study is not a conventional x-ray image, but rather a number, or **T-score**, that relates the measured bone density to normal values. In the laboratory, bone health is indicated by serum levels of calcium, phosphorus, and alkaline phosphatase. Conditions that cause metabolic breakdown of bone typically cause elevated alkaline phosphatase levels and altered calcium and phosphorus levels. However, these tests are not sensitive for osteopenia and the type of osteoporosis that occurs in postmenopausal women.

Osteopenia occurs normally with aging. Bone mineral density reaches its peak in the early 30s and begins to decline after this point. In women, there is a direct relationship between estrogen levels and bone mineralization. After menopause, when estrogen production by the ovaries ceases, bone resorption by osteoclasts far outstrips bone mineralization, with a net decrease in bone strength. By definition, osteoporosis is present when the bone mineral density is less than 2.5 standard deviations less than normal. Whereas most osteoporosis occurs in postmenopausal women, it may occur in older men, in patients on long-term corticosteroid therapy, and in those subject to prolonged bed rest. Persons with large bones are less affected than are persons with small bones, and physically active people, especially those who engage in weight-bearing activities such as jogging, hiking, weight-lifting, or stair climbing, develop osteoporosis at a slower rate.

No single specific cause for osteoporosis has been identified. Obviously, estrogen is necessary for maintaining bone, and lack of exercise induces resorption of bone simply because it is not being used. However, lack of dietary calcium and interference in normal calcium metabolism by diseases such as chronic renal failure, hyperparathyroidism, excess corticosteroids, hyperthyroidism, inadequate intake of vitamin D, and certain intrinsic diseases of bone such as Paget disease can all result in osteoporosis. Risk factors include smoking, eating disorders, female sex, white or Asian race, and other diseases the patient may have that affect bone, such as rheumatoid arthritis. Once developed, reversion back to normal bone thickness is very difficult if not impossible to achieve. Therefore, prevention of the development of the disease is most important and this must be done years (decades) before the disease is likely to become manifest. Therapies that have been directed at this goal include increased calcium intake, vitamin D supplements, estrogens in menopausal women, testosterone in men with low levels, exercise, bisphosphonates (agents that inhibit bone resorption by osteoclasts), and calcitonin (a thyroid hormone that also inhibits bone resorption). Unfortunately, in most instances, preventive treatment is not employed and complications are treated as they develop.

The most common complications of osteoporosis are compression fractures of vertebrae and hip fractures. Vertebral disease is associated with pain and height reduction. Hip fracture is a severe acute illness that is often fatal or leads to permanent disability, particularly in frail older women.

BOX 21–13   Osteoporosis

Causes

Aging

Reduction in sex steroids

Corticosteroids

Immobilization of bone

Lesions

Thin, weak bone

Manifestations

Back pain

Fractures

Low bone mineral density by dual-energy x-ray absorptiometry

Normal calcium, phosphorus, alkaline phosphatase

Osteomalacia and Rickets

Osteomalacia and rickets are relatively rare conditions characterized by softening of bone. They differ from osteoporosis in that there is inadequate deposition of calcium and phosphorus, leaving an excess of the protein matrix of the bone. Osteomalacia is the adult form characterized by bone softening. **Rickets** is the childhood form with both softening and decreased growth of bones. The majority of cases are secondary to poor intake or poor utilization of vitamin D, with consequent improper deposition of calcium and phosphorus in bone. This is why vitamin D was introduced as a supplement in milk many years ago. In children, untreated rickets leads to markedly deformed bones. Osteomalacia in adults may cause fractures. Serum levels of calcium, phosphorus, and alkaline phosphatase are abnormal.

BOX 21–14   Osteomalacia and Rickets

Causes

Vitamin D deficiency due to inadequate diet or malabsorption

Lesions

Bone matrix without calcium present

Manifestations

Soft flexible bones

Fractures

Deformity and retarded bone growth (rickets)

Degenerative Arthritis

This very common disease is also called **degenerative joint disease** and osteoarthritis. It occurs most often in the middle-aged to older adult and is estimated to be present in 20 million persons in the United States. The main manifestations are joint stiffness and often pain. The lesion consists of erosion of the articular joint cartilage, with subsequent deformity of the cartilage and of the bone, resulting in stiffness and decreased motion. New growth of bone at the margins of the joint leads to so-called lipping (**osteophytes**), which further limits movement of the joint (**Figures 21–14B** and **21–15**). Degenerative joint disease is more common in women and typically involves the weight-bearing joints and the distal finger joints (**Figure 21–16A**). This pattern of involvement, plus a typical x-ray picture, helps distinguish degenerative from rheumatoid arthritis. Degenerative arthritis is likely to develop with time in injured joints or joints subject to undue stress, such as might occur with congenital dislocation of the hip or a knee that has been subject to athletic injuries.

Rheumatoid Arthritis

Rheumatoid arthritis is an autoimmune disease that can affect various organ systems in the body, most commonly the joints. The joint lesions, characterized by pain, stiffness, and deformity, are caused by inflammation of the

BOX 21-15   Degenerative Arthritis

Causes

Aging

Joint injury or deformity

Lesions

Destroyed articular cartilage

New bone formation with "lipping"

Manifestations

Pain

Decreased mobility of joint

Enlarged joint

Bone and cartilage changes by x-ray

synovial lining. As the inflammation extends on to the joint surface, it destroys cartilage and produces a layer of granulation tissue called a **pannus**, which induces destruction of the underlying cartilage and resorption of bone. Eventually, the entire joint surface may be destroyed and replaced by fibrous tissue, resulting in ankylosis, or joint rigidity. Morphologically, the joint lesion consists of a low-grade chronic inflammation of the synovial lining and joint surface, with destruction of the joint cartilage, fibrosis around the joint, and osteoporosis of the surrounding bone resulting from disuse (**Figure 21–14C**).

Rheumatoid arthritis is three times more common in women than in men and the overall prevalence is nearly 2% of the population. The onset is usually in the third to sixth decades of life. The disease varies in severity from mild joint stiffness to severe cases having distortion and ankylosis of many joints, with almost total loss of function. Usually, the arthritis is symmetrical, meaning the same joint on both sides of the body is affected, and it begins in small joints such as the metacarpal–phalangeal joints and can later involve large joints such as the ankles, elbows, and knees. Involvement of the metacarpal-phalangeal joints leads to characteristic outward (ulnar) deviation of the fingers (**Figure 21–16B**). Many patients with severe rheumatoid arthritis also have chronic inflammation and vasculitis involving other organs such as the heart, muscle, lungs, skin, and blood vessels.

As with most autoimmune diseases, the exact etiology of rheumatoid arthritis is not known. Genetic susceptibility and environmental factors are both thought to play a role. Most people with rheumatoid arthritis have antibodies against a particular region on the immunoglobin G (IgG) molecule; in other words, they produce an antibody against an antibody. The abnormal antibody is called rheumatoid factor. The resultant immune complexes form in serum and synovium, but they are not thought to be critical in stimulating the inflammatory response. Rheumatoid factor can be measured in serum and is a marker of disease activity, but it can also be present in other diseases and even in individuals without rheumatoid arthritis.

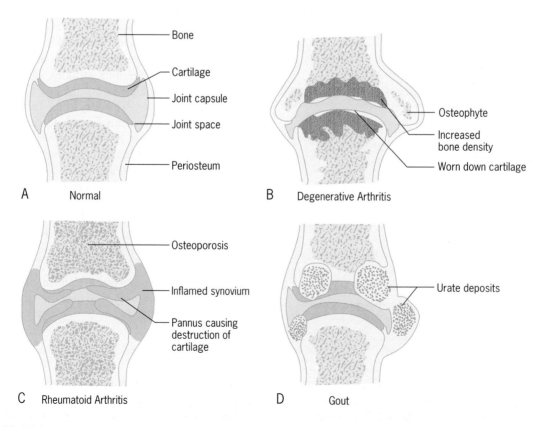

FIGURE 21–14 Schematic representation of normal joint (**A**), lesions of degenerative arthritis (**B**), rheumatoid arthritis (**C**), and gout (**D**).

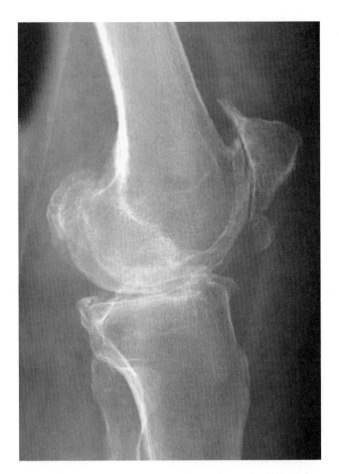

FIGURE 21–15 Degenerative joint disease of the knee, lateral x–ray. The joint spaces, or the spaces between the tibia, femur, and patella are narrowed and the edges of the bones are blurry, indicating erosion and reactive sclerosis of the articular surfaces of the bone. The contour of the patella is quite irregular and large osteophytes, or "spurs," are growing from its edges. (Courtesy of Dr. Kirkland W. Davis, MD, Department of Radiology, University of Wisconsin School of Medicine and Public Health.)

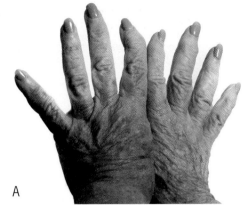

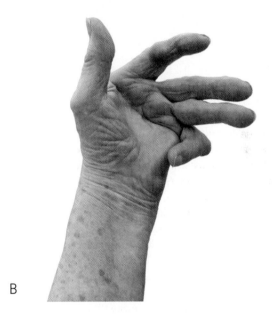

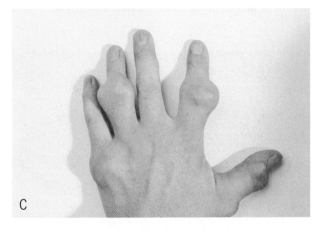

FIGURE 21–16 Hand changes in advanced cases of various types of arthritis. **A.** Degenerative arthritis. (© Laurin Linder/ShutterStock, Inc.) **B.** Rheumatoid arthritis. (© Peterfactors/Dreamstime.com) **C.** Gout. (© GIRAND/GJM/age fotostock)

Joints affected by rheumatoid arthritis are swollen, warm, and painful. The disease usually develops over months and years, with gradual involvement of additional joints. The disease can also wax and wane, with periods of severe arthritis followed by periods of remission. Treatment is primarily symptomatic, aimed at reducing pain and inflammation. Corticosteroids and methotrexate, which decrease immune reactions, and antagonists of tumor necrosis factor (TNF) are effective, but make the patient susceptible to infection. Heat, splints, and exercise also confer temporary relief. Severe joint deformities can be corrected by surgically replacing them with prostheses.

Juvenile arthritis occurs very early in life and may be extremely severe. **Ankylosing spondylitis** is an inflammatory arthritis predominantly involving the spine and sacroiliac joints. Long considered a variant of rheumatoid arthritis because the lesions are histologically similar, it is now considered to be a separate disease because

it occurs in young men, tests negative for rheumatoid factor, has a strong association with the inherited HLA-B27 antigen, and has a familial tendency. The deformity of the spine with stooped posture often leads to severe disability. Treatment usually consists of nonsteroidal anti-inflammatory agents (NSAIDs) and physical therapy.

BOX 21–16   Rheumatoid Arthritis

Causes
Autoimmune reaction
Lesions
Pannus
Resorption of articular cartilage and underlying bone
Manifestations
Pain, swelling, immobility of joint
Joint deformity
Positive tests for rheumatoid factor
Changes seen by x-ray

Gout

Abnormal metabolism of uric acid results in **gout**. Excess uric acid is deposited in many tissues, particularly joints, causing painful arthritis. In the chronic stage, these urate deposits accumulate to form **tophi** (**Figures 21–14D, 21–16C,** and **21–17**). Formerly, gout was called the "disease of kings" because it can be caused by excess consumption of wine and red meat, and it was associated with a gluttonous lifestyle. Gout occurs almost exclusively in men older than the age of 30 years and clinically manifests with bouts of painful arthritis. The joint classically affected is the metatarsal–phalangeal joint at the base of the large toe. Other joints affected include the fingers, wrists, ankles, and knees. Treatment of acute gout involves NSAIDs; chronically, lifestyle modifications and various pharmaceutical agents that promote the excretion of uric acid or inhibit its production (allopurinol) are used.

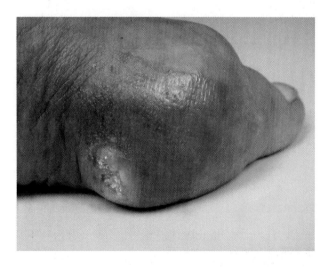

FIGURE 21–17 Gout. This is a left big toe affected by gout. The skin at the inferior of the metatarsal–phalangeal joint has broken down, and white granular material—the tophus—is extruding from the defect. The tophus is composed of urate crystals. (© GIRAND/BSIP/age fotostock)

BOX 21–17   Gout

Causes
Genetic
Consumption of alcohol, meat
Lesions
Tophi in joints and soft tissue
Manifestations
Sudden joint pain (acute stages)
Deformity of joints with masses from tophi (chronic stage)
Mostly in adult men
Elevated serum uric acid

Ganglion

A **ganglion** is a smooth cystic swelling that arises from joint capsules, most commonly on the wrist. Ganglion cysts are often associated with continued trauma and may be painful, although they usually arise insidiously as a simple swelling. Surgical removal may be undertaken if the ganglion is bothersome to the patient.

BOX 21–18   Ganglion

Causes
Unknown
Lesions
Outpouching of synovial lining into soft tissue
Manifestations
Fluctuant lump on back of wrist

Hyperplastic/Neoplastic Diseases

There are many types of neoplasms and nonneoplastic tumors of bone, cartilage, joints, and tendon sheaths. Most are rare and are not discussed here. The most common malignant tumors are metastatic cancers from sites such as the breast, lung, prostate, and kidney, as well as multiple myeloma and lymphomas. The most common primary malignant neoplasms of bone—osteosarcoma and Ewing sarcoma—are diseases of children and young adults. Paget disease of bone is a peculiar hyperplastic disease.

Paget Disease of Bone

Paget disease, or **osteitis deformans**, is a localized or multifocal enlargement of bone of unknown cause that affects about 2% of the population, typically in persons older than 40 years of age. It may be related to paramyxovirus infection. Initially, the affected bone may be more porous, but there is a gradual haphazard bony proliferation leading to some deformity of the bone and occasionally to pathologic fracture. High serum alkaline phosphatase reflects the active bone remodeling, but there is no defect in calcium and phosphorus metabolism. Most patients are asymptomatic. Rarely, osteosarcoma may develop in the lesion.

Osteosarcoma

Osteosarcoma is a malignant bone-forming tumor arising in bone. It is the most common malignant tumor of bone in children, but it also occurs in older adults. In the latter, it usually arises in the context of some other disease, such as Paget disease or long-standing osteomyelitis, or in the field of prior irradiation. Osteosarcoma arises most commonly at the ends of long bones; 50% of these tumors occur around the knee (**Figure 21–18**). Most patients present with a bony mass that is often painful and can undergo pathologic fracture. There is usually no evidence of metastasis at the time of presentation, but occult metastases are probably present because amputation alone is followed by overt metastases and death in 80% of patients. Aggressive radiation and chemotherapy before the lesion is removed, followed by additional chemotherapy, have achieved a cure rate of more than 60%.

BOX 21–19   Osteosarcoma

Causes
Unknown
Radiation
Paget disease of bone
Lesions
Sarcoma with bone production
Manifestations
Mass in bone
Pathologic fracture
Usually children and young adults
Lung metastases

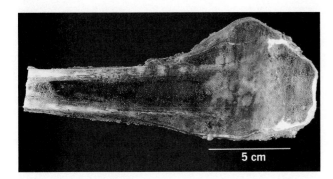

FIGURE 21–18 Osteosarcoma. This is the proximal tibia of a skeletally immature individual (you can still see the remnant of the cartilaginous epiphyseal plate running across the tibia at the right of the image). The normal marrow cavity in the diaphysis at the left is red and granular, reflecting the hematopoietic tissue and numerous thin bony trabeculae in the marrow, and the normal cortical bone is thick and white. As you follow the cortical bone from the left (distal) to the right (proximal), it first expands and then disappears as it is invaded and destroyed by the solid neoplastic growth that fills the metaphysis and destroys the epiphyseal plate.

Organ Failure

The main function of the skeletal system is to maintain support and mobility for everyday activity. Injury or disuse of major joints and fractures of weight-supporting bones is likely to lead to considerable incapacity of movement. Extensive severe arthritis or widespread bone metastases may confine patients to a wheelchair or bed.

Practice Questions

1. A 48-year-old man is tall and thin, and has a dislocated eye lens and an unusual heart murmur. Three other close family members have a similar physical appearance. His diagnosis is most likely
   A. osteogenesis imperfecta.
   B. achondroplasia.
   C. Marfan syndrome.
   D. torticollis.
   E. rheumatoid arthritis.

2. Following an automobile accident, x-ray examination of a 20-year-old woman shows a fracture in the middle of her right femur that separates the two segments of bone. This is an example of
   A. an open fracture.
   B. a comminuted fracture.
   C. a compression fracture.
   D. a complete fracture.

3. The woman in question 2 has her femur placed in a cast. After 3 months, healing of the femur, as evidenced by x-ray, is nearly complete, but she experiences a series of low-grade fevers and develops a sinus tract in the skin of the femur that drains pus. Most likely, she has developed
   A. osteomyelitis.
   B. osteoporosis.
   C. osteomalacia.
   D. acute arthritis.

4. A 77-year-old woman slips on the ice in front of her home and fractures her left hip. At the hospital, her physician goes over her records and notices that she has lost 2 inches in height over the past 8 years. Her symptoms are classic for
   A. osteomyelitis.
   B. osteoporosis.
   C. osteomalacia.
   D. Paget disease.

5. Degenerative arthritis is differentiated from rheumatoid arthritis in a 55-year-old woman by all of the following except which one?
   A. X-ray examination
   B. Laboratory tests
   C. Which joints are affected
   D. Signs of inflammation

6. A 55-year-old, overweight truck driver complains to his physician of severe low back pain with sciatica. Of the following, the more likely cause of his condition is
   A. muscle spasm.
   B. sprained ligaments.
   C. vertebral fracture.
   D. herniated intervertebral disc.

7. A 78-year-old woman falls on the ice and breaks her femur. X-ray examination and subsequent biopsy of the fracture site reveal metastatic tumor. This is an example of which of the following types of fracture?
   A. Pathologic
   B. Open
   C. Comminuted
   D. Complete

8. Rheumatoid factor is an antibody directed against
   A. the pannus.
   B. immunoglobulin G.
   C. the synovium.
   D. joint cartilage.

Skeletal Muscle and Peripheral Nerve

OBJECTIVES

1. Name the two major divisions of muscle disease in terms of pathogenesis.
2. Relate how laboratory tests and procedures (e.g., creatine kinase, electromyography, muscle biopsy) are helpful in evaluation of a person with muscle disease.
3. List the causes, lesions, and major manifestations of each of the specific muscle and nerve diseases listed in this chapter.
4. Compare the signs and symptoms of neurogenic muscle disorders with those of myopathic disorders.
5. Understand why it is important to separate dystrophic, inflammatory, and neurogenic causes of muscle weakness.
6. Be able to define and use in context the terms in bold print in this chapter.

KEY TERMS

actin
amyotrophic lateral sclerosis
congenital myopathy
creatine kinase
diabetic neuropathy
diplopia
Duchenne muscular dystrophy
dystrophin
dystrophy
electromyography
fascicle
Guillain-Barré syndrome (GBS)
muscle biopsy
muscle fiber

myasthenia gravis
myelin sheath
myopathic disease
myosin
myotonia
myotonic dystrophy
nerve biopsy
neurofibroma
neurogenic disease
nodes of Ranvier
paralysis
polymyositis
rhabdomyosarcoma
Schwannoma
spindles
weakness
Werdnig-Hoffman disease

Review of Structure and Function

Skeletal muscle is the largest organ in the body and utilizes about 10% of the body's oxygen in the resting state but as much as 80% or more with intense exercise. All skeletal muscles are separated into bundles called **fascicles**, which are enclosed in connective tissue. Fascicles are in turn composed of individual **muscle fibers** (cells), each of which courses the entire length of

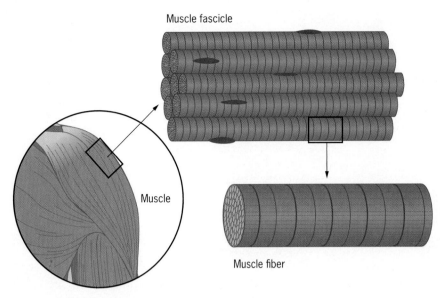

Muscle fascicle

Muscle

Muscle fiber

FIGURE 22–1 Schematic representation of skeletal muscle, with a fascicle and an individual fiber. Each muscle fiber courses the entire length of the muscle. The alternating light and dark bands are called striations and can be seen by light microscopy.

the muscle (**Figure 22–1**). Muscle fibers are innervated by branches of axons from anterior horn neurons in the spinal cord. In muscles that need fine discriminatory movements, such as the eye, one neuron may innervate as few as four to six muscle fibers; by comparison, in large muscles used for strength and weight bearing (gluteus or quadriceps), one neuron may innervate 2,000 or more muscle fibers. Muscle maintains its tone by a complex system of nerves that wrap around special fibers (**spindles**) and send information regarding the degree of muscle contraction back to the spinal cord neurons. Chemically, muscle is composed primarily of two proteins, **actin** and **myosin**, which are filaments arranged alternately in parallel rows. These filaments slide back and forth beside each other, thereby performing the contraction and relaxation processes.

The overlapping of the filaments delineates the I and the A bands, which can be seen by light microscopy as striations (Figure 22–1).

Muscle fibers are divided into types I and II on the basis of their histochemical reactions (**Figure 22–2**). These types also correspond somewhat to physiologic properties. For example, type I fibers are more used for slow, sustained contractions, whereas type II fibers contract more quickly. Type II fibers respond to exercise by hypertrophy and to disuse by atrophy. In humans, the two fiber types are evenly distributed throughout all muscles, but in many animals an individual muscle may be composed entirely of one fiber type. For example, in domestic birds such as chickens, the dark muscles (leg, thigh) consist entirely of type I fibers, while the light muscles (wings, breast) are all type II fibers.

Peripheral nerves run from the spinal cord to organs, including muscles, where they receive either sensory input for return to the spinal cord or brain or deliver a signal to skeletal muscle to contract. Some nerves belong to the autonomic nervous system. Sensory autonomic nerves transmit sensations from internal organs, and motor autonomic nerves send signals to smooth muscle such as in the vascular system, the intestinal tract, and the uterus. Autonomic nerve axons are characteristically unmyelinated, whereas regular motor and sensory nerves contain a **myelin sheath** composed of several layers of lipid membranes wrapped around the axon with periodic constrictions called **nodes of Ranvier**. Axons and myelin sheaths are sustained by Schwann cells (**Figure 22–3**). Both myelin sheaths and axons can regenerate if damaged. Typically, axons regenerate by splitting into several smaller axons and grow at a slow, finite rate back to their end organ. When myelin sheaths

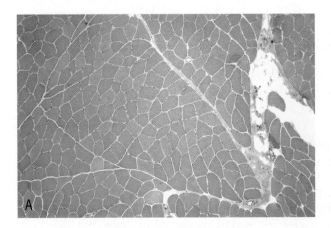

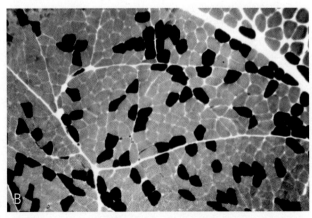

FIGURE 22–2 Cross section of muscle fibers. **A.** Routine hematoxylin and eosin stained section. Each individual muscle fiber has abundant pink cytoplasm. Nuclei are present around the periphery of each cell. **B.** Skeletal muscle stained with the enzyme ATPase to demonstrate type I and II fibers. (Courtesy of Dr. M. Shahriar Salamat, Department of Pathology and Laboratory Medicine, University of Wisconsin School of Medicine and Public Health.)

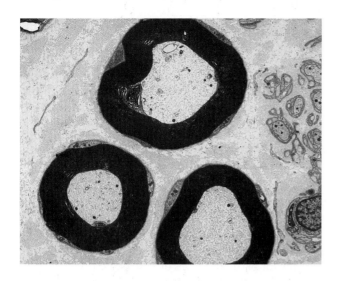

FIGURE 22–3 Cross section of part of a nerve by electron microscopy. The large, dense, dark circles are the myelin sheaths that encircle axons. On the right edge of the image are several unmyelinated axons. They are wrapped around by Schwann cells, and Schwann cell nuclei are also present as large, elongated, gray structures with black granules on the periphery of the myelinated axons. (Courtesy of Dr. M. Shahriar Salamat, Department of Pathology and Laboratory Medicine, University of Wisconsin School of Medicine and Public Health.)

regenerate, they usually do not contain as many lipid wrappings as formerly existed.

The location where the nerve inserts into the muscle is called the neuromuscular junction and is composed of a complex, folded membrane. Acetylcholine is released by the nerve fiber, depolarizing the membrane and thus leading to contraction of the muscle.

Most Frequent and Serious Problems

Probably the most common affliction of muscle is simply weakness with or without muscle atrophy. This may occur as a part of a generalized disease such as cancer or any disease that results in prolonged immobilization. Muscular dystrophies are important muscle diseases because they are often inherited and, consequently, genetic counseling becomes an important aspect of disease prevention. The most frequently occurring and most severe dystrophy is Duchenne muscular dystrophy. Whenever there is disease of the nervous system, there will also be associated muscle weakness. Therefore, victims of traumatic nerve injuries, neoplasms, strokes, and many other nervous system diseases will all display muscle weakness. Trauma may result in muscle weakness from either muscle destruction or nerve damage.

Disruptions in peripheral nerve function constitute neuropathies and can result in various types of sensory loss or weakness if motor fibers are primarily involved. Inflammatory neuropathies are not common, but can be severe. The most important type of infectious neuropathy worldwide is leprosy. Diabetics commonly acquire

peripheral neuropathies that can be severe and difficult to treat. Hereditary, motor, and sensory neuropathies can occur by themselves or be associated with other diseases. A variety of biologic toxins, industrial chemicals, heavy metals such as lead and arsenic, and drugs can result in toxic neuropathies. Some of the most common offending drugs are ethanol and acrylamides. Peripheral nerve tumors are rare, but occasionally Schwannomas or neurofibromas arise from the Schwann cells in peripheral nerves. These are commonly associated with the disease called neurofibromatosis.

Symptoms, Signs, and Tests

Weakness is the common denominator of muscle disease, whether it be primary disease of muscle (myopathic) or secondary to disease of the nervous system (neurogenic). The pattern of weakness often affords the physician an important clue as to the type of muscle disease present. For example, muscular dystrophies most often involve proximal muscle groups, whereas diseases of nerves are more likely to result in atrophy and weakness of the more distal parts of the extremities. If weakness persists for any length of time, the muscle will become atrophic, irrespective of the cause of the disorder, simply because of disuse. Conversely, atrophy of muscle obviously results in weakness. Pain is occasionally associated with muscle disease and when present often signifies muscle inflammation.

Although the presence of muscle disease is often obvious because of weakness and atrophy, many times the patient's symptoms may be nondescript or vague. In such cases, certain laboratory tests both aid in the diagnosis of muscle disease and help quantify the degree of muscle damage. **Creatine kinase** is an enzyme normally involved in the metabolism of muscle that is present in the serum in increased quantities following many disorders that damage muscle. It is usually more elevated in myopathic than in neurogenic disorders, and the degree of elevation of this enzyme roughly parallels the extent of muscle damage. **Electromyography** can also help to separate intrinsic muscle disorders from neurogenic muscle disorders and to quantify the extent of muscle damage. Electromyography is accomplished by inserting a needle into a muscle and recording the electrical activity. The most reliable means of separating myopathic from neurogenic causes of muscle disease is **muscle biopsy**, a procedure that is easily performed on most muscles. The major differences between neurogenic and myopathic muscle disorders are summarized in **Table 22–1**.

The peripheral nerve status of a patient is assessed first by a good neurologic examination in which the various sensory modalities such as touch, pain, temperature, and two-point discrimination are tested. Motor neuron integrity is assessed by examining the patient for weakness in the various muscle groups supplied by particular nerves. Electrophysiologic nerve conduction tests can determine the speed and amplitude of an impulse conducted along

TABLE 22-1	Comparison of Normal, Myopathic, and Neurogenic Muscle Disorders		
	Normal	**Myopathic**	**Neurogenic**
Symptoms or signs	None	Proximal weakness, possible pain	Distal weakness, often in a nerve distribution; possible sensory loss
Electromyography	No spontaneous activity in muscle	Asynchronous spontaneous activity	Synchronous activity of small amplitude
Serum enzyme (creatine kinase)	Normal	Often markedly elevated	Mildly elevated or normal
Biopsy	Normal fiber configuration	Variable size of fibers; degenerative fibers; possible fibrosis	Atrophic fibers in small groups

an axon that can help in identifying whether damage to a nerve is primarily directed at the axon or at the myelin sheath. More definitive evaluation can be obtained by a **nerve biopsy**. Commonly, the sural nerve in the lower leg is examined because sacrifice of this nerve does not harm the patient. However, the sural nerve is predominantly sensory, and if motor function is to be evaluated, a muscle biopsy is usually necessary. The most important direct examination of peripheral nerve is by electron microscopy because this can determine whether the damage is to the axon or the myelin sheath, whether there is inflammation present, whether the unmyelinated nerves are involved, and what the status of the nerve vasculature is.

Specific Diseases
Genetic/Developmental Diseases

Numerous types of primary muscle degeneration are collectively called dystrophies. Because many of the more common types of dystrophy are genetically determined, we consider the entire group under developmental rather than under degenerative disorders, keeping in mind that the exact cause of some types of dystrophy is undetermined.

Dystrophy literally means poor nutrition and was originally applied to muscle disorders thought to be of simple cause and not caused secondarily by disease of the nerves. Today there are many diseases termed dystrophic that have various causes. Many are hereditary with onset at an early age. Others are definitely hereditary but do not become manifest until adult life. Still others do not appear to be hereditary at all. Dystrophies are classified according to the pattern of muscle involvement—group(s) of muscles affected—or according to the type of microscopic lesion. Different dystrophies initially show slightly different lesions, but eventually all lead to muscle atrophy with replacement of muscle by adipose and fibrous tissues. Most of the dystrophies involve proximal muscles of the extremities and the pelvis and shoulder girdles in preference to distal muscles of the extremities. There is no known cure for any of the dystrophies, and all follow a variable but fairly predictable course. Therapy must be supportive. By light microscopy, most dystrophies show variable fiber size, fiber splitting, increased

amounts of connective tissue, and large rounded fibers (**Figure 22-4**). Other microscopic findings are more specific for particular types of dystrophy.

Duchenne Dystrophy

The most common and serious of the dystrophies is Duchenne dystrophy, which is inherited as a sex-linked recessive disorder with an incidence of 1 in 3,500 male births, and which affects males within the first few years of life, giving them an expected life span of only 12 to 20 years. The Duchenne gene encodes for a muscle protein called **dystrophin** that normally links the cytoskeleton of the muscle cell to the extracellular matrix. Mutations in the gene result in dystrophin deficiency with consequent loss of stability and breakdown of the muscle fiber. As in most myopathic conditions, the weakness is predominantly of the proximal muscle groups. Boys with Duchenne dystrophy characteristically develop "pseudohypertrophy" of the calves, in which the calves appear large and muscular but are actually replaced by adipose tissue (**Figure 22-5**). The heart muscle may also be involved in this disease. A less severe variety of the disease is referred to as Becker dystrophy. The diagnosis of Duchenne dystrophy is based on typical age of occurrence, family history, and findings of intrinsic muscle disease (myopathic) by electromyography, genetic analysis, enzyme tests, and muscle biopsy. The biopsy shows disruption, loss of both type I and type II muscle fibers with replacement by connective tissue, and absence of dystrophin by immunostaining.

BOX 22-1 Duchenne Muscular Dystrophy

Causes
Sex-linked recessive inheritance
Lesions
Disrupted fibers
Replacement of muscle by adipose and fibrous tissue
Manifestations
Occurrence in males
Enlarged calves
Progressive weakness
Possible heart involvement

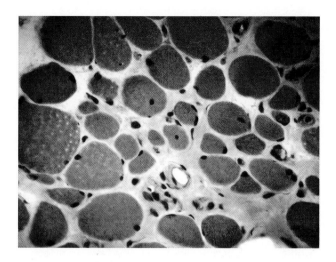

FIGURE 22–4 Dystrophic muscle. (Compare to Figure 22–2A.) Note the excess connective tissue between the nerve fibers, marked variation in fiber size, and large, rounded fibers. Nuclei are centrally (rather than peripherally) located in some fibers.

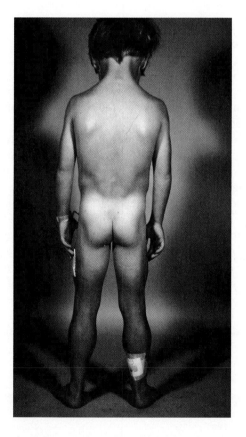

FIGURE 22–5 Duchenne muscular dystrophy. Note the "pseudohypertrophy" of the calves.

Myotonic Dystrophy

Myotonic dystrophy is an autosomal dominant disease associated with muscle weakness and a characteristic inability to release contraction (**myotonia**). Patients with myotonic dystrophy will shake hands with someone and then be unable to let go. Patients with myotonic dystrophy also may have cataracts, frontal balding, heart disease, and gonadal atrophy. Type I fibers are preferentially involved by atrophy, splitting, and encasement in fibrous tissue. In many fibers, nuclei migrate to the center of the fiber. The electromyographic findings are very characteristic in this disease. Patients may lead a long life but are often quite disabled.

BOX 22–2   Myotonic Dystrophy
Causes
Autosomal dominant inheritance
Lesions
Disrupted fibers
Replacement of muscle by adipose and fibrous tissue
Manifestations
Myotonia
Cataracts
Heart disease
Gonadal atrophy
Progressive weakness

Hereditary Motor and Sensory Neuropathies

This group of hereditary motor and sensory neuropathies includes neuropathies associated with familial amyloid and with porphyria, both uncommon diseases. Most cases of hereditary motor and sensory neuropathy, however, are those that used to be called Charcot-Marie-Tooth disease (peroneal muscular atrophy). This uncommon disease usually presents in childhood with progressive muscle atrophy of the calf and subsequent orthopedic problems related to the foot. It is not life threatening but can result in considerable morbidity because of the crippling effect. The disease is usually inherited as an autosomal recessive trait with the affected gene located on chromosome 17.

Other Dystrophies

Other, less common dystrophies named by site of involvement include limb–girdle dystrophy (limbs, pelvic and pectoral girdles) (**Figure 22–6**), facioscapulohumeral (face, scapula, and humerus), and oculopharyngeal. More recently discovered dystrophies, which are often called **congenital myopathies**, are named according to histologic appearance of the muscle. These include nemaline myopathy, in which small threadlike rods are found in the muscle; central core disease, in which each fiber has a central, pale-staining area on cross section; and central nuclear myopathy, in which the muscle fiber nuclei are in the center of the fiber instead of at the normal, peripheral position. These disorders are all manifested as variable degrees and types of weakness.

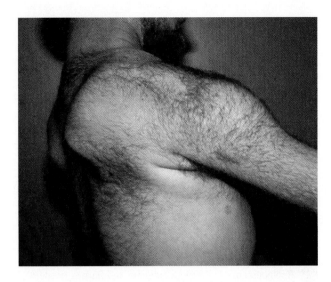

FIGURE 22–6 Limb–girdle muscular dystrophy. Note the winging of the scapula and atrophy of the deltoid muscle.

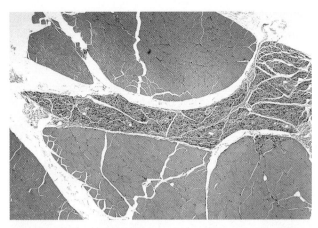

FIGURE 22–7 Neurogenic atrophy. Normal skeletal muscle fibers are present at the left and right of the image. The fibers in the center are small and angulated. (Courtesy of Dr. M. Shahriar Salamat, Department of Pathology and Laboratory Medicine, University of Wisconsin School of Medicine and Public Health.)

Inflammatory/Degenerative Diseases

Neuroscience practitioners commonly divide diseases of muscle into myopathic types, in which there is primary affliction of muscle, and neurogenic types, in which the muscle affliction is secondary to disease of the nerves that innervate the muscle. The muscular dystrophies are one group in the myopathies category. Other types of myopathic disorders include all those conditions in which muscle weakness follows another disease process, such as immunologic disease, vascular disease, neoplasia, or metabolic disease.

Autoimmune Diseases

Polymyositis is an autoimmune inflammatory disease that affects skeletal muscle in preference to other organs and is characterized by a lymphocytic infiltrate. A similar lymphocytic infiltration of muscle fibers is seen in other autoimmune diseases such as systemic lupus erythematosus and rheumatoid arthritis. These diseases, collectively referred to as autoimmune inflammatory myopathies, produce muscle weakness, often accompanied by pain and tenderness and elevation of serum creatine kinase. Autoimmune inflammatory myopathies can often be successfully treated with corticosteroids because these drugs are antilymphocytic in addition to being anti-inflammatory. Paradoxically, muscle weakness and atrophy can also result from corticosteroid therapy in susceptible persons.

Neurogenic Disorders

As alluded to previously, any affliction of peripheral nerve or spinal cord motor neurons results in muscle weakness and wasting. Acceptable treatment demands the separation of nervous system disease from that of primary muscle disease. Histologically, muscles that are atrophic secondary to lesions of the nervous system show a characteristic pattern of atrophy in which atrophic fibers have sharply angulated contours and occur in groups (**Figure 22–7**). The group occurrence is because adjacent fibers are all innervated by the same axon.

In addition to laboratory tests, helpful clues to the presence of neurogenic disease include the pattern of muscle involvement and the presence of sensory symptoms such as decreased pain. For example, muscle weakness in the distribution of a motor nerve or loss of sensation in the same area as the weakness would indicate a neurogenic disorder. In addition, disease of nerves tends to affect the more distal muscles in the extremities first. Treatment of neurogenic muscular diseases consists of dedicated physical therapy to prevent irreversible atrophy and fibrosis of muscle and contracture of joints. The most common neurogenic disorder of muscle is that which is secondary to peripheral nerve injury. Other important primary neurogenic diseases that severely affect muscle are Werdnig-Hoffman disease in infants and amyotrophic lateral sclerosis in adults.

BOX 22–3 Neurogenic Disorders

Causes

Peripheral nerve disruption or spinal cord anterior horn cell degeneration

Lesions

Angular atrophy of fiber in groups

Manifestations

Weakness in distribution of peripheral nerve or spinal cord involvement

Weakness often distal

Amyotrophic Lateral Sclerosis

Amyotrophic lateral sclerosis (ALS, or Lou Gehrig disease) is a sporadic disease with a prevalence rate of approximately 5 per 100,000 people, which means that there may be 15,000 cases in the United States. The disease may occur at any age, but rarely occurs before the age of 20 years or after the age of 70 years. There is a 2:1 male:female ratio and approximately 10% of cases are familial. The clinical symptoms of ALS are muscle weakness, predominantly symmetrical and usually in the distal extremities. The weakness progresses to involve the whole body, including areas supplied by the cranial nerve nuclei. Occasionally, the disease may begin with bulbar (brain stem) involvement, usually starting with atrophy of the tongue. A noteworthy feature of the disease is the fasciculations, which are small vermiform movements seen under the skin or on the tongue of patients with the disease. These small movements are attributed to the irritation of dying neurons. The course of ALS is usually relentless and without remission. The average duration of the disease is 3 years, but may be prolonged. Without cortical motor neuron and corticospinal tract involvement, the disease process is referred to as spinomuscular atrophy. The result of ALS is the degeneration and eventual loss of motor neurons in the spinal cord, medulla, and cortex, accompanied by degeneration of the corticospinal tracts. **Werdnig-Hoffman disease** is an analogous disease of dying motor neurons but one that occurs in infants and small children.

Myasthenia Gravis

Myasthenia gravis is characterized by a progressive decrease in muscle strength associated with activity and a return of strength after rest. It is an autoimmune disease affecting the junction of nerve endings with muscle (neuromuscular junction), so it does not fall clearly into either of the myopathic or neurogenic categories discussed earlier. In myasthenia gravis, antibodies against the acetylcholine receptor are present in the serum of most affected persons, resulting in degeneration of the receptor. Consequently, the nerve impulse, which is normally transmitted by acetylcholine, is ineffectively transferred to the muscle, resulting in progressively weaker muscle contractions.

The initiating cause of the autoantibody production is not known. In many cases, the disease is associated with a neoplasm of the thymus. The onset of myasthenia gravis is usually insidious. Almost any muscle may be affected; however, half of the patients with this disease have **diplopia** (double vision) as a first symptom because of frequent involvement of extraocular muscles. Myasthenia gravis runs a course of years but is ultimately fatal in most cases because of slowly developing atrophy of muscles, especially those required for respiration.

The course of the disease may be improved by use of anticholinesterase drugs. Normally, cholinesterase degrades acetylcholine; anticholinesterase drugs slow this process, thus making more acetylcholine available to initiate muscle contraction. If a thymoma is found by chest x-ray, its removal may be associated with clinical improvement.

BOX 22–4 Myasthenia Gravis

Causes

Autoimmune reaction

Lesions

Biochemical defect without initial histologic change

Atrophy of muscle—late

Manifestations

Decreased muscle strength with activity

Diplopia often first symptom

Associated thymoma in many cases

Metabolic Myopathies

Many metabolic conditions can result in muscular weakness. Some of these are inherited, such as the glycogen storage diseases, lipid metabolism disorders, and familial periodic paralysis. Other metabolic disorders are situational, such as myopathy caused by excessive alcohol intake or uremia. The inherited metabolic myopathies may surface in childhood or adulthood depending on the relative amounts of key enzymes in the patient's system. In familial periodic paralysis, the patient may become profoundly weak within a matter of minutes because of poorly understood fluctuations in serum potassium. These episodes can occur irregularly throughout a patient's life. Metabolic myopathies are diagnosed by history and selected tests. The muscle biopsy may be helpful in some, such as glycogen storage disease, in which glycogen is actually seen in the muscle.

Acute Inflammatory Demyelinating Polyradiculoneuropathy (Guillain-Barré Syndrome)

Guillain-Barré syndrome (GBS) occurs in 1 to 2 persons per 100,000 population yearly in the United States. The disease is usually characterized by a rapid paralysis starting in the peripheral limbs and advancing to affect more proximal muscle functions including respiration. More than half of the cases of GBS appear to be triggered by an acute influenza-like illness from which the patient has just recovered. This indicates that the disease is probably an immune phenomenon triggered by T cells and antibodies directed against a virus that cross-react with nerve tissue. This hypothesis is supported by experiments in which lymphocytes transferred from the GBS lesions of human patients to animals can produce the disease. Other cases follow surgical procedures or vaccinations.

Diabetic Neuropathy

Diabetic neuropathy can occur in any patient with diabetes. It is the most common cause of neuropathy in developed countries and its prevalence is reaching the same magnitude in undeveloped countries. Diabetic neuropathy typically involves distal nerves and can be symmetrical or asymmetrical. Patients usually display decreased sensation in their hands and feet without significant motor abnormalities. Because these patients have diminished pain sensation in their extremities, combined with compromised microvasculature associated with this disease, they are predisposed to ulcers that heal poorly. The autonomic nerves are also affected in a high proportion of diabetic patients with neuropathies.

Hyperplastic/Neoplastic Diseases

Rhabdomyosarcoma is a rare primary malignant neoplasm of skeletal muscle. Metastases of carcinomas to skeletal muscle are uncommon; sarcomas will occasionally spread through skeletal muscle. **Neurofibromas** and Schwannomas are more common tumors arising anywhere along the course of peripheral nerves. They are usually benign but may rarely be malignant. A familial disease—neurofibromatosis—made manifest by a plethora of these tumors, especially under the skin, was brought to public attention by the "elephant man."

Organ Failure

A single muscle or group of muscles may fail (**paralysis**) because of focal dystrophic, traumatic, neurogenic, or inflammatory involvement. Simultaneous failure of most of a person's muscle mass may be acute or chronic. Acute paralysis of all muscles follows administration of curare-like drugs, which block the neuromuscular junction. These drugs are often used during operative procedures when complete muscle relaxation is required. Acute paralysis of muscle may also follow rapidly progressive peripheral nerve diseases in which there is generalized inflammation of nerves or nerve roots. Chronic muscle failure is the end result of any neurogenic or myopathic disorder and consists of replacement of muscle by fibrous and adipose tissues. Whether acute or chronic, muscle failure eventually affects the diaphragm and intercostal muscles, and the patient will succumb to respiratory paralysis and pneumonia.

Practice Questions

1. Skeletal muscle is composed of two proteins called
   A. actin and myosin.
   B. myosin and creatine.
   C. actin and myelin.
   D. creatine and myelin.
2. Which of the following statements about skeletal muscle is false?
   A. Each muscle fiber is innervated by multiple nerves.
   B. Each muscle fiber is as long as the entire muscle.
   C. Each muscle fiber contains contractile and structural proteins.
   D. Muscle fibers are divided into type I and type II fibers on the basis of their histochemical staining patterns.
3. Which of the following is *not* true of Duchenne dystrophy?
   A. It is sex-linked.
   B. It involves the heart.
   C. It involves hands and feet.
   D. It involves a mutation in the dystrophin gene.
4. Which of the following is associated with a thymic tumor?
   A. Werdnig-Hoffman disease
   B. Guillain-Barré syndrome
   C. Myasthenia gravis
   D. Myotonic dystrophy
5. Nerve involvement in which of the following diseases is primarily sensory?
   A. Amyotrophic lateral sclerosis
   B. Diabetic neuropathy
   C. Myasthenia gravis
   D. Werdnig-Hoffman disease
6. Which of the following diseases is *not* autoimmune?
   A. Myasthenia gravis
   B. Guillain-Barré syndrome
   C. Polymyositis
   D. Duchenne dystrophy

Central Nervous System

OUTLINE

OBJECTIVES

1. Name the difference between a focal and a generalized neurologic deficit.
2. List the causes of increased intracranial pressure. Relate why increased intracranial pressure is dangerous.
3. Describe the diagnostic tests utilized in diagnosing central nervous system disease, including cerebrospinal fluid analysis, angiography, electroencephalogram, computed tomography, and magnetic resonance imaging.
4. List the causes, lesions, and manifestations of each specific disease listed in this chapter.
5. Compare developmental brain malformations with developmental brain destructive lesions in terms of pathogenesis and clinical expression.
6. Compare meningitis with encephalitis in terms of pathogenesis, location of lesion, and clinical expression.
7. State how rabies should be suspected, diagnosed, and treated.
8. Describe the relationship between cerebrovascular accidents and atherosclerosis.
9. State which cells in the brain are most vulnerable to anoxia as a consequence of cerebrovascular accidents.
10. Explain why a patient who recovers from a brain concussion should be closely watched.
11. Name the differences between epidural and subdural hematomas in terms of pathogenesis and development of symptoms.
12. Compare Alzheimer disease with Parkinson disease in terms of age of onset, symptoms, and brain changes.
13. Give three reasons why Creutzfeldt–Jakob disease is so feared.
14. Explain how congenital hydrocephalus differs from acquired hydrocephalus in terms of pathogenesis and clinical expression.
15. Give the reason why almost all patients with brain tumors should be operated on.
16. Define and be able to use in context all the words in headings and in bold print throughout the chapter.

KEY TERMS

Alzheimer disease
anencephaly
aneurysm
aphasia
astrocyte
astrocytoma
blood–brain barrier

brain injury
brain stem
cerebellum
cerebral palsy
cerebrospinal fluid
cerebrovascular accident
cerebrum

choroid plexus
circle of Willis
cognitive function
coma
computed tomography
    (CT scan)
concussion
contrecoup lesion
contusion
coup lesion
Creutzfeldt–Jakob
    disease (CJD)
dementia
destructive brain lesion
diffuse Lewy body disease
Down syndrome
dura
dysesthesia
electroencephalogram (EEG)
encephalitis
epidural hematoma
epilepsy
foramen magnum
glioblastoma
gray matter
hemiparesis
hydrocephalus

Lewy body
malformation
medulloblastoma
meninges
meningioma
meningitis
meningomyelocele
multiple sclerosis (MS)
myelitis
Negri bodies
neuron
oligodendroglia
paresis
paresthesia
Parkinson disease
penetration
pia-arachnoid
pituitary adenoma
positron emission
    tomography (PET scan)
prion
rabies
reflexes
spina bifida
spinal cord
subdural hematoma
white matter

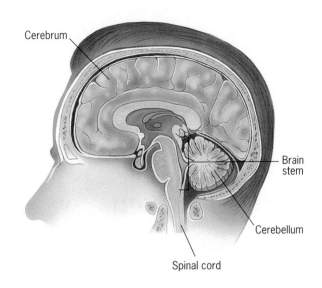

FIGURE 23–1 Parts of the central nervous system.

Review of Structure and Function

The central nervous system (CNS) consists of the brain and spinal cord (**Figure 23–1**). The brain consists of the **cerebrum**, **cerebellum**, and **brain stem** (midbrain, pons, and medulla). The cerebrum consists of an outer layer of **gray matter** (cortex), deep gray matter, and **white matter** (**Figure 23–2**). The cortex is replete with neurons that are employed for intellectual (cognitive) functions as well as for sensory and motor functions above the vegetative level. The deep gray matter consists of groups of neurons such as the thalamus and basal ganglia that perform functions similar to the cortex, albeit at a much more primitive level.

The white matter is composed primarily of axons and their myelin sheaths. Brain axons are long processes of neurons that connect with neurons in other parts of the brain and spinal cord. Axons of spinal cord neurons innervate skeletal muscles. Thus, a voluntary thought generated from neurons of the cerebral cortex can control movement of skeletal muscles. Of course, some axons convey sensory impulses in the opposite direction, from the spinal cord to various parts of the brain. The cerebellum, which is situated in the posterior inferior aspect of the skull, is responsible for coordination of motor functions. The brain stem is a relay between the brain and the **spinal cord** and is also a control center for heart rate, respiration rate, sleep and wakefulness, integration of eye movements, and other functions.

The brain is covered by **meninges**, which include an outer, tough membrane called the **dura**, which is next to the skull, and an inner lace-like membrane, the **pia-arachnoid**, which lies directly over the cortex. Meninges also form a continuous covering over the spinal cord.

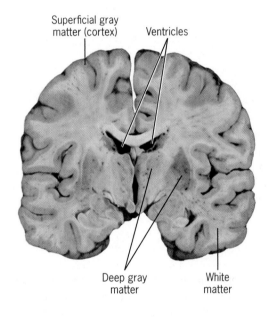

FIGURE 23–2 Coronal section of the brain. (Courtesy of Dr. M. Shahriar Salamat, Department of Pathology and Laboratory Medicine, University of Wisconsin School of Medicine and Public Health.)

Cerebrospinal fluid is utilized for metabolic exchange, as an excretory vehicle, and as a means to absorb pressure changes in the central nervous system. The cerebrospinal fluid is formed in the ventricles of the brain by secretion from the **choroid plexus** and by filtration through the ependyma. It flows from the three ventricles in the anterior part of the brain, through a narrow aqueduct, to the area of the brain stem (medulla). At this point, it passes out of the ventricular system and percolates between the layers of the pia-arachnoid membrane, bathing the brain and spinal cord before being absorbed back into veins.

Most of the blood flows to the brain through the two internal carotid arteries anteriorly and the paired vertebral arteries posteriorly. The carotid arteries supply blood to the bulk of the cerebrum, whereas the vertebral arteries supply blood only to the brain stem, cerebellum, and posterior part of the cerebrum (occiput). Although the vertebral arteries carry much less blood than the carotids do, they supply the vital areas in the brain stem, including cranial nerve nuclei and control centers for respiration and consciousness. These vessels all interconnect at the base of the brain, forming the **circle of Willis** (Figure 23–8). Consequently, occlusion of one major artery to the brain may not necessarily result in deprivation of blood to its area of distribution because blood can be "borrowed" from other arteries via the circle of Willis. The major arteries branch into smaller arteries as they course through the pia-arachnoid membrane and eventually penetrate the cortex and deeper structures.

The anatomy and physiology of the capillaries in the brain differ from those in the rest of the body. The brain capillaries are constructed to function in such a manner as to prevent passage of many substances into the brain that can easily reach tissues in other organs. This selective exclusion of substances is termed the **blood–brain barrier**. For example, certain antibiotics will not pass the barrier and consequently are not useful in the treatment of brain infections. The actual site of the blood–brain barrier is the endothelium, but the astrocytes lying just outside of the capillaries give signals to the endothelium, which help to govern the passage of molecules between the blood and the brain. The capillaries entering the choroid plexus are different from those in the brain parenchyma; thus, some drugs that cannot enter the brain parenchyma may enter the cerebrospinal fluid. However, this blood–cerebrospinal fluid barrier does not allow indiscriminate passage of all drugs.

Microscopically, the important cellular constituents of the brain stem and spinal cord are the **neurons, astrocytes**, and **oligodendroglia**. Neurons are the large cells found in gray matter that conduct nervous impulses. Their efferent processes (axons) may extend for long distances in gray and white matter. Their short afferent processes (dendrites) connect to other neurons through synapses. Astrocytes with their spider-like processes provide structural support to the central nervous system. Astrocytes also regulate the blood–brain barrier and tissue electrolytes. When the brain is injured, astrocytes proliferate, much like fibroblasts, to form a glial scar composed of glial processes but lacking collagen. Oligodendroglia manufacture and maintain the myelin sheath that surrounds and protects axons and dendrites.

Most Frequent and Serious Problems

The major diseases of the brain are cerebrovascular accidents (strokes), traumatic injuries, infections (meningitis, encephalitis, and abscess), Alzheimer disease, and neoplasms. Strokes are the third leading cause of death in the United States. Developmental disorders and degenerative diseases such as multiple sclerosis, Parkinson disease, and senile dementia also are significant. Headaches and epilepsy are very important in terms of prevalence and morbidity but may be manifestations of a variety of diseases.

Symptoms, Signs, and Tests

The most common presenting symptoms of central nervous system disease are headache, diminution or loss of a motor function, sensory loss, seizures, and disturbances in intellectual or memory capabilities.

The neurologic examination of a patient presenting with one or more of these symptoms includes examination of the motor and sensory systems and testing of cognitive function. The motor system examination involves observation of the patient's gait, posture, and symmetry of muscle mass, as well as testing for muscle strength, coordination, and quality of reflexes. Abnormalities of any of these parameters could be caused by lesions of the cerebrum, cerebellum, spinal cord, peripheral nerves, or muscle. Examination of the sensory system entails eliciting a careful history of abnormal sensations (**dysesthesias** and **paresthesias**) and testing for diminished or absent sensory perception on various areas of the body by means of pinprick or application of heat, cold, or vibration. Lesions causing abnormalities of sensation may be located in the peripheral nerves, spinal cord, or cerebral cortex. Testing of **reflexes** is an important part of a neurologic examination. A decreased reflex may indicate a lesion in the corresponding peripheral nerve, with resultant inability to either transmit the sensory impulse back to the spinal cord or to transmit the motor impulse out to the muscle. A hyperactive reflex, such as an exaggerated knee jerk, represents an intact nerve between the knee and the spinal cord, albeit without the modifying control normally mediated by the central nervous system. Testing of **cognitive** (memory, intellect) **functions** of the cerebral cortex entails asking the patient to repeat special phrases and perform arithmetic tasks. Other aspects of the neurologic examination may include tests for the integrity of the cranial nerves, observations of abnormal movements, and specific tests for the ability to perform coordinated movements.

The neurologic examiner attempts to categorize the findings as focal (referable to a specific area of nervous system involvement) or generalized (involving integrated functions of the whole brain). Examples of focal signs or symptoms are **hemiparesis** (weakness of one side of the body), localized areas of sensory deprivation, abnormalities of one or two cranial nerves, or localized headaches. Examples of generalized signs and symptoms are intellectual impairment, generalized headaches, stupor, or loss of consciousness (**coma**). One of the major causes of generalized signs and symptoms is increased intracranial pressure. Because the brain is enclosed in a rigid skull, an increase in volume anywhere within the cranial cavity will rapidly cause a generalized increase in pressure throughout the entire brain. This effect follows the development of any mass lesion in the cranial cavity, such as a neoplasm, hematoma, abscess, or localized edema surrounding a lesion. The increased intracranial pressure may also be the result of generalized edema secondary to diffuse infection. The only major opening in the skull is the **foramen magnum** (the opening for the spinal cord), and the substance of the brain tends to be pushed toward this foramen as a consequence of any increased intracranial pressure (**Figure 23–3**). As the cerebrum is forced into the space where the cerebellum lies, the oculomotor nerve becomes pinched, resulting in pupillary dilation on the same side as the lesion. This affords the physician a valuable clue as to the side of the brain lesion. The downward and backward excursion of brain substance toward the foramen magnum results in hemorrhage into the brain stem, with coma and rapid death resulting from involvement of respiratory and activating centers if the pressure is unrelieved. The treatment of increased intracranial pressure is removal of any space-occupying lesion. In addition, steroid drugs and osmotic agents, such as mannitol, may help relieve brain edema by drawing interstitial and intracellular fluid back into the vascular system.

The most important laboratory examination utilized in the evaluation of central nervous system disease is the analysis of **cerebrospinal fluid**. Cerebrospinal fluid is usually obtained by inserting a needle into the lumbar pia-arachnoid space in a sitting or reclining patient. As the fluid is being withdrawn, the pressure is measured with a manometer to detect elevations in intracranial pressure. The fluid is then examined under the microscope for the presence of leukocytes, red blood cells, neoplastic cells, and microorganisms. Chemical determinations are made for protein and sugar. Serologic tests are utilized for the detection of syphilis and other microorganisms, including viral agents. If an infectious agent is suspected, the fluid is cultured.

Several radiologic procedures are used in evaluation of the patient with a neurologic lesion. Skull x-rays are used to detect fractures of the skull. A skull fracture connotes an injurious force of sufficient magnitude to also damage the underlying brain. A patient presenting with a localized lesion in the brain often undergoes angiography. Radiopaque dye is injected into the appropriate artery (most often carotid) and a simultaneous x-ray is taken to look for abnormal distribution or distortion of vessels in the region of a lesion such as a neoplasm, abscess, or hematoma. Angiograms are also utilized to demonstrate vessel occlusion in the patient with a cerebrovascular accident and to find the site of rupture of an intracranial aneurysm.

Computed tomography (CT scan) is used extensively to study the brain, ventricles, and subarachnoid spaces. Plain CT scans allow evaluation of ventricular size, the presence of blood, or an infarct. Intravenous contrast material may be injected to detect a brain tumor that has sufficient vascular supply to become enhanced. Magnetic resonance imaging (MRI) produces even better images than a CT scan but is not always available—especially in smaller medical centers.

Positron emission tomography (PET scan) also renders an image of the brain. In addition, because of the injection of radioisotopes, this technology can assess metabolic and chemical activity in the brain.

The **electroencephalogram (EEG)** is a device for evaluating electrical activity simultaneously in various areas of the brain. Normal neurons discharge electrically in certain known patterns. Abnormalities in patterns denote neuronal disturbance, which may be predictive of injury in specific areas. Patients with seizures may have violent focal disturbances in neuronal electrical activity, thereby localizing the site where the seizure originates. A damaged area in the brain may generate abnormal electrical activity by EEG even when the disturbance is not of sufficient magnitude to cause a clinical seizure. The patient with generalized signs and symptoms may show diffuse EEG abnormalities. The EEG is also used to determine if brain death has occurred in some patients who are in a deep coma.

Specific Diseases
Genetic/Developmental Diseases

Developmental abnormalities are more important in the brain than in any other single organ, with the possible exception of the heart. Persons with brain developmental abnormalities may live for many years with very little functional deficit or may be quite retarded and require constant nursing care. Developmental abnormalities of the central nervous system are usually divided into malformations and destructive brain lesions.

Malformations

Malformations are the result of deleterious forces acting upon the embryonic or fetal brain roughly within the first half of gestation. Malformations may be mediated genetically or may be the result of infection or hypoxic or

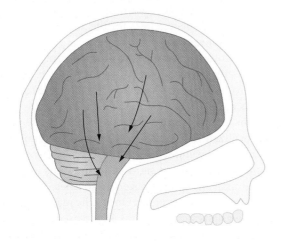

FIGURE 23–3 Forces resulting from increased intracranial pressure pushing the brain into the foramen magnum.

traumatic insult to the brain. Further brain development following an insult early in gestation will result in abnormal brain structure (malformation). Individuals with brain malformations are often severely retarded mentally, unable to care for themselves, and, consequently, confined to hospitals. Other persons with brain malformations function at various levels in society.

Down syndrome is an example of a malformation caused by a chromosomal abnormality. Affected persons have three copies (trisomy) of chromosome 21; they vary widely in intellectual capabilities. The structural abnormalities of the brain in Down syndrome are not striking and consist of abnormal variation in brain shape and location of neurons.

One of the most common malformations is **spina bifida,** in which the posterior arches and spines of some vertebrae are absent. This defect is often discovered incidentally on x-rays, but if severe, a **meningomyelocele** results. Meningomyelocele is a defect in the spinal column through which spinal cord and meninges protrude into the skin of the back. The cause of meningomyelocele is not known. It may result in severe paralysis of the legs but is compatible with life. **Anencephaly** is a severe malformation in which the entire forebrain is missing. Infants with anencephaly are stillborn or die soon after birth. Hydrocephalus may also result from a malformation that occludes the flow of cerebrospinal fluid. Hydrocephalus is discussed later in this chapter.

BOX 23–1   Malformations

Cause

Chromosomal abnormality or embryonic injury

Lesions

Abnormally formed white and/or gray matter

Manifestations

Often mental retardation

Destructive Brain Lesions

Destructive brain lesions occur in the last half of gestational life or during the first 2 years after birth. Because the brain is reasonably well formed during the second half of gestation, injuries at this time result in destructive lesions with actual loss of brain substance in various areas. Most destructive lesions occur at the time of labor and delivery or in the neonatal period in premature infants and are the result of anoxia from prolonged and difficult labor or respiratory distress following delivery. Infections, especially meningitis, may also cause destructive brain lesions. Destructive brain lesions vary greatly in severity. Most patients have motor problems (weakness or incoordination), although one-third or more also are mentally retarded. Clinically, some patients with destructive brain lesions are referred to as having **cerebral palsy,** which is defined as a

nonprogressive condition manifested by motor retardation and sometimes accompanied by mental retardation. Malformations may also be a cause of cerebral palsy, but more often the mental retardation they cause overshadows the motor retardation. External influences such as maternal diet, drugs, radiation, and toxins can adversely affect brain development. The severity of the defect depends on the stage of development at the time of insult.

BOX 23–2   Destructive Brain Lesions

Cause

Fetal injury in last half of pregnancy or at birth

Lesions

Destruction of white and/or gray matter

Manifestations

Motor handicaps with some mental retardation (cerebral palsy)

Inflammatory Diseases

Numerous infectious diseases involve the brain preferentially. Some of the more common processes and diseases are discussed in this chapter, whereas others, such as central nervous system syphilis, poliomyelitis, and HIV infection, are covered in the chapter on infectious diseases. The more common manifestations of degenerative diseases of the brain and spinal cord are also discussed in this section.

Meningitis

Meningitis means inflammation of the pia-arachnoid and is most often caused by bacteria. Meningitis most commonly occurs by itself but may be associated with other infections, such as pharyngitis or pneumonia. The onset is usually abrupt, and the major signs and symptoms are fever, headache, neck rigidity, and pain caused by muscle spasm from nerve irritation. *Escherichia coli* and group B streptococci cause the majority of cases of meningitis in newborn infants, while *Haemophilus influenzae* and *Neisseria meningitides* cause the majority of cases of meningitis in small children.

Streptococcus pneumoniae and *N. meningitides* are often the cause of meningitis in older children and adults. *Neisseria* meningitis is especially important because it can occur in epidemics. In all cases of meningitis, bacteria usually gain access to the brain and spinal cord via the blood. The diagnosis of acute meningitis is made on the basis of cerebrospinal fluid findings of neutrophilic leukocytes, decreased glucose, and the presence of organisms. Treatment consists of immediate antibiotic therapy. If treatment is not immediate or is inadequate, the presence of the bacteria and the leukocytes will result in alterations to or breakdown of the blood–brain barrier, leading to edema with consequent increased intracranial pressure and death of the patient. The lesion of acute meningitis is mainly that of purulent exudate in the subarachnoid space. Less commonly, bacteria settle in the brain parenchyma rather than the meninges, forming an abscess that behaves as an expanding mass lesion and, if untreated, is almost always fatal.

Chronic meningitis may be caused by tuberculosis or several types of fungal organisms, the most common being *Cryptococcus neoformans.* The inflammatory cells in chronic meningitis are predominantly monocytes and lymphocytes rather than neutrophils, and the disease often smolders at the base of the brain for weeks to months, gradually affecting more and more cranial nerves at their point of exit from the brain. If a patient does not die from acute or chronic meningitis, there is always a danger of developing hydrocephalus from the obliteration of the subarachnoid space by fibrous tissue, with resultant failure to absorb cerebrospinal fluid. Chronic meningitis can also accompany Lyme disease, histoplasmosis, and blastomycosis.

> **BOX 23–3   Meningitis**
>
> **Cause**
>
> Bacterial or fungal entry into the CNS, usually via the blood
>
> **Lesions**
>
> Acute or chronic inflammation of the pia-arachnoid
>
> **Manifestations**
>
> Headache
>
> Neck rigidity and pain
>
> Fever
>
> Coma
>
> Neutrophils in spinal fluid
>
> Possible hydrocephalus

Encephalitis

Encephalitis refers to a more or less diffuse inflammation of the brain. It is usually caused by viral infections. Bacterial, fungal, and protozoal infections usually affect the meninges or cause localized abscesses rather than encephalitis. Many viral encephalitides in the United States are mosquito-borne and occur in epidemics in the warm months of the year. Common types include St. Louis, equine, West Nile, and Venezuelan encephalitis. Patients with any of these viral encephalitides usually present with generalized signs and symptoms of irritability, drowsiness, and headache. Specific diagnosis depends on culture and identification of the viral agent from the cerebrospinal fluid by serologic testing. In contrast to bacterial infections, viral encephalitis is usually accompanied by a cerebrospinal fluid lymphocytosis. There is no specific treatment for these diseases, and patients either die, recover fully, or recover with variable neurologic deficit.

Herpes simplex virus type I also can cause an encephalitis. The same virus that causes oral blisters in susceptible persons may, on rare occasions, invade the brain and result in severe destruction of large areas of the brain, most often the temporal lobes.

HIV can cause a primary encephalitis, and when HIV progresses to AIDS, encephalitis secondary to toxoplasma or cytomegalovirus is common.

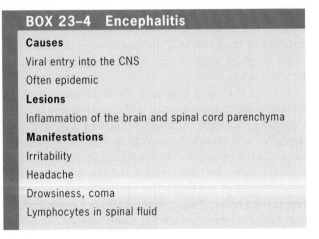

> **BOX 23–4   Encephalitis**
>
> **Causes**
>
> Viral entry into the CNS
>
> Often epidemic
>
> **Lesions**
>
> Inflammation of the brain and spinal cord parenchyma
>
> **Manifestations**
>
> Irritability
>
> Headache
>
> Drowsiness, coma
>
> Lymphocytes in spinal fluid

Rabies

Although death from **rabies** occurs only rarely in the United States, it is such a feared disease that virtually every animal bite raises a concern for rabies. The reservoir of the virus is in wild animals, especially foxes, raccoons, skunks, and certain types of bats. These animals may transmit the disease to domestic pets, which in turn transmit the virus to humans via bites. The virus travels up the peripheral nerve to the brain, and once the brain is infected, death is practically inevitable. Symptoms are pain at the bite site, fever, malaise, and vomiting, progressing to delirium and painful laryngeal spasm when attempting to drink (hydrophobia). The incubation period is proportional to the distance from the bite to the brain. After a bite by a domestic or wild animal, if there is any indication that the animal might have rabies, treatment of the victim with antirabies immune globulin as well as vaccination should begin immediately. A pet should be watched closely for 12 days; if the animal is still alive and well after 12 days, it is unlikely that it has rabies. Veterinarians and other animal workers are usually prophylactically immunized. If a person is bitten by a wild animal, especially one that displays abnormal behavior, every attempt should be made to locate the animal and submit it to an appropriate laboratory analysis for rabies. Rabies analysis consists of inoculating mice with brain tissue from the suspected animal plus a search for the viral inclusion bodies of rabies in the neurons of the suspected animal. These inclusion bodies, called **Negri bodies**, are found in the cytoplasm of neurons by light microscopy and by immunofluorescence, in which fluorescent-labeled antibodies are directed against the inclusions on tissue section and visualized with a microscope having an ultraviolet light source.

Myelitis

Myelitis is an infection of the spinal cord. Poliomyelitis is a specific infection of the gray matter of the spinal cord. The poliomyelitis virus preferentially destroys the gray matter of the cord, killing the anterior horn motor neurons with resultant paralysis. Poliomyelitis is no longer the dreaded disease that it was prior to 1960 because of successful immunization programs.

Vascular Disease and Trauma

Cerebrovascular Accident (Stroke)

A stroke is a sudden neurologic deficit caused by either vascular occlusion from thrombosis or embolism or from hemorrhage into the brain. The majority of **cerebrovascular accidents** (CVAs) are caused by emboli, which separate from a thrombus in a large vessel such as the carotid artery (**Figure 23–4**) or perhaps the heart. The embolus then travels distally, where it lodges in a brain vessel and results in an infarct. Most thrombi initially form because the endothelium of the vessel in which they arise has been damaged by atherosclerosis. Consequently, the common denominator of most cerebrovascular accidents is atherosclerotic vascular disease. This is why cerebrovascular accidents become increasingly prevalent in older adults.

Whether from emboli or thrombi, vascular occlusions result in infarcts in the brain tissue supplied by the affected vessel. The damaged brain tissue loses function within minutes and becomes soft and necrotic within a few days. Later, tissue is lost from the area, leaving a cystic cavity (**Figures 23–5** and **23–6**).

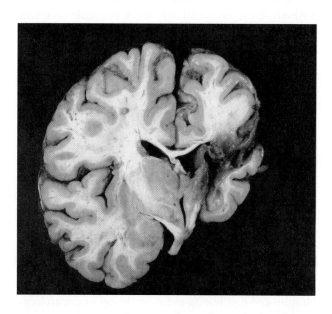

FIGURE 23–5 Coronal section of a cerebrum with an old infarct in the distribution of the middle cerebral artery. The dead tissue has been resorbed, resulting in gross asymmetry of the brain.

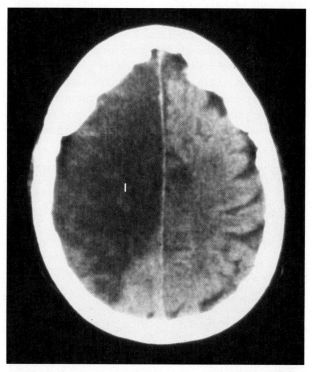

FIGURE 23–6 CT scan of large hemispheric infarct (I). (Courtesy of Dr. Patrick Turski, Department of Radiology-MRI, University of Wisconsin School of Medicine and Public Health.)

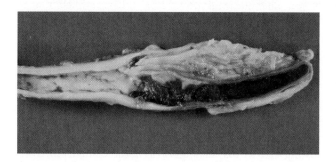

FIGURE 23–4 A thrombus fills the lumen of this carotid artery in a patient who died of a massive brain infarct.

The middle cerebral artery is the largest cerebral artery, and it is most often occluded by emboli because it is a direct continuation of the carotid artery. Occlusion of the middle cerebral artery is important because this artery supplies the part of the cortex controlling motor function. Involvement of the motor cortex produces weakness (**paresis**) or paralysis on the opposite side of the body. If the dominant side of the brain (the side that primarily controls speech and motor function, usually the left side) is involved, the patient will also have **aphasia** (impaired language function). The chronic neurologic deficits following a cerebrovascular accident are referable to the region of infarct.

Cerebrovascular accidents involving the vertebral arteries or their branches may also cause paralysis because of injury to motor fibers in the brain stem coursing between the brain and the spinal cord. Large cerebrovascular accidents in the brain stem usually kill the patient because of interruption of the nervous centers that control respiration.

Cerebrovascular accidents are also caused by rupture of vessels and bleeding into the brain (brain hemorrhage). The ruptured vessel has usually been weakened by arteriosclerosis, most often in a patient with hypertension. The signs and symptoms of a brain hemorrhage depend on its location and size, but up to half of the patients with large brain hemorrhages die within hours because the accumulation of blood displaces adjacent tissue (**Figure 23–7**) and rapidly elevates the intracranial pressure.

A third important cause of stroke is ruptured saccular **aneurysm**. Saccular (berry) aneurysms occur predominantly in the vicinity of the circle of Willis, where vessels branch (**Figures 23–8** and **23–9**). They are saccular outpouchings of vessels resulting from deficiencies in the blood vessel wall. The reasons for development of these aneurysms are poorly understood. Saccular aneurysms are present in 2–5% of the population, but most do not rupture. A disproportionate number of ruptured aneurysms occur in women—particularly those who

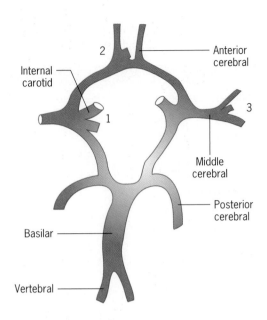

FIGURE 23–8 Circle of Willis and three most frequent locations of aneurysms.

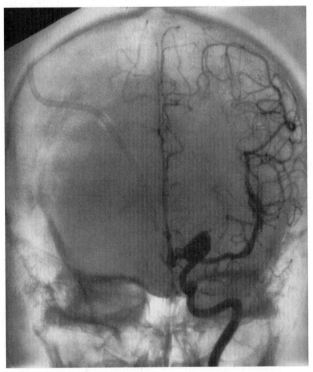

FIGURE 23–9 Carotid angiogram demonstrating radiopaque dye in a saccular aneurysm of the middle cerebral artery.

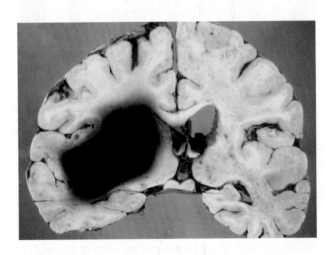

FIGURE 23–7 Large hypertensive hemorrhage in deep gray matter with displacement of adjacent brain tissues.

smoke cigarettes—in the third and fourth decades of life. When they do rupture, blood is spilled into the subarachnoid space and can be detected in the cerebrospinal fluid. Consequently, examination of the cerebrospinal fluid following a stroke may distinguish a ruptured aneurysm from the other important causes of strokes.

Overall, up to one-third of the patients with a cerebrovascular accident die, one-third are left with a serious

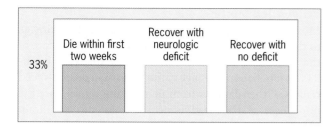

FIGURE 23–10 Prognosis for stroke patients.

neurologic deficit, and one-third recover with minimal or no brain damage (**Figure 23–10**). The individual's prognosis depends on the amount of brain involved and the quality of supportive care received. Many persons sustain small infarcts that never result in neurologic deficit because they occur in noncritical, so-called silent areas of the brain. Little can be done to reverse the damage done by a cerebrovascular accident, but much can be done with good physical therapy to rehabilitate the patient who has sustained a cerebrovascular accident. In persons who sustain a cerebrovascular accident caused by an embolus, the symptoms can often be reversed, and permanent damage avoided, if they are treated with embolus-dissolving plasminogen activators within 60–90 minutes of onset.

When the brain is damaged by ischemia following a cerebrovascular accident, the neurons die within minutes to hours and are never replaced. The oligodendroglia are likewise very vulnerable to injury and readily die following ischemia. The astrocytes proliferate rapidly and repair the injury structurally by forming a scar (glial scar). The astrocytes and their processes are the central nervous system analogue of fibroblasts and connective tissue. Monocytes enter from the blood after injury and aid in clearing away the debris.

BOX 23–6   Cerebrovascular Accident

Cause

Occlusion or rupture of a brain blood vessel

Lesions

Brain infarct

Brain hemorrhage

Manifestations

Sudden paralysis of opposite side of body

Possible aphasia

Possible loss of consciousness

Vascular occlusion by angiography

Trauma

The brain is especially vulnerable to injuries resulting from high-speed transportation. The more common types of **brain injuries** include concussion, contusion, epidural hemorrhage, subdural hemorrhage, and penetrating

injury. Patients who have sustained head trauma may have a concussion and recover completely, only to lapse into coma several hours later. The usual reason for late deterioration is that a subdural or epidural bleed developed immediately following the injury but did not affect the patient until a critical amount of blood accumulated. For this reason, any patient who has had sufficient head trauma to sustain a concussion should be watched closely for 12 to 24 hours.

Concussion

Concussion is a momentary loss of consciousness and loss of reflexes following head trauma, with amnesia for the traumatic event and complete recovery. No structural damage can be detected in the brain.

BOX 23–7   Concussion

Cause

Cranial trauma

Lesions

None

Manifestations

Momentary loss of consciousness

Momentary loss of reflexes

Amnesia of the event

Contusion

Contusions are bruises of the surface of the brain sustained at the time of traumatic impact. Contusions occurring on the same side of the brain as the trauma are termed **coup lesions**, whereas those on the opposite side are **contrecoup lesions**. If the head is in motion at the time of impact, the contrecoup lesion often is larger than the coup lesion because the force of the blow is magnified as it is transmitted to the opposite side. Contusions result in hemorrhages from small blood vessels in the brain. These hemorrhages cause further vessel occlusion and consequent edema, rendering the patient vulnerable to the sequelae of increased intracranial pressure.

BOX 23–8   Contusion

Cause

Trauma to head or back

Lesions

Bruises of cortex at the site of the trauma (coup) or

Small hemorrhages opposite the site of trauma (contrecoup)

Manifestations

Increased intracranial pressure

Epidural Hematoma

Epidural hemorrhage occurs between the dura and the skull (**Figure 23–11**). It is associated with severe trauma in which the skull is usually fractured. Because an artery

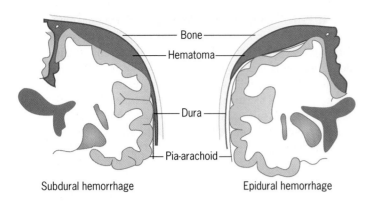

Subdural hemorrhage   Epidural hemorrhage

FIGURE 23–11 Comparative locations of epidural and subdural hemorrhages.

is ruptured (middle meningeal), the blood accumulates rapidly, and the patient will die within hours unless the hematoma is removed by an operation. Often the patient with an epidural hematoma sustains a concussion followed by a lucid interval prior to the onset of the signs of increased intracranial pressure.

BOX 23–9   Epidural Hematoma

Cause

Traumatic rupture of a dural artery

Lesions

Rapid accumulation of blood between the dura and the skull

Manifestations

Rapid increase in intracranial pressure

Subdural Hematoma

Subdural hematoma is a collection of blood beneath the dura (Figure 23–11). It is a common sequela of head injury and is the result of rupture of veins on the dorsum of the brain. Because this bleeding is venous, the blood does not accumulate as rapidly as in epidural hemorrhage and consequently is not quite as life threatening, although usually the blood must be removed by a surgical procedure to prevent compression of the underlying brain. Subdural hematomas are relatively more common in infants and older persons and often are discovered in patients who have no history of trauma. Infants have thin-walled veins and in older adults, the brain shrinks away from the skull, allowing torsion and tearing of veins when there is brain movement with relatively mild trauma.

BOX 23–10   Subdural Hematoma

Cause

Traumatic or atraumatic rupture of a vein between the dura and the pia-arachnoid

Lesions

Slow accumulation of blood beneath the dura

Manifestations

Slow increase in intracranial pressure

Penetrating Injuries

Most **penetrating** injuries are from bullets. The damage to the brain from a bullet is proportional to the square of the velocity of the bullet; consequently, high-speed bullets do much more damage to the brain than do low-speed bullets. Other dangers from penetrating injuries are the impaction of fractured bone splinters into the brain plus the strong likelihood of introducing infection into the open wound.

Penetrating and crushing injuries of the spinal cord are very common and if severe may result in complete paralysis of the body below the lesion. A very common form of spinal cord injury is herniation of the cushioning material (disc) between vertebrae. Spinal cord injuries are often surgical emergencies.

Degenerative Diseases

Multiple Sclerosis

Multiple sclerosis (MS) is a common disease that affects many young and middle-aged adults throughout the world, primarily in northern hemispheric countries. There are at least 100,000 persons in the United States with multiple sclerosis at any one time, and there is a slightly higher incidence among women than men. The basic lesion is focal loss of the myelin sheath (demyeli-nation), which appears to render axons incapable of properly transmitting a nervous impulse. Because this loss of myelin can occur anywhere in the brain or spinal cord, the symptoms may vary considerably from one patient to another. Visual impairment is usually present to some degree because multiple sclerosis preferentially affects the optic nerves as well as the tissue surrounding the brain ventricles and the spinal cord. The cause of multiple sclerosis is not known, although it is strongly suspected to be a virus or an immunologic reaction to a virus in persons who have a genetic predisposition. The disease span is usually 5 to 25 years, with the course of the disease alternately remitting and relapsing. The patient eventually becomes quite debilitated from muscle weakness. The diagnosis is made on

---

BOX 23–11   Multiple Sclerosis

Cause

Unknown, probably virus and/or immune reaction

Lesions

Focal loss of myelin randomly throughout the brain and spinal cord

Manifestations

Visual impairment

Motor weakness

Relapsing course

Increased spinal fluid protein, MRI changes

the basis of clinical history and physical findings that support a multifocal neurologic deficit plus the findings of increased immunoglobin G (IgG) protein in the cerebrospinal fluid. The lesions can be seen using MRI (**Figure 23–12**).

Creutzfeldt–Jakob Disease

Creutzfeldt–Jakob disease (CJD) is the human prototype of a group of diseases in animals and humans that result in brain degeneration and have been referred to as "slow virus" diseases. "Mad cow" disease, allegedly acquired by eating infected beef in the United Kingdom, is a form of CJD. Persons who are afflicted with CJD become rapidly demented and usually die within 4–6 months after diagnosis with severe brain degeneration. A characteristic electroencephalogram often renders the diagnosis, but sometimes brain biopsy is necessary.

CJD is rare in its occurrence but, similar to rabies, strikes fear in the public disproportionate to its incidence. It is not caused by a virus at all but appears to be the result of transformation of a normal brain protein into an abnormal configuration allowing it to replicate. The abnormal protein (called a **prion**) then builds up in the brain and is associated with severe degeneration of the gray matter characterized by the formation of multiple vacuoles referred to as spongiform degeneration. CJD can be transmitted to animals by direct inoculation of brain tissue from a person with the disease. In fact,

the disease can be transmitted after the affected brain tissue has been immersed in formaldehyde solution for years, accounting for part of the fear of the disease. Transmission by simple contact is rare or nonexistent because persons exposed to patients with CJD, including spouses, do not acquire the disease. A few known transmissions in humans have been via organ or tissue transplants. The importance of CJD is that it represents a remarkable type of protein proliferation, apparently undirected by either DNA or RNA, and the protein with its ability to replicate can be transmitted. There are familial varieties of CJD, each being associated with mutations in the prion gene. There is no known cure or effective treatment.

Senile Dementia

Dementia means a decrease in cognitive function, usually accompanied by loss of memory for recent events. Senile dementia is a descriptive term for a condition of older persons who have poor memory for recent events, pick at their clothes, get lost easily, and are often irritable. The degree of dementia in a patient is proportional to the loss of substance in the frontal lobes, the region of the brain that is associated with higher cognitive function. The loss of substance may be the result of trauma or stroke (infarct), but it is most often secondary to generalized atrophy and degeneration of the neurons in the gray matter (**Figure 23–13**).

When dementia is accompanied by certain microscopic brain changes, it is **Alzheimer disease**; this disease accounts for more than 60% of cases of chronic dementia. Alzheimer disease is ordinarily a disease of the aged but occasionally affects persons in their 40s. Characteristic silver-staining neuritic plaques and neurofibrillary tangles, as well as an abnormal protein called amyloid, are found in the cerebral cortex and allow the neuropathologist to diagnose Alzheimer disease. A large number of plaques, tangles, and amyloid are found in the hippocampal formation in the temporal lobes,

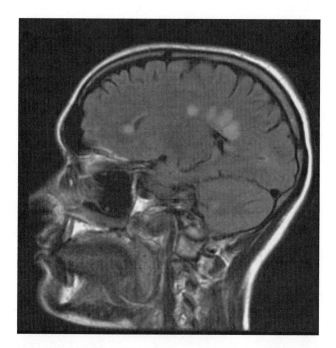

FIGURE 23–12 Magnetic resonance image of brain in midline section (sagittal), demonstrating multiple plaques (light areas) of multiple sclerosis in the white matter. (Courtesy of Dr. Patrick Turski, Department of Radiology-MRI, University of Wisconsin School of Medicine and Public Health.)

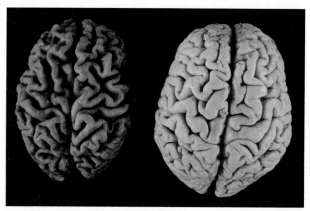

FIGURE 23–13 Atrophic brain of Alzheimer disease (left) compared to normal brain (right).

explaining the loss of recent memory associated with the disease. It is not known what causes neurons to degenerate resulting in Alzheimer disease, and there is no real effective treatment. The social impact of this disease is significant. It is estimated that currently there are more than 5 million persons with Alzheimer disease in the United States; with an increasing population of older persons, there may be as many as 8 million cases by the year 2020. A significant increase in the quantity and quality of resources necessary to care for these patients will be needed. These resources include more and better training of healthcare professionals in the home and nursing home care of these patients. Dementia may also accompany numerous metabolic conditions such as uremia or electrolyte and fluid imbalance. Many of these types of dementia are reversible.

BOX 23–12   Senile Dementia

Causes

Alzheimer disease

Other organic brain diseases

Lesions

Brain atrophy

Diffuse loss of neurons in the cerebral cortex

Manifestations

Poor recent memory

Irritability

Lapses in social restraints

Parkinson Disease

Parkinson disease is caused by degeneration of certain portions of the extrapyramidal (involuntary) motor system, especially the substantia nigra nucleus in the midbrain. A characteristic inclusion called the **Lewy body** is present in degenerating substantia nigra neurons. Parkinson disease usually, but not always, affects older people and results in tremors at rest, masklike

---

BOX 23–13   Parkinson Disease

Cause

Unknown

Lesions

Degeneration and depigmentation of nuclei in the brain stem

Lewy bodies

Manifestations

Tremor (resting)

Rigidity of muscles

Shuffling gait

Possible dementia

---

facial expression, shuffling gait, and rigidity of skeletal muscles. Many older people appear to have minor degrees of Parkinson disease, and roughly 50% of persons with Parkinson disease also have some degree of dementia. Treatment of Parkinson disease with L-dopa results in some symptomatic relief in about half of the patients.

A related disease is **diffuse Lewy body disease** because Lewy bodies are found in neurons throughout the brain; the brains of these patients also show changes of Alzheimer disease.

Hydrocephalus

Hydrocephalus literally means "water brain," and it may occur congenitally or arise at any time after birth from a variety of causes. In hydrocephalic individuals, the ventricles enlarge (**Figure 23–14**) secondarily to a block in the flow of cerebrospinal fluid at some level. The most common type of congenital hydrocephalus is stenosis (closure) of the aqueduct between the third and fourth ventricles. As the ventricles expand with accumulated cerebrospinal fluid, the head may enlarge enormously. In older children and adults, the causes of hydrocephalus are more often tumors that block the flow of cerebrospinal fluid and meningeal scarring secondary to meningitis or hemorrhage, with consequent failure of cerebrospinal fluid to be reabsorbed into the venous system. In older children and adults, the head does not usually enlarge because the skull is well formed; rather, the increased pressure from the accumulated fluid in the ventricles

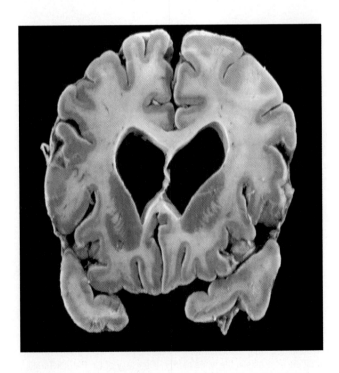

FIGURE 23–14 Hydrocephalus. Compare the size of the ventricles to those in Figure 23–2.

causes pressure atrophy of the surrounding white and gray tissue, resulting in mental deterioration. If the increased pressure is not relieved, the brain may herniate toward the foramen magnum. Pressure may be relieved by placement of a tube that acts as a shunt between the ventricles and the veins, heart, or peritoneal cavity.

BOX 23–14   Hydrocephalus (Congenital)

Cause

Usually from failure of the aqueduct of Sylvius to properly open

Lesions

Enlarged brain ventricles from the pressure of increased spinal fluid

Manifestations

Enlarged head

Mental and motor deterioration

BOX 23–15   Hydrocephalus (Acquired)

Cause

Scarring of the meninges or blockage of a ventricle

Lesions

Enlarged brain ventricles from the pressure of increased spinal fluid

Manifestations

Normal-sized head

Mental and motor deterioration

Epilepsy

Epilepsy is a condition of recurrent seizures. Seizures are focal and/or generalized disturbances of neuronal electrical activity, which may be manifested by abnormal movements or sensations and loss of reflexes, memory, or consciousness. There are many different types of epilepsy; its development may follow recovery from trauma or central nervous system infections or may be induced by malformations or neoplasms of the brain. In most cases, persons with epilepsy have a lifelong history of seizures without a known cause. Seizures may also be caused by more acute conditions such as electrolyte imbalance, high fever, uremia, and eclampsia. Seizure activity in persons with epilepsy is usually controlled with barbiturates or phenytoin-type drugs.

Hyperplastic/Neoplastic Diseases

Brain Neoplasms

Neoplasms of the brain and spinal cord are not as neatly separated into benign and malignant varieties as are tumors elsewhere. The reason is that small, slowly growing tumors of the brain that would be benign in other locations may readily disrupt vital functions in strategic

---

BOX 23–16   Epilepsy

Causes

Usually unknown

Old trauma

Previous infection

Malformations

Neoplasms

Lesions

Glial scar

Neoplasm or malformation

Manifestations

Intermittent seizures

Abnormal electroencephalogram

---

locations such as the brain stem, killing the patient. Other benign brain tumors may occur in deep areas of the brain where the surgeon cannot gain access to them without destroying adjacent vital brain structures.

Brain tumors are the second most common neoplasms occurring in children (leukemias are first). Two-thirds of brain tumors in children occur in the posterior fossa, predominantly in the cerebellum. Conversely, two-thirds of brain tumors in adults occur in the anterior parts of the brain, in the white matter of the hemispheres.

The most common presenting signs and symptoms in patients with brain tumors are those of increased pressure because of the mass lesion, often with accompanying edema. Generalized symptoms such as headaches, vomiting, blurred vision, and seizures may all result from increased intracranial pressure, while focal signs may accompany brain tumors, depending on where the tumor arises.

The treatment of brain tumors almost always entails an operation because some of the tumor tissue needs to be examined to establish a histologic diagnosis. In general, if a tumor is of a slow-growing type, the surgeon will attempt to remove as much of it as possible. In contrast, if a tumor appears to be malignant, the surgeon will sample enough tissue to establish a definitive diagnosis and then treat the patient further with radiation and/or chemotherapy.

The most common brain tumors are those arising from astrocytes. Slower-growing types are called **astrocytomas**. The fast-growing malignant type is called a **glioblastoma** (**Figure 23–15**). Glioblastomas are the most common brain tumor in adults and usually result in death within a year or two following diagnosis. As the tumors grow, they produce an expanding, poorly defined mass. Almost no patients survive. Unfortunately, astrocytomas can evolve into glioblastomas. Brain tumors arising from oligodendroglia, ependymal cells, and neuronal cell lines occur but are less common.

The second most common brain tumor is the **meningioma**, a benign neoplasm that arises from the dura and is slow growing and well circumscribed without infiltration of surrounding brain (**Figure 23–16**). Because most meningiomas arise from the dorsum (top) of the head, the surgeon can usually excise the entire tumor, and the patient's prognosis is good. If a meningioma arises at the base of the brain, however, the surrounding vital structures such as hypothalamus, brain stem, and blood vessels make surgical excision much more difficult, and the prognosis is correspondingly worse.

Pituitary tumors (**adenomas**) are also common and likewise are difficult to remove because of location. Some pituitary adenomas secrete growth hormone, resulting in gigantism or acromegaly. One of the most important brain tumors in children is the **medulloblastoma**, which arises in the cerebellum from primitive cells that are neuronal precursors. These tumors are malignant but do respond well to radiation therapy, and 30–40% of patients now survive.

Metastatic tumors to the brain are common. They usually are removed only if there is just one focus of metastasis and the patient is in sufficiently good health to withstand the surgical procedure. Tumors of the spinal cord are much less common than brain tumors.

BOX 23–17 Brain Neoplasms
Cause
Unknown
Lesions
Neoplastic mass
Edema at periphery of mass
Manifestations
Increased intracranial pressure
Focal neurologic deficits depending on tumor site

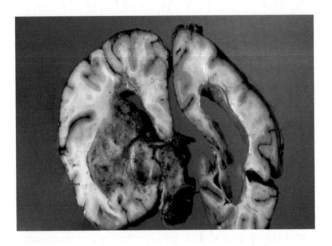

FIGURE 23–15 Glioblastoma. A large, pink, tan and hemorrhagic mass is infiltrating the left side of the brain. It is displacing the midline to the right and impeding the outflow of the ventricles so that the right ventricle is greatly dilated and the remainder of the tissue on the right markedly atrophic due to the resultant hydrocephalus.

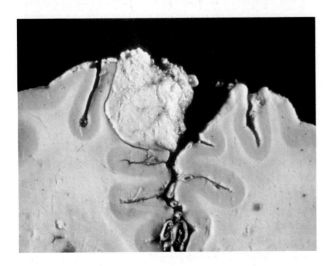

FIGURE 23–16 Meningioma arising from the dura, with displacement but no infiltration of the brain.

Organ Failure

Because the brain is a composite of numerous groups (nuclei) of neurons with partially related functions, any group of neurons may fail, resulting in a focal neurologic deficit. Generalized brain failure results from diffuse brain disease and places the patient in a vegetative state, incapable of performing basic mental or motor functions (coma). The patient in coma is alive because of the continuing function of the brain stem, which is often the last part of the brain affected by diffuse disease. Coma may be reversible if structural damage to the brain has not taken place. In many areas of the United States, a patient is considered legally dead if two successive electroencephalograms taken 24 hours apart both show complete absence of electrical activity in the brain, irrespective of the status of the heart. Interpretation of the death of the patient by demonstrating death of the brain is somewhat controversial and poses ethical as well as legal dilemmas. Other criteria for determining brain death should include body temperature and reflex responses determined by neurologic examination. Because barbiturates may cause decreased or absent electrical activity in the brain that is reversible, blood levels of these substances should also be measured before pronouncing brain death.

Practice Questions

1. Meningitis is best diagnosed using which of the following tests?
   A. Cerebral spinal fluid analysis
   B. Angiography
   C. Electroencephalogram
   D. MRI

2. Of the following, which is the most common cause of meningitis in the newborn?
   A. *Cryptococcus neoformans*
   B. *Escherichia coli*
   C. *Neisseria meningitides*
   D. West Nile virus

3. Overall, most cases of encephalitis are transmitted by
   A. mosquitoes.
   B. flies.
   C. human contact.
   D. fecal contaminants.

4. Most cerebrovascular accidents result from
   A. thrombi.
   B. ruptured aneurysms.
   C. brain hemorrhage.
   D. emboli.

5. A 76-year-old man falls, and his head hits the sidewalk. He does not lose consciousness but 4 hours later begins to feel dizzy with right-sided weakness. He is taken to the ER for examination and no skull fracture is found. Which of the following conditions does he most likely have?
   A. Subdural hematoma
   B. Concussion
   C. Epidural hematoma
   D. Contusion

6. The abnormal protein associated with Creutzfeldt–Jacob disease is
   A. amyloid.
   B. prion.
   C. Lewy body.
   D. immunoglobulin.

7. A 9-year-old boy experiences gradual onset of headaches, nausea, and loss of balance. A mass is found in his cerebellum by MRI, a biopsy is taken for tissue diagnosis, he is treated with radiation therapy, and he is doing well 3 years later. Which of the following did he most likely have?
   A. Astrocytoma
   B. Meningioma
   C. Medulloblastoma
   D. Glioblastoma

Mental Illness

OUTLINE

OBJECTIVES

1. Discuss why mental or psychiatric disorders are, or are not, functional disorders.
2. Explain how the roles of psychiatrists, psychologists, and social workers differ.
3. Name the six mental illnesses that account for the most first admissions to mental hospitals.
4. Name the disorders that account for 80% of long-term mental illness hospitalizations.
5. Cite the age range at which the major mental illnesses most frequently begin.
6. List the factors that predispose individuals to suicide.
7. List the major psychiatric emergencies.
8. Explain how the psychiatric history and mental status examination differ from the usual medical history and physical examination.
9. List seven major categories of manifestations of psychiatric illness and the terms that are used to define the specific manifestations in each category.
10. List the criteria used to classify the major categories of mental illness.
11. Compare the causes, lesions (if any), and major manifestations of the specific diseases discussed in this chapter.
12. Describe how schizophrenia and bipolar disorder differ.
13. Describe how symptoms suggestive of, but not due to, organic lesions may create medical problems.
14. Be able to define and use in context all the words in headings and bold print throughout the chapter.

KEY TERMS

acrophobia
agoraphobia
alcohol use disorder
anorexia nervosa
anxiety disorder
Asperger syndrome
attention-deficit/hyperactivity
    disorder (ADHD)
autism spectrum disorder
biopsychosocial model
bipolar disorder
bulimia nervosa
claustrophobia
conversion disorder
cultural formulation
dementia
depression
generalized anxiety disorder
    (GAD)
intellectual disability
major depressive disorder
malingering

mania
mental disorders due to a
    another medical condition
obsessive–compulsive
    disorder (OCD)
panic disorder
personality disorder
post-traumatic stress
    disorder (PTSD)
psychiatrist
psychologist
psychosis
psychosomatic
schizophrenia
sleep disorder
social phobia
social worker
sociopathic
somatic symptom disorders
substance use disorder
suicide

Nature of Mental Illness

Mental disorders are those that affect behavior, emotion, and cognition. Mental disorders can be severe, disabling, and even life-threatening conditions. They often are amenable to treatment, including measures such as psychotherapy and psychotropic medications. Accurate diagnosis of mental disorders is important for determining the prognosis and appropriate treatment strategy. The *Diagnostic and Statistical Manual of Mental Disorders* (DSM) defines mental disorders in terms of diagnostic criteria, specifically a combination of psychiatric symptoms and functional impairment.

While the DSM refers to "mental disorders" (implying a distinction from "physical disorders"), it is abundantly clear that the substrate of mental illness is the brain. Mental disorders have bidirectional relationships with neurologic disorders, cardiac disease, and endocrine disorders. In addition, various substances have psychotropic properties. Behavioral interventions have also been shown to result in changes in brain metabolism. Thus it is important to avoid a false dichotomy between mental illness and physical illness.

The **biopsychosocial model** postulates that illness arises from a complex interplay among biological, psychological, and social factors. The formulation posited by this model describes how the patient's illness arose in terms of biological, psychological, and social factors. These factors may be predisposing (they put the patient at risk of developing illness), precipitating (they are the proximal cause of the illness or its exacerbation), perpetuating (they prevent the illness from resolving), or protective (they have decreased the severity of illness or are preventing relapse). Both the DSM diagnoses and the biopsychosocial formulation lead to the development of a treatment plan.

The role of culture is increasingly being recognized in the development and progression of mental illness. According to DSM, *culture* refers to knowledge, concepts, rules, and practices that are learned and transmitted across generations. Cultural aspects of mental illness can be assessed using **cultural formulation**.

Healthcare specialists who deal primarily with mental disorders include psychiatrists, psychologists, and social workers. **Psychiatrists** are physicians who are trained to diagnose and treat psychiatric illness. **Psychologists** usually hold advanced degrees in psychology and are concerned with the study of normal and abnormal behavior. Psychologists often play a role in diagnosis of subtle psychiatric illnesses by administering specific psychological tests. They may also be involved in psychological or behavioral aspects of treatment of patients. **Social workers** are especially concerned with the social and physical environments of patients with psychiatric illness, just as they are with patients having organic disease. Psychiatric illnesses often are first detected by primary care practitioners.

Most Frequent and Serious Problems

Mental illnesses are common, with a lifetime prevalence of approximately 25%, and may be severe and disabling. Four of the 15 most disabling disorders (as measured by years of living with disability in the 2010 World Health Organization [WHO] Global Burden of Disease study) in the world are mental illnesses: **major depressive disorder**, anxiety disorders, drug use disorders, and alcohol use disorders. **Suicide**, the most devastating consequence of mental illness, is the most common cause of violent death worldwide (49%), eclipsing the number of fatalities attributable to both homicide (31%) and war (19%). Psychiatric disorders often arise early in life, disrupting a person's education, capacity for meaningful work, and ability to build and sustain relationships.

Depressive and bipolar disorders include major depressive disorder, dysthymic disorder, and bipolar disorder; together, they account for 10% of medical costs worldwide. These disorders are characterized by a disturbance of mood accompanied by a manic or depressive syndrome that is not due to any other physical or mental disorder. In major depressive disorder, patients experience recurrent episodes of low mood and loss of interest, whereas bipolar disorder also consists of episodes of mania (inappropriately elevated mood). The lifetime prevalence of major depressive disorder is 18% and of bipolar disorder is 2–3%.

Approximately one in four Americans has one or more **anxiety disorders**, which generally are characterized by excessive or irrational fear or worry. These disorders include panic disorder, generalized anxiety disorder, post-traumatic stress disorder, obsessive–compulsive disorder and social phobia.

Schizophrenia, another common severe psychiatric disorder, affects approximately 1% of the population. Schizophrenia—a disorder of thought processes and perceptions—usually includes hallucinations (sensory perceptions in the absence of associated environmental stimuli) and delusions (fixed false beliefs that cannot be explained on the basis of the patient's cultural or spiritual background). It usually begins between 15 and 25 years of age in men and between 25 and 35 years of age in women.

Substance use disorders are very common, are highly comorbid with other psychiatric disorders, and result in significant medical and functional problems. Alcohol use disorder is the most common psychiatric disorder and accounts for approximately 100,000 deaths per year in the United States.

A **personality disorder** is an enduring pattern of maladaptive traits that are inflexible and pervasive across a broad range of situations and that cause significant distress or impairment. Typically, the pattern is stable and of long duration, with onset in adolescence or early adulthood. The presence of a personality disorder typically complicates the diagnosis and management of other psychiatric conditions.

Anorexia nervosa often is associated with a poor outcome and has a mortality rate of at least 10%, typically due to starvation, electrolyte imbalance, or suicide. Its essential features are that the individual refuses to maintain a minimally normal body weight, is intensely afraid of gaining weight, and exhibits a significant disturbance in the perception of the size or shape of his or her body. **Bulimia nervosa** is characterized by binge eating and compensatory methods (e.g., purging) to prevent weight gain; its course is generally less severe than that of anorexia nervosa.

Sleep disorders include obstructive sleep apnea (wherein inadequate pulmonary ventilation results in frequent awakenings during sleep), restless legs syndrome (a subjective sensation of inability to keep still that interferes with falling asleep), and period limb movement disorder (regular jerking movements during sleep). Insomnia also is a very common symptom of psychiatric disorders.

Many medical disorders present with psychiatric symptoms. A classic mimic is hypothyroidism, which shares many symptoms with major depressive disorder, including low energy, excessive sleep, and weight gain. Consequently, the evaluation of psychiatric symptoms (discussed later in this chapter) typically includes a medical assessment to rule out common neurologic, endocrine, cardiac, pulmonary, rheumatologic, and infectious diseases.

Suicide may be associated with acute or chronic environmental stress, substance use disorders, psychiatric disorders (especially major depression, bipolar disorder, borderline personality disorder, and schizophrenia), or chronic illnesses (especially chronic lung diseases or illnesses in which chronic pain is a major factor). The rate of completed suicides in the United States is approximately 13 per 100,000 per year, with more than 30,000 suicides occurring each year. Women are more likely to attempt suicide, but men are 3–4 times as likely as women to complete suicide. In the United States, suicide is the eighth leading cause of death overall, but the second leading cause of death in the 15- to 24-year-old group. Three to five attempts are made for every suicide committed, depending on the underlying psychiatric diagnosis.

Psychiatric emergencies in addition to suicidality include delirium (sudden change in mental status due to infectious, toxic, or metabolic etiology), alcohol and sedative–hypnotic withdrawal, mania, and psychosis. Patients with panic attacks may also present to emergency rooms, often because the symptoms of such an attack mimic cardiac and pulmonary emergencies (e.g., chest pain, shortness of breath).

Symptoms, Signs, and Tests

Mental illnesses are manifested by a wide range of symptoms, subjective feelings, and behaviors, the majority of which are not specifically pathologic when viewed in isolation. Because the symptoms are nonspecific and because many are known to be associated with medical and neurologic illnesses, a complete physical examination and screening laboratory tests are essential components of a psychiatric evaluation. X-rays of the chest, brain magnetic resonance imaging (MRI), electroencephalogram (EEG), personality testing, and neuropsychological testing (to assess cognition) are often a part of a thorough psychiatric evaluation. Hormonal studies may be important to rule out pituitary, thyroid, or adrenal disease with psychiatric manifestations.

As in physical illnesses, a detailed history is essential and is usually obtained from family members as well as the patient. The mental status examination, a specific component of the psychiatric evaluation, is of great value in differentiating between organic and non-organic mental diseases. The mental status examination includes evaluation of (1) orientation to time, place, and person; (2) memory, both recent and remote; (3) intellectual functions, including general fund of information and arithmetic ability; (4) judgment; (5) mood and affect, (6) speech pattern; and (7) delusions and hallucinations.

Rating scales can provide standardized measures of the severity of symptoms. For example, the nine-item Patient Health Questionnaire (PHQ-9) is used to screen for and diagnose major depressive disorder.

Table 24–1 classifies and defines many of the manifestations of mental illness. It should be remembered that many of these symptoms and signs are experienced by normal people. When they are disproportionately intense or prolonged in relation to their stimulus or when they significantly interfere with the individual's ability to function in and gain gratification from his or her environment, they may indicate an abnormal mental state. Symptoms such as anxiety and depression are experienced by almost everyone at certain times. Not infrequently, an individual's symptoms are more troublesome to others than they are to the person with the symptoms.

Specific Diseases

The classification of mental illness is based on several major parameters, including intelligence (for intellectual disability), presence or absence of brain lesions, ability to correctly interpret reality, and duration of the condition. Below-normal intelligence occurring before age 18 is referred to as **intellectual disability**; the acquired loss of intellectual capacity after age 18 is termed **dementia**. Mental changes associated with demonstrable brain lesions are termed **mental disorders due to another medical condition**. The ability to correctly interpret reality is the fundamental consideration in separating psychoses from nonpsychotic illnesses. Some psychiatric disorders are episodic and recurrent (e.g., major depressive disorder, bipolar disorder), whereas others are chronic with acute exacerbations (e.g., schizophrenia).

TABLE 24–1	Types of Manifestations of Psychiatric Illness

Disturbances of consciousness
- Confusion: lack of orientation of time, place, or person
- Delirium: bewildered, restless

Disturbances of affect
- Euphoria: feeling of well-being inappropriate to apparent events
- Depression: feeling of sadness inappropriate to apparent events
- Grief: sadness appropriate to a loss (e.g., death of relative)
- Anxiety: feeling of apprehension with or without a precipitant
- Irritability: excessive sensitivity and response to stressful stimuli
- Lability: rapid shifts in affect

Disturbance of motor behavior
- Compulsion: uncontrollable impulse to perform an act
- Hyperactivity: restless, aggressive
- Hypoactivity: slowed psychological and physical function

Disturbance of thought processes
- Disorganization: lack of logical coherence
- Flight of ideas: rapid shifting of ideas, often with pressured speech

Disturbance of thought content
- Delusion: false belief that cannot be corrected by reasoning
- Hypochondria: exaggerated concern over health not based on physiologic disease
- Obsession: recurrent thought, feeling, or impulse
- Phobia: exaggerated fear of a specific situation
- Suicidal ideation: thought, intent, and/or plan to harm self
- Homicidal ideation: thought, intent, and/or plan to harm others

Disturbance of perception
- Hallucinations: false sensory perceptions not associated with real stimuli
- Illusions: false sensory perceptions of real stimuli

Disturbances of cognition
- Amnesia: partial to total inability to recall past experiences
- Aphasia: loss of ability to comprehend language (sensory aphasia) or verbalize (motor aphasia)
- Agnosia: inability to recognize and interpret sensory impressions
- Paramnesia: falsification of memory by distortion of recall
- Intellectual disability: developmental lack of intelligence that interferes with social and vocational performance
- Dementia: loss of intellectual capacity occurring after developmental period and secondary to neurologic disease

The American Psychiatric Association has established criteria for the classification of mental illnesses in its *Diagnostic and Statistical Manual of Mental Disorders* (DSM). Although other classification systems exist (e.g., International Classification of Diseases [ICD]), the DSM is the most widely accepted system. Some general comments are in order before proceeding with a discussion of specific categories.

Emotional disorders may be associated with medical illnesses in several ways. First and most common is the emotional response of an individual to a physical illness or injury. While one would consider this a normal, if not expected, reaction, the severity of symptoms, usually depression and/or anxiety, may vary considerably, depending on such factors as the person's basic personality, prior level of activity, and seriousness of the illness. Often the symptoms are of sufficient intensity and persistence to justify a diagnosis of transient situational disturbance. Second, mental illness may occur secondary to a neurologic, cardiac, pulmonary, endocrine, or rheumatologic disorder (mental disorder due to another medical condition). Third, certain physical illnesses are called psychophysiologic disorders because of their frequent association with emotional disturbances. In most instances, the nature of the association between emotional disturbance and physical illness is poorly understood (i.e., the causal relationship is not clear). Thus, this term is no longer generally used. Of note, whereas the DSM refers to "mental disorders" (implying a distinction from "physical disorders"), it is abundantly clear that the substrate of mental illness is the brain. Thus, one should avoid the false dichotomy between mental illness and physical illness.

In addition to considering the possible relationship of the patient's mental illness to medical or neurologic disease, it is also important to judge whether the patient is psychotic. Psychosis entails altered perceptions (hallucinations), illogical beliefs (delusions), and illogical thinking (loose associations). Most psychoses fall into the categories of schizophrenia and mood disorders. Psychosis may also be due to medical illness (e.g., neurosyphilis, CNS tumor), use of illicit substances (e.g., cocaine, hallucinogens), or medication side effects (e.g., steroids).

Another important point to be made about the classification of mental illnesses is that most symptoms are not specific to any particular category. This is particularly true of depression and anxiety, which commonly occur with many different types of mental illness. For example, depression, one of the most common and important symptoms, may be associated with medical illness (e.g., hypothyroidism), schizophrenia, mood disorders, substance use disorders, and transient situational disturbances.

Depressive and Bipolar Disorders

The group of illnesses including depressive and bipolar disorders is broadly referred to as mood disorders because they are characterized by alteration of mood. **Mania** is a euphoric or irritable, hyperactive state, whereas **depression** is a sad or melancholy state with either decreased activity or agitation. The most common mood disorders are major depressive disorder and **bipolar disorder** ("bipolar" refers to alternating depression and mania). The lifetime prevalence of major depressive disorder in the United States is 18%, whereas for bipolar disorder it is 2%. Mood disorders are episodic with good recovery between episodes, although emerging evidence indicates that subtle symptoms may persist.

A major depressive episode is diagnosed when at least five of the following symptoms occur for at least two weeks and cause functional impairment: depressive mood, loss of interest or enjoyment (anhedonia), fatigue, changes in appetite, changes in sleep, suicidal ideation, psychomotor agitation or retardation, poor concentration, and feelings of worthlessness or helplessness. Typically, a patient with major depressive disorder will experience multiple major depressive episodes over the course of his or her lifetime.

A manic episode includes elevated or irritable mood and at least three of the following symptoms occurring for at least one week and causing functional impairment: grandiosity, decreased need for sleep, pressured speech, racing thoughts, distractibility, increased activity, and excessive involvement in pleasurable activities. Patients with bipolar disorder must have at least one manic episode, but typically will have multiple manic and depressive episodes; the episodes may become more frequent over time. Both major depressive episodes and manic episodes may be accompanied by psychosis, including hallucinations, paranoia, somatic delusions, religious delusions, or grandiose delusions.

The etiology of depression is unclear, although it has been associated with a number of biological factors. First-degree relatives of probands with depression are 2–3 times more likely to have depression than controls; the heritability of depression has been estimated to be between 31% and 42%. Polymorphisms of the *5-HTTPR*, *BDNF*, and *COMT* genes also have been associated with depression. Neuroimaging studies implicate hypoactivity in the frontal cortex and hyperactivity in the hippocampus and activity in the pathophysiology of depression as causative factors. The monoamine hypothesis of depression states that disruptions in the functioning of serotonin, norepinephrine, and dopamine systems may result in depression. Abnormalities in neuroendocrine function, especially the hypothalamic–pituitary–adrenal (HPA) axis, have long been associated with depression; for example, approximately half of patients with depression do not experience the normal suppression of endogenous cortisol expected with exogenous administration of cortisol. Increasing attention is being paid to the role of neuroplasticity—that is, the ability of neurons to form and prune connections as a substrate for learning; depression may be due to failure of plasticity, and treatments of depression may work by promoting neuroplasticity.

Family studies, twin studies, adoption studies, and genome-wide scans indicate a clear genetic component to bipolar disorder. First-degree relatives of patients with bipolar disorder are 7 times more likely to develop bipolar disorder than control subjects, and heritability is estimated to be between 73% and 93%. As yet, no specific genetic polymorphism has been reliably associated with bipolar disorder. Neuroimaging findings in some studies of bipolar disorder include enlarged ventricles, increased deep white matter lesions (especially in the frontal lobes), decreased gray matter in parts of the limbic system, increased metabolism in the anterior cingulate cortex, and decreased metabolism in the prefrontal cortex. Patients with bipolar disorder have been found to

have dysfunction of the HPA axis, specifically elevated cortisol levels due to impaired central glucocorticoid signaling. Bipolar disorder is particularly sensitive to sleep and sleep disturbance: sleep deprivation and travel-related changes in time zone have been associated with the onset of mania.

Effective treatments for major depressive disorder include antidepressant medications (which have serotonergic, noradrenergic, and/or dopaminergic mechanisms of action), psychotherapy (especially cognitive-behavioral therapy and interpersonal psychotherapy), phototherapy (for depression with a seasonal component), physical exercise, and electroconvulsive therapy. It is critical to distinguish between major depressive disorder and bipolar disorder, as the latter requires different management: mood stabilizers (specifically, lithium, antiepileptic drugs, and antipsychotics), careful management of sleep and daily rhythms, and electroconvulsive therapy. Unfortunately, both illnesses may become chronic and treatment refractory.

Anxiety, Obsessive–Compulsive, Trauma-Related, and Stressor-Related Disorders

The anxiety disorders are characterized by symptoms such as exaggerated or inappropriate feelings of tension and nervousness, phobia, insomnia, obsession, or compulsiveness, in which one symptom usually dominates and in which there is no evidence of psychosis or of reaction to a transient situation. Anxiety disorders frequently co-occur with mood disorders and substance use disorders.

Sigmund Freud originally used the term *neurosis* not only to indicate a specific disease process, but also to indicate unpleasant symptoms in a person with nonpsychotic mental illness. Modern nosology identifies the following anxiety disorders: **panic disorder**, characterized by repeated bouts of severe anxiety (i.e., panic attacks); **generalized anxiety disorder (GAD)**, or chronic worry that is difficult to control; **obsessive–compulsive disorder (OCD)**, or recurrent intrusive thoughts accompanied by compensatory behaviors; **post-traumatic stress disorder (PTSD)**, referring to hyperarousal, reexperiencing, and avoidance of psychologically painful stimuli following a traumatic event (e.g., combat, rape); **social phobia**, or anxiety in social settings; and specific phobias.

Most anxiety disorders have their average age of onset in early adulthood, usually before the age of 30. The lifetime prevalence of GAD is 4–7%, the prevalence for panic disorder is 2–3% of women and 0.5–1.5% of men, and the prevalence of OCD is 2–3%.

Anxiety symptoms occur to some degree in everyone and may be found in patients with other mental illnesses such as psychoses or personality disorders. Thus anxiety symptoms are not necessarily specific. In anxiety disorders, the patient is usually aware that the symptoms are irrational but is unable to control them. Consequently, this group of mental illnesses does not reflect a thought disorder as do the psychotic illnesses. In addition, persons with anxiety disorders maintain the ability to distinguish external reality from internal processes; reality impairment (referred to as "cognitive distortions") remains isolated to the symptom itself and does not, as in psychotic illnesses, pervade the individual's total awareness.

People with phobias persistently avoid specific objects, activities, or situations because of irrational fears. Patients with **agoraphobia** avoid being alone, whereas patients with social phobia avoid specific social situations due to overconcern about humiliation and embarrassment. Common specific phobias involve animals (particularly reptiles, insects, and rodents), tight places (**claustrophobia**), high places (**acrophobia**) and blood.

Panic attacks involve sudden, short-lived, severe anxiety reactions without the patient being certain when the attack will occur. Symptoms relate to sudden autonomic nervous system discharge, which produces dyspnea, palpitations, chest pain, choking, dizziness, paresthesias, hot and cold flashes, sweating, trembling, and fear.

OCD involves senseless and repetitive thoughts (obsessions), such as violence, contamination, and doubt, or compulsions to perform an act, such as hand washing, counting, checking, or touching, accompanied by a desire to resist such activity. However, attempts to resist the compulsion are accompanied by tension and anxiety.

In individuals with acute stress disorder and PTSD, the normal stress response is amplified and generalized to situations that would typically not evoke such a response. The risk of developing PTSD is proportional to the severity and type of trauma; overall, 14% of individuals who experience a psychologically significant trauma go on to develop PTSD.

Treatment usually consists of antidepressant medications, sedative–hypnotic medications (in some cases), and cognitive-behavioral psychotherapy.

Schizophrenia

Psychosis is a syndrome in which behavior is seriously disorganized and contact with reality is impaired. Schizophrenia is a common cause of psychosis and a disproportionate cause of disability. It affects approximately 1% of the population—a rate that is surprisingly constant around the world. The core features of schizophrenia include delusions and hallucinations. Alterations in mood and behavior are also prominent in schizophrenia, and patients with this disease often are ambivalent, display inappropriate emotional responses, and can become either aggressive (when acutely psychotic) or withdrawn. The symptoms of schizophrenia include three types: (1) positive symptoms: hallucinations and delusions; (2) negative symptoms: flattened affect, avolition, alogia (inability to speak), and poor interpersonal interactions; and (3) cognitive symptoms: problems with working memory, organization, and planning.

The cause of schizophrenia is unknown. The familial tendency suggests a poorly defined, possibly multiple-gene, genetic influence in schizophrenia. Potential environmental influences may include starvation and infection: pregnant women undergoing food deprivation or experiencing influenza in the second trimester are more likely to have children with schizophrenia than are women without such exposure. Numerous biochemical, structural, and neurophysiologic abnormalities have been demonstrated in patients with schizophrenia, none of which have been proved to be causative. These include abnormalities in neuronal migration, enlarged cerebral ventricles (present in approximately half of patients with schizophrenia), abnormal dopamine metabolism, abnormal hippocampal functioning, eye tracking abnormalities, inadequate gating of auditory stimuli, and abnormal connectivity among cortico-striatal-thalamic functional networks. Early use of cannabis and chronic, severe use of stimulants have both been associated with higher risk of schizophrenia. Genetic inquiries have identified various other polymorphisms associated with schizophrenia, each of which likely makes a small contribution to the risk of developing schizophrenia.

Schizophrenia usually has its onset in late adolescence and early adulthood, with fewer new cases occurring in middle age. The severity of the disease varies considerably. Some patients are able to maintain employment while being treated on an outpatient basis, whereas others require hospitalization. In general, schizophrenia is a chronic disabling illness that results in social and occupational decline. The early course of the illness, referred to as the prodrome, is characterized by cognitive changes (e.g., drop in IQ), social withdrawal, depression, and anxiety. The prodrome lasts for months to years before the illness moves into its active phase of psychosis and functional decline. The course after the active phase is highly variable: some individuals enter a residual phase of minimal symptoms and only mildly impaired functioning, others have a chronic, severe course, and still others have intermediate outcomes. The residual phase may be punctuated by acute exacerbations due to nonadherence to treatment, substance use, or natural course of the illness. It is estimated that one-third of individuals have fairly good outcomes, another third have moderate outcomes, and the final third have poor long-term prognoses.

The predominant modes of medical therapy for schizophrenia include antipsychotic medications (which typically have dopaminergic and serotonergic properties), cognitive therapy, psychosocial rehabilitation, and family psychoeducation.

Substance-Related and Addictive Disorders

Substance use disorders are highly comorbid with other psychiatric disorders—in particular, mood, anxiety, and psychotic disorders. Substance use disorders result in significant medical complications, psychosocial dysfunction, and burden to society.

Alcohol use disorder is the most common psychiatric disorder; other important substances of abuse include tobacco, stimulants (cocaine, amphetamines), opioids (both heroin and prescription narcotics), sedative–hypnotics, hallucinogens (e.g., phencyclidine), inhalants, and cannabis. Approximately 450,000 people die each year in the United States due to the consequences of tobacco use, whereas 100,000 die each year from alcohol use.

Substance use disorders consist of some combination of the following: difficulty controlling substance use, unsuccessful efforts to reduce substance use, craving, recurrent use despite interpersonal problems or physical hazards, tolerance (need for increased amount of the substance to achieve the intended effect, or diminished effect with continued use of the same amount of the substance), and withdrawal (physiologic effects of not taking the substance). Alcohol withdrawal is a potentially life-threatening condition that can result in delirium, hallucinations, and seizures.

Psychosocial interventions are the mainstays of treatment of substance use disorders, although medications have also been found to be helpful in the treatment of alcohol use disorder (naltrexone, acamprosate, topiramate, and disulfiram) and opioid use disorder (naltrexone, buprenorphine, and methadone).

Personality Disorders

A personality disorder is an enduring pattern of maladaptive traits that are inflexible and pervasive across a broad range of situations and that cause significant distress or impairment. Typically, this pattern is stable and of long duration, with onset in adolescence or early adulthood. The various types of personality disorders are defined in approximate order of frequency in **Table 24–2**. There is ample overlap of these categories. Disorders formerly called **sociopathic** or psychopathic are now considered antisocial personality disorders. Personality disorders should be distinguished from personality changes that may occur in certain neurologic conditions, such as Alzheimer disease and traumatic brain injury.

Neurodevelopmental Disorders

It is estimated that one in five children will have some form of mental illness during any given year. Children are susceptible to many of the disorders mentioned previously (in particular, mood disorders, anxiety disorders, and substance use disorders), but are also uniquely vulnerable to autism, attention-deficit/hyperactivity disorder, and various causes of intellectual disability.

Intellectual disability consists of deficits in intellectual and adaptive functioning; these deficits have an onset before age 18 but usually are present from birth. The prevalence of intellectual disability is approximately 1%. The cause is unknown much of the time. Known causes include prenatal infectious diseases, such as rubella, toxoplasmosis, cytomegalic inclusion disease, and syphilis; neonatal meningitis or encephalitis; Down syndrome; metabolic disease such as hypothyroidism and phenylketonuria; brain damage from perinatal diseases such as erythroblastosis fetalis, birth injury, and anoxia at birth; and external agents such as trauma, carbon monoxide poisoning, and lead poisoning.

TABLE 24–2	**Personality Disorders**
Disorder	**Characteristics**
Histrionic	Excitability, emotional instability, overactivity, self-dramatization
Dependent	Need overtly expressed, compliant, eager to perform for others, clinging, immature
Avoidant	Withdrawn, overly sensitive, shy, low self-esteem
Antisocial	Lack of loyalty to individuals, groups, or society; selfish, irresponsible, impulsive, lack of guilt, violation of rules; formerly referred to as sociopathic or psychopathic personality disorder
Obsessive–compulsive	Overly conscientious, overly meticulous, perfectionistic; distinguished from obsessive–compulsive disorder by not being distressing to the individual
Paranoid	Hypersensitive, rigid, unwarranted suspicion, jealous, excessive self-importance
Narcissistic	Grandiose sense of self-importance, exhibitionism, preoccupation with fantasies of unlimited success, power, brilliance, or beauty
Borderline	Unstable self-image, chronic feelings of emptiness and suicidal ideation, volatile relationships characterized by shifting between idealization and devaluation, impulsivity
Schizoid	Detachment from social relationships, does not desire or enjoy close relationships
Schizotypal	Eccentric behavior, abnormalities of thinking, may be on a spectrum with schizophrenia

Depressive and anxiety disorders (e.g., social anxiety disorder, generalized anxiety disorder) are fairly common in childhood, with suicide rates escalating dramatically in adolescence. Psychotic disorders are uncommon in childhood, although schizophrenia and bipolar disorder may begin in late childhood and adolescence. **Autism spectrum disorder** is a pervasive developmental disorder that usually starts before 36 months of age and is marked by deficits in social communication and social interaction, along with restricted, repetitive patterns of behavior, interests, or activities. Patients also may have accompanying intellectual impairment or language impairment. **Asperger syndrome** is considered to be a part of the autism spectrum; with this disorder, intelligence is intact but there are problems with communication and behavior.

Attention-deficit/hyperactivity disorder (ADHD) is common in children and adolescents, with a prevalence of approximately 5% in children (and 2.5% in adults). ADHD includes either inattention symptoms (e.g., difficulty sustaining attention and organizing tasks) or hyperactivity–impulsivity symptoms (e.g., fidgeting, running and talking excessively, interrupting frequently), or both. Treatment with dopaminergic stimulants is typically effective and well tolerated.

Other mental illnesses affecting children and adolescents include learning disorders, oppositional defiant disorder, substance use disorders, and conduct disorder (which may be a precursor to antisocial personality disorder).

Mental Disorders Due to Another Medical Condition

The essential feature of this category of disorders is mental disturbance due to disease of the brain or widespread alteration of brain function due to an underlying medical or neurologic problem. A mental disturbance may also be due to a substance or toxin (substance-induced mental disorder). The psychiatric diagnostic process—especially when a patient presents with new-onset psychiatric symptoms or a decompensation in chronic, stable symptoms—includes an evaluation of the possibility of a medical or substance-induced etiology of the symptoms. It is extremely important to recognize medical causes of mental disorders because treatment in such cases is likely to be very different than that of primary psychiatric disorders.

Acute changes in mental status are typically due to substance intoxication or withdrawal, although they also may occur in response to neurologic conditions such as epilepsy, ischemic stroke, traumatic brain injury, and subarachnoid hemorrhage. In vulnerable populations (e.g., older adults), infections or electrolyte disturbance may result in an acute change. Substances commonly associated with acute changes include alcohol (either intoxication or withdrawal), sedative–hypnotics, hallucinogens, stimulants (and other dopaminergic agents), and corticosteroids.

Chronic changes in mental status may manifest as dementia, personality change, psychosis, or mood symptoms and are most commonly due to progressive neurologic disorders such as Alzheimer disease, Parkinson disease, Huntington disease, cerebrovascular disease, and CNS neoplasm. Alzheimer disease, a diffuse atrophy of the brain with loss of neurons of unknown cause, accounts for most cases of chronic irreversible dementia. Its course is slowly progressive, with survival of 6–12 years.

Repeated cerebral infarcts may produce dementia in some individuals but are a much less common cause of dementia than Alzheimer disease. Vascular dementia is more likely to be associated with a stepwise progression and findings that indicate focal neurologic damage.

Many other brain diseases and metabolic intoxications, such as acidosis, uremia, and hepatic failure, can present with mental disturbances. Some symptoms and signs of psychosis due to medical conditions or substances may overlap with other causes of psychosis (e.g., schizophrenia), but the more common signs and symptoms of organic psychoses are delirium (mental confusion, disorientation, abnormal emotions, and altered consciousness) and dementia (loss of the intellectual processes, such as memory, reasoning, judgment, and problem solving, and the loss of the higher aspects of personality).

Somatic Symptom Disorders

The common feature of **somatic symptom disorders** is the prominence of somatic symptoms associated with significant distress and impairment. These disorders include somatic symptom disorder (excessive thoughts, feelings, or behaviors related to one or more somatic symptoms), illness anxiety disorder (preoccupation with having or acquiring a serious illness), **conversion disorder** (involuntary loss of a specific function suggestive of neurologic illness, such as paralysis, loss of voice, blindness, anesthesia, or incoordination), and factitious disorder (falsification of physical or psychological signs or symptoms, associated with deception even in the absence of obvious external rewards). The term **malingering** (technically not a mental illness) is used if the symptoms are produced to avoid an obvious external circumstance, such as conscription into the military.

Somatic symptom disorder and conversion disorder are distinguished from factitious disorder and malingering in that the symptoms suggestive of physical illness are not under voluntary control. The complaints, which are frequently referred to as **psychosomatic**, may take the form of headache, fatigue, palpitations, fainting, nausea, loss of sensation, paralysis, blindness, vomiting, abdominal pain, bowel troubles, allergies, and menstrual and sexual difficulties. In its fully developed form, a patient with somatic symptom disorder will have a lifelong pattern beginning in the teenage period of seeking medical evaluation, being hospitalized, and even having unnecessary surgery. This disorder is more common in women and is often associated with use of many potentially addicting prescription drugs obtained from multiple physicians and pharmacies. Pain, often the dominant symptom, accounts for the most common types of drugs obtained by these patients.

It is important to recognize that psychosomatic complaints may be dominant symptoms in other mental illnesses, especially depression and schizophrenia; however, the other features of these diseases will also be present. Another problem is that the expression of complaints associated with physical illness varies greatly among individuals; thus the diagnosis of physical illness may be delayed in persons with frequent psychosomatic complaints or in those who do not readily express pain.

Sleep–Wake Disorders

The most common disorders of sleep are sleep apnea and restless legs syndrome—an irresistible urge to move the limbs that results in disturbed sleep, periodic limb movements during sleep, and narcolepsy (which is likely caused by a genetic deficiency of hypocretin, an HPA peptide). It should be noted, however, that sleep disruption (insomnia or hypersomnia) are very common in psychiatric disorders, including mood disorders, anxiety disorders, and psychotic disorders. Substances (alcohol and nicotine, in particular) and behavioral patterns are often implicated in the onset and maintenance of sleep difficulties. A careful history and studies of oxygen saturation, air flow, respiratory effort, eye and jaw muscle movement, and heart and brain electrical activity (collectively called polysomnography) can help distinguish among the causes of sleep disturbance.

Practice Questions

1. What is the most common cause of violent death?
   A. Suicide
   B. War
   C. Homicide
   D. Accidental poisoning
2. Which of the following is a thought disorder resulting in distortion of reality?
   A. Conversion disorder
   B. Panic disorder
   C. Schizophrenia
   D. Mania
3. What is the most common serious psychiatric disorder on an overall basis?
   A. Schizophrenia
   B. Alcohol abuse
   C. Malingering
   D. Anxiety
4. Alternating depression and hyperactivity is a symptom of which of the following disorders?
   A. Psychosis
   B. Personality disorders
   C. Somatic symptom disorders
   D. Mood disorders

GENERAL REFERENCE

American Psychiatric Association. *Diagnostic and Statistical Manual of Mental Disorders*, 5th ed. Washington, DC: American Psychiatric Association; 2013.

Endocrine System

OUTLINE

OBJECTIVES

1. Review the anatomy and function of the endocrine organs.
2. Name the syndromes related to excess or deficiency of adrenocorticotropic hormone, growth hormone, antidiuretic hormone, thyroid hormone, parathyroid hormone, glucocorticoids, catecholamines, mineralocorticoids, and insulin.
3. Describe the general principles of diagnosis of endocrine diseases, including the role of laboratory analysis.
4. List signs and symptoms of hyposecretion and hypersecretion of the pituitary, thyroid, parathyroid, adrenal, and pancreatic islet hormones.
5. Name and describe the most common diseases of the endocrine organs.
6. Name and describe the neoplasms of the endocrine system.
7. Compare and contrast type 1 and type 2 diabetes mellitus.
8. Describe the acute and chronic complications of diabetes mellitus.
9. Be able to define and use in context all terms and words in headings and in bold print in this chapter.

KEY TERMS

acromegaly
Addison disease
adenoma
adrenal cortex
adrenal gland
adrenal medulla
adrenocorticotropic hormone (ACTH)
androgens
antidiuretic hormone
anterior pituitary adenoma
Cushing syndrome
diabetes insipidus
diabetes mellitus
diabetic ketoacidosis
endocrine system
epinephrine
follicle-stimulating hormone (FSH)
follicular carcinoma
gigantism

glucagon
glucocorticoid
glucose tolerance test
goiter
Graves disease
growth hormone (GH)
Hashimoto thyroiditis
hemoglobin A1$_c$
hormone
hypercalcemia
hyperparathyroidism
hyperthyroidism
hypoglycemia
hypothalamus
hypothyroidism
insulin
insulinoma
iodine
islets of Langerhans
luteinizing hormone (LH)
medullary carcinoma

melanocyte-stimulating
    hormone (MSH)
microangiopathy
mineralocorticoids
multiple endocrine
    neoplasia 1 (MEN1)
multiple endocrine
    neoplasia 2 (MEN2)
myxedema
neuroblastoma
ovary
oxytocin
pancreatic neuroendocrine
    neoplasia
panhypopituitarism
papillary thyroid carcinoma

paraneoplastic syndrome
parathyroid
paresthesia
pheochromocytoma
pituitary
placenta
polydypsia
polyuria
prolactin
testis
tetany
thyroid
thyroid adenoma
thyroid-stimulating
    hormone (TSH)
vasopressin

Review of Structure and Function

The **endocrine system** includes those organs, or tissues within organs, that secrete their cellular products into the bloodstream. The products of the endocrine cells are **hormones**, which exert their influence on tissues of the body remote from their site of origin. Major endocrine organs or tissues include the **hypothalamus**, posterior and anterior **pituitary** gland, **thyroid** gland, **parathyroid** glands, **adrenal cortex** and **adrenal medulla**, **islets of Langerhans**, ovaries, testes, and placenta (**Figure 25–1**). The hormones produced at each of these sites and their effects are listed in **Table 25–1**.

Hormones are essential to health because they regulate metabolism, growth, and development. The anterior pituitary produces *trophic* hormones, or hormones that stimulate growth and development in other tissues. Some of the anterior pituitary hormones are intermediates that stimulate hormone production in other endocrine organs: **adrenocorticotropic hormone (ACTH)**, **thyroid-stimulating hormone (TSH)**, **follicle-stimulating hormone (FSH)**, and **luteinizing hormone (LH)**. Others act directly on target tissues: **melanocyte-stimulating hormone (MSH)**, **growth hormone (GH)**, and **prolactin**. Production of hormones by the anterior pituitary is controlled by the hypothalamus. The hypothalamus is a portion of the brain that monitors hormone levels in the blood and secretes releasing or inhibitory factors to control the production of pituitary hormones. This control mechanism is illustrated in **Figure 25–2**.

Posterior pituitary hormones, like hormones from the remainder of the endocrine organs, act directly on target tissues. The posterior pituitary does not produce the hormones it releases. **Oxytocin**, which stimulates uterine contractions during labor, and **vasopressin** (also called **antidiuretic hormone** [ADH]), which regulates blood pressure, are produced elsewhere in the brain and stored in the posterior pituitary.

The ovaries, testes, and placenta are discussed in other chapters and so are not elaborated on here again. In addition, there are numerous other hormones, not mentioned in Table 25–1, such as those of the gastrointestinal tract, which are beyond the scope of this text.

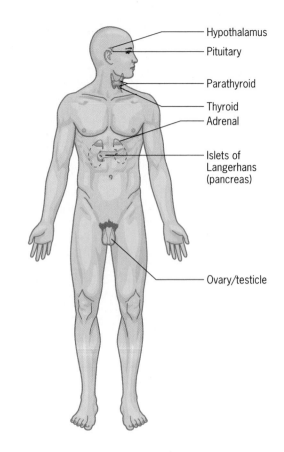

FIGURE 25–1 Endocrine organs and tissues.

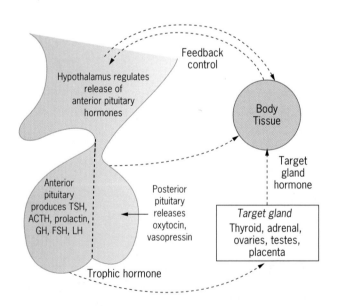

FIGURE 25–2 Negative feedback control mechanisms for hormones governed by the hypothalamus and anterior pituitary. A stimulating hormone of the hypothalamus causes increased production of the corresponding anterior pituitary hormone, which, in turn, causes the target organ to produce its hormone. The target organ's hormone inhibits the production of stimulating hormone by the hypothalamus, thus shutting off the stimulation until blood levels of the target organ's hormone drop.

TABLE 25-1 Site of Origin and Effects of Hormones

Site	Hormone (Synonyms, Abbreviations)	Effect
Anterior pituitary	Adrenocorticotropic hormone (corticotropin, ACTH)	Stimulates production of glucocorticoids by adrenal cortex
	Melanocyte-stimulating hormone (MSH)	Stimulates pigment production in skin
	Growth hormone (somatotropin, GH)	Promotes growth of body tissues
	Thyroid-stimulating hormone (thyrotropin, TSH)	Stimulates production and release of thyroid hormones
	Follicle-stimulating hormone (FSH)	Initiates maturation of ovarian follicles
		Stimulates spermatogenesis
	Luteinizing hormone (LH)	Causes ovulation and stimulates ovary to produce estrogen and progesterone
		Stimulates androgen production by interstitial cells of testis
	Prolactin	Stimulates secretion of breast milk
Hypothalamus	Releasing hormones	Act on anterior pituitary to cause release of specific hormones
	Inhibitory hormones	Act on anterior pituitary to cause inhibition of release of specific hormones
Posterior pituitary	Antidiuretic hormone (vasopressin, ADH)	Causes conservation of body water by promoting water resorption by renal tubules
	Oxytocin	Stimulates smooth muscle contraction in breast to aid in milk ejection
Thyroid	Thyroxine (tetraiodothyronine, T_4)	Increases rate of cellular metabolism
		Nutritional effects on brain and other organs
	Triiodothyronine (T_3)	Same as thyroxine
	Calcitonin	Promotes retention of calcium and phosphorus in bone
Parathyroid	Parathyroid hormone (parathormone, PTH)	Regulates metabolism of calcium and phosphorus
		Promotes resorption of calcium and phosphorus from bone
Adrenal cortex	Glucocorticoids	Antagonizes effects of insulin
		Inhibits inflammatory response and fibroblastic activity
	Mineralocorticoid, mainly aldosterone	Promotes retention of sodium by renal tubules
	Androgens	Masculinization
Adrenal medulla	Catecholamines (epinephrine and norepinephrine)	Regulation of blood pressure by effects on vascular smooth muscle and heart
Islets of Langerhans	Insulin	Promotes utilization of glucose and lipid synthesis
	Glucagon	Promotes utilization of glycogen and lipid
Ovaries	Estrogens	Cause development of female secondary sex characteristics
		Necessary to maintain menstrual cycle and pregnancy
	Progesterone	Preparation of endometrium for implantation and maintenance of pregnancy
Placenta	Human chorionic gonadotropin (HCG)	Maintains corpus luteum and progesterone production in pregnancy
	Human placental lactogen	Stimulates growth of breasts and has growth hormone–like effects
Testes	Testosterone	Causes development of male secondary sex characteristics

Most Frequent and Serious Problems

Diabetes mellitus is the most common endocrine disease. It is estimated to affect 10% of adults and is the seventh leading cause of death in the United States. Before death, diabetes incurs significant morbidity by way of complications, including renal failure requiring dialysis, blindness, neuropathy, and deep skin ulcers often necessitating amputation of an affected digit or limb. It is estimated that the total cost incurred by diabetes every year, including the cost of medical care as well as indirect cost of time lost from work because of disability, is $175 billion in the United States alone. In addition, the incidence of diabetes is rising at an alarming rate, in developed as well as in developing countries.

Hyperfunction and hypofunction of the thyroid gland are also quite common, affecting up to 5% of the population, and women more so than men. The thyroid may become enlarged with either condition. An enlarged thyroid is called a **goiter**. **Hyperparathyroidism** is not uncommon and is usually caused by parathyroid adenomas. **Cushing syndrome**, caused by excess corticosteroids (glucocorticoids), is most commonly induced by the administration of corticosteroids for treatment of various illnesses (e.g., systemic lupus erythematosus, rheumatoid arthritis) or for the prevention of organ transplant rejection. Neoplasms of endocrine organs are relatively uncommon. The most common of them is thyroid cancer, which is unusual in that it tends to affect a younger population than cancers generally do: the median age at diagnosis is 49 years, and it can develop as early as the teenage years.

Symptoms, Signs, and Tests

Most endocrine disorders manifest by symptoms related to underproduction or overproduction of a hormone. The diagnosis depends on matching the patient's symptoms and signs with hormone dysfunction and with laboratory confirmation of excess or deficiency of a particular hormone. For example, overproduction of insulin decreases blood glucose levels and the patient presents acutely with measurable **hypoglycemia** manifested by hunger, pallor, shakiness, and decreased ability to perform mental tasks. All these manifestations result from the body's cells being unable to perform metabolic tasks because of the lack of glucose. Conversely, too little insulin, as occurs with diabetes mellitus, leads to elevated blood glucose levels, and the patient presents with **polyuria**, or excessive urination, and **polydipsia**, or excessive drinking. These symptoms occur because the kidney attempts to rid the body of the excess glucose and requires water to do so. The resultant loss of water leads to dehydration and thirst. Laboratory demonstration of excess glucose in the blood establishes the diagnosis of diabetes mellitus. In similar ways, symptoms caused by excess or deficiency of other hormones present with symptoms referable to the effect of the hormone in the body. These symptoms are mentioned in the discussion of diseases of specific endocrine organs later in this chapter.

The only endocrine gland accessible to physical examination is the thyroid gland. Enlargement of the gland can be nodular or diffuse. Localized nodules, cysts, and masses can be felt as well as diffuse hypertrophy, or goiter. Neoplasms of other endocrine organs are detected by the effects of the mass, by the effects of hormones produced by the neoplasm if it is functional, or by hypofunction if the neoplasm replaces the normal glandular tissue. In addition, neoplasms can be detected by radiologic techniques, including computed tomography (CT) scan, ultrasound, and magnetic resonance imaging (MRI).

The major means of diagnosing aberrations in the function of endocrine glands is by laboratory analysis of blood or urine for the hormones or their breakdown products. The levels of these proteins can be quantitated and compared to "normal" measures. These include thyroid hormone, parathyroid hormone (PTH), steroid hormones, catecholamines and their breakdown products, and the stimulatory hormones released by the pituitary (GH, ACTH, LH, FSH, TSH, and prolactin). Indirect assessment of endocrine function can be accomplished by measuring blood or urine chemicals that are affected by a particular hormone. For instance, the presence of too little insulin can be inferred by finding too much glucose in the blood and urine. The status of the parathyroid glands can be evaluated by measurements of blood and urine calcium and phosphorus levels because the metabolism of these substances is regulated by parathyroid hormone. Except for measurement of electrolytes and glucose, these laboratory tests are not done routinely or for screening purposes. They are performed when signs, symptoms, or radiologic findings suggest that an endocrine abnormality may be present.

Specific Diseases

Diseases of the endocrine system are usually related to underproduction or overproduction of a particular hormone or to neoplasia within the endocrine gland. In this chapter, we deviate from the general chapter outline we have been using and classify diseases by endocrine organ. The names of the conditions caused by deficiency or excess of the various hormones are given in **Table 25–2**. Because the list of hormones is long, and the diseases caused by excesses and deficiencies twice that, only the most common diseases are discussed here.

Diseases of the Pituitary Gland

Panhypopituitarism

Destruction of the anterior pituitary gland leads to **panhypopituitarism**. The most common causes of this rare condition are neoplasms of the pituitary that are large enough to destroy the gland, postpartum pituitary necrosis, and surgical removal of the pituitary for treatment of tumors. The pituitary is hyperplastic during pregnancy and thus more susceptible to infarction caused by an episode of hypotension as a result of excess hemorrhage during childbirth. Postpartum infarction of the pituitary gland is called *Sheehan syndrome*. Persons with panhypopituitarism have atrophy of the thyroid, adrenal cortex, and gonads because the trophic or stimulatory hormones TSH, ACTH, GH, LH, and FSH are no longer produced. This results in hypothyroidism, adrenal insufficiency, decreased libido or secondary sex

TABLE 25-2 Diseases Associated with Deficiency and Excess of Various Hormones

Hormone	Hormone Deficiency	Hormone Excess
Adrenocorticotropic hormone	Addison disease	Cushing syndrome
Growth hormone	Pituitary dwarfism	Gigantism; acromegaly
Vasopressin (antidiuretic hormone)	Diabetes insipidus	Syndrome of inappropriate ADH secretion (SIADH)
Thyroid hormones	Hypothyroidism	Hyperthyroidism
Parathyroid hormone	Hypoparathyroidism	Hyperparathyroidism
Glucocorticoids	May occur as part of Addison disease	Cushing syndrome
Mineralocorticoids	May occur as part of Addison disease	Conn syndrome (hyperaldosteronism)
Insulin	Diabetes mellitus	Hypoglycemia

characteristics, and growth retardation, depending on the age of onset. Women with postpartum panhypopituitarism additionally are not able to breastfeed their infants because the breasts are not stimulated to produce milk by prolactin. Although lethal if not treated, panhypopituitarism is readily treated by dietary replacement of trophic hormones.

> **BOX 25-1 Panhypopituitarism**
>
> **Causes**
> Pituitary neoplasms
> Postpartum hypotension (Sheehan syndrome)
> Surgical removal
> Infection
> Gene defects
> **Lesions**
> Infarct, replacement, or pressure atrophy of pituitary
> Inflammation
> **Manifestations**
> Decreased sexual function
> Hypothyroidism
> Adrenocortical insufficiency
> Decreased pigmentation
> Decreased lactation
> Decreased growth in children

Gigantism and Acromegaly

Excess growth hormone (GH) leads to enlargement of all tissues, although bone enlargement is the most prominent clinical finding. In children with open growth plates, bones can grow longer as well as wider, leading to **gigantism**. In adults, excess GH causes thickening of soft tissue and bones, a condition called **acromegaly**. Patients suffer early debilitation because of bone and joint disease

and die prematurely of cardiac dysfunction. Patients with acromegaly have large hands and prominent, coarse facial features (**Figure 25–3**). Gigantism and acromegaly are caused by pituitary adenomas that secrete GH, and are treated by removal of the neoplasm, by drugs that

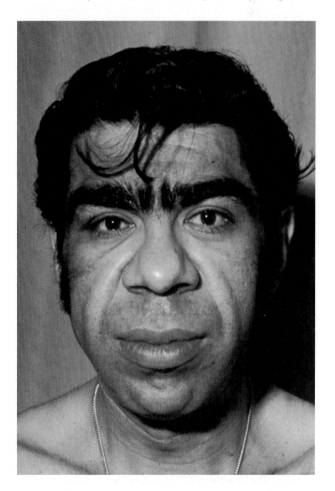

FIGURE 25–3 Acromegaly. A large face with coarse facial features is characteristic of chronic growth hormone excess in adults. (Courtesy of Dr. Don Schalch, Division of Endocrinology, University of Wisconsin School of Medicine and Public Health.)

inhibit GH secretion (somatostatin analogues), or by radiation to decrease the size of the neoplasm.

Diabetes Insipidus

Destruction of the posterior pituitary and/or hypothalamus leads to decreased release of vasopression (antidiuretic hormone). This results in failure of water reabsorption in the kidney. The resultant excess urination leads to excess thirst, so the symptoms of **diabetes insipidus** resemble those of diabetes mellitus: polyuria and polydypsia. Diabetes insipidus is very rare and is usually caused by infiltrative processes such as neoplasms, infections such as meningitis, head injury, and, sometimes, surgical operations in the area of the hypothalamus or pituitary gland. Because hormone replacement is available, the prognosis of the condition depends on its underlying cause.

Pituitary Neoplasms

Adenomas of the anterior pituitary are the most common tumors affecting the pituitary gland. Many pituitary adenomas do not secrete enough hormone to produce endocrine effects. Instead, they grow slowly and eventually compress the optic nerve to produce visual field defects. Functioning pituitary adenomas usually produce only a single hormone and can cause gigantism, acromegaly, Cushing syndrome, lactation, or amenorrhea, depending on the cell type of the neoplasm. Pituitary tumors usually occur in adults. They can be cured if they can be removed, but surgical removal is often difficult because of the proximity of surrounding vital structures. Some adenomas can be managed by drugs that suppress hormone secretion and may even cause the tumor to shrink.

Diseases of the Thyroid Gland

The thyroid gland, consisting of two lobes connected by a narrow strip of tissue (Figures 25–1 and **25–4**), lies in the neck anterior and lateral to the trachea. It consists of acini that secrete a colloid substance containing thyroid hormones (**Figure 25–5**). Calcitonin-secreting C cells

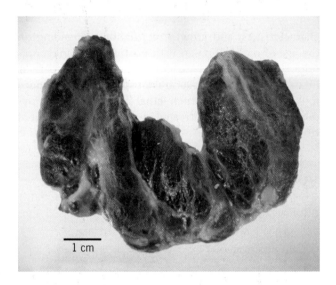

FIGURE 25–4 Thyroid gland. Gross appearance. The gland is composed of right and left lobes connected across the midline by the isthmus.

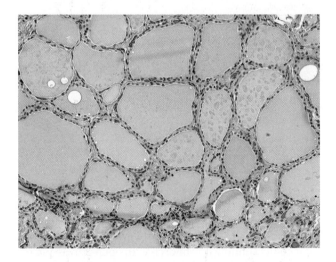

FIGURE 25–5 Thyroid gland. Microscopic appearance. Follicles are composed of central, homogeneous colloid containing thyroid hormone precursors, and a peripheral cuff of epithelial cells that produce the hormone.

are present in the stroma but are not conspicuous on routine histologic sections. Idiopathic hypothyroidism, Hashimoto thyroiditis, Graves disease, nodular goiter, adenoma, and papillary carcinoma are the most common diseases of the thyroid gland.

Hypothyroidism

Hypothyroidism is much more commonly caused by destruction or atrophy of the thyroid gland than it is by deficient production of thyroid-stimulating hormone by the pituitary. The production of thyroid hormone requires **iodine**, a necessary dietary supplement. Iodine deficiency is the most common cause of hypothyroidism worldwide. In the United States, the most common cause of hypothyroidism is an autoimmune process called **Hashimoto thyroiditis**, in which lymphocytes gradually destroy thyroid epithelial cells. They are primed to attack the thyroid by antibodies generated against thryoidal antigens such as thyroglobulin and thyroid peroxidase, proteins used in the synthesis of thyroid hormone. Lymphocytes flood the thyroid and form prominent lymphoid aggregates and follicles (**Figure 25–6**). In the early stages of Hashimoto thyroiditis, the thyroid gland is usually symmetrically enlarged but maintains normal function. As the thyroid cells are destroyed, they are replaced by fibrosis, and signs and symptoms of hypothyroidism gradually set in.

The results of hypothyroidism are similar regardless of the cause of the disease. Because the normal action of thyroid hormone is to stimulate cellular metabolism, thyroid deficiency results in slowing of the metabolism. Patients present with slow muscular responses,

including slow speech and dull reflexes, constipation, and slow heart rate; they feel cold much of the time, gain weight, lose hair, and have a sallow complexion, dry hair, and dry skin. Patients with prolonged hypothyroidism may develop deposits of mucopolysaccharides in skin, muscle, and viscera, producing a doughy edema called **myxedema**. Diagnosis of hypothyroidism is suspected from the clinical findings and confirmed by one or more laboratory tests that indicate a low level of circulating thyroid hormone and an elevated TSH level.

Other diseases that cause hypothyroidism include rare infectious or inflammatory conditions, drugs such as amiodarone or lithium that interfere with normal iodine use by the thyroid, genetic diseases that affect the synthesis of thyroid hormone, or deliberate destruction of the thyroid by medical or surgical means to treat hyperthyroidism or cancer. The severity of hypothyroidism varies greatly among patients, and diagnosis depends on careful consideration of laboratory data and clinical observations. In most cases, little can be done about the cause, but replacement therapy with thyroid hormone is effective in accelerating the patient's metabolism and reversing the symptoms.

BOX 25–4   Hypothyroidism

Causes

Iodine deficiency

Hashimoto thyroiditis (autoimmune thyroiditis)

Treatment of hyperthyroidism

Drugs

Surgery

Genetic conditions

Lesions

Destruction, atrophy, fibrosis of thyroid gland

Lymphocytic infiltration (thyroiditis)

Manifestations

Goiter (in some cases)

Decreased activity, intolerance to cold, weight gain, bradycardia

Constipation, hair loss, dry hair and skin, sallow complexion

Myxedema

Decreased thyroid hormone levels

Increased TSH

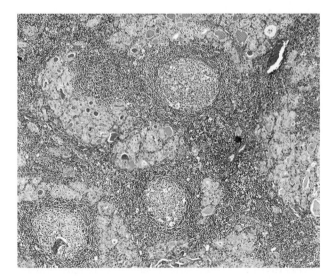

FIGURE 25–6 Hashimoto thyroiditis. The small, dark blue spots are lymphocytes that are destroying the follicular epithelial cells and forming lymphoid follicles, so the tissue vaguely resembles a lymph node with germinal centers.

Hyperthyroidism

Hyperthyroidism, also called thyrotoxicosis, can be caused by a functional thyroid adenoma or multinodular goiter, but the most common cause is another autoimmune disease, called **Graves disease**. This is

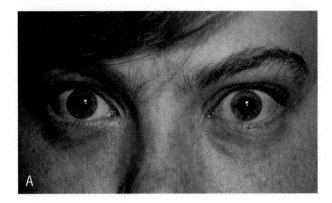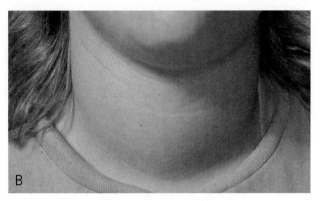

FIGURE 25–7 Graves disease. **A.** Exophthalmos is characterized by a wide-eyed, staring gaze. **B.** Diffuse swelling of the neck due to goiter. (Courtesy of Dr. Don Schalch, Division of Endocrinology, University of Wisconsin School of Medicine and Public Health.)

caused by stimulation of the thyroid by an antibody that mimics TSH, binding to the TSH receptor on the thyroid epithelial cell surface and inducing it to release thyroid hormone. The thyroid gland is usually diffusely enlarged, may be infiltrated by lymphocytes, and secretes thyroid hormone even though TSH production by the pituitary is suppressed by the high levels of circulating thyroid hormone. Graves disease is characterized by the triad of diffuse goiter, ophthalmopathy, and dermopathy (**Figure 25–7**). It generally affects patients between 20 and 40 years of age, is 10 times as common in women as in men, and affects up to 2% of the population in the United States.

Manifestations of hyperthyroidism reflect heightened metabolic activity: increased heart rate and palpitations, weight loss despite increased appetite, flushed skin and intolerance to heat, tremor, hyperactivity, diarrhea, insomnia, increased bone turnover, and psychiatric manifestations such as emotional lability and anxiety. The increased metabolic activity associated with hyperthyroidism can lead over time to heart failure, muscle degeneration (thyrotoxic myopathy), and bone fractures.

The ophthalmopathy and dermopathy of Graves disease are not seen in other conditions that cause hyperthyroidism. The eye changes are caused by swelling of the soft tissues of the orbit, leading to protrusion of the eye (exophthalmos) and weakness of the eye muscles. The skin changes consist of localized raised thickening of the skin of the anterior of the legs, called pretibial myxedema.

Measurement of the level of thyroid hormone and TSH in the blood is used to diagnose hyperthyroidism. Treatment of hyperthyroidism may involve drugs to suppress thyroid function or reduction of thyroid tissue by surgical removal or administration of radioactive iodine. Because iodine is selectively taken up by thyroid tissue, radioactive damage incurred by radioactive iodine can be safely limited to the thyroid.

BOX 25–5   Hyperthyroidism

Causes

Graves disease

Toxic nodular goiter

Thyroid neoplasms (some)

Lesions

Diffuse hyperplasia and lymphocytic infiltration (Graves disease)

Multiple functioning nodules or solitary neoplasm

Manifestations

Enlarged and/or nodular thyroid

Tremor, nervousness, emotional lability, anxiety, diarrhea

Increased heart rate, palpitations, flushed skin, heat intolerance, weight loss

Muscle weakness, heart failure, bone fractures

Increased circulating thyroid hormone

Exophthalmos, dermopathy in Graves disease

Thyroid Neoplasms

An adenoma is a discrete, encapsulated neoplasm that can arise in the background of otherwise entirely normal thyroid tissue. Similar-appearing nodules are found in some nodular goiters, and carcinoma can mimic adenoma in its localized, nodular growth. Thyroid nodules are therefore biopsied to determine the likelihood of their being benign or malignant, and they are removed if there is a reasonable suspicion of carcinoma. Most of the nodules that are surgically removed turn out to be prominent nodules in a multinodular goiter or adenomas. Occasionally, adenomas are functional, producing excess thyroid hormone that results in hyperthyroidism. This is also a reason for surgical removal.

The category "thyroid carcinoma" encompasses three groups when classified on the basis of clinical presentation, prognosis, and treatment. A highly aggressive variant, *anaplastic carcinoma*, diffusely infiltrates the structures of the neck and is not curable by any modality. Fortunately, this is very rare. **Medullary carcinoma** arises from the calcitonin-secreting cells that reside in the connective tissue of the thyroid gland. Sporadic medullary carcinoma is rare; it is most commonly seen in multiple endocrine neoplasm syndromes, discussed later. Most of the thyroid carcinomas are well differentiated and tend to be curable by a combination of surgery and treatment with radioactive iodine. Histologically, these are classified as **papillary carcinoma** (**Figure 25–8**), which accounts for about 75–85% of cases of thyroid carcinoma, and **follicular carcinoma**, which accounts for about 20%.

The strongest known risk factor for the development of well-differentiated thyroid cancer, particularly the papillary variant, is exposure to ionizing radiation. In the first half of the 20th century, before the harmful effects of radiation were appreciated, many children received radiation treatment for benign conditions such as acne, scalp ringworm, or tonsillitis. These children, as well as people who were exposed to radioactive fallout from nuclear power plant disasters and the atomic bombs dropped in Japan at the close of World War II, had a much higher incidence of thyroid cancer than the general population. Cessation of radiation therapy for benign conditions of the head and neck has not led to a decrease in incidence rates in the United States, however. To the contrary, the incidence of well-differentiated thyroid cancer has actually been increasing for the past two decades or so. This rise in numbers is not just because more small cancers are detected as a result of better imaging modalities: the incidence of both large and small cancers is increasing. About 75% of thyroid cancers occur in women, and in women, thyroid cancer is currently the seventh most common malignancy.

Prognosis for well-differentiated thyroid cancer is excellent: 5-year survival is close to 100%. Even very small (less than 1 cm) cancers can spread to lymph nodes, but lymph node metastasis does not portend as grim a prognosis as in other cancers. One of the strongest predictors of survival is age: patients younger than 45 years of age have a much better prognosis than do patients older than 45 years. This is why for patients younger than 45 years there are only two stages of well-differentiated thyroid cancer: thyroid cancer without and with distant metastasis.

Thyroid cancers usually come to attention by causing a palpable nodular growth in the thyroid. Occasionally, it presses on the underlying trachea to give the sensation of neck fullness or choking; grows into the surrounding tissue to impinge on the laryngeal nerves, causing hoarseness or vocal cord paralysis; or spreads to lymph nodes, causing them to swell. Increased CT imaging also detects thyroid nodules that may not have been detected by physical examination. Thyroid carcinomas typically do not cause symptoms of excess production of thyroid hormone. The diagnosis can be established by fine-needle aspiration (FNA) of the nodule under ultrasound guidance. This is very accurate in diagnosing papillary thyroid carcinoma, but it is not possible to distinguish between a follicular thyroid carcinoma and an adenoma by way of FNA. When the results are equivocal, the nodule should be excised and examined by a pathologist for evidence of cancer.

BOX 25–6   Thyroid Cancer

Risk Factors

Radiation exposure

Family history

Multiple endocrine neoplasia (medullary thyroid cancer)

Lesions

Nodule with papillary, follicular, or medullary histology; anaplastic carcinoma grows rapidly and extensively throughout the neck

Enlarged lymph nodes in the neck if the cancer has spread

Manifestations

Palpable nodule

May cause neck compression or impinge on laryngeal nerve if large

Detection of nodule by CT or ultrasound

Fine-needle aspiration and pathology to confirm diagnosis

Diseases of the Parathyroid Glands

Typically, there are four parathyroid glands located on the posterior superior and posterior inferior surfaces of each lobe of the thyroid gland (Figure 25–1), but their number and location are notoriously variable. The parathyroid glands are tiny, each usually weighing no more than 0.2 gram. The parathyroid epithelial cells secrete parathyroid hormone, also called parathormone or PTH, which regulates the balance of calcium and phosphorus in the body by stimulating the release of calcium from bone, increasing renal absorption of calcium, enhancing calcium absorption from the gastrointestinal tract, stimulating

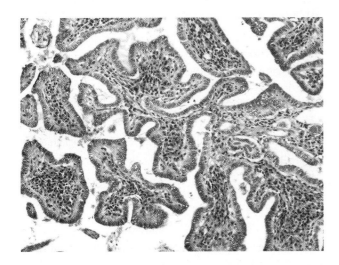

FIGURE 25–8 Papillary thyroid carcinoma.

the activation of vitamin D in the kidneys, and inhibiting renal absorption of phosphorus. It is integral to building and maintaining bone. Hypoparathyroidism is very uncommon because all four glands have to be removed or destroyed to result in complete absence of parathormone production. If it does occur, the main complications are not caused by aberrant bone mineralization, but rather by the effect of decreased calcium in the blood. Calcium is necessary for several intracellular processes, among them muscle contraction. Hypocalcemia manifests with neuromuscular irritability: **paresthesia** (a tingling sensation) around the mouth and in the fingers, muscular irritability and **tetany** (prolonged contraction of the muscle after a single stimulus), and convulsions. Treatment consists of calcium supplementation and a synthetic vitamin D derivative.

Hyperparathyroidism

Hyperparathyroidism is a relatively common disease, affecting about 100,000 people in the United States every year. The condition can be mild and go undetected for a long time. Primary hyperparathyroidism occurs when the production of parathormone by the parathyroid glands is not controlled by normal feedback mechanisms. Most cases of primary hyperparathyroidism are caused by a benign neoplasm, or adenoma, growing in a single parathyroid gland. Other causes are diffuse hyperplasia of all four glands and, rarely, a parathyroid carcinoma. Secondary hyperparathyroidism occurs with conditions associated with low serum calcium, most often chronic renal failure or vitamin D deficiency. The low serum calcium induces the parathyroid glands to crank up parathormone production. Secondary hyperparathyroidism may, if it is chronic and not controlled, degenerate to tertiary hyperparathyroidism. In this condition, the parathyroid glands produce parathormone even after serum calcium is regulated (e.g., by exogenous administration of calcium and vitamin D). Of the three types of hyperparathyroidism, primary hyperparathyroidism is by far the most common.

Regardless of the cause of the disease, excess parathyroid hormone causes increased breakdown of bone, increased absorption of calcium by the intestine, increased reabsorption of calcium by the kidney, and increased loss of phosphorus in the urine. The net effect is to increase serum calcium and decrease serum phosphate. **Hypercalcemia** is nowadays usually detected on routine bloodwork. It rarely becomes severe enough to cause symptoms, but if symptoms do develop, they are generally nonspecific: fatigue, depression, and aches. Asymptomatic hypercalcemia must be further investigated with more lab tests to establish the diagnosis because several other important diseases can present in this manner. Elevated serum PTH confirms the diagnosis of parathyroidism. To treat the patient, however, it must be determined whether the hyperparathyroidism is primary or secondary.

Before screening tests were available and patients presented with advanced disease, the classic symptom complex of hyperparathyroidism was described as "stones, bones, abdominal groans, and psychic moans." The excess calcium in the serum and excess secretion of phosphorus by the kidneys result in the precipitation of calcium into stones. As calcium and phosphorus leach from the bone, it becomes thin and prone to fracture. The vertebrae are the bones that most commonly fracture in this condition. The bone lesions are characterized by the presence of giant multinucleated osteoclasts (bone-resorbing cells) and fibrosis, sometimes with cyst formation (osteitis fibrosa cystica). "Abdominal groans" refers to abdominal pain caused by constipation, indigestion, or sometimes more severe conditions, such as acute pancreatitis. "Psychic moans" refers to diverse mental disorders including depression, memory loss, and psychosis. There are other complications as well, including heart failure and abnormal glucose metabolism. The wide range of findings underscores how essential careful regulation of serum calcium is to cell homeostasis in all the tissues of the body.

The treatment of hyperparathyroidism depends on its underlying cause. A solitary adenoma can be surgically removed. Diffuse primary hyperparathyroidism is treated by removing all parathyroid tissue and reimplanting a small amount under the skin in the forearm so that it will continue to produce the essential hormone. Secondary and tertiary hyperparathyroidism involve calcium replacement therapy in addition to treatment of the chronic renal failure or other disease that is causing low serum calcium levels.

BOX 25–7 Hyperparathyroidism

Causes

Primary (adenoma, hyperplasia, carcinoma)

Secondary (chronic renal disease, vitamin D deficiency)

Tertiary (long-standing secondary hyperparathyroidism)

Lesions

Nodule or diffuse hyperplasia of parathyroid gland(s)

Resorption of bone

Renal calculi

Manifestations

Increased serum calcium, decreased serum phosphate, increased serum PTH

Flank pain from renal calculi

Bone pain and pathologic fracture

Abdominal pain from constipation, indigestion, pancreatitis

Neuromuscular and neuropsychiatric disturbances

Heart failure

Diseases of the Adrenal Glands

The two adrenal (or suprarenal) glands are located deep within the abdomen, embedded in adipose tissue above each kidney (Figures 25–1 and **25–9**). The adrenal glands are composed of two embryologically and functionally very distinct tissues. The cortex consists of epithelial cells that synthesize and secrete **glucocorticoids, mineralocorticoids**, and **androgens**, while the neural-derived chromaffin cells of the medulla secrete hormones involved in control of the vascular system, primarily **epinephrine** (adrenaline) (**Figure 25–10**). Because the cortex produces three different hormones with three very different effects, six diseases can occur just from overproduction or underproduction of these hormones.

The most common of these is hypercortisolism, called Cushing syndrome. In addition, all three hormones can be markedly reduced if the entire adrenal cortex tissue is damaged. This occurs in Addison disease. Because most of the diseases of the adrenal cortex are very rare, only Addison disease and Cushing syndrome are discussed here. The adrenal medulla usually comes to medical attention when it develops a neoplasm.

Addison Disease

Addison disease is characterized by insufficient production of all the adrenocortical hormones as a result of destruction of adrenal cortical tissue. In the United States, the most common cause is autoimmunity, and it may occur in conjunction with autoimmune damage to other endocrine organs, such as the parathyroid glands, thyroid, and islet cells of the pancreas. Tuberculosis of the adrenal glands was formerly the most common cause. Despite the important roles of the adrenocortical hormones in maintaining electrolyte balance, controlling the immune system, and regulating sexual function, the onset of symptoms in Addison disease is gradual and the symptoms are nonspecific, so the diagnosis can be overlooked. Symptoms include fatigue, anorexia, nausea, weight loss, fainting because of hypotension or hypoglycemia, loss of body hair, and depression. In addition, the skin may take on a bronze color because decreased serum cortisol causes increased production of ACTH by the pituitary, and the precursor of ACTH is also the precursor to melanocyte-stimulating hormone. Laboratory tests show low cortisol levels and high ACTH levels, as well as electrolyte imbalances (hyperkalemia, hyponatremia). Symptoms may become acute and life threatening, with vomiting, diarrhea, weakness, and hypotension. Acute insufficiency is likely to be precipitated by stress or infection. Immediate treatment with glucocorticoids and intravenous fluids containing salt and sugar is needed. Exogenous replacement of corticosteroids, mineralocorticoids, and androgens is the mainstay of treatment for this disease.

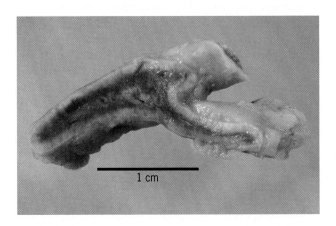

FIGURE 25–9 Gross appearance of the adrenal gland (cross section). The cortex is a thin strip of golden yellow tissue running around the circumference of the irregularly shaped gland. The medulla is the translucent gray tissue in the center of the gland.

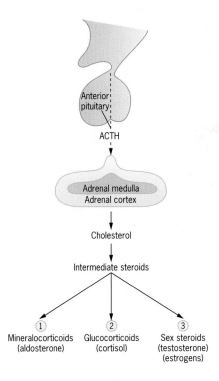

FIGURE 25–10 Derivation of the three main classes of steroids produced by the adrenal cortex. The most important or most representative of each class are in parentheses. Sex steroids are also produced by the gonads. The adrenal medulla produces epinephrine.

BOX 25–8   Addison Disease
Causes
Autoimmune destruction of the adrenal cortex
Tuberculosis
Other rare causes
Lesions
Lymphocytic infiltration and atrophy of adrenal cortex
Other manifestations depending on underlying cause—for example, granulomata with tuberculosis
Manifestations
Increased skin pigmentation
Nonspecific symptoms: fatigue, hypotension, hypoglycemia, nausea, vomiting, and others
Acute decompensation with stress

Cushing Syndrome

Cushing syndrome is the result of excess corticosteroids, predominantly glucocorticoids, regardless of whether the imbalance is caused by excessive stimulation of the adrenals by ACTH, primary overproduction by the adrenals, ectopic production of ACTH by a tumor (e.g., by small cell carcinoma of the lung), or exogenous administration of corticosteroids. The most common cause is iatrogenic, or induced by the use of corticosteroids in the treatment of other diseases.

The clinical manifestations of Cushing syndrome illustrate the wide-ranging effects of cortisol on the body's metabolism and immune system. The most obvious effect of Cushing syndrome is a peculiar "central" obesity limited to the face (**Figure 25–11**), trunk, and upper back (the so-called moon faces and buffalo hump). Cortisol induces breakdown of tissues including muscle, skin, and bone. Proximal muscle weakness, fragile skin that bruises easily and heals poorly, and osteoporosis are common. Cortisol increases circulating glucose by stimulating gluconeogenesis, but it also inhibits uptake of glucose by cells, so patients develop diabetes.

The primary reason to give cortisol as a therapeutic agent is to inhibit the body's immune system—for example, to decrease the inflammation in autoimmune disorders. The flip side of this is that the patient becomes immune suppressed and therefore develops infections easily and clears them poorly. Some patients taking cortisol develop severe mental disturbances, including depression and psychosis. Other manifestations include hypertension, hirsutism (increased body hair), and menstrual abnormalities.

Cushing syndrome usually develops slowly, and signs and symptoms may be quite subtle at first. In iatrogenic cases, the cause is evident. In other cases, laboratory tests can be used to determine whether the cause is excess cortisol production by the adrenal or excess ACTH production by the pituitary. It would appear that such serious complications would sharply curtail the use of exogenous steroid therapy. Yet, for many diseases, steroids are by far the most effective treatment and the positive effects on the patient's health outweigh the negative effects, which often can be countered or minimized by other medications.

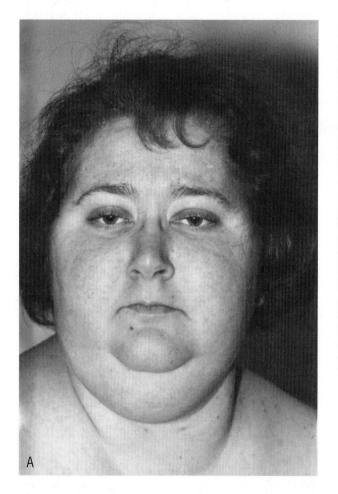
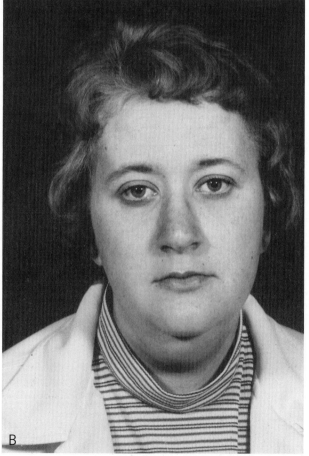

FIGURE 25–11 Cushing syndrome. **A.** Facial obesity and swelling of Cushing syndrome. The woman was discovered to have a cortisol-producing adrenal adenoma. **B.** The same woman after removal of the adenoma.

BOX 25-9 Cushing Syndrome

Causes

Iatrogenic (exogenous steroids taken therapeutically)

Increased pituitary production of ACTH

Cortisol-secreting adrenal adenoma or carcinoma

ACTH-secreting carcinoma

Lesions

Pituitary or adrenal adenoma, carcinoma

Diffuse hyperplasia of adrenal cortex (if there is excess ACTH secretion)

Atrophy of adrenal cortex (if ACTH production is suppressed by excess cortisol)

Manifestations

Obesity of face, trunk, and upper back

Easy bruising of skin, poor healing, striae

Hypertension

Hyperglycemia

Osteoporosis leading to fractures

Hirsutism

Psychosis

Muscle weakness

Adrenal Medullary Neoplasms

Neoplasms of the adrenal medulla are fortunately very rare, but they are so striking in their manifestations that they warrant special mention. **Pheochromocytoma** is a neoplasm of the chromaffin cells of the adrenal medulla that produces catecholamines in an unregulated fashion. Catecholamines—epinephrine and norepinephrine—are the primary hormones of the sympathetic nervous system, and the hormones released in the so-called "fight or flight" response. Continuously elevated catecholamines increase vascular tone and thereby cause hypertension and have direct stimulating effects on the heart, which over time can lead to heart failure. Periodic bursts of catecholamines released from these tumors give patients episodes of severe headache, flushing, sweating, palpitations, anxiety, and tremors. Measurement of a catecholamine breakdown product, vanillylmandelic acid (VMA), in the urine is helpful in diagnosis. The patient's blood pressure has to be aggressively treated prior to and during surgery because sudden release of large amounts of catecholamines during surgery can result in potentially lethal elevations in blood pressure.

The other interesting neoplasm of the adrenal medulla is **neuroblastoma**, which is one of the most common malignancies in children. This arises from neural crest cells, which normally develop into ganglion cells of the sympathetic nervous system. In neuroblastoma, the malignant cells appear "arrested" at various stages of their development: in some tumors, they are very primitive appearing, while in others, there are variable numbers of recognizable ganglion cells. The prognosis of this tumor depends on its degree of differentiation, its stage, the age of the patient (infants tend to have a longer survival than do children), and various molecular features such as chromosomal and genetic abnormalities. With adequate treatment, the 5-year survival varies from 40–80% depending on the age of the patient.

Diseases of the Pancreatic Islets of Langerhans

Myriads of small clusters, or islets, of endocrine cells that develop from pancreatic ductules are scattered throughout the pancreas. Various cell types in the islets secrete different hormones—**glucagon** (alpha cell), **insulin** (beta cell), somatostatin (delta cell), and pancreatic polypeptide (PP cell). Diabetes mellitus is the major disease related to abnormal hormone production by the islets.

Diabetes Mellitus

The effect of diabetes mellitus on diverse organs and tissues has already been discussed in different chapters of this text. Nephropathy, retinopathy, coronary artery disease, and small vessel disease causing nonhealing ulcers and blindness are the most common complications of this disease. Unfortunately, diabetes is very prevalent. An estimated 8% of the U.S. population has diabetes. Prevalence varies by age: the older the population, the more diabetic patients there are. It also varies considerably by race, so that, in comparison to the 8% overall prevalence rate, the prevalence among American Indians and blacks is 14%, and in some American Indian populations it even rises to a staggering 30%. In many of these populations, people expect to develop diabetes as a natural consequence of aging. In addition, incidence rates of diabetes have been rising alarmingly over the past two decades, in concert with the rise in obesity. Diabetes is now the seventh leading cause of death in the United States.

Diabetes mellitus is a disease in which there is a persistent state of hyperglycemia and loss of glucose homeostasis. The utilization of glucose by cells requires insulin, a hormone normally produced by the beta cells in the pancreatic islets. In diabetes, the effect of insulin on cells is diminished, either because there is a decrease in its production or because the cells are resistant to its effects. These two mechanisms of disease are the basis of distinction between the two types of diabetes mellitus: type 1 and type 2 (**Table 25–3**). In type 1 diabetes, the pancreatic islets are destroyed, so there is an absolute deficiency of insulin production. In type 2 diabetes, cells are resistant to insulin: they are not stimulated to take up glucose even though insulin is present. These two types have formerly been called by various different names. Type 1 used to be called insulin-dependent and juvenile diabetes, in contrast to non-insulin-dependent and adult-onset diabetes (type 2). It is now known that children can develop type 2 diabetes and adults can be

TABLE 25–3	Comparison of Type 1 and Type 2 Diabetes	
	Type 1	**Type 2**
Age	Usually in children or young adults	Usually after age 40, and incidence increases with age
Onset	Generally abrupt	More often insidious
	Often diagnosed after infection	Patients often obese
	Diabetic ketoacidosis	Nonketotic coma resulting from dehydration
Treatment	Insulin	Diet, exercise, oral medications; insulin may be required in severe cases
Complications	Occur early, often severe	Full range of complications may be present at diagnosis
Insulin levels	Low or absent	Frequently normal or high

diagnosed with type 1 diabetes, and patients with severe type 2 diabetes are also often insulin dependent, so it is now preferred to discuss diabetes in terms of types rather than with the other descriptors.

Both types have a multifactorial etiology involving both genetic and nongenetic factors. Neither type exhibits a Mendelian inheritance pattern, but both have a strong genetic basis. Type 1 is strongly associated with HLA haplotypes. The genes conferring increased risk in type 2 diabetes are not well worked out, but there is a concordance rate in monozygotic twins of around 50%, and it very often runs in families, while type 1 diabetes has more of a sporadic occurrence. An immunologic or viral injury has been postulated for type 1 diabetes, though again, the exact nature of the injury leading to pancreatic islet cell destruction is not known. For type 2 diabetes, diet and exercise clearly play a role in the etiology and treatment of the disease. Obesity is the strongest risk factor for the development of type 2 diabetes. The rates of obesity and diabetes have been rising in parallel, and there is strong scientific evidence that obesity induces insulin resistance. Even mildly obese people have some degree of insulin resistance, even if this is not accompanied by yet clinically detectable hyperglycemia. The obesity epidemic is now of such magnitude that even children are being diagnosed with type 2 diabetes.

Type 1 diabetes is an autoimmune disease. Lymphocytes attack antigens on the beta cells and destroy them. There is therefore an absolute deficiency in insulin production. The disease becomes clinically apparent when insulin production is diminished by at least 90%. In contrast, in type 2 diabetes the cells of the body do not respond normally to insulin, they are resistant to its effects, and, although insulin is present, glucose is not taken up by the cells but remains in circulation. In response to persistent hyperglycemia, the beta cells actually increase their insulin production. Over time, the islet cells can "burn out," resulting in insulin deficiency.

Other factors linked with diabetes are pregnancy, infections, and corticosteroid therapy. Each of these is associated with "stress" and increased circulating steroids. Steroids antagonize the effect of insulin on cells, so patients develop hyperglycemia even though insulin production is normal. Gestational diabetes, or diabetes that develops during pregnancy, usually reverses after delivery of the baby, but women who developed gestational diabetes are at greater risk of developing type 2 diabetes later in their lives.

The clinical manifestations of diabetes mellitus are initially caused by the hyperglycemia itself. Excess glucose in the filtrate of the kidney renders the filtrate hyperosmolar, so it retains water. This leads to the symptoms of polyuria and polydypsia: the patient urinates frequently and is excessively thirsty because of the diuresis induced by excess glucose molecules in the glomerular filtrate. Also, because glucose is not transported into cells, they rely on alternative sources of energy, primarily lipids. The by-products of lipid metabolism are acetoacetic acid and beta-hydroxybutyric acid. These acids are produced more rapidly than they can be cleared by peripheral tissues and the kidneys, so ketoacidosis results. The state of **diabetic ketoacidosis** is characterized by dehydration and acidosis in the setting of severe hyperglycemia. This is a medical emergency. Treatment revolves around rehydration and administration of insulin. Diabetic ketoacidosis typically develops in type 1 diabetes, but it may also develop in patients with advanced type 2 diabetes who have developed insulin insufficiency. Patients with type 2 diabetes are more likely to develop hyperosmolar nonketotic coma as a result of severe dehydration.

Glucose is utilized by every tissue in the body and is necessary for cells' optimal function. Conditions that reflect impaired glucose metabolism are generalized weakness, increased tendency to infection, and poor wound healing. Long-term complications of diabetes, regardless of type, occur as a result of persistent hyperglycemia. These usually arise about 10–20 years after the onset of diabetes, but their rate of development is variable and strongly correlated with the degree to which serum glucose is controlled by medications or insulin. Vascular injury, especially of endothelial cells, underlies these complications, but its pathogenesis is quite complex and, as yet, not entirely understood. It appears to involve a combination of inflammatory mediators, changes in extracellular matrix, and impaired ability to withstand oxidative stress. The end result is accelerated atherosclerosis in large vessels, leading to increased incidence of atherosclerotic heart disease and stroke, and narrowing of small vessels, or **microangiopathy**, with resultant impaired perfusion of tissues such as the skin, retina, and kidneys. Microangiopathy is not reversible, not even with exercise and diet. Its deleterious effects account for most of the morbidity associated with diabetes.

Most diabetics die from the effects of atherosclerosis, just as does the general population. In contrast to patients without diabetes, however, diabetics develop atherosclerosis and its complications at a younger age. Though macrovascular disease is the most common cause of death, the microangiopathy is the major cause of morbidity. Vascular complications have been discussed in detail in other chapters. Suffice it to enumerate them, from head to toe: stroke; blindness; neuropathy with effects as disparate as paresthesias, loss of pain sensation, and paralysis of the stomach and bladder; myocardial infarction; mesenteric ischemia and bowel infarction; nephropathy leading to chronic renal failure and dialysis dependence; increased susceptibility to infection and poor wound healing; sexual dysfunction; and gangrene of the toes and feet that can progress to osteomyelitis and necessitate amputation.

Type 1 diabetes is usually diagnosed when a child is noted to drink excessively and to urinate frequently, including nighttime urinations with bed wetting. Similar symptoms may bring an adult in to see the doctor, but adults are usually screened for hyperglycemia before symptoms occur. The diagnosis of diabetes mellitus is made on the basis of laboratory studies. The normal fasting plasma glucose level is less than 100 mg/dL. Any abnormal result should be followed with additional tests. **Glucose tolerance tests** assess the ability of the cells to utilize glucose. After fasting, the patient is given a standardized glucose solution to drink, and the blood glucose is measured 2 hours later. Excessive glucose indicates impaired glucose tolerance. The third test that is used is the **hemoglobin A1$_c$**. Glucose in the blood sticks to red blood cells: in medical lingo, red blood cells become glycosylated. Hemoglobin A1$_c$ is a measure of the percentage of glycosylated red blood cells. Because red blood cells live for about 120 days, hemoglobin A1$_c$ gives an impression of the average glucose level in the blood over the past 4 months. Elevated levels are indicative of a persistent hyperglycemic state.

Treatment of diabetes depends on the underlying cause. Patients with type 1 diabetes require insulin. There are many different types of insulin preparations: long-acting, short-acting, ultra-short-acting. Implantable pumps can now administer insulin without the need for additional needle sticks. Still, adequate control of blood glucose requires frequent—four or more times a day—monitoring of glucose levels, which requires both needle pricks of the finger and expensive glucose strips ($10–$30 for a 12-day supply). The first line of treatment for type 2 diabetes is weight control with diet and exercise. Even a modest decrease in weight has favorable effects on insulin resistance. Unfortunately, most patients are not able to control their disease adequately with lifestyle modifications. Medications work in various ways. Metformin, one of the most common medications used, decreases glucose production by the liver and increases peripheral glucose utilization. Sulfonylureas stimulate insulin production by the islet cells. Other medications increase insulin sensitivity or decrease the absorption of glucose in the gastrointestinal tract. A serious side effect of these medications is inadvertent induction of hypoglycemia. Adequate medical therapy helps avoid serious, severe, acute complications of hyperglycemia, ketoacidosis, and dehydration and delays the development of microangiopathy and its myriad manifestations.

Treatment additionally requires understanding the natural history of the disease and being vigilant for the development of complications. This means taking additional measures to protect the heart and kidneys (e.g., antihypertensive drugs, angiotensin-converting enzyme [ACE] inhibitors, lipid-lowering drugs), frequent monitoring of eye and kidney function, and meticulous foot care to avoid the development of diabetic ulcers.

Currently, no treatments restore insulin production or reverse insulin resistance entirely. However, newer treatment modalities are promising to offer patients more freedom from the heightened vigilance required to control blood glucose levels. Pancreas transplantation and the newer technique of islet cell transplantation reintroduce functioning islet cells in patients with absolute insulin deficiency. Drawbacks to the former technique include the need for continuous immunosuppression, the difficulty of detecting rejection of the pancreas, and limited organ donors; however, the benefit for those in whom the graft survives is tremendous. Glucose levels are normal, young women have even had successful pregnancies without requiring additional glycemic control, and vascular complications do not develop. If complications have already developed at the time of transplantation, these cannot be reversed, but they can be stabilized. Another treatment modality that is being developed involves a glucose monitor implanted under the skin that communicates with a portable insulin pump, which automatically calculates insulin requirements and delivers the appropriate dose. With this system, glucose can be monitored continuously, and insulin doses microadjusted, with a near-physiologic degree of control.

Pancreatic Neuroendocrine Tumors

Any of the cells of the islets can undergo clonal expansion, resulting in a **pancreatic neuroendocrine neoplasm**. These are very rare, accounting for only about 5% of pancreatic neoplasms. They usually come to clinical attention when a mass is noted in the pancreas on a CT scan performed for other purposes. Occasionally, they can produce one of the pancreatic hormones in an unregulated fashion, causing symptoms of hormone excess. The most common functional pancreatic neuroendocrine neoplasm is an **insulinoma**, a neoplasm of the beta cells that produce insulin. It manifests with symptoms of hypoglycemia: episodes of headache, lethargy, blurred vision, confusion, stupor, and loss of consciousness. The symptoms are relieved by eating. The behavior of pancreatic neuroendocrine tumors is difficult to predict. Surgical removal of small tumors confined to the pancreas is usually curative. Larger ones and those that have spread to the lymph nodes are more likely to recur.

Endocrine Syndromes

Multiple Endocrine Tumor Syndromes

There are at least two syndromes in which tumors of several endocrine organs occur in family members. **Multiple endocrine neoplasia 1 (MEN1)** is an autosomal dominant disease in which affected patients develop hyperplasia of the parathyroid glands and tumors of the islet cells of the pancreas and/or anterior pituitary. These are usually benign tumors that come to attention by increased hormone production. They develop in patients at a younger age than in the general population and they tend to be more aggressive; thus, affected patients tend to die young. The underlying gene defect is in a gene called *MENIN*. Its protein product, menin, is widely distributed in the body, but its function has not yet been elucidated. **Multiple endocrine neoplasia 2 (MEN2)** is characterized by the early development of medullary thyroid carcinoma. There are three variants of MEN2, characterized by the occurrence of different manifestations in conjunction with the medullary thyroid carcinoma. These include pheochromocytomas, a Marfanoid body habitus, parathyroid hyperplasia, and mucosal neuromas. All variants of MEN2 are autosomal dominant, and the gene defect involves the *RET* proto-oncogene. Screening for mutations in children in affected families can prevent the development of potentially lethal medullary thyroid carcinoma because the thyroid gland can be removed prophylactically.

Ectopic Hormone-Producing Cancers

Endocrine cells are widely distributed throughout the body in tissues that are not primarily thought of as endocrine organs. Cancers arising from these cells can produce hormones. Small cell carcinoma of the lung is the most strongly associated with ectopic hormone production, particularly antidiuretic hormone and ACTH. Hormone production may be the initial manifestation of cancer. For example, a patient may present with Cushing syndrome features, with a workup revealing a normal anterior pituitary gland and a nodule in the lung. Ectopic hormone production by a neoplasm is called a **paraneoplastic syndrome**.

Organ Failure

Failure of each of the major endocrine organs has been mentioned under hypofunction in the preceding sections. Acute failure that is life threatening occurs with lack of parathyroid hormone, adrenocorticosteroids, and insulin. Failure of the pituitary and thyroid lead to more gradual changes that are usually detected, diagnosed, and treated by administration of the deficient hormone before there are lethal consequences.

Practice Questions

1. The pituitary gland is sometimes called the master gland of the body. This is because it
   A. directly regulates growth and metabolism.
   B. is the largest endocrine gland.
   C. is under positive and negative feedback control.
   D. produces hormones that affect the rate of synthesis and release of other hormones.
   E. is located in the brain.

2. A patient has persistent hypercalcemia. This is demonstrated to result from an endocrine abnormality. The endocrine organ most likely involved is situated
   A. in the retroperitoneum.
   B. in the brain, above the optic chiasm.
   C. straddling the trachea.
   D. in the neck, on either side of the midline.
   E. in the pancreas.

3. The most common malignancy of endocrine organs is
   A. thyroid carcinoma.
   B. parathyroid carcinoma.
   C. pancreatic neuroendocrine neoplasm.
   D. paraneoplastic syndrome.
   E. pheochromocytoma.

4. Many diseases of endocrine organs come to attention by producing symptoms of excessive or deficient hormone production. It is desirable to detect such diseases before they produce symptoms, however, because the effects may not be reversible. Methods of detection include all of the following except which one?
   A. Direct physical examination of the thyroid gland
   B. Routine laboratory analysis of serum electrolytes and calcium
   C. Routine screening for fasting blood glucose levels
   D. Routine screening for cortisol and ACTH levels

5. Hashimoto thyroiditis and Addison disease are usually caused by
   A. tumors.
   B. infections.
   C. defective genes.
   D. autoimmunity.

6. Cushing syndrome can manifest with which of the following constellations of symptoms?
   A. Heart palpitations, weight loss despite increased appetite, exophthalmos
   B. Weight gain, particularly in the abdomen, face, and upper back; easy bruising and susceptibility to infection; and fractures of the vertebral bone
   C. Bone fractures, abdominal pain, and kidney stones
   D. Episodes of palpitation, sweating, tremors, and headache
   E. Polyuria, polydypsia, and dehydration

7. Which of the following malignancies occurs exclusively in children?
   A. Medullary thyroid carcinoma
   B. Papillary thyroid carcinoma
   C. Neuroblastoma
   D. Pheochromocytoma
   E. Multiple endocrine neoplasia

8. The main difference between type 1 and type 2 diabetes mellitus is that
   A. type 1 diabetes occurs primarily in children whereas type 2 diabetes does not affect children.
   B. type 1 diabetes requires insulin for treatment whereas individuals with type 2 diabetes never become insulin dependent.
   C. in type 1 diabetes islet cells are destroyed whereas in type 2 diabetes there is no change in the islets.
   D. type 1 diabetes is caused by an absolute deficiency of insulin whereas type 2 diabetes is caused by insufficiency of glucagon.
   E. type 1 diabetes is caused by an absolute insufficiency of insulin whereas type 2 diabetes is caused by decreased peripheral utilization of glucose.

Multiple Organ System Diseases

The purpose of this section is (1) to discuss groups of diseases that frequently involve more than one organ system and (2) to provide a broader overview of some of the diseases that have been encountered in the previous section. The first four chapters in this section are organized by cause or causative mechanisms (infections, immune reactions, physical injury, chemical injury). The final chapter reviews diseases caused by undernutrition and overnutrition.

Infectious Diseases

OUTLINE

Infection and the Body's Defense Mechanisms
Symptoms, Signs, and Tests
Specific Diseases
Practice Questions

OBJECTIVES

1. Name the classes of microorganisms that cause infection.
2. Describe the various ways in which microorganisms can interact with their host.
3. List the body's major defenses against infection by microorganisms.
4. List and describe different causes of immune compromise in humans.
5. Appreciate the effectiveness of public health interventions and vaccinations in decreasing the transmission and incidence of infectious diseases.
6. Discuss the local and systemic symptoms and signs of inflammation secondary to infection.
7. Recognize and describe some of the common laboratory techniques used in the diagnosis and treatment of infectious disease, and know the most effective means of definitive identification of bacterial, viral, and helminthic infections.
8. Know the definition of the terms *opportunistic infection*, *zoonotic infection*, and *emerging infectious disease*, and list examples of each.
9. Define what is meant by "pyogenic infection," and list some of the common infectious agents that cause pyogenic infections.
10. Know what an "exotoxin" is, identify some of the common diseases caused by exotoxins, and recognize how the treatment of these diseases differs from the treatment of other bacterial diseases.
11. Recognize the diseases of childhood for which immunizations are available.
12. Describe the route of transmission, pathogenetic mechanism, epidemiology, and treatment of infection by human immunodeficiency virus (HIV).
13. Define *antigenic shift*, and describe how it complicates the development of effective vaccinations against some common and serious viral infections.
14. Name some of the infectious organisms that are known to cause cancer, and identify the infections they cause in humans.
15. Compare primary and secondary systemic fungal infections in terms of common organisms causing each, condition of the respective hosts, and type of inflammatory response elicited by each.
16. Name and describe some of the more common protozoal and helminthic infections.
17. Describe what prion protein is and how it differs from the other infectious agents described in this chapter.
18. Define and be able to use in context all words and phrases in bold print throughout the chapter.

KEY TERMS

abscess	anthrax
acquired immune system	antibiotic susceptibility
AIDS	test
anaerobic bacteria	antigenic shift

bacteremia
bacteria
bacterial toxins
botulism
candidiasis
carrier
cellulitis
chickenpox
Chlamydia
cholera
commensal organism
culture
diphtheria
emerging infectious
    disease
enteric bacteria
fungus
gas gangrene
giardiasis
Gram stain
helminth
Herpes simplex viruses
human immunodeficiency
    virus (HIV)
human papilloma viruses
immunization
impetigo
indigenous flora
infection
infectious mononucleosis
inflammatory response
innate immune
    system
interferon
latent period
leprosy
Lyme disease
malaria
measles
methicillin-resistant
    Staphylococcus aureus
    (MRSA)
Mycoplasma

mycotic infection
necrotizing fasciitis
nucleic acid sequencing
opportunistic infection
parasite
pathogen
pinworm
plague
polio
primary fungal
    infection
prion protein
protozoa
pus
pyogenic bacteria
reportable infection
Rickettsia
rubella
saprophyte
schistosomiasis
secondary infection
serologic test
shingles
Staphylococcus aureus
streptococci (alpha- and
    beta-hemolytic)
structural barrier
symbiotic organism
tapeworms
tetanus
toxic shock syndrome
toxoplasmosis
trachoma
trichinosis
tularemia
undulant fever
upper respiratory tract
    infection
vaccination
vector
vertical transmission
viruses
zoonotic infection

Infection and the Body's Defense Mechanisms

Microorganisms are ubiquitous. They live in environments in which nothing else will grow, such as the deepest oceanic waters, boiling mineral springs, stratospheric dust, arctic ice, and acidic wastewaters from mineral mines. The total biomass of bacteria on earth is estimated to be equal to that of plants. Unwittingly, we live in very close relation to millions of different types of microorganisms from birth on—in the air we breathe, the water we drink, and the food we eat. Our entire body is a biome: more than 1,400 different types of bacteria live in our belly buttons alone, and the number of bacteria in the gut is 10 times the number of total cells in the body! Our mouths, skin, and respiratory, reproductive, and digestive tracts not only harbor microorganisms, but many essential human functions, such as digestion and

absorption, actually depend on them. Given the number of microorganisms we are continuously and directly in contact with, the number that actually cause disease is ridiculously small—although for the student first exposed to them in an introductory text, the list seems very large, indeed. Microorganisms that cause diseases in humans fall into several classes of small, predominantly single-cell organisms: bacteria, fungi, protozoa, viruses, and multicellular helminths (parasitic worms). Prions are another type of infectious agent, unusual in that they do not consist of living organisms but rather comprise misfolded proteins that can induce disease.

This introductory section is broken into three parts. In the first, the various ways in which microbes interact with their hosts is discussed. In the second, the mammalian host's mechanisms of defense against invasive organisms or infectious agents are briefly described. In the third, a very brief overview of the most prevalent diseases, in the United States and worldwide, is presented. After this background, we present infectious diseases grouped by the type of organism or infectious agent that causes them. This discussion is not meant to be comprehensive. Only those microorganisms that cause widespread disease or are illustrative of certain pathogenic properties are mentioned. Also, some specific infections or infectious organisms, such as tuberculosis, viral hepatitis, and *Helicobacter pylori*, are discussed in detail in organ-specific chapters, so they are not included here.

Microbe–Host Interactions

The organisms that live in or on a host (such as a human) are called **indigenous flora**. Indigenous organisms can further be described as **commensal**, meaning they simply live in or on the host without doing harm but also not necessarily contributing to the host's well-being, or **symbiotic**, meaning they contribute to the host's health while deriving protection, nutrition, or some other benefit from the host. The human skin and mouth contain millions of commensal organisms, and the human gut contains several symbiotic ones that perform essential digestive functions that the cells of the gastrointestinal tract cannot do, such as break down complex sugars. Some microorganisms, especially bacteria, specialize in biodegrading organic material, such as dead plants and animals. Such microorganisms are called **saprophytes**.

When microorganisms cause disease by elaborating a toxin or gaining entrance to host tissue, they are called **pathogens**. Any disease directly caused by pathogens is an **infection**. The word "infection" also is used to describe the process of organisms gaining entry to the body regardless of whether disease becomes manifest. In this chapter, "infection" will be used synonymously with "infectious disease."

Microorganisms can have different interactions with their hosts, depending on circumstances. For example, *Clostridium perfringens* is an indigenous member of the colonic flora. After death of the host animal, it becomes a saprophyte and participates in the postmortem degradation of tissues. *C. perfringens* may become a pathogen in a live host either by releasing potent toxins or by invading necrotic tissue.

Certain microorganisms can survive for a long period within the host without causing overt signs of infection. This period in which the organism is present in the host but the host does not show signs of infection is called the **latent period**. *Herpes simplex* virus lies latent in nerve ganglia until it is stimulated to reactivate, when it causes painful cold sores on the lips. Another example is the protozoan *Plasmodium*, which lies in an inactive form in liver cells and is periodically shed into the blood to cause the symptoms of malaria. People who harbor a latent infection are **carriers** of the disease, whether or not they are symptomatic. → Typhoid

Many members of the indigenous flora can become pathogenic when the host's immune system is breached—for example, when the skin commensal organism *Staphylococcus aureus* gains entry into a wound to cause a wound infection. Most infectious agents, however, require some method of spreading from person to person, or **vector**, to survive. Routes of spread include the six "Fs": contaminated *food* and water, dirty *fingers*, *fecal* contamination, the bite of *flies* or other insects, transmission of body *fluids*, either directly through sexual contact or indirectly via aerosolized droplets (coughing, sneezing), and *fomites*, inanimate objects such as blankets or handkerchiefs that are impregnated with the infectious organism. Specific pathogens usually require a specific vector for transmission. For example, malaria is spread via the bite of a particular species of mosquito: it cannot be transmitted via coughing or contact with contaminated feces. Cholera, in contrast, is transmitted via fecally contaminated water and does not require an insect vector.

Pathogens usually show a predilection for infecting specific tissue types. For example, some species of the bacteria *Neisseria* live on mucous membranes in the genital tract, whereas other preferentially infect the meninges.

A **parasite** is an infectious agent that requires the host to perform some essential function for it. The most obvious parasites are helminths, such as schistosomes, which derive their nutrition by helping themselves to meals of their host's blood. Viruses are parasitic because they cannot replicate on their own: they require the hosts' replicative machinery to transcribe their genetic material and create proteins from it. Some bacteria, such as *Chlamydia*, are intracellular parasites: they cannot reproduce outside the haven of the infected cell.

The Body's Defense Mechanisms

The most obvious protection against invasion by foreign organisms is the presence of **structural barriers** between the host and the environment, such as the skin and mucous membranes of the gastrointestinal tract and lungs. When these are intact, which they are most of the time, tight junctions between the cells, inhospitable secretions, thick layers of mucus, and the presence of indigenous flora prevent extraneous pathogens from gaining entry. To pass through these barriers, potentially infectious organisms have to either (1) make use of transient breaches in the barrier (e.g., the virus causing HIV/AIDS gets through tiny tears in mucous membranes during sexual intercourse), (2) have mechanisms by which they can withstand harsh environments (e.g., the bacterium causing gastritis can live in the acidic mucus of the stomach), or (3) be able to actively penetrate the barrier (e.g., the parasite causing schistosomiasis burrows through the skin to gain entry into the host's bloodstream).

The second major line of defense is the **inflammatory response**, which protects against microorganisms that have penetrated structural barriers. The inflammatory response is a stereotypical response that is provoked by any injury or foreign substance that damages tissue or is recognized as intrusive. Structural barriers and the inflammatory response are part of the **innate immune system**.

The third major line of defense, the **acquired immune system**, requires previous or prolonged exposure to the offending agent and enhances the effectiveness of the inflammatory process. The immune defense mechanism consists of two distinctive systems: the *humoral system*, in which antibodies in the blood recognize specific, foreign substrates in the body and prime the inflammatory system to attack these, and the *cellular immune system*, in which the defense reaction is mediated by lymphocytes.

When the immune system is weakened or deficient, the host becomes susceptible to infections by organisms that usually do not cause disease. These so-called **opportunistic infections** can be caused by fungi, bacteria, viruses, or parasites. Numerous conditions or diseases may weaken the immune system. Many of these are actually caused by medical interventions: aggressive antibiotic therapy alters the indigenous flora, allowing overgrowth of pathogenic organisms; bone marrow transplant for leukemia or lymphoma causes profound neutropenia; chemotherapy for cancer suppresses the ability of the bone marrow to produce white blood cells; organ transplant recipients have pharmacologically induced depression of the immune system to prevent rejection of the transplanted organ; and treatment with steroids (e.g., for autoimmune diseases) interferes with optimal functioning of the immune system. In addition, pregnancy and underlying diseases, such as diabetes or concurrent infections, alter or weaken the immune system, as do malnutrition and fatigue. Developing fetuses do not have a functioning immune system, but fetuses and newborns are protected against infectious diseases by maternal antibodies before and after birth until about the age of 18 months. Children do not develop a robust immune system until approximately 2 years of age. Fetuses, newborns, and infants are therefore vulnerable to development of severe infections. Some familial diseases induce a profound immunocompromised state because of a genetic inability to produce proteins or enzymes critical to the function of the inflammatory or immune systems. Opportunistic infections are therefore important concerns in the general population, not just in those persons with HIV/AIDS.

A list of organisms that commonly cause opportunistic infections in humans is given later in this chapter in **Table 26–7**. The number of opportunistic infections has increased in the past several decades because the powerful drugs used to prevent organ rejection or to treat cancer commonly suppress bone marrow and the immune system, thereby decreasing the patient's ability to produce white blood cells and antibodies. Immunocompromised patients, such as those with advanced cancer or AIDS, often succumb to opportunistic infections.

Antibodies are highly effective in neutralizing certain bacterial toxins such as tetanus toxin and diphtheria toxin, in enhancing phagocytosis of bacteria, and in preventing dissemination of certain viruses such as rabies virus and polio virus. Immune sera—sera that are loaded with premade antibodies against a specific foreign invader—are available for selected diseases when conditions warrant their use. For example, antirabies serum can be administered after a non-immunized person has been bitten by a rabid animal. The production of antibodies by the immune system can be induced by **immunization**, also called **vaccination**, which primes the immune system to recognize particular foreign antigens and immediately produce antibodies to them in case of reexposure. Immunization protects against many infectious diseases of childhood, sexually transmitted diseases, and certain infectious diseases that are more common in vulnerable populations, such as veterinarians (e.g., rabies) and human healthcare workers (e.g., hepatitis B virus). Immunization of infants has dramatically decreased the incidence and thereby the morbidity and mortality of infectious diseases of childhood, such as whooping cough, diphtheria, and measles. Smallpox has remarkably been eliminated by a worldwide immunization initiative. As effective as they are, massive immunization campaigns are difficult to coordinate and administer on a worldwide scale: this is why only one disease has ever been completely eradicated, even though vaccinations against so many are available.

The most effective means of preventing infectious disease is by avoiding exposure to pathogens. Public health efforts revolving around sanitation, such as preventing human and animal wastes from getting into the water supply, have been instrumental in reducing the transmission of waterborne diseases, such as cholera, hepatitis A, and viral gastroenteritis. Improving living conditions, particularly the overcrowding of the urban poor and incarcerated individuals, reduces the transmission of airborne pathogens, such as tuberculosis. Simple technological interventions, such as putting mosquito netting around beds and draining stagnant waters, reduces the transmission of many insect-borne diseases, such as malaria. The use of condoms is the most effective way of preventing transmission of venereal diseases, including HIV/AIDS, during sexual intercourse. And the simple ritual of hand washing before touching a patient is the most effective—and unfortunately all too often ignored—means of reducing transmission of microorganisms in the healthcare setting. Despite the remarkable advances made in the pharmaceutical treatment of infectious diseases, and given the often severe morbidity, if not mortality, that can be caused by them, "an ounce of prevention is worth a pound of cure" is still the best adage for managing infectious diseases.

Most Frequent and Serious Infectious Diseases

Most infectious diseases are acute, meaning of sudden onset and short duration. Very few chronic illnesses are due to infection—the notable exceptions being tuberculosis, syphilis, HIV/AIDS, and helminth infestations. Respiratory infections, including upper respiratory infections, pneumonia, and bronchitis, account for more than 80% of acute infections. Most of these diseases are either treated at home, with rest and fluids, or on an outpatient basis, with antibiotics. Because most of these infections are self-limited or easily treated, they are not of much concern to public health authorities. In contrast, infectious diseases that are associated with significant morbidity or even mortality do need to be reported to state or federal public health authorities. **Table 26–1** shows the relative frequency of **reportable infections** in the United States.

Of the reportable infections, chlamydia is by far the most common. In fact, sexually transmitted diseases in general are the most common reportable infectious diseases in the United States: there are more than 1.7 million new cases of chlamydia, gonorrhea, and syphilis in this country every year. This count does not include cases of human papillomavirus (HPV), which is the cause of genital warts and cervical cancer; *Herpes simplex* virus (HSV), the cause of genital herpes; or other potentially sexually transmitted diseases such as hepatitis B and C. HPV and HSV infections do not need to be reported, and there are modes of transmission of HBV and HCV other than sexual, so they are not counted as "sexually transmitted."

Worldwide, infectious diseases count among the top 10 leading causes of death. These conditions include diarrheal diseases of infancy (caused by microorganisms in contaminated food and water), HIV/AIDS, tuberculosis, lower respiratory infections (pneumonia), and malaria.

TABLE 26-1	Number of New Cases of Reportable Infectious Diseases in the United States

Disease	Number of Cases
Chlamydia	1,412,791
Gonorrhea	321,849
Salmonellosis	51,887
Syphilis, all stages	46,042
HIV diagnoses	35,266
Lyme disease	33,097
Pertussis (whooping cough)	18,719
Streptococcus pneumoniae, invasive	17,138
Giardiasis	16,747
Shigellosis	13,352
Tuberculosis	10,528
Cryptosporidiosis	9,250
Rocky Mountain spotted fever	2,802
Malaria	1,724
Hepatitis A	1,398
Meningococcal disease	759
Mumps	404
Typhoid fever	390
Measles (rubeola)	220
Toxic shock syndrome	168
Botulism	153
Brucellosis	79
Hansen disease (leprosy)	82
Cholera	40
Tetanus	36
Trichinosis	15
Rabies, human	6
Plague	3
Psittacosis	2

Data from *Morbidity and Mortality Weekly Report.* Centers for Disease Control and Prevention. Public Health Service, Vol. 60, No. 53, July 5, 2013.

Most of these deaths could be prevented through public health interventions, including sanitation, clean drinking water, improvement of living conditions in urban slums, greater use of condoms, and prevention of the transmission of mosquito-borne diseases.

In the United States, "influenza and pneumonia" are the only infectious diseases that make the list of top 10 causes of death: they are in position nine. Influenza is a viral disease caused by any of numerous strains of viruses, and pneumonia is caused by several different types of infectious agents, mostly bacteria. Both of these diseases tend to disproportionately affect the very young or elderly, especially the elderly who are debilitated due to some other disease, such as dementia or cancer. Influenza can be deadly all on its own, but lethal pneumonia is typically a secondary process in a patient who is ill for some other reason.

Increasingly, it is recognized that some infectious diseases are implicated in the development of neoplasia. For example, infection with the bacterium *Helicobacter pylori*, the causative agent of gastritis, is very closely correlated with the development of gastric lymphoma, as well as gastric adenocarcinoma. Human papillomavirus is the causative agent of cervical cancer. Infection with certain parasites that colonize the bile ductular system predisposes patients to the development of cholangiocarcinoma, which is quite prevalent in parts of Asia. New correlations between infectious agents and neoplasms are continually coming to light through biomedical research. The exact pathophysiologic mechanism involved in the development of cancer in the setting of infectious diseases has not been worked out, but it is clear that infectious organisms have a greater impact on health than we had once thought.

Symptoms, Signs, and Tests

Infectious diseases rarely have distinctive clinical presentations. Most present as nonspecific syndromes, characterized by fever, rapid pulse, muscle aches, and a feeling of tiredness and ill health, or *malaise*. Because infectious diseases elicit an inflammatory response, they are accompanied by the cardinal signs of inflammation—heat, redness, swelling, and pain—at the site of infection. Physical examination may be sufficient for diagnosis. For example, the rash of measles or chickenpox is distinctive, as is the parotid swelling of mumps. Abnormal excretions or secretions, such as diarrhea or rhinitis (nasal discharge), indicate the site of infection, as does the location and quality of pain. For example, a gnawing or burning pain in the upper abdomen that persists for many weeks could be due to infection by *H. pylori*, while sharp, severe abdominal pain in the right lower quadrant that is accompanied by anorexia is likely due to appendicitis.

The most common tests that are used to identify a disease as infectious are not specific. Measurement of body temperature detects fever, which occurs with most bacterial, viral, and rickettsial infections, but rarely also with noninfectious diseases. Elevated white blood cells counts usually accompany infectious diseases: elevated neutrophils with bacterial diseases, elevated lymphocytes with some viral diseases, and elevated eosinophils with parasitic diseases. The presence of fever in association with elevated white blood cell counts is highly suggestive of an infectious disease and needs to be followed up with more specific laboratory tests.

Microscopic examination of blood or tissue smears with or without staining is of diagnostic value. **Gram stains** of bacterial preparations are used to identify gram-positive (blue-staining) and gram-negative (red-staining) bacteria and to subdivide them into *coccal* (round) and *bacillary* (elongated) forms. This information is often sufficient to start antibiotic treatment while results of culture, genetic testing, and susceptibility testing are pending. Smears without Gram stain are also generally useful in identifying the larger, more varied types of organisms, including fungi, protozoa, and eggs of helminths.

Direct **culture** of organisms from a lesion or **nucleic acid sequencing** by polymerase chain reaction are the most definitive tests. Culture is most commonly used for bacteria, and it is also the method of choice for diagnosis of many fungal diseases. Recently, considerable progress has been made in developing rapid and highly accurate tests for microorganisms, especially viruses, which rely on detection of specific RNA or DNA sequences. Indeed, molecular testing is replacing culture for the detection of viruses. Helminths and most protozoa are not cultured, but rather are identified by direct microscopic examination. Most specimens for bacterial cultures are taken from the throat, urine, sputum, and purulent lesions. When indicated, blood and spinal fluid cultures may be taken to look for infection involving the blood and meninges, respectively.

Pathogens isolated in culture can be tested for their **susceptibility** to selected antibiotics so that the most appropriate therapy can be administered. This is done by culturing bacteria on special agar plates that are impregnated with different concentrations of antibiotics (**Figure 26–1**). The areas in which the bacteria fail to grow identify antibiotics and antibiotic concentrations that will most likely inhibit their growth in the patient from which they were isolated, while the areas in which bacterial colonies do form contain antibiotics that are not effective against them.

In some instances, specific antibodies can be used to detect organisms in samples obtained by swabbing or scraping a lesion. For example, antibodies to group A streptococci attached to latex particles can be mixed with material from a throat swab: agglutination of the particles is interpreted as streptococcal pharyngitis. This is a very rapid and useful test to determine whether a patient with a sore throat should be treated with penicillin. Another technique involves the use of fluorescent-tagged antibodies mixed with a tissue sample and examined under a fluorescent microscope. This technique can be used for rapid diagnosis of *Herpes simplex* type 1 and 2 infections, *Legionella* pneumonia, and urethritis due to *Chlamydia*.

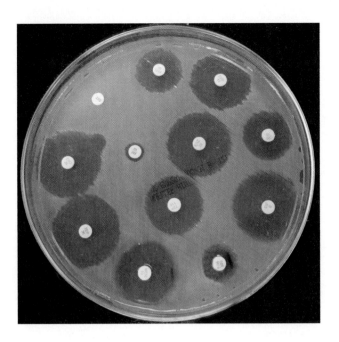

FIGURE 26–1 Antibiotic susceptibility test. Discs impregnated with different antibiotics are placed on an agar plate on which bacteria are incubated. A clear space around a disc means that particular antibiotic exerts a growth-inhibitory effect on the bacteria.

Immunologic reactivity of the host to an infection can be evaluated by measurement of serum antibodies or by skin testing to assess cellular immunity. In either case, the positive result simply indicates previous exposure to the organism; it may not mean active disease is present. Furthermore, antibodies or skin reactivity may not be present in early stages of a disease. Tests for antibodies in the patient's serum are called **serologic tests**. Serology is commonly employed for the diagnosis of syphilis, systemic fungal disease, and several other bacterial, viral, and parasitic diseases. Skin tests are most commonly employed as a screening test for tuberculosis.

Specific Diseases
Bacterial Infections

Bacteria are unicellular microbial agents that contain DNA and all the subcellular mechanisms required to live and reproduce, including the ability to synthesize energy and protein and the ability to protect themselves from the environment. As already mentioned, humans harbor millions of bacteria on the skin, in the oral and nasal cavities, the anterior urethra, the genital tract, and throughout the intestinal tract. These constitute the body's indigenous flora. Bacteria cause disease when they grow in abnormal locations or in abnormal numbers. The host tissues' homeostatic mechanisms need to be disrupted before the bacteria can gain entry to abnormal locations or overgrow their usual location. For example, broad-spectrum antibiotics (antibiotics that are effective against a wide variety of bacteria) severely disrupt the indigenous flora of the gut by eradicating a large number of the bacteria that live there. This diminishes the growth inhibitory effects of the indigenous flora on the intestinal bacterium *Clostridium difficile*, which can overgrow the gut and cause potentially lethal destruction of the mucous membrane of the colon. Bacteria can also populate and overgrow accumulated secretions when body passageways are blocked. Common **secondary infections** include abscesses, pneumonia, and wound infections. **Table 26–2** lists common sites of obstruction and the resulting types of infection.

The presence of dead tissue is another potent factor predisposing the patient to develop secondary bacterial infection. Dead tissue is a growth medium for bacteria and lacks a blood supply that would bring in phagocytes and antibodies to clear the offending organism. Diabetic foot ulcers, which consist of tissue that has become necrotic because of poor blood supply, are a common site of bacterial infection. Open wounds, such as burn wounds, readily become infected if the tissue is not routinely debrided, kept sterile, and protected against environmental contamination.

Defective mechanical barriers in the lungs, intestine, nasal sinuses, genitourinary tract, and skin may allow bacteria access to the body's tissues. Bacteria can remain localized at the site of entry, or they can gain access to the circulation and disseminate throughout the body. An example of a localized infection is an **abscess**, a collection of dead tissue, phagocytes, and bacteria that is walled off first by fibrin and then fibrous tissue. When bacteria gain entry into the bloodstream, a condition called **bacteremia**, they can travel to other tissues and infect these as well. For example, clumps of bacteria initially infecting heart valves can break off into the bloodstream and be carried to the kidneys, spleen, liver, and other organs, where the bacteria establish new foci of infection. Bacteremia is a serious complication of infectious disease and must be treated aggressively to prevent the development of septic shock.

Bacteria interact with the host's inflammatory and immune systems in many different ways. Some bacteria have a very thick wall that prevents their destruction by phagocytosis (e.g., *Mycobacterium tuberculosis*, the causative agent of tuberculosis). Some have short hair-like processes that allow them to attach very securely to host tissues (e.g., *Escherichia coli*, the most common causative agent of urinary tract infection). Some bacteria produce enzymes that enable them to dissolve interstitial tissue, so they are able to spread rapidly through tissues (e.g., staphylococci). Other bacteria are not harmful in and of themselves, but produce **toxins** that have harmful effects. For example, *Clostridium botulinum*, which can contaminate foods that are improperly canned, produces a toxin that paralyzes nerve synapses, called botulinum toxin. Ingestion of the toxin is what causes the deadly disease known as **botulism**. Administration of antibiotics alone is not sufficient to treat the disease: even in the absence of the bacterium, the circulating toxin can exert its lethal effect on nerve synapses.

The discussion of bacteria in the ensuing pages does not reflect a unifying taxonomy, but is practical, in that the categories are useful for grouping bacteria that have similar effects (e.g., "pyogenic bacteria"), affect similar organs (e.g., "sexually transmitted diseases"), or are similarly transmitted (e.g., "zoonotic diseases"). **Pyogenic bacteria** are those that produce an exuberant acute inflammatory reaction that results in the production of **pus**, or a collection of dead tissue, bacteria and phagocytes. **Anaerobic bacteria** are those that do not require oxygen for growth and, therefore, are not detected by routine culture media. **Zoonotic infections** are ones that are acquired from an animal host.

Pyogenic Bacterial Infections

Staphylococcal Infections

The genus *Staphylococcus* constitutes a large variety of gram-positive, round bacteria (cocci) that elicit an inflammatory reaction productive of copious amounts of pus. Staphylococcal species can cause a wide variety of infectious manifestations, including **impetigo** (a superficial infection of the skin), skin abscesses (called *furuncles* and *carbuncles*), pneumonia, food poisoning, and endocarditis. Most skin abscesses are caused by staphylococci. Of the several varieties of staphylococci, the most virulent is **Staphylococcus aureus**. *S. aureus* is a member of the indigenous flora of the respiratory tract and skin. It can enter the body by any route and infect any organ, but it has a particular propensity to cause skin and deep soft-tissue abscesses.

In the past, *S. aureus* infection was easy to treat with standard antibiotic therapy. In recent decades, however, a strain of *S. aureus* has emerged that is resistant to therapy with penicillin, methicillin, and other antibiotics. This strain is called **methicillin-resistant S. aureus (MRSA)**. Infection with MRSA can produce

TABLE 26–2 **Sites of Obstructions and Associated Infections**

Site of Obstruction	Type of Infection
Sebaceous gland	Furuncle and acne
Eustachian tube	Otitis media
Nasal sinus openings	Sinusitis
Bronchus	Pneumonia
Urethra	Cystitis
Ureter	Pyelonephritis
Bile ducts	Cholangitis
Appendix (fecalith)	Acute appendicitis

very severe, systemic infections that are difficult to treat, because the bacterium is so resistant to antibiotics. MRSA has become such a problem in hospitals that special precautions must be taken to prevent its transmission. Usually, MRSA is not more virulent than regular *S. aureus*, but because it is so difficult to treat, infection can spread rapidly and lead to severe tissue destruction and death. MRSA may be introduced to hospitalized patients via urinary catheters, IV catheters, and surgical wounds, and it can cause surgical wound infections, urinary tract infections, pneumonia, and bloodstream infections. Debilitated patients are at greater risk of developing the infection. In the community setting, MRSA most commonly causes a skin infection that initially resembles a boil, but can rapidly progress to widespread tissue destruction, a condition called **necrotizing fasciitis**. In the late 1970s, there was a nationwide outbreak of a severe illness affecting women using a hyperabsorbent tampon. The illness was called **toxic shock syndrome** and was traced to a strain of *S. aureus* that produced a powerful exotoxin that was absorbed through the vaginal wall, resulting in shock. That type of tampon was taken off the market, but toxic shock syndrome still occurs on rare occasions. It is treated by removal of the source of the infection, fluid replacement, and antibiotic therapy.

Streptococcal Infections

Unlike the group of staphylococci, of which there is one main pathogen of humans, the genus *Streptococcus* consists of numerous species that can cause infections in humans. Streptococci are commensal organisms in humans, inhabiting the skin, mouth, upper respiratory tract, and intestine. They are classified according to their ability to cause changes in red blood cells in agar. **Alpha-hemolytic streptococci** cause oxidation of iron in the red blood cells, turning the agar green. *Streptococcus pneumoniae*, also called *Pneumococcus*, and *viridans* streptococci are members of this group. **Beta-hemolytic streptococci** cause complete destruction of the red blood cells in agar. The streptococci of the beta-hemolytic group are further classified according to carbohydrates on their cell walls. Of these, group A and group B beta-hemolytic streptococci are the most important. All streptococcal infections must be treated early with antibiotics and surgical debridement (if there is extensive tissue destruction) to prevent bacteremia, sepsis, and death.

Alpha-Hemolytic Streptococci

Streptococcus pneumoniae (*Pneumococcus*) is a member of the indigenous nasopharyngeal flora and is the most common cause of pneumonia, otitis media, and meningitis. In the past *Pneumococcus* was highly susceptible to penicillin and related antibiotics, but there has been a marked increase in infections involving antibiotic-resistant strains in recent years, resulting in a major change in the

management of pneumococcal diseases. A vaccine against *Pneumococcus* is available and highly recommended for children, the elderly, immunocompromised individuals, and patients who do not have a spleen (the spleen cleans blood of bacteria and destroys these organisms before they can disseminate through the body). *Viridans* streptococci are part of the indigenous flora of the mouth and are the most common cause of dental caries. These organisms occasionally get into the bloodstream, usually during dental work, from whence they can colonize

---

BOX 26–1   Staphylococcal Infections

Cause

Staphylococcus aureus

MRSA

S. aureus toxin

Lesions

Abscesses (furuncles, carbuncles)

Pneumonia

Endocarditis

Necrotizing fasciitis

Septicemia

Bacterial overgrowth on tampon

Enteritis

Manifestations

Redness, swelling, heat, pain

Fever

Leukocytosis

Purulent drainage

Toxic shock syndrome

Food poisoning

BOX 26–2   Alpha-Hemolytic Streptococcal Infections

Cause

Streptococcus pneumoniae (*Pneumococcus*)

Viridans streptococci

Lesions

Pneumonia, otitis media, sinusitis (rarely: endocarditis, meningitis)

Dental caries, endocarditis superimposed on damaged heart valves

Manifestations

Heat, redness, swelling, pain at site of infection

Fever

Leukocytosis

Positive blood culture

Secondary effects, such as heart murmur (destruction of cardiac valves in endocarditis)

damaged heart valves and slowly destroy them. Patients undergoing dental treatment must be asked whether they are aware of having heart valve disease because routine administration of antibiotics prior to dental manipulation effectively prevents infection of the heart valves.

Beta-Hemolytic Streptococci

Group A beta-hemolytic streptococci can cause a wide variety of infectious diseases, either by direct effects of the bacteria themselves, by expression of an exotoxin, or by delayed, immunologic mechanisms. The most common group A beta-hemolytic strain is *Streptococcus pyogenes*. This organism can spread rapidly through tissues and through lymphatic vessels. Acute pharyngitis (strep throat) is the most common disease caused by group A streptococci. *Scarlet fever* is an uncommon systemic streptococcal infection so named because the effect of one of the bacteria's toxins on blood vessels is to produce a scarlet rash. Group A streptococci can also cause impetigo, cellulitis (an infection of soft tissue), and necrotizing fasciitis. Immunologically mediated sequelae that do not become evident until weeks after the initial infection has subsided include rheumatic fever and poststreptococcal glomerulonephritis. Some strains of group A beta-hemolytic streptococcus can cause life-threatening invasive infections by elaborating an exotoxin. Symptoms include bacteremia, severe soft-tissue damage, and shock (streptococcal toxic shock syndrome).

Group B beta-hemolytic streptococci are part of the indigenous flora of the rectum and vagina and, less commonly, the throat. They can infect the fetus *in utero* or during birth and cause pneumonia, sepsis, or meningitis in the baby. For prevention of this potentially devastating infection, women are screened for rectal and vaginal colonization in the third trimester of pregnancy and, if positive, treated with antibiotics when labor begins. Group B beta-hemolytic streptococci can also cause skin infections and sepsis, particularly in the elderly.

Gram-Negative Rods

Gram-negative bacilli, or rod-shaped bacteria, constitute the majority of bacteria in the gut. These enteric bacteria include species of *Escherichia* (e.g., *E. coli*), *Klebsiella*, *Enterobacter*, *Serratia*, and *Proteus*. Some closely related organisms (*Pseudomonas*, *Salmonella*, *Shigella*, and *Yersinia*) are not universally present, so persons harboring them either have active infection or are carriers. Different strains of *E. coli* are found in virtually everyone's intestinal tract, while only a small percentage of people will harbor one or more types of the other organisms. Many enteric bacteria can produce disease only if they invade body tissues, and all are especially pathogenic in debilitated patients. A specific strain of *E. coli* is a common cause of meningitis in newborns. *Pseudomonas aeruginosa*, found in soil and water, commonly contaminates wounds and is characteristically associated with green pus. *Pseudomonas* and *Klebsiella* also cause severe necrotizing pneumonia. *Pseudomonas* is an increasingly common cause of hospital-acquired infections. Patients with bacteremia from gram-negative enteric organisms often lapse into severe shock, which is elicited by toxin in the bacterial cell wall. This type of shock is referred to as "endotoxic" or "gram-negative" shock and has a 30% to 50% mortality rate.

BOX 26–3   Beta-Hemolytic Streptococcal Infections

Cause

Group A streptococci (*S. pyogenes*)

Group A strep toxin

Group B streptococci

Lesions

Acute pharyngitis (strep throat), scarlet fever, impetigo, cellulitis, necrotizing fasciitis

Streptococcal toxic shock syndrome

Pneumonia, meningitis, sepsis of newborn

Manifestations

Heat, redness, swelling, pain at site of infection

Fever

Leukocytosis

Rapid destruction of soft tissues (necrotizing fasciitis)

Toxic shock

Remote, immunologically mediated (group A strep): rheumatic fever, glomerulonephritis

---

BOX 26–4   Gram-Negative Enteric Bacterial Infections

Cause

Escherichia

Klebsiella

Pseudomonas

Enterobacter

Others (*Shigella*, *Salmonella*, *Yersinia*)

Lesions

Enteric infection

Wound infection

Peritonitis

Necrotizing pneumonia (*Pseudomonas*, *Klebsiella*)

Meningitis in newborns (*E. coli*)

Abscess

Manifestations

Heat, redness, swelling, pain at site of infection

Diarrhea

Fever

Leukocytosis

Endotoxic (gram-negative) shock

Other Important Pyogenic Bacterial Infections

Neisseria meningitidis, a small, gram-negative, intracellular diplococcus (double sphere), causes endemic and epidemic meningitis, especially in adolescents and young adults. About 10% of people harbor this bacterium in the throat, and it is transmitted via saliva—in other words, through kissing or other close contact. The disease usually starts with pharyngitis and fever, like any other kind of upper respiratory illness, and then progresses to photophobia (sensitivity to light), a stiff neck, and altered mental status. Myocarditis and disseminated intravascular coagulation are more rare but serious complications. Untreated, the infection can rapidly progress and cause increasing central nervous system impairment as the meninges swell secondary to the inflammation. The bacteria can gain access to the bloodstream, causing bacteremia or septicemia, and produce a toxin that impairs the ability of the heart to circulate blood. If the patient does not die, s/he is likely to develop hearing loss or brain damage. A vaccine is available against meningococcal meningitis. It is typically given to children just before they become teenagers, and a booster shot given a few years later. As college students are among the susceptible population, they should all be vaccinated against *N. meningitides*.

Legionella pneumophila is a gram-negative bacterium that lives in water reservoirs and cooling units for air conditioners. It was discovered when it caused a severe epidemic of pneumonia at an American Legion convention in Philadelphia in 1976—hence the names *Legionella* and "Legionnaire's disease." The lesions are mainly confined to the lung and occur only when large numbers of organisms are inhaled. The disease is more common in summer and can be acquired in the community or in the hospital. It is easily treated with antibiotics.

Bacterial Infections Mediated by Exotoxins

There are two types of toxins released by bacteria: exotoxins are proteins produced by bacteria, and endotoxins are proteins within bacterial cell walls that are released during the infectious process. The most well-known effect of an endotoxin is "endotoxic shock," which occurs with infection by gram-negative (usually enteric) bacteria. In this section, the effects of exotoxins are discussed (see **Table 26–3**).

Bacteria of the genus *Clostridium* are notorious for producing exotoxins. *C. tetani* is found in soil and, because it is anaerobic, can grow deep in necrotic tissue—for example, in wounds that are contaminated by soil and not debrided of dead tissue. The toxin produced by *C. tetani* diffuses throughout the body and stimulates the nerve–muscle junction, causing painful contraction of skeletal muscles. This condition is called **tetanus**, or, informally, "lockjaw." Death is caused by paralysis of the muscles of respiration. The organisms themselves are confined to the wound, so debridement of necrotic tissue helps prevent the development of tetanus. Furthermore, tetanus can be prevented by an inoculation of tetanus toxoid to stimulate antibody production against the toxin. Every person should be immunized against tetanus in childhood and receive booster immunizations every 10 years.

Clostridium botulinum, the cause of botulism, secretes a powerful exotoxin that paralyzes the body's muscles by blocking the nerve–muscle junction, leading to rapid death from respiratory failure. *C. botulinum* proliferates and produces toxin in improperly canned vegetables and meats. Adequate sterilization of canned foods prevents the disease.

Several types of clostridial organisms cause **gas gangrene**, the most common being *C. perfringens*. *C. perfringens* lives in the soil and gastrointestinal tract

TABLE 26–3 Selected Exotoxin-Producing Bacteria

Bacterium	Source	Disease
Clostridium tetani	Soil; wound infection	Tetanus: painful contraction of skeletal muscles, paralysis
Clostridium botulinum	Improperly canned foods	Botulism: neurotoxicity, paralysis
Clostridium perfringens	Soil, gastrointestinal tract; wound infection	Gas gangrene: extensive destruction of tissues
Corynebacterium diphtheriae	Epidemic respiratory infection	Diphtheria: pseudomembrane and laryngeal swelling blocking respiratory tract Distant effects including myocardial and peripheral nerve damage
Vibrio cholerae	Water contaminated by feces from an infected person	Cholera: severe and profuse diarrhea leading to dehydration
Bacillus anthracis	Infected domestic animals Spores in soil Biological warfare	Anthrax: severe tissue destruction and bleeding

and can colonize deep wounds. As the organisms break down proteins in the dead tissue, they produce a foul-smelling gas. The resultant tissue distention by the gas compresses blood vessels, which in turn induces more tissue anoxia and tissue necrosis. *C. perfringens* also produces enzymes that destroy adjacent tissues and cause even more tissue necrosis. Primary treatment is aimed at breaking this perpetual cycle by thorough debridement of wounds. In addition, antibiotics directed against the bacteria, antitoxins directed against the necrotizing enzymes, and oxygen therapy to inhibit growth of the bacteria are helpful. Gas gangrene most commonly occurs after severe wounds but may also occur in the uterus following traumatic, nonsterile abortions.

The deadly childhood disease **diphtheria** is caused by the bacterium *Corynebacterium diphtheriae*. It colonizes the back of the throat and produces a toxin that interferes with protein production by the host's cells. The infection causes a local superficial necrotizing reaction in the pharynx, which results in dead cells, phagocytes, and bacteria plastering together and forming a thick pseudomembrane over the back of the throat. The laryngeal swelling and pseudomembrane can obstruct the opening to the trachea, resulting in severe respiratory distress and, eventually, death. In addition, the toxin is released into the blood, where it exerts distant effects on various tissues, including the heart. If the patient does not die from obstruction of the respiratory tract, long-term sequelae such as myocarditis, resulting in congestive heart failure, and peripheral nerve degeneration, resulting in paralysis, can occur. The disease can be prevented by immunization against the toxin. In patients who are not vaccinated, the disease can be ameliorated by administering both antibiotics, to clear the bacterial infection, and synthetic antitoxin, to counteract the effect of the diphtheria toxin.

The last outbreak of **cholera** in the United States occurred in 1911, but this disease causes more than 100,000 deaths every year worldwide. *Vibrio cholerae*, which is extremely infective, is transmitted via the fecal–oral route. Outbreaks of cholera occur in overcrowded camps and slums with poor sanitation. The toxin produced by *V. cholerae* causes an imbalance in the electrolytes in the gastrointestinal tract, leading to severe diarrhea and death due to rapid dehydration. Treatment with oral electrolyte and fluid replacement therapy can be life-saving, and co-administration of antibiotics shortens the course of the disease.

Anthrax is caused by the bacterium *Bacillus anthracis*. Humans are not the usual host of this bacterium but are exposed to it through contact with infected livestock or inhalation of bacterial spores that can survive in dirt for decades. *B. anthracis* is not at all a common cause of disease in the United States, but it has been

developed and, unfortunately, been used as a biological weapon by various governments. In 2001, anthrax spores were sent through the U.S. Postal Service to several journalists and members of Congress, resulting in five deaths. Just a few grams of the spores are sufficient to cause widespread infection and death. The spores are inhaled and eventually gain access to the bloodstream, where they produce three powerful toxins that result in uncontrollable tissue destruction and bleeding. Eradication of the bacterium with antibiotics does not necessarily cure the disease because the toxin continues to circulate in the blood in lethal levels. An antibody that can neutralize the toxins has only recently been developed.

Zoonotic Bacterial Diseases

Zoonotic diseases are transmitted from animals or animal vectors to humans. Usually, humans are not the primary reservoir for the infectious agent, so infection depends on contact with pathogen's natural host. In some cases, such as pulmonic plague, the infectious agent can readily spread from human to human after the initial human infection does occur. These are rare causes of illness in the United States, but can be very serious if not identified and treated in time to prevent complications. Zoonotic diseases can be caused by all classes of infectious agents, including bacteria, viruses, protozoa, helminths, and prions, but bacteria are the most common source. **Table 26–4** lists the more common zoonotic diseases discussed in this text.

Lyme disease is caused by infection with *Borrelia burgdorferi*, which is carried by a variety of small (1–3 mm) deer tick adults or larvae. The site of the tick bite can be identified by a small "bull's eye" or targetoid lesion on the skin, but this lesion is often missed if it is in an inapparent location, such as behind the ear. The bite can also be accompanied by fever and lymphadenopathy. In the second stage of the disease, the organisms spread throughout the body, resulting in skin lesions, muscle pain, arthritis, lymphadenopathy, cardiac arrhythmias, meningitis, and severe lethargy. The third stage occurs 2 to 3 years after initial infection and is characterized by severe arthritis and encephalitis. The latter manifests as sleepiness, personality change including tearfulness and irritability, and cognitive problems including memory loss, among others. Lyme disease is one of the purported causes of "chronic fatigue syndrome." It appears to be increasing in incidence, given that as many as 50% of deer ticks in the northeastern United States are infected with *B. burgdorferi*. There are numerous endemic regions in the United States. Treatment with tetracycline can be effective if initiated in the first stage of the disease.

Salmonella bacteria are contracted from animals, primarily by eating undercooked pork and poultry or

TABLE 26–4	Examples of Zoonotic Diseases		
Disease	**Causative Agent**	**Transmission**	**Disease Characteristics**
Bacteria			
Lyme disease	*Borrelia burgdorferi*	Via ticks, from wild deer	Three stages: "targetoid" skin rash, systemic spread, severe arthritis and encephalitis
Salmonellosis	*Salmonella* sp.	Ingestion of undercooked pork, poultry, eggs	Gastroenteritis with profuse, watery diarrhea
Plague	*Yersinia pestis*	Via fleas, from rodents	Bubonic (skin necrosis), pneumonic (lung involvement), and hemorrhagic manifestations
Tularemia	*Francisella tularensis*	Via ticks, from rabbits or rodents	Skin lesions, lymphadenopathy, fever, pneumonia
Brucellosis	*Brucella* sp.	From dairy animals (meat, milk, or direct contact)	Undulant fever: waxing and waning fever, malaise
Typhus	*Rickettsia prowazekii*	Lice	Chills, cough, delirium Rash Photophobia, headache Muscle and back pain
Rocky Mountain spotted fever	*Rickettsia ricketsii*	Tick (natural host)	Fever, rash Infection of blood vessels throughout the body, resulting in damage to brain and nerves (paralysis, hearing loss), and gangrene of fingers or entire limbs
Viruses			
Rabies	Rabies virus	Bite of rabid animal	Encephalitis
Prion protein			
Creutzfeldt–Jakob disease	Prion protein	Ingestion of meat with abnormal prion protein	Neurodegeneration

raw eggs. This bacterium causes an enteritis characterized by severe, profuse diarrhea that can be deadly in infants, the elderly, and immunocompromised individuals. Periodic epidemics of **plague** repeatedly decimated the European population in the Middle Ages. Isolated cases of plague continue to occur in the United States, and more severe outbreaks occur in developing nations. The causative bacterium, *Yersinia pestis*, is transmitted from rodents via the bite of fleas. In the human host, it is transported to lymph nodes, where it rapidly reproduces, causing the "bubos" or swelling of lymph nodes from which bubonic plague gets its name. This form of plague additionally is characterized by necrosis of the fingers, toes, and nose, and by hemorrhagic vomiting. In pneumonic plague, the bacteria gain access to the lungs and can be transmitted from one human to another via coughing or sneezing. Improvement of living conditions, primarily eradication of fleas from human habitations, effectively prevents the epidemic outbreak of plague.

Rickettsia are small, fragile bacteria that grow only within the cells of the host. Infections by *Rickettsia* are rare but serious zoonotic diseases. Transmission requires an insect vector, such as lice (typhus) or ticks (Rocky Mountain spotted fever). *Rickettsia* are quite susceptible to antibiotics. The challenge in treating rickettsial infections is making the diagnosis early enough because early symptoms of infection are mild and nonspecific, but established infection can be lethal. *Rickettsia* preferentially attack the endothelial cells of blood vessels. The ensuing hemorrhage leads to skin rashes, which is one of the defining signs of the infection. Ehrlichiosis and anaplasmosis are newly recognized infections caused by a rickettsial-like organism acquired through tick bites that are being encountered with increasing frequency in the United States. They are characterized by fever, thrombocytopenia, and lymphadenopathy, but do not produce a rash.

Other bacterial zoonotic diseases that can affect humans include tularemia and brucellosis. **Tularemia** is an uncommon disease caused by *Francisella tularensis* infection. The bacterium is contracted from a wild animal reservoir, especially muskrats and rabbits, via direct contact or tick bites. Tularemia can cause pneumonia as well as a severe systemic infection, but is usually responsive to tetracycline treatment. Brucellosis is a chronic systemic disease, often referred to as **undulant fever** because of the waxing and waning of febrile episodes in the patient. It is caused by various species of the *Brucella* genus. These bacteria are harbored in cows, sheep, hogs, and goats, and human disease is acquired by ingestion of infected meat, unpasteurized dairy products, or by contact with an infected animal. The organisms live intracellularly in macrophages, which spill the organisms into the bloodstream every few days to cause the febrile episodes.

Other Important Bacterial Infections

Anaerobes in the lower alimentary tract and in the mouth outnumber aerobes by more than 1,000 to 1. They can cause abscesses, wound infections, or any other kind of infection resembling those associated with *E. coli* or staphylococci. When they overgrow, they often produce foul-smelling gases that aid in their detection, or toxins that mediate the inflammatory injury.

Mycobacterium leprae, a tuberculosis-like organism, causes **leprosy**. The bacteria preferentially invade skin and peripheral nerves, causing palpable lumps of granulomatous inflammation over the nerves. Over the course of many years, physical disfigurement results from the breakdown of tissue that has lost its nerve supply. Leprosy is uncommon but does occur in the United States, particularly in southern states. The availability of effective drugs for treatment has obviated quarantine for prevention of transmission of this disease.

Mycoplasma are bacteria that do not possess rigid cell walls. *Mycoplasma pneumoniae* is the primary cause of atypical pneumonia, which does not present with the typical symptoms of fever, malaise, and chest pain, but rather may smolder for many weeks with low-grade symptoms such as coughing, shortness of breath, and fatigue. Because the patient usually feels well enough to attempt to go about daily activities, atypical pneumonia also is called "walking pneumonia." It tends to affect children and adolescents. *Mycoplasma genitalium* and *Ureaplasma urealyticum* are other mycoplasmal organisms; they cause nongonococcal urethritis.

Chlamydia are obligate intracellular parasites, meaning they lack the ability to survive in the absence of a host-derived energy system and, therefore, must gain entry into host cells. Overall, chlamydial genitourinary infections are the number one reported communicable disease in the United States (see Table 26–1). Different species of *Chlamydia* can also cause inclusion conjunctivitis, pneumonia in newborns, trachoma, and psittacosis. **Trachoma** is a chronic, progressive conjunctivitis that leads to blindness. *C. trachomatis* is spread mainly by flies in rural areas of the world, and is the leading cause of blindness in sub-Saharan Africa and parts of Asia and South America. *C. psittaci* is transmitted from birds, especially imported pet birds, to humans and can cause pneumonitis and generalized disease.

Viral Infections

Viruses essentially consist of encapsulated genetic material: they do not have the ability to create their own energy and they cannot replicate by themselves. Viruses proliferate by being taken up by a host cell, integrating their genetic material into the host cell's DNA, and then reassembling themselves as the viral genes and proteins are produced along with the host's. When the host cell cytoplasm is packed with assembled viral particles, the cell membrane ruptures, spilling the newly formed viral particles into the surrounding tissue or into the blood, where they can infect other cells.

Viruses are so small that they are invisible with standard light microscopy, and can be seen only at higher magnifications, with electron microscopy. Visualization of the viral particles is not a standard method of detection or diagnosis of viral illness: serologic tests for specific viral antigens are much more effective. Some viruses aggregate into inclusion bodies that can become visible in the nucleus or cytoplasm of cells (**Figures 26–2** and **26–3**) with standard light microscopy, and this is a helpful finding that prompts further, more specific testing for particular viruses.

The routes of transmission of viruses are similar to those of bacteria: they can be spread between people via aerosolized secretions (influenza), sexual contact (HPV, HIV), direct skin contact (chickenpox), or maternal–fetal transmission (HIV, hepatitis B virus), as well as via insect vectors (West Nile virus, yellow fever), and contaminated food and water (Hepatitis A virus, polio virus). Certain viruses have predilections for infecting certain types of cells. For example, the human immunodeficiency virus (HIV) preferentially infects lymphocytes, the West Nile virus preferentially affects tissues of the central nervous system, and HPV affects cells of squamous epithelia. Unlike many bacteria, viruses do not have a predilection for overgrowing injured or necrotic tissue.

Viral infections usually elicit an initial inflammatory reaction, accompanied by the usual signs of infection—namely, fatigue, fever, and malaise. Blood work can show normal white blood cell counts, but often the number of lymphocytes is elevated more than other types of white blood cells. An acute inflammatory reaction with pus production does not occur. The primary white blood cell involved in reactions to viral infections is the lymphocyte, and the virus is eliminated by a combination of T-cell–mediated cytotoxic reactions against virally infected cells, causing death of the host cell and therefore inhibition of the production of new viral particles, and

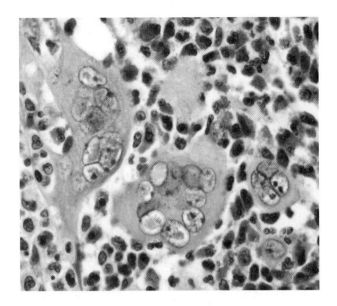

FIGURE 26–2 *Herpes simplex* virus–infected cells. The cells are multinucleate, the nuclei are large, and many of the nuclei contain amorphous pink material that represents condensed viral proteins.

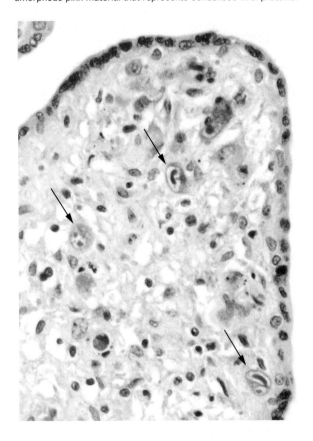

FIGURE 26–3 Cytomegalovirus. Arrows point to three large cells with irregular nuclei, each with oddly shaped inclusions, in a placental villus. The fetus died in utero of overwhelming cytomegalovirus infection involving the lungs and brain.

production of antibodies, which enhance recognition of viruses and virally infected cells by the immune system. In addition, virally infected cells produce a protein called **interferon**, which suppresses protein synthesis in neighboring cells, thereby "interfering" with the replication of viral particles once they are released from the originally infected cell.

Viral diseases do not respond to antibiotic therapy. Consequently, treatment revolves around supportive measures such as rest, adequate hydration, and alleviation of fever. Interferon is used to suppress viral replication in some diseases (e.g., hepatitis C). Pharmaceutical antiviral agents are available for a few viruses, but they are not as reliably effective against viruses as antibiotics are against bacteria. Even the drugs currently used to treat HIV infection merely inhibit viral replication; they do not eradicate the virus from the body altogether.

The immune system elaborates antibodies to viruses after the initial exposure, but it is unfortunately often the initial exposure that has serious, even lethal, effects. Immunizations are particularly powerful in preventing the development of serious viral disease by priming the immune system to develop antibodies to specific viral antigens, so that when and if infection does occur, the viruses can rapidly be eliminated before they elicit the manifestations of the disease. Many serious viral diseases of childhood, including polio, mumps, and measles, are now preventable with vaccinations.

Some viruses are totally eliminated from the body by the host's immune system after the initial infection, while others remain harbored in tissues for the life of the individual (**Figure 26–4**). For example, the hepatitis B and C viruses can do extensive damage in the liver and are never eliminated by the immune system. Other viruses can remain latent for long periods of time. Latent infections may become reactivated in immunocompromised individuals (e.g., cytomegalovirus) or as a consequence of aging (e.g., the virus that causes chickenpox reactivates in elderly people to cause the painful skin outbreak called **shingles**), or they may result in the development of a completely different disease. For example, Epstein-Barr virus, the cause of **infectious mononucleosis**, stays latent in B lymphocytes, and while it never reactivates in immunocompetent individuals to cause another bout of "mono," it is known to cause the development of some cancers.

Viral illnesses range from acute, self-limited, and rarely serious ones (as long as adequate supportive care is available), like the "common cold" or "intestinal flu," to lethal infections, such as HIV/AIDS. The most common viral disease overall is the "common cold," which is caused by several different types of viruses. The most common deadly viral disease worldwide is, of course, HIV/AIDS, which is the leading cause of death in many developing countries, and the sixth leading cause of death in people between the ages of 25 and 34 in the United States. On the continuum of severity between the common cold and HIV lie scores of viral diseases that cause varying degrees of morbidity, from cold sores due to *Herpes simplex* virus (HSV), to prolonged malaise and fatigue due to infectious mononucleosis (Epstein-Barr virus), to destructive liver disease caused by hepatitis B and C viruses.

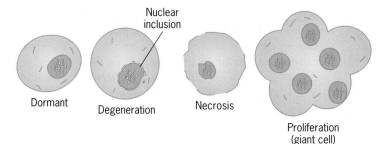

Nuclear inclusion

Dormant Degeneration Necrosis

Proliferation (giant cell)

FIGURE 26–4 Possible reactions of cells to viral infection.

Several of the epidemic scourges of history were caused by viruses. *Smallpox*, which decimated the Native American population when European settlers brought it to the New World, has been eradicated throughout the world by international public health initiatives. This virus is highly contagious and causes a rash much like that associated with chickenpox, although when it heals it leaves deep, pitted scars. Focal necrotizing lesions occur in many organs, especially the lungs and intestinal tract, leading to death in 10% to 20% of cases. *Influenza* is an upper respiratory tract infection that has a high mortality rate, particularly among children and the elderly. Influenza outbreaks occur yearly, primarily in the late fall through early spring. This infection is highly transmissible through respiratory secretions (coughing, sneezing). The symptoms of influenza range

from those of a head cold with malaise, sore throat, headache, and fever to severe muscular aches and pains, nausea and vomiting, and pneumonia. A vaccination against the most prevalent strains of the virus is manufactured each year, and all vulnerable populations should be immunized annually. In addition, the virus is easily killed by exposure to soap, so frequent hand washing reduces its transmission. While even with these measures the death toll per year approaches 100,000. The pandemic of 1918, in which the symptoms of flu had a rapid onset and were accompanied by hemorrhages from the nose, ears, mouth, and intestines, killed tens of millions of people.

Viral Diseases of Childhood

Nowadays, the vaccination schedule for common infectious diseases of childhood is more familiar to the primary care nurse or physician taking care of children than are the actual clinical manifestations of these diseases. Thankfully, because of vaccinations, these diseases rarely come to clinical attention—in fact, the diagnosis stands a chance of being delayed or even missed because the manifestations of the diseases (**Figure 26–5**) are so rarely seen that they are not routinely recognized. Where once virtually every child developed **measles** and mumps in

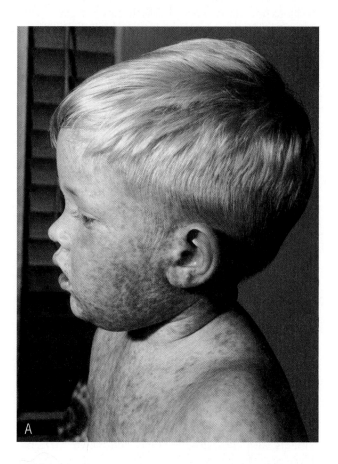

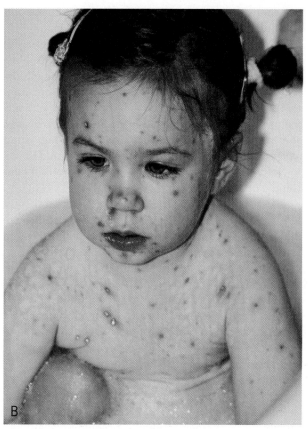

FIGURE 26–5 A. Macular rash of measles. (Courtesy of CDC.) **B.** Papular rash of chickenpox. (© Dagfrida/ShutterStock, Inc.)

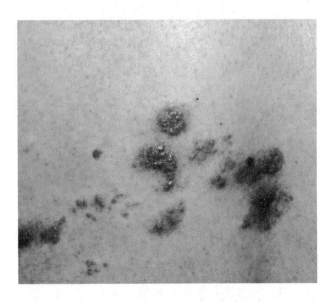

FIGURE 26–6 Shingles. (© Stephen VanHorn/ShutterStock, Inc.)

periodic outbreaks of the disease, now the CDC reports fewer than 1,000 cases of each of these infections in the United States every year (Table 26–1). While **polio** routinely swept across cities in the summer months, leaving dead and paralyzed children in its wake, not a single case of polio has been reported in the United States since 1979. Indeed, because of massive and concentrated public health efforts, the incidence of polio has dropped precipitously throughout the world.

Table 26–5 lists the common infectious diseases of childhood for which vaccinations are available. Note that three of these infections are actually bacterial (whooping cough, *Haemophilus influenzae*, and diphtheria) but are listed in the table for the sake of completeness. All of these diseases are potentially deadly, some more so than others. Polio is a crippling, if not always lethal disease, while mumps is a very mild illness in children. The diseases tend to be more severe if contracted in adulthood.

Most of the diseases listed in Table 26–5 are transmitted via the respiratory route—in other words, through inhalation of aerosolized particles. The notable exception is polio, which can also be transmitted via the fecal–oral route and colonizes the gastrointestinal tract as well as the mouth and throat. Many of these diseases can also be transmitted across the placenta to a developing fetus and cause death of the fetus (miscarriage) or congenital birth defects. The most notorious of these is **rubella**. If a non-immune mother is infected with rubella virus during the first trimester of her pregnancy, the virus can cross the placenta and infect the developing fetus, resulting in miscarriage or severe birth defects including deafness, eye defects, heart defects, mental retardation, autism, and growth delay. Women seeking to become pregnant and newly pregnant women are routinely screened for immunity against rubella.

Once a person has been infected with one of these viruses, antibodies confer lifetime immunity. The exception to this rule is varicella zoster virus (VZV), which causes **chickenpox** in childhood. Once the initial infection is cleared, VZV can lie dormant in nerve cell bodies for many decades. In older individuals, it can then reactivate and travel along the nerve to cause a very painful vesicular rash on the skin, called shingles (**Figure 26–6**). The vaccine against chickenpox may not protect against shingles, as the immunity imparted by the vaccine generally wanes with age. However, a more concentrated form of the vaccine can be given to adults that does protect against shingles.

Human Immunodeficiency Virus

The **human immunodeficiency virus** (HIV) is the cause of AIDS, and one of the leading causes of death in the world. Worldwide, there are approximately 34 million HIV-positive people, mostly in sub-Saharan Africa and Asia. In the United States, there are 1.1 million HIV-positive people, 50,000 people were newly diagnosed with AIDS in 2011, and 15,500 people died of AIDS that year. More than 30 million people have died worldwide in the AIDS epidemic, 600,000 of them in the United States.

The acronym **AIDS** stands for "acquired immunodeficiency syndrome." AIDS is diagnosed when an HIV-positive patient has a very low CD4+ T-cell count or develops infections or neoplasms that are associated with this type of immune deficiency, such as disseminated fungal infections, Burkitt lymphoma, or Kaposi sarcoma. The disease is characterized by a very long latent period of 2 to 8 years or more between the initial infection and the manifestation of AIDS. Generalized lymphadenopathy, fever, weight loss, diarrhea, and a decreased level of CD4+ T lymphocytes precede the development of AIDS.

The first cases of AIDS occurred in the United States in the early 1980s. It was soon recognized that HIV is transmitted both sexually and by direct inoculation through the use of contaminated needles and transfusion of infected blood products. Within 2 to 12 weeks after exposure, an acute clinical illness develops characterized by fever, night sweats, lymphadenopathy, rash, myalgias, arthralgias, headache, and persistent lethargy. Mood changes, irritability, diarrhea, and anorexia may also be seen. However, the initial illness is usually thought to be just another "cold" by affected individuals, and not recognized as caused by HIV. Some HIV-infected persons never develop the initial illness. While the virus is proliferating in the body's T cells over the course of the next several years, the patient has no indication that s/he is infected. AIDS is heralded by persistent generalized lymphadenopathy, followed by fevers, weight loss, diarrhea, fatigue, night sweats, and encephalopathy with dementia, the latter occurring in 60% to 90% of all patients with clinical AIDS. Once full-blown AIDS has developed, the prognosis for long-term survival is very poor. The list of opportunistic infections that can affect

TABLE 26–5 Infectious Diseases of Childhood for Which Vaccinations Are Available

Disease	Transmission	Symptoms	Complications or Long-Term Sequelae	Fatality Rate
Virus				
Measles (rubeola)	Respiratory	Conjunctivitis Photophobia Rash, beginning behind the ears and over the face, then spreading over the entire body Cough, fever	Otitis media Pneumonia Corneal ulceration or scarring Ear infections Encephalitis (usually fatal)	Approximately 3/1,000 in the United States; approximately 30% in underdeveloped nations with inadequate supportive care and in immunocompromised individuals
Rubella (German measles)	Respiratory (childhood) Intrauterine (congenital)	Child: Mild rash, fever, lymphadenopathy Fetus: Intrauterine infection causes miscarriage or serious birth defects	Congenital rubella syndrome: deafness, congenital heart defect, and eye abnormalities (e.g., cataract), among others	Childhood disease: rarely causes death; Intrauterine infection: miscarriage or severe birth defects (50%)
Varicella zoster (chickenpox)	Direct contact of blisters or contaminated clothing, blankets Respiratory Very rarely, congenital	Malaise, fever Blistering and itchy rash Disease more severe in adults, pregnant women, immunocompromised individuals	Secondary bacterial infections in the blisters Reactivation in adulthood: shingles Can lead to severe, generalized infection (heart, liver, kidneys)	Most deaths occur in adults and in immunocompromised individuals Infection during pregnancy: 10–20% risk of maternal pneumonia and up to 40% maternal mortality
Mumps	Respiratory	Malaise, fever Painful swelling of parotid glands In adult men, inflammation of the testes	Scarring and atrophy of testes causing infertility	Rarely causes death
Polio	Fecal–oral	90% of patients have no symptoms Fever, malaise Stiff neck Muscle weakness Signs of neurologic injury	Paralysis	5–10% due to paralysis of respiratory muscles Fatality is higher in adults
Bacteria				
Whooping cough (*Bordetella pertussis*)	Respiratory	Paroxysmal coughing with inspiratory whooping Can last for weeks to months	Secondary to violent coughing: vomiting, subconjunctival hemorrhages, rib fractures, hernia, pleural rupture, and pneumothorax Pneumonia Encephalopathy Seizures	Especially severe in infants (1% fatality)
Haemophilus influenzae disease (*Haemophilus influenzae* type b) (Hib)	Respiratory	Meningitis Pneumonia Otitis media Epiglottitis Cellulitis Infectious arthritis	Brain damage Hearing loss	3–6% fatality in children; higher in elderly
Diphtheria (*Corynebacterium diphtheriae*)	Respiratory Direct contact with nasal discharge, saliva, tears	Fever, chills Fatigue Pharyngitis Difficulty breathing Bloody nasal discharge Lymphadenopathy	Toxin-mediated damage to heart (heart failure) and nerves (paralysis)	5–10% fatality

patients with compromised immune systems is long, and includes diseases caused by bacteria (e.g., *Mycobacterial* species, salmonellosis), viruses (e.g., cytomegalovirus, *Herpes simplex* virus infection), and fungal organisms (toxoplasmosis, *Pneumocystis jirovecii* pneumonia, candidiasis, cryptococcosis, histoplasmosis, coccidioidomycosis). In addition, patients with AIDS can develop neoplasms that are exceedingly rare in the general population, such as Kaposi sarcoma, an aggressive neoplasm of the blood vessels in the skin.

The symptoms of AIDS and its complications are related to depression of the immune system, particularly the cellular immune system. HIV infects cells by attaching to a receptor present on cell surfaces called CD4 (**Figure 26–7**). Although found on many types of cells, the CD4 receptor is most prevalent on T-helper (CD4+) lymphocytes, and these become the primary repository of infection. Lymphocytes are replenished by the bone

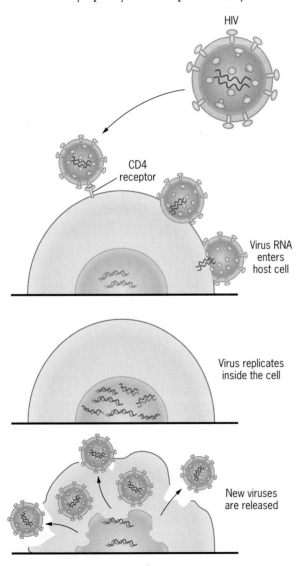

FIGURE 26–7 Schematic diagram of internalization of HIV by way of CD4 receptor on certain cells, replication of viral genetic material in the cell's nucleus, and release of new viral particles through death of the host cell.

HIV

CD4 receptor

Virus RNA enters host cell

Virus replicates inside the cell

New viruses are released

marrow. Even as the CD4+ T cells are destroyed by the replicating virus, the bone marrow can keep up their production for many years. Eventually, however, the viral burden becomes so high that the bone marrow is overwhelmed in attempting to keep up with production, and the number of CD4+ T cells in the blood begins to drop. CD4+ T cells are critical in orchestrating the immune response, particularly the activity of B lymphocytes, so eventually both cellular and antibody-mediated immunity are compromised. In this setting, opportunistic organisms are easily able to infect the patient and produce devastating disease.

HIV infection can be diagnosed with very high reliability by routine laboratory tests. Diagnosis requires two tests. Within a few weeks to months after the initial infection, HIV antibodies appear in the patient's serum. The first test, called an ELISA test, detects these antibodies. The ELISA test is easy to administer and relatively inexpensive, so it is suitable for use as an initial screening tool. However, it can yield falsely positive results. Positive results of the ELISA test need to be followed up with a more definitive test, called Western blot. This combination of tests can identify whether a patient is infected with HIV, but it does not help monitor therapy or predict the development of complications. Patients who are HIV positive are followed by routine quantification of their circulating CD4+ T cells and the "viral load." Concentrations of more than 500 CD4+ T cells per microliter of blood usually are sufficient to maintain a normal immune response; anything less than this number, however, is cause for concern. Counts less than 200 CD4+ T cells per microliter are part of the definition of AIDS. The concentration of HIV RNA circulating in the peripheral blood is the viral load. High viral loads correlate with low CD4+ T-cell counts, and predispose the HIV-positive individual to the development of opportunistic infections. Both viral load and CD4+ T-cell count are used to monitor therapy.

Prior to the development of opportunistic infections, HIV-positive patients develop some nonspecific signs and symptoms. Lymph nodes throughout the body become enlarged, a condition called "generalized lymphadenopathy." Biopsy of the lymph nodes simply shows an increase in the number of lymphocytes within them. Patients also experience generalized wasting due to loss of adipose tissue and organ atrophy. The organisms causing opportunistic infections in HIV-positive patients are not specific for AIDS: they also occur in patients whose immune systems are compromised for other reasons. The neoplasms that are associated with AIDS, such as Burkitt lymphoma and Kaposi sarcoma, also are driven by infection: Burkitt lymphoma by EBV and Kaposi sarcoma by one of the herpes viruses. These neoplasms usually do not develop in patients who are immunocompromised for other reasons.

HIV is aggressively tested for in blood products, so there is no longer any risk of transmission via blood transfusions. In the early years of the epidemic, homosexual men and intravenous drug users made up the largest proportion of people with HIV in the United States. As the epidemic progressed and infection became more prevalent, heterosexual intercourse became a much more common route of transmission than male homosexual intercourse. Women became disproportionately affected by HIV, in developing nations as well as in the United States. Moreover, the virus can be transmitted from mother to child, either while the fetus is developing in the uterus, during delivery (the most common route of infection), or from infected breast milk. The risk of **vertical transmission** (from mother to child) can be reduced to less than 2% with appropriate intervention, but if the mother has no access to therapy, as is the case in most of the developing world, vertical transmission can be as high as 40%. Approximately 3.3 million of the total number of people infected worldwide in 2011 were children, more than 90% of whom contracted the disease during the fetal and neonatal periods.

As yet there is no vaccine against HIV, although many potential candidates are in clinical trials. HIV is treated with various antiviral drugs: at least three different types of antiviral agents are needed to keep the viral load at undetectable levels in the blood. This combination of drugs called "highly active antiretroviral therapy" (HAART). The drugs target specific proteins that HIV requires to replicate, such as protease, reverse transcriptase, and integrase. They do not eliminate the virus, but rather slow its replication so substantially that life expectancy is extended by decades. In addition, reduction of the viral load through use of HAART reduces vertical transmission and transmission via sexual contact.

The most effective way of preventing AIDS is to prevent transmission of HIV altogether. This is, of course, easier said than done. The primary means to prevent transmission include testing of blood products before use, elimination of the use of potentially contaminated needles by drug users, protection of an unborn or newborn child of an HIV-positive mother, and prevention of contact of infected semen with mucosal surfaces. Sexual intercourse is by far the most common mode of transmission. The virus is present in macrophages in the semen of male carriers and can gain access to male or female sexual partners through the anal, vaginal, or cervical mucosa during intercourse. The transmission rate is higher with anal intercourse. Male-to-female transmission is much more likely than female-to-male transmission. Condoms provide the most effective protection against sexual transmission. Puritanical religious injunctions against the use of condoms and subsequent prohibition of access to them, and local or cultural prejudices against their use, have created strong resistance to their universal acceptance. Thus, the AIDS epidemic rages on as costs for treatment, prevention, and research continue to escalate.

BOX 26–5   Human Immunodeficiency Virus Infection

Cause

Human immunodeficiency virus

Lesions

Decreased CD4+ T lymphocytes

Manifestations

Positive ELISA test

Positive Western blot test

Nonspecific wasting, lymphadenopathy

Opportunistic infections

Dementia

Kaposi sarcoma, other neoplasms

Upper Respiratory Tract Infections

Numerous viral agents can cause a "sore throat," ranging from the innocuous ones causing the common cold (rhinovirus, adenovirus), to the potentially deadly influenza virus. **Upper respiratory tract infections** are often accompanied by other, generalized signs of infection, including fever, chills, muscle aches and pains, anorexia, fatigue, and malaise. Some of the viruses causing upper respiratory tract infections, such as respiratory syncytial virus (RSV), can cause serious complications, such as bronchitis and pneumonia, in children, the elderly, and immunocompromised individuals. Others have secondary effects in other organs—for example, coxsackievirus can cause myocarditis.

The agent of infectious mononucleosis, or "mono," is the Epstein-Barr virus (EBV), one of the human herpesviruses. This disease characteristically affects teenagers and young adults. It appears that the older the patient, the more devastating the disease manifestations are. Mono is transmitted via respiratory secretions—hence its moniker the "kissing disease." Generally, it starts with a sore throat and extreme tiredness, like any other "cold," but then progresses to splenomegaly and lymphadenopathy, and sometimes even acute hepatitis. Worst of all, the symptoms persist for several weeks. Some patients are ill for many months. In fact, mono can cause the symptoms of "chronic fatigue syndrome" in about 10% of patients—namely, severe fatigue that interferes with daily activities and can be accompanied by muscle and joint pain, headaches, lymphadenopathy, and post-exertional malaise. The peripheral blood in patients with infectious mononucleosis will show increased numbers of lymphocytes, many of which have an atypical appearance. Serum from these patients will react on a glass slide with horse red blood cells, causing them to agglutinate. This is the basis of the Mono Spot test, which is used to diagnose the disease.

The success of vaccinations in reducing or, in the case of smallpox, entirely eradicating, viral diseases begs the question of why we do not have a vaccine for the "common cold." The solution to the common cold is obviously not as simple as one would wish. As already mentioned, multitudes of viruses can cause such respiratory infections, so developing and administering a vaccine against any one virus may not be very cost-effective. Additionally, many of these viruses are able to undergo **antigenic shifts**, meaning they can subtly alter the composition of their proteins so the immune system no longer responds to them. Antibodies produced against the virus, due to either vaccinations or prior exposure, are therefore no longer capable of recognizing the altered protein, so immunity against the virus is lost. The most serious of the upper respiratory viral infections, influenza, is caused by one such highly mutable virus. Every year, international epidemiological investigations are undertaken to allow scientists to predict which strains of virus are most likely to sweep across the world and cause outbreaks of influenza. Vaccines are developed against only these strains, and susceptible people (the elderly, infants and children, healthcare workers, immunocompromised patients, and patients with underlying illness) are encouraged to be vaccinated against these most prevalent strains on an annual basis. As yet, scientists have not discovered a method of circumventing viruses' ability to undergo antigenic shifts.

BOX 26–6   Infectious Mononucleosis

Cause

Epstein–Barr virus

Lesions

Pharyngitis

Lymphadenopathy

Splenomegaly

Hepatitis

Manifestations

Malaise

Weakness

Sore throat

Enlarged lymph nodes

Chronic fatigue

Atypical lymphocytes in the peripheral blood

Positive Mono Spot test

Viral Infections of the Skin and Mucous Membranes

Herpes simplex virus types 1 and 2 produce a variety of infections. HSV type 1 mostly causes oral and skin lesions and is transmitted by direct contact. HSV type 2 mostly causes genital lesions and is transmitted by sexual contact. After the initial infection with HSV, the virus lies dormant in nerves and occasionally reactivates to cause vesicular lesions on or near the lips. These lesions are called "cold sores" or "fever blisters" because reactivation of the virus is often precipitated by febrile illness. While the outbreaks tend to be localized, HSV type 1 can cause a severe and often fatal encephalitis, and HSV type 2 can be transmitted during vaginal delivery if the mother has active genital lesions, thereby causing a fatal disseminated neonatal infection. Administration of acyclovir is highly effective in ameliorating the course of primary *Herpes simplex* infection and may be life-saving in encephalitis or disseminated infection of the neonate.

More than 50 genetically distinct **human papillomaviruses** can cause benign and neoplastic lesions of squamous epithelium, including the skin, esophagus, larynx, and pharynx, and the vulvar, vaginal, and ectocervical lining. Benign lesions caused by HPV include common skin warts (verruca vulgaris); warts on the soles of the feet, called plantar warts (verruca planus); venereal warts (condyloma acuminata); and laryngeal polyps. These lesions can grow to large sizes, can be painful (especially plantar warts), and, if numerous or very large, can interfere with respiration (nasopharyngeal and laryngeal warts). Different strains of HPV cause neoplastic lesions, ranging from dysplasia to invasive carcinoma, in the genital tract and posterior oropharynx. It is important to remember that the strains of HPV causing benign lesions are different from those causing neoplastic lesions.

Emerging Viral Diseases

An **emerging infectious disease** is an infectious disease that has never been seen before in humans, or an established infectious disease that is suddenly becoming more prevalent. The concern with emerging infectious diseases is that the causative organism could potentially develop the ability to easily spread between humans, causing morbidity and mortality on a massive scale, like the epidemic infectious diseases of the past (e.g., plague, influenza, smallpox). In the 1980s, HIV/AIDS was an emerging disease: very rare cases of a mysterious wasting illness causing immune dysfunction were reported in far-flung areas of the world in the prior decades, but it was not until the infection spread at an alarming rate in the 1980s that it came to epidemiologic attention.

Most emerging diseases are viral and zoonotic. It is thought that HIV originated from a similar virus in primates, but then underwent an antigenic shift to be able not only to infect humans but also to spread between humans. Diseases that are currently under intense scrutiny for signs that they are developing into emerging diseases include *avian* and *swine influenza viruses*, which are contracted from fowl and pigs, respectively, especially when these are in close contact with humans; *viral hemorrhagic fevers* such as those caused by Ebola and Marburg virus; and *severe acute respiratory syndrome (SARS)*, caused by a coronavirus, which in 2003 spread alarmingly from China, where it caused the largest number of deaths, to more than 30 countries in the course of a few months. The animal reservoir of the latter two infectious diseases is not yet conclusively known. While most emerging diseases are viral, several well-known bacterial and fungal diseases have also been scrutinized by epidemiologists for signs of reemergence, including multidrug-resistant tuberculosis, cholera, plague, and tularemia.

Fungal Infections

Fungi are eukaryotic organisms that constitute a biological kingdom separate from plants, animals, and bacteria. Some fungi, such as mushrooms, are multicellular; most are unicellular and microscopic. Fungi are most ubiquitous in soil and dead matter, but they also live as commensal or symbiotic organisms in the human digestive tract, oropharynx, skin, and vagina. Unicellular fungi exist in two forms, depending on their environment: either *yeast* (bud) or *hyphal* (stem) forms. An infection by a fungus is called a mycosis or a **mycotic infection**.

Commensal fungi can cause disease if they overgrow their local environment. Superficial fungal infections of the skin, such as athlete's foot and ringworm, can persist for months to years. Various species of *Candida* live in the oropharynx and can overgrow to cause mucocutaneous **candidiasis**, particularly in patients with diabetes, patients on prolonged antibacterial therapy, and immunocompromised patients. Overgrowth of *Candida* can also occur in the female genitalia, causing a "yeast" infection. While these infections tend to be mild and easily controlled with simple interventions, fungi contracted from the environment can cause serious systemic diseases. Fungal organisms are also common causes of opportunistic diseases in immunocompromised individuals.

The prevalence of mycotic infections varies by geographic region (**Figure 26–8**). Because fungal organisms tend to live in soil and degrading organic matter, and because systemic fungal infections are contracted from the environment, it stands to reason that different fungal infections are seen in different areas of the world. Moreover, farmers, archaeologists, and other people working intimately with the soil, and spelunkers and bird fanciers, who are exposed to bat and bird droppings, are at increased risk for developing mycotic infections.

Primary Systemic Fungal Infections

Fungi usually enter the body via the respiratory route. Because they cannot always be cleared by acute inflammation or by antibody-mediated reactions, they tend to elicit a granulomatous response. Fungal organisms can survive in the granulomas for considerable periods of time. If the patient is immunocompromised, either reactivated disease or initial infection can cause a more serious and potentially lethal disease. Some of the **primary fungal**

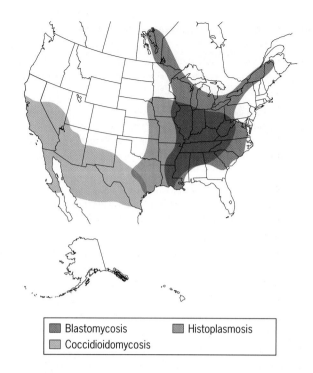

| Blastomycosis | Histoplasmosis |
| Coccidioidomycosis | |

FIGURE 26–8 Geographic distribution of disease-causing fungi in the United States. (Courtesy of CDC.)

infections in the United States are listed in **Table 26–6**. These diseases share the common features of proliferation of fungi in the yeast phase (**Figure 26–9**) and transmission via exposure to contaminated soil. The diseases are not directly transmissible from one infected human to another. All these diseases can either affect the whole body or be concentrated in one organ (**Figure 26–10**).

In addition to causing an acute disease, systemic fungal infections can follow a slow, protracted course. Some of these infections resemble tuberculosis in that they manifest with a chronic cough, wasting, night sweats, and low-grade fevers. They also resemble tuberculosis in causing granulomatous disease in the lungs. Diagnosis depends on culturing the organism, demonstrating antibodies to the particular organism in the patient's serum by serologic tests, or detecting a specific antigen or genetic sequence of the organism by more sophisticated serologic and genetic tests. The majority of fungal infections in immunocompetent individuals do not require pharmacologic treatment. In immunocompromised patients, aggressive treatment with antifungal agents and supportive measures are required to minimize the tissue destruction and prevent fatal complications.

Opportunistic Infections

Not all opportunistic infections are caused by fungal organisms (**Table 26–7**); however, fungal organisms are the most common causes of opportunistic infection. Opportunistic fungal infections usually occur with the fungus in the hyphal phase (**Figure 26–11**) and elicit an

TABLE 26–6 Common Primary Systemic Fungal Infections in the United States

Disease and Organism	Disease Manifestations
Histoplasmosis *Histoplasma capsulatum*	• Primary: usually subclinical infection, or flu-like illness, with cough • Disseminated: infection of lungs, liver, eyes (retina), and generalized lymphadenopathy
Coccidioidomycosis *Coccidioides immitis*	• Primary: subclinical infection, or flu-like illness with rash and joint pain • Chronic: meningitis, arthritis • Disseminated: infection of any organ system, including skin, meninges, urinary tract, heart, bone, joints
Blastomycosis *Blastomyces dermatitidis*	• Acute: flu-like illness with fever, headache, joint and muscle pain; pneumonia • Chronic: low-grade fever, productive cough, weight loss, night sweats; can present with inflammation in bone, larynx, skin, prostate • Disseminated: acute respiratory distress syndrome, CNS involvement, including meningitis and brain abscesses
Cryptococcosis *Cryptococcus neoformans*	• Acute: most people experience no symptoms; pneumonia • Disseminated (in immunocompromised individuals): CNS infection (headache, mental status changes); infection of skin, bone, eyes, joints

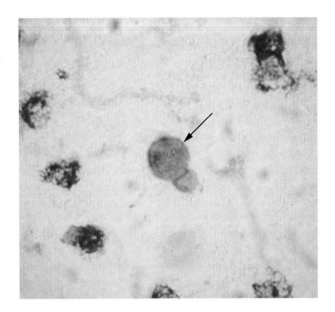

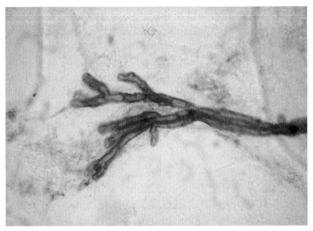

FIGURE 26–11 *Aspergillus fumigatus* in hyphal phase. (Courtesy of Dr. Carol Spiegel, Department of Pathology and Laboratory Medicine, University of Wisconsin School of Medicine and Public Health.)

FIGURE 26–9 *Blastomyces dermatitidis* (arrow) in yeast phase. (Courtesy of Dr. Carol Spiegel, Department of Pathology and Laboratory Medicine, University of Wisconsin School of Medicine and Public Health.)

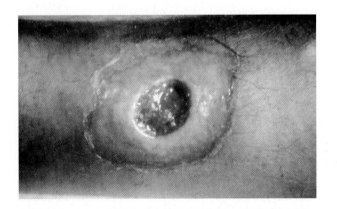

FIGURE 26–10 *Blastomyces* skin ulcer.

acute inflammatory response rather than a granulomatous one. The inflammatory response therefore resembles that of pyogenic bacteria and results in extensive tissue destruction. In severely ill patients, many of these fungi can gain entry in the blood vessels. This phenomenon, which is called angioinvasion, is almost invariably fatal. The fungus *Rhizopus* (Mucor) can attach to blood vessel walls in the brain or lungs, causing microthrombi that obstruct the passage of blood and lead to infarction of the downstream tissue. Other angioinvasive fungal species travel through the blood to distant sites, setting up separate foci of infection in disparate tissues.

Treatment of opportunistic infections requires first and foremost a high index of suspicion—in other words, knowing that the patient is immunocompromised for whatever reason, and then knowing which kinds of infectious agents are most likely to cause disease in patients with

TABLE 26–7	Common Opportunistic Infections		
Infectious Organism	**Vulnerable Patients**	**Site of Involvement**	**Disease or Complications**
Fungus			
Candida	Diabetes	Mouth, tongue	Thrush
	Burns	Skin and soft tissue	Superficial and deep wound infections
	Neutropenia	Severe, disseminated infection	Abscesses, thrombophlebitis, endocarditis, shock and disseminated intravascular coagulation
	HIV/AIDS	Mouth, tongue, esophagus, vagina	Localized overgrowth; rarely causes invasive disease
Aspergillus	Cystic fibrosis	Lungs	Allergic reaction to fungus in lungs
	AIDS Chemotherapy Neutropenia Steroid therapy	Systemic	Invasive aspergillosis: lung, heart valves, brain
Rhizopus (Mucor)	Diabetics	Sinus Orbit Brain	Rhinocerebral mucomycosis (tissue necrosis, encephalitis, cerebral infarctions)
	Neutropenia Steroids Burns	Lungs	Hemorrhagic pneumonia and pulmonary infarcts
Pneumocystis jirovecii	AIDS	Lungs	Pneumonia
Cryptococcus neoformans	AIDS	Lung Meninges Brain	Meningoencephalitis
Virus			
Cytomegalovirus (CMV)	Neonate (intrauterine infection)	CNS	Mental retardation
HIV	HIV/AIDS	Eye Gastrointestinal tract	Retinitis Esophagitis Colitis
Bacteria			
Clostridium difficile	Patients taking broad-spectrum antibiotics	Colon	Toxic megacolon
Mycobacterium avium complex (MAC)	AIDS	Lungs Gastrointestinal tract	Tuberculosis-like illness, with fever, fatigue, weight loss Cough, chest pain Diarrhea, abdominal pain Can disseminate to bone marrow
Protozoa			
Toxoplasma gondii	AIDS Neonate (if mother is infected during pregnancy)	Central nervous system	Encephalitis
Cryptosporidium	AIDS	Digestive system	Chronic diarrhea or cholera-like diarrhea

particular types of immune suppression. Antifungal and antiviral agents usually need to be given intravenously, in the hospital setting, accompanied by supportive measures including fluids, antipyretics, and drugs that can enhance the function of the heart and lungs in cases of severe, disseminated disease. Opportunistic infections are a common cause of death in immunocompromised patients, regardless of the reason for the depression of the immune system.

Protozoal Diseases

Protozoa are unicellular organisms that have a nucleus and intracellular structures, are motile (can move around), and subsist on other organisms (e.g., bacteria) for food. They tend to live in water and soil, and some have complex life cycles that allow them to alternate between proliferative and dormant forms, depending on the harshness of the environment. Dormant *cysts* can survive for a long time without water or food, while proliferative *trophozoites* are fully active, feeding and reproducing. When they cause infection, protozoa behave as parasites: they require the mammalian host to complete a part of their life cycle. In some instances, this requires not only getting into the host but also entering the host's cells. Most protozoans that cause disease in humans are intracellular parasites.

Protozoa can cause infections in a variety of tissues and of a wide range of severity in humans (**Table 26–8**). At the most benign end, infection with *Trichomonas vaginalis* can cause vaginal itching and lower urinary tract infection, but is rarely associated with significant morbidity. More seriously, **giardiasis** (caused by *Giardia lamblia*), which is transmitted via the fecal–oral route, causes severe gastroenteritis in areas of the world where the water supply is infected, and **malaria**, which is caused by a small protozoan that invades and destroys red blood cells, is the fifth leading cause of death in low-income countries.

Some of the protozoa causing diseases in humans are transmitted via an arthropod intermediate, such as mosquitoes or flies. An example is malaria. There are four types of malaria, caused by four different protozoal species: *Plasmodium falciparum*, *P. vivax*, *P. ovale*, and *P. malariae*. All are transmitted by varieties of Anopheles mosquitoes, mainly in sub-Saharan Africa. In the past, malaria was prevalent in North America as well, primarily along the eastern and southern coastal areas and throughout the central states. In the late 1940s, massive eradication programs were undertaken to drain swampy areas in which mosquitos tend to breed, and to spray DDT, a

TABLE 26–8 Some of the More Common Protozoal Diseases in Humans

Disease	Organism	Transmission	Site of Infection	Manifestations
Trichomoniasis	*Trichomonas vaginalis*	Sexual	• Vagina	• Itching, discharge
Giardiasis	*Giardia lamblia*	Fecal–oral	• Intestines	• Diarrhea • Abdominal pain • Nausea • Dehydration • Constipation • Gas production
Amebiasis	*Entamoeba histolytica*	Fecal–oral	• Intestines • Liver	• Diarrhea • Dysentery • Liver abscesses
Malaria	*Plasmodium* sp.	Mosquito bite	• Red blood cells	• Paroxysm (alternating coldness, rigor, and fever) • Symptoms referable to all organ systems, including joint pain, respiratory distress, convulsions
Trypanosomiasis (Chagas disease)	*Trypanosoma cruzi*	Bite and feces of "kissing bug"	• Heart • Esophagus	• Cardiomyopathy • Dilation of esophagus
Toxoplasmosis	*Toxoplasma gondii*	Fecal–oral Contaminated meat	• Brain	• Congenital: stunted CNS development • Immune compromised: mental status changes, seizures, encephalitis
Leishmaniasis	*Leishmania* sp.	Sandfly	• Skin • Mucous membranes • Visceral organs	• Skin ulcers • Nasopharyngeal ulcers • Lymphadenopathy • Hepatosplenomegaly • Can infect all tissues of the body, including bone marrow, kidneys, testes
Cryptosporidiosis	*Cryptosporidium parvum*	Fecal_oral	• Small intestine	• Diarrhea

highly toxic insecticide, throughout rural areas. DDT was later banned for agricultural use because of its devastating effect on the environment, but it is still used for malaria control in endemic areas. Eradication and control of the infection in the areas in which malaria is still endemic revolve around use of insecticide-impregnated mosquito netting around beds and spraying the interior of rural homes with insecticides. Massive malaria-control interventions, prophylactic drugs, and timely administration of medical care to malaria patients have led to a worldwide decrease in the number of deaths due to malaria in recent years. Nevertheless, this infection remains one of the top causes of death, primarily in children.

The bite of a *Plasmodium*-infected mosquito results in the release of the motile form of the protozoa, called a sporozoite, into the blood of the victim. Being motile, sporozoites easily travel through the bloodstream and invade hepatic cells, where they multiply. When the hepatocyte is filled to bursting, it spills thousands of copies of the asexual and nonmotile form of the protozoa, or merozoites, into the blood, from where they invade red blood cells. The merozoites replicate in the red blood cells and are released from them in cyclic waves that are concomitant with clinical symptoms of chills, fever, severe headaches, sweating, and profound malaise. Anemia, renal failure, pulmonary edema, and diarrhea can all occur acutely. The parasite can bind to the endothelium of cerebral microvessels, resulting in clogging of the vessels and subsequent hemorrhages, cerebral edema, and neuronal death. Finally, the protozoa can go into a dormant phase in hepatocytes, only to reawaken some time later and start the cycle all over again. Adults are relatively resistant to cerebral malaria, but after repeated bouts of infection they typically develop fibrotic, pigmented livers and spleens.

Malaria is diagnosed in suspected patients by microscopic examination of blood smears for the parasite in red blood cells. Serum antibodies can be detected by serology but do not distinguish between current or past infection. Treatment ranges from orally administered antibiotics in an outpatient setting, to hospital admission, triple-drug therapy, and close monitoring for the development of respiratory depression and seizures.

While one is unlikely to encounter malaria in the United States (except in a patient who has come from areas of the world in which malaria is still endemic), **toxoplasmosis** is a protozoal infection that is quite prevalent. In fact, it is estimated that one-third of the human population is infected by *Toxoplasma gondii*. In most patients, *Toxoplasma* causes no symptoms at all, but in immunocompromised individuals and neonates (see Table 26–7), it can cause severe, life-threatening illness. *T. gondii* organisms are found in the soil and are harbored in small animals. They complete their life cycle in the domestic cat. Most infections in humans are caused by exposure to cat feces, such as when emptying litter boxes. Pregnant women are counseled to avoid litter boxes because transmission of the organism across the placenta can have devastating teratogenic effects on the brain of the fetus. Toxoplasmosis is the "T" in the acronym "TORCH" infections, which are infectious causes of severe fetal anomalies.

Helminth Infections

Helminths comprise the parasitic worms—namely, the *roundworms* and the *flatworms* (**Figure 26–12**). Globally, the biggest burden of helminthic infection is in poor countries. School-age children are particularly susceptible to infection by parasitic worms. The parasitic worms derive their nutrition from their host, so helminth infections not only pose an additional caloric and nutritional burden on already marginally fed or underfed populations but also cause anemia, fatigue, stunted growth and development, impaired cognition, and diminished physical fitness. Co-infection with worms and other agents of infectious diseases discussed in this chapter, including HIV and *Plasmodium*, is extremely common. When there is co-infection, the two organisms often have synergistic effects, meaning each aggravates the disease course or manifestations of the other.

Diagnosis of helminth infections is most commonly made by detecting bits and pieces of worm or their eggs in a sample of fecal material examined microscopically. Laboratory analysis of blood work may reveal eosinophilia, as helminth infections generally elicit an immune response rich in eosinophils. More specific laboratory tests, such as antigenic tests, are used to identify some worms that are difficult to differentiate microscopically.

Most worms are internalized in humans from contaminated food and water, and then proliferate in the

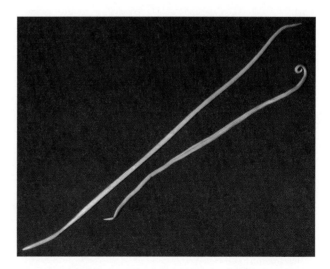

FIGURE 26–12 Two Ascaris lumbricoides nematods (roundworms). The larger of the two is the female of the species while the normally smaller male is on the right. Adult female worms can grow over 12 inches in length. (Courtesy of the CDC.)

gastrointestinal tract. Worms have complex life cycles, and have natural reservoirs outside the human host. For example, **schistosomiasis** is caused by members of a genus of flatworm whose life cycle goes through various stages within and without the human host. Schistosome eggs are shed into water from a human host's fecal or urinary stream and hatch upon contact with water. The resultant embryonic worms infect freshwater snails, replicate, and begin to mature within the snail before being shed again into the water. In that medium, they penetrate human skin and travel through the host's venules to the lungs, then to the liver, and finally to mesenteric and hemorrhoidal veins, where the now mature worms begin to produce eggs. The eggs penetrate the intestine or urinary bladder and are shed via feces or urine to start the cycle over again, while the parents stay in the veins for years, continually producing eggs. The worms feast on red blood cells, so patients develop anemia, and the eggs that do not make it into the intestine or bladder are carried by the blood into the liver or the bladder wall, where they incite an inflammatory reaction that over the course of many years destroys these organs and incites the development of liver and bladder cancer.

Helminth infections range from mild, innocuous although unpleasant infestations, to diseases that cause significant morbidity and mortality (**Table 26–9**). The common **pinworm** belongs to the former category: *Enterobius vermicularis* (pinworm) causes annoying anal itching but otherwise does not cause serious disease. These small white worms are rapidly spread among members of a family by direct contact if hand hygiene is not good. They most often cause symptoms in children, and can sometimes be seen crawling about the anal orifice where they lay their eggs at night. Cellophane tape can be used to cleanly pick the eggs from the anus for easy microscopic diagnosis. A much more serious disease is **trichinosis**, caused by the roundworm *Trichinella spiralis*. This organism is acquired through ingestion of inadequately cooked meat, especially pork, because the larval stage of this worm encysts in the animal's muscles (**Figure 26–13**). After humans eat the meat, the larvae mature and produce more larvae, which disseminate and encyst in the muscles of the human host. Just about any muscle can be affected in humans, including the heart. Patients develop severe muscle pain, fever, and marked eosinophilia in the blood. Occasional deaths result from involvement of heart or respiratory muscles.

Tapeworms are a type of flatworm that are typically picked up from ingestion of undercooked meat or fish and then take up residence in the host's gastrointestinal tract. Common symptoms include abdominal pain and diarrhea. The larvae of the pork tapeworm *Taenia solium*, called cysticerca, can invade the intestinal wall and disseminate to other organs, including the brain. Neurocysticercosis can manifest with seizures, headache, confusion, gait imbalance and hydrocephalus. The dog tapeworm *Echinococcus granulosus* also causes

TABLE 26–9 Some of the Diseases Caused by Helminths

Organism	Disease	Route of Infection	Infected Organ(s)	Disease Manifestations
Schistosoma sp.	Schistosomiasis (Bilharzia)	Infected water, across the skin	• Skin • Liver • Bladder • Intestine • Kidney • CNS	• Chronic disease • Anemia, malnutrition • Destruction of liver: portal hypertension • Cystitis and ureteritis, progressing to bladder cancer
Enterobius vermicularis	Pinworm	Fecal–oral	• Intestine	• Anal itching
Trichinella spiralis	Trichinosis	Undercooked meat (pork)	• Muscle • Heart	• Muscle pain
Taenia solium	Cysticercosis	Undercooked meat (pork)	• Brain	• Encysted larvae in brain cause seizures, headaches
Echinococcus granulosus	Echinococcosis	Food contaminated by dog feces	• Liver	• Hydatid cysts
Ascaris lumbricoides	Ascariasis	Fecal–oral	• Lung • Intestine	• Pneumonitis • Intestinal obstruction
Trichuris trichuria (whipworm)	Trichuriasis	Fecal–oral	• Intestine	• Abdominal pain • Anemia • Appendicitis • Rectal prolapse
Wuchereria bancrofti (and others)	Filariasis	Mosquito bites	• Lymphatic system	• Lymphatic obstruction, lymphedema, elephantiasis

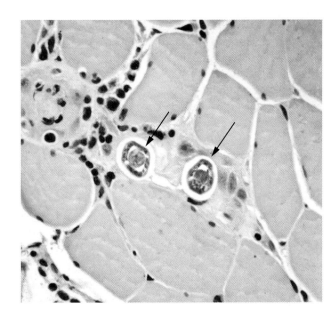

FIGURE 26–13 *Trichinella* larvae encysted in skeletal muscle.

encystment of larval organisms in tissues. These cysts, called *hydatid cysts*, can become very large. Treatment involves surgically opening the cyst and evacuating its contents, taking care not to spill them into the surrounding tissues.

Prion Protein

A very unusual and poorly understood infectious agent is **prion protein**. This protein normally exists on cell membranes, but in its abnormal form is misfolded and induces other prion proteins to undergo a shape change so they resemble the misfolded form. The misfolded prion proteins attach to one another and accumulate within cells. While every tissue in the body can harbor the misfolded protein, accumulation of it within cells of the central nervous system causes symptoms and, eventually, death. In humans, the most common manifestation of prion protein infection is Creutzfeldt–Jakob disease. Similar diseases, collectively called *transmissible spongiform encephalopathy*, occur in sheep, cows, and deer, and it is thought that humans can acquire this type of encephalopathy through ingestion of infected meat. In all affected animals, including humans, the disease is rapidly progressive, consisting of a decline in mental function, inability to stand, loss of interest in food, and, over the course of weeks to months, death.

This chapter has provided a survey of infectious diseases, briefly discussing the characteristics of bacteria, viruses, fungi, protozoa, helminths, and prion protein, providing examples of the more common infectious agents or ones that are illustrative of particular processes, and listing characteristics of many infectious agents and diseases in tables throughout. The chapter is quite long, yet the reader has been given only a small glimpse into the multifaceted world of infectious agents, their life cycles and pathogenetic mechanisms, the diseases they produce, and the immune response to them. Infectious agents causing diseases in particular organ systems are discussed in later chapters, and it is hoped that with this brief introduction the subsequent discussions will be made more relevant and understandable. The websites of the Centers for Disease Control and Prevention (CDC) and the World Health Organization (WHO) are excellent resources for anyone interested in more in-depth discussions of the organisms briefly described in this chapter.

Practice Questions

1. An organism that transmits a pathogen to a human or animal is termed a(n)
   A. carrier.
   B. saprophyte.
   C. vector.
   D. protozoan.
   E. arthropod.

2. Which of the following is the most common reportable infection in humans in the United States?
   A. AIDS
   B. Gonorrhea
   C. Hepatitis
   D. Chlamydia
   E. Upper respiratory tract infection

3. In humans, 80% of all infections occur in which organ system?
   A. Respiratory
   B. Gastrointestinal
   C. Urinary tract
   D. Skin

4. A 26-year-old woman develops skin abscesses that are resistant to treatment with methicillin. What is the most likely pathogen?
   A. *Staphylococcus aureus*
   B. *Escherichia coli*
   C. *Haemophilus influenzae*
   D. Group A streptococcus

5. What is an emerging infectious disease?
   A. An infectious disease that is showing initial manifestations in a patient
   B. An infectious disease that is newly described in a population or increasing in incidence
   C. An infectious disease that requires emergency measures to bring it under control
   D. Usually an opportunistic infection
   E. Usually caused by bacteria

6. Which of the following common diseases of childhood is not caused by a virus?
   A. Whooping cough
   B. Mumps
   C. Chickenpox
   D. Rubella
   E. Measles

7. A 19-year-old woman complains of a sore throat, weakness, and lethargy developing over 2 weeks. Her physician finds an enlarged spleen and lymph nodes. Her laboratory examination reveals atypical lymphocytes. What is most likely to be her diagnosis?
   A. Cytomegalovirus disease
   B. AIDS
   C. Herpes simplex infection
   D. Infectious mononucleosis
   E. Histoplasmosis

8. Which of the following is most likely to be an opportunistic fungal infection?
   A. Histoplasmosis
   B. Rhizopus
   C. Coccidioidomycosis
   D. Blastomycosis

Immunologic Diseases

OUTLINE

OBJECTIVES

1. Define and describe antigens and antibodies.
2. Compare B lymphocytes and T lymphocytes in terms of function.
3. List the major functions of each of the five classes of immunoglobulins.
4. Describe the four major types of allergy and give examples of each.
5. Describe the tests or procedures described in this chapter that are helpful in evaluation of a patient with allergy or immune deficiency (e.g., serum electrophoresis, serum immunodiffusion, immunofluorescent tests, ANA test, skin tests, complement fixation test, Coombs test).
6. List the causes, lesions, and major manifestations of each of the specific immune diseases discussed in this chapter.
7. Compare deficiencies of the immunoglobulins from those of the T-cell immune system.
8. Compare hay fever and asthma in terms of cause, lesions, manifestations, and complications.
9. Understand how transfusion reactions are diagnosed and how they are prevented.
10. Describe the basic lesion common to the delayed hypersensitivity diseases.
11. Define and use in context all terms in bold print in this chapter.

KEY TERMS

adaptive immune system
agammaglobulinemia
allergy
anaphylactic-atopic allergy
anaphylaxis
angioedema
antigen
antigen-presenting
  cell (APC)
antinuclear antibody (ANA)
Arthus-type hypersensitivity
asthma
autoimmune disease

B lymphocyte
blood transfusion reactions
complement
contact dermatitis
cross-matching
cytotoxic T cells
cytotoxic-type
  hypersensitivity
delayed hypersensitivity
direct Coombs test
electrophoresis
eosinophilia
epitope

erythroblastosis fetalis
glomerulonephritis
graft-versus-host disease
hapten
hay fever
hypersensitivity reaction
hypogammaglobulinemia
IgA
IgD
IgE
IgG
IgM
immune complex
immune surveillance
immunity
immunodiffusion
immunofluorescence
immunoglobulin
immunohistochemistry
indirect Coombs test
innate immunity
major histocompatibility complex (MHC)
memory cells
natural killer (NK) cells
opsonization
plasma cells
polyarteritis nodosa
rheumatoid factor (RF)
secondary response
serum sickness
status asthmaticus
systemic lupus erythematosus
T-helper cells
T lymphocytes
T suppressor cells
Type I allergy
Type II allergy
Type III allergy
Type IV allergy
typing
urticaria

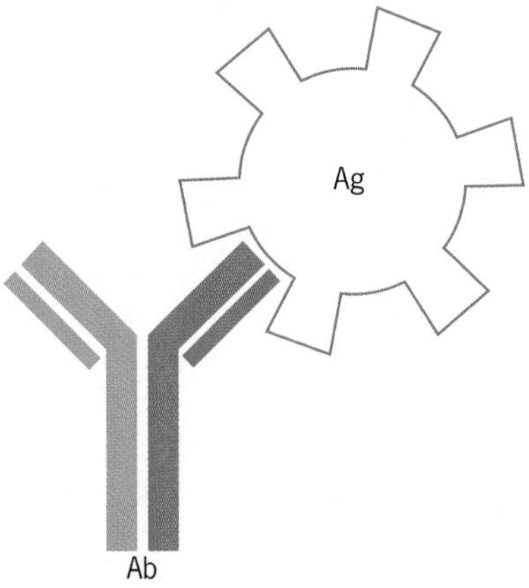

FIGURE 27–1 Schematic representation of antigen (Ag) with epitope, and antibody (Ab).

Review of Structure and Function

Immunity is a term that means the resistance to or protection from an individual's environment. Certain forms of protection, such as the skin and the inflammatory response, are considered **innate immunity** and are discussed in other chapters. The **adaptive immune system** is an internal chemical system whose purpose is to enhance specific reactivity to materials (predominantly proteins) that are foreign to the body. The innate and adaptive immune systems are linked in a way that allows general protective responses to become more specific to the offending agent. This chapter is devoted to the adaptive immune system.

Material recognized as foreign by the immune system is called an **antigen**. The site on the antigen to which an antibody binds is called an **epitope**. One antigen can have several epitopes. Most antigens are introduced from outside of the body, but some are altered endogenous materials that are treated as if they were foreign. The immunologic system recognizes antigens by producing antibodies or specialized lymphocytes specific for each antigen (**Figure 27–1**). Large foreign particles, such as bacteria, contain several antigens (with possibly many epitopes) and may elicit the production of several different antibodies. Also, several different foreign chemicals or materials may contain the same antigen; for example, some persons have the same antigen in heart muscle that exists in group A streptococci.

Antigens are classified as either complete or incomplete. Complete antigens both induce immune responses and react with the antibodies produced by the immune response. Incomplete antigens can react with antibodies but cannot induce an immune response unless chemically coupled to another antigen. Incomplete antigens are also called **haptens**. Antibodies are produced within the cytoplasm of **plasma cells**, which are derived from lymphocytes. Antibodies produced by plasma cells are released into the blood, where they circulate freely as part of the gamma globulin fraction of serum proteins and are called **immunoglobulins**. The lymphocytes that are capable of developing into plasma cells to produce immunoglobulins are called **B lymphocytes** or B cells. B cells originate from lymphoid tissue of the gastrointestinal tract and bone marrow.

A second type of lymphocyte is the **T lymphocyte** or T cell, so named because its production is programmed by the thymus. T lymphocytes and B lymphocytes are similar morphologically in ordinary tissue sections; specialized tests are required to distinguish them. They are both capable of recognizing specific epitopes on antigens.

There are several known functions of T cells, and subtypes of T cells are named to reflect their function. Some **T-helper cells** physically deliver information about antigens to B cells to aid B cells in the production of antibodies, whereas other T cells primarily aid macrophages in carrying out delayed hypersensitivity functions. **T suppressor cells** suppress other T cells to down-regulate the immune response and suppress B cells to prevent the production of excess antibody; they also prevent the production of antibodies to the body's own tissues. **Cytotoxic T cells** can directly kill other cells that process foreign or altered antigens, such as neoplastic cells or cells infected with viruses. Another class of lymphocytes, **natural killer (NK) cells**, destroy other cells in the absence of any known antigenic stimulation, possibly by reacting with glycoproteins on the target cells' surface. It is hypothesized that the body continually develops neoplastic cell lines, but that NK cells destroy these neoplastic cells before they can accumulate to form neoplasms. This type of police action by NK cells is termed **immune surveillance**. There is probably some overlap in function of each of the T-cell types.

Antigens are usually broken down (processed) and then presented to T cells by macrophages, dendritic cells, or other specialized cells collectively called **antigen-presenting cells (APCs)**. The antigen is cradled on the APC surface by special **major histocompatibility complex (MHC)** molecules (**Figure 27–2**). Once a T cell with a specific receptor for a particular antigen acknowledges the antigen, it will either help program a group of B cells to produce antibody, suppress the production of antibody, or directly kill a foreign cell, depending on whether it has helper, suppressor, or cytotoxic function. The concept of specific antigenic receptors on T cells implies that there must be countless different T cells in the normal body to accommodate the almost infinite number of potential antigens. This indeed appears to be the case and is a very functional aspect of immunity because if the possibility of T-cell cross-reactivity with different antigens were great, then the possibility of self-reactivity would also be great, resulting in autoimmune phenomena.

In addition to their role in the regulatory mechanisms already outlined, T cells work in cooperation with B cells in other ways to increase the specificity of the immunoglobulin to the antigen. T cells also elaborate numerous cytokines with various functions in acute and chronic inflammation, including recruitment of other cells.

About 10 days after the first encounter with an antigen, antibodies become detectable. Subsequent encounters with the same antigen are associated with a more rapid production of antibodies called the **secondary response**. Certain lymphocytes serve as **memory cells**, which means that they are long-lived and are programmed to proliferate rapidly after a second encounter with that antigen.

Immunoglobulins carry out their function in several ways, depending on the structure of the antigen and the class of antibody involved. Immunoglobulins are divided into five classes (IgA, IgG, IgM, IgD, and IgE) based on their biologic properties and major differences in their protein structure. IgG and IgM, the most common, are schematized in **Figure 27–3**.

IgG, the most abundant immunoglobulin, can combine with antigens such as bacterial exotoxins to neutralize their activity, or it can adhere to antigens on the surface of larger foreign materials such as bacteria to promote their phagocytosis by leukocytes, a process called **opsonization**. IgG is particularly important for infants, who have an immature immune system. IgG antibodies are transmitted across the placenta to the fetus from the mother; thus, the infant is protected during its first 6 months of life from diseases previously encountered by the mother. The combination of IgG with antigen sometimes employs another reaction, called complement activation. **Complement** is a group of special serum proteins that often take part in antigen–antibody reactions. Activation of complement is a complex series of enzymatic reactions that has at least three important effects: proteins are produced that may lyse (rupture) cells, mediators are released that may in turn cause release of histamine from mast cells, and chemotactic agents are

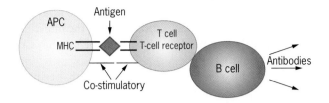

FIGURE 27–2 Antigen presentation. The antigen-presenting cell (APC) cradles the antigen in the peptide arms of the MHC molecule, allowing engagement by the T-cell receptor. The T cell then passes information about the antigen to the B cell. Co-stimulatory molecules from both cells have to be engaged for the T cell to pass on the complete message. If the MHC is class II, it will engage a T-helper cell; if it is class I, it will engage a cytotoxic T cell.

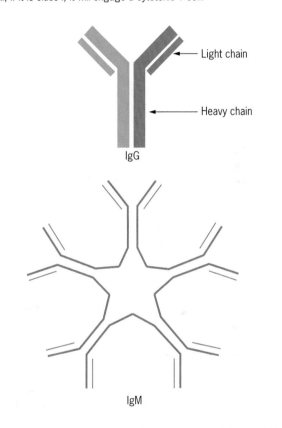

FIGURE 27–3 Basic structures of immunoglobulins G (IgG) and M (IgM). IgM is the equivalent of five IgG molecules.

produced that may attract leukocytes. The first effect can destroy cells that are recognized as foreign; the other two effects initiate the vascular and cellular components of acute inflammation, respectively.

IgM antibodies are noteworthy for their large size, which is five times that of IgG antibodies (referred to as a pentamer) (Figure 27–3). IgM antibodies do not readily pass into the tissues or across the placenta. They develop more quickly than do IgG antibodies following antigenic stimulation, and they are important in controlling bacteria that enter the bloodstream and in agglutination (clumping) of large foreign substances such as incompatible red blood cells. IgM antibody reactions may also activate complement.

IgA is noteworthy because it is secreted into body fluids such as tears, milk, saliva, bronchi, and the intestinal tract, where it may interact with antigens before they can enter the body's tissues.

IgE acts in a very specific manner. IgE becomes attached to basophils in the bloodstream and mast cells in tissues. When antigen reacts with IgE on the surface of basophils or mast cells, the cells release vasoactive substances such as histamine. IgE reactions are often associated with increased numbers of eosinophils in tissue and blood, presumably because antigens binding IgE release chemotaxins for eosinophils.

IgD serves as an antigen receptor on the surface of mature B cells (along with IgM).

Thus, immunoglobulins can protect the body from antigenic foreign materials in a variety of ways, including precipitating or neutralizing the chemical action of small foreign materials, agglutinating larger foreign materials so that they can be phagocytosed, and lysing foreign cells (**Figure 27–4**). Immunoglobulins can also initiate an acute inflammatory reaction to control the spread of and destroy certain foreign agents, and they can combine with foreign substances on body surfaces to prevent their entry into the body.

The MHC genetically controls the expression of both self and foreign antigens on cell surfaces of most cells in the body. This system in humans is located on genes in the sixth chromosome and is very similar to the ABO blood system in which different individuals express different red cell surface antigens. Just as it is important to ensure that transfused blood is given to recipients who are of the same ABO type as the donor, so organ transplants such as kidney, skin, or bone marrow must share similar MHC antigens between donor and recipient. If the antigens are not similar, the recipient's immune system will recognize a transplanted organ as foreign and produce antibodies and/or cytotoxic T cells to destroy

it. Conversely, donor lymphocytes, transplanted with an organ into an incompatible host, can, under certain circumstances, mount an attack against the recipient's tissues. This phenomenon is referred to as **graft-versus-host disease**.

T cells cannot process an antigen unless it is presented to the T cells in conjunction with products of the MHC, referred to as HLA molecules. For example, a macrophage presenting an antigen to a T cell must carry on its surface, combined with the foreign antigen, certain HLA proteins that the T cells can recognize as similar to their own. Otherwise, the T cell cannot recognize the antigen as foreign. This is referred to as MHC restriction (Figure 27–2). The reasons for this restriction are not entirely known, but it likely serves as a link in programming B cells to produce antibodies.

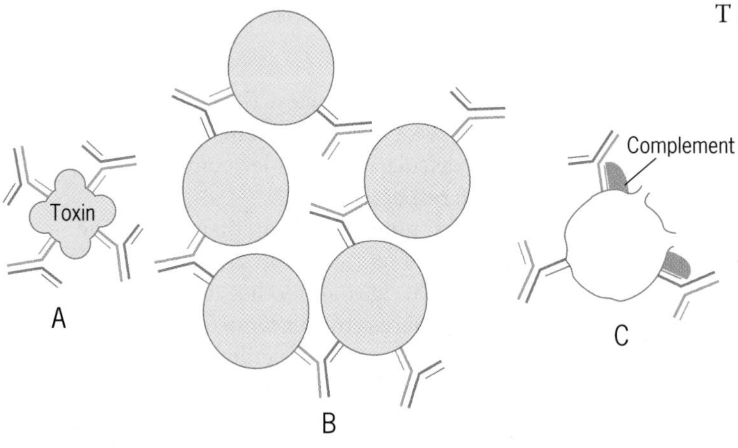

Classification of Immunologic Diseases

Immune reactions are generally protective and helpful. However, in certain circumstances, they can be more harmful than helpful, in which case they produce disease. Immune diseases fall into two major categories: immune deficiency diseases, in which there is too little response to foreign agents, and **allergy** or **hypersensitivity reactions**, in which there is too much response to antigens. The term *hypersensitivity* is slightly broader than the term *allergy* and may include some exaggerated responses that are not antigen–antibody mediated or are of unknown cause. Hypersensitivity reactions to the body's own components mediated by lymphocytes and/or antibodies are called autoimmune diseases.

Immune deficiency diseases are subdivided into inherited and acquired forms and into deficiencies of the T-cell and B-cell immune systems, or both.

The four major types of allergy (hypersensitivity) are divided on the basis of mechanisms. The first three types involve immunoglobulins, and the fourth type involves T lymphocytes.

Type I allergy, called **anaphylactic-atopic allergy**, includes those reactions mediated by IgE antibody and involves release of vasoactive chemicals from tissue mast cells or blood basophilic leukocytes (**Figure 27–5**). The reaction occurs within minutes; hence, it is sometimes designated as immediate hypersensitivity. It is virtually the same reaction as the initial stage of the acute inflammatory reaction.

Type II allergy, called **cytotoxic-type hypersensitivity**, involves destruction of host cells either by agglutination and phagocytosis or by lysis of the cell membrane as a consequence of complement fixation (**Figure 27–6**). Red blood cells are commonly targets of this type of hypersensitivity, and the antigens are either the red blood cell membrane itself or a foreign chemical, such as a drug, that adheres to the red

FIGURE 27–4 Neutralizing **(A)**, agglutination **(B)**, and lysing **(C)** actions of immunoglobulins.

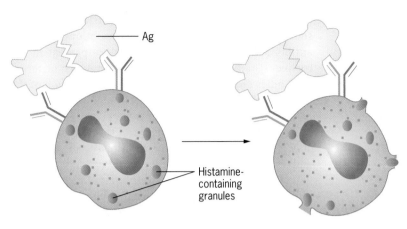

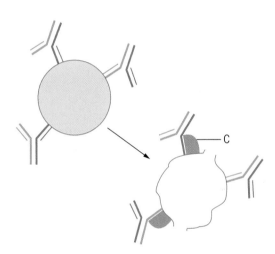

FIGURE 27–5 Pathogenesis of type I allergic reaction. Antigen reacts with antibody attached to mast cells by cross-linking two IgE molecules (or receptors) to cause release of histamine from granules.

FIGURE 27–6 Type II allergic reaction with lysis of red blood cells. Antibody reacts with cell-surface antigens, resulting in complement fixation (c) and cell lysis.

cell membrane as a hapten. The reaction may be either immediate or prolonged.

Type III allergy, called **immune complex** or **Arthus-type hypersensitivity**, is defined as a complement-mediated reaction to precipitates of antigen and antibody (antigen–antibody complexes). The antigen–antibody complexes lodge in vessel walls, and the activation of certain inflammation-inducing components of complement (C3a, C5a) results in release of vasoactive substances from mast cells and attraction of polymorphonuclear leukocytes to the site (**Figure 27–7**). The acute inflammatory reaction takes several hours to develop and may be prolonged if the amount of antibody is small. Excess of antigen over antibody is required to produce the reaction because complete binding of all

antigens by antibodies inhibits complement activation.

Type IV allergy, called **delayed hypersensitivity** or cell-mediated hypersensitivity, is the harmful destruction of tissue by T lymphocytes and macrophages (**Figure 27–8**). Lymphocyte-mediated reactions are slow to develop, usually requiring 1 to 2 days to reach a peak—hence the name *delayed hypersensitivity*.

The mechanism of many diseases likely comprises two or more of the four types of hypersensitivity. Moreover, there are numerous other allergic diseases that cannot be subclassified on the basis of mechanism because the mechanism is not known. Many autoimmune diseases and drug reactions fall into the unclassified category.

The principal criteria that separate allergic from non-allergic reactions to foreign substances are as follows:

1. The initial reaction in an allergic disease requires approximately 10 days, the time required for antibody production; subsequent responses recur immediately for immunoglobulin-mediated allergies and in 1 to 2 days for cell-mediated allergies. The reaction time for nonallergic responses to

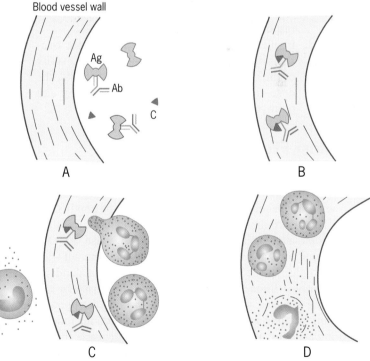

FIGURE 27–7 Pathogenesis of type III allergic reaction. Antigen and antibody form complexes (**A**) in the presence of excess antigen. The complexes are deposited in the vessel wall and fix complement (**B**). Activated components of complement cause release of vasoactive materials from mast cells and chemotaxis of polymorphonuclear leukocytes (**C**). The end result is acute inflammation and destruction of the vessel wall (**D**).

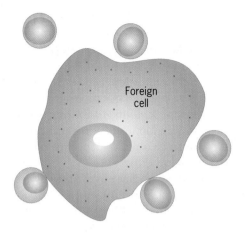

FIGURE 27–8 Pathogenesis of type IV allergic reaction. Sensitized T lymphocytes attack foreign cells.

foreign materials is constant and dependent on the nature of the offending agent rather than on an allergic mechanism. For example, chemical injuries may be immediate, inflammatory reactions may take several hours, and hyperplastic responses may take days to weeks or more.

2. Allergic diseases tend to occur only in selected susceptible individuals, while other foreign substances tend to affect people without bias. Multiple genetic and environmental factors appear to be involved in the selected susceptibility to allergens (antigens). Most people have the protective responses, but a few have the harmful responses to antigens.

3. In allergic diseases, there is usually a poor relationship between dose of allergen and severity of the reactions, whereas with other agents, the dose–injury relationship is more often linear and quite predictable.

Most Frequent and Serious Problems

Among type I hypersensitivity reactions, atopic allergies are most frequent, affecting about 10% of the population. The most common example is hay fever (allergic rhinitis). Atopic allergies are chronic reactions because they are caused by exposure to antigens in the environment—for example, ragweed pollen, house dust, or animal danders. Allergic asthma, another atopic reaction caused by the same antigens, affects approximately 3% of the population. Anaphylactic reactions are acute reactions following a distinct reexposure to an antigen. Urticaria (hives) is a common form and may be the result of food allergy or drug reaction. A more severe and immediately life-threatening form of type I hypersensitivity is anaphylactic shock, a condition in which vasoactive substances are released systemically. Drugs and insect stings are the most common causes of anaphylactic shock.

The most common types of cytotoxic (type II) hypersensitivity reactions are **transfusion reactions**, in which antibodies to transfused blood cells are present in the recipient, and erythroblastosis fetalis, in which maternal antibodies cross the placenta to cause destruction of the infant's red blood cells.

Immune complex hypersensitivities (type III) are both common and very complicated, and they vary considerably in terms of the exact mechanisms, tissue involved, and severity. Frequent types are serum sickness, which is usually a drug reaction, and some types of glomerulonephritis. Cryoglobulinemia associated with hepatitis C is a common immune complex disorder that causes vasculitis and glomerulonephritis. Glomerulonephritis associated with lupus erythematosus is most likely an immune complex hypersensitivity reaction with DNA/anti-DNA antibodies found in glomerular tissue.

Allergic contact dermatitis is the most common type of delayed hypersensitivity (type IV) reaction, and poison ivy is the most common specific cause. Graft rejection, following a skin graft or renal transplant, is an example of delayed hypersensitivity in which the donor and recipient tissue antigens are incompatible.

Immune deficiencies are much less common than allergies are. Inherited immune deficiencies, whether of the B-cell or T-cell immune systems, are rare but particularly significant because they lead to repeated, severe infections in the first few years of life and are often fatal. Acquired immune deficiencies are more common than inherited forms and vary in severity from mild to severe. Causes include disseminated hematopoietic diseases such as leukemia or lymphoma, cancer chemotherapy, and immunosuppressive drug therapy, which is used to protect transplanted organs from being rejected as foreign tissue. Acquired immune deficiency syndrome (AIDS) is a frequent result of T-helper cell immunodeficiency caused by HIV infection.

Symptoms, Signs, and Tests

The clinical manifestations of immune disease are quite varied and often unique to the specific types of diseases as well as to the organ system involved. Consequently, clinical manifestations are discussed in relation to specific diseases.

Many laboratory tests have been devised to aid in the diagnosis of immune diseases. The amount of gamma globulin in the blood can be measured by **electrophoresis** of serum (**Figure 27–9**). Immunoglobulin and complement (C3, C4) levels can be measured by nephelometry, which uses the principle of scattered light. The five specific types of immunoglobulin are usually measured by **immunodiffusion** tests in which prepared antibodies are reacted against IgG, IgA, IgM, IgE, and IgD. The reaction product precipitates in a gel medium and can then be stained and measured. These tests are most

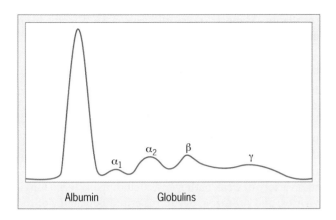

FIGURE 27–9 Normal serum proteins as measured by serum electrophoresis test.

important in the evaluation of relative and absolute immune deficiencies.

The components of complement can also be measured by immunodiffusion. A decreased level of complement is inferential evidence that a type II or III reaction has taken place.

The most important tests for diagnosing type I anaphylactic-atopic allergies are skin tests, in which a suspected antigen, such as a drug, house dust, cat hair, seafood, dander, or ragweed pollen, is injected into the skin. Allergy to a specific antigen is manifested immediately as a small inflammatory reaction at the site of injection. Hundreds of different antigens have been isolated and can be used for such skin tests.

Cytotoxic (type II reactions) antibodies on erythrocytes are demonstrated by the **direct Coombs test** in which antihuman gamma globulin is added to a test tube

of washed erythrocytes. If the erythrocytes have been coated with cytotoxic or other antibodies, they will agglutinate upon addition of the antihuman gamma globulin (**Figure 27–10**). The **indirect Coombs test** detects serum antibodies having the potential to react with erythrocytes. In this test, the patient's serum is first incubated with another person's erythrocytes in a test tube to allow the antierythrocyte antibodies to coat the erythrocytes. The test then proceeds in the same fashion as the direct Coombs test. Similar tests are less commonly performed to demonstrate antibodies to white cells or platelets.

Immune complex (type III) diseases are often diagnosed on the basis of history plus the clinical picture of the disease. However, the deposition of antigen–antibodies and complement in tissues may be tested for by **immunofluorescence**. In this test, a section of tissue (biopsy) from a diseased organ is overlain with fluorescent-tagged antibodies to specific immunoglobulin or complement. The fluorescent-tagged antibody will form a complex with the deposited immunoglobulin or complement (usually in vessels) and fluoresce a bright yellow-green color under special blue light (**Figure 27–11**). This test is used routinely on kidney biopsies to separate the various types of glomerulonephritis.

Testing for antigens in tissue is also accomplished by **immunohistochemistry**. A section of tissue is placed on a glass slide and overlain with antibodies that bind to the suspected antigen. The antibodies are "tagged" with a chemical expressing a specific visible color (chromogen). The presence of the antigen can then be visualized by light microscopy.

Delayed (cell-mediated) hypersensitivity to microorganisms such as occurs in tuberculosis and fungal diseases can be evaluated by skin tests in which the antigen (killed microorganisms) is injected into the skin and,

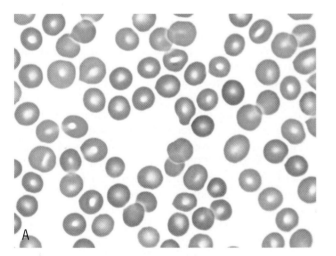
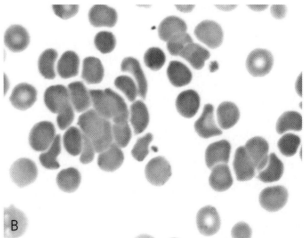

FIGURE 27–10 Agglutination. **A** shows red blood cells as they normally appear on a smear: as individual units, separate from one another. (Courtesy of Dr. David Yang, Department of Pathology and Laboratory Medicine, University of Wisconsin School of Medicine and Public Health.) In **B**, red blood cells are clumped together because antibodies in the recipient's serum have reacted to antigens on the surface of the donor's red blood cells. If this were to happen *in vivo*, the patient would suffer rapid and severe hemolysis. (Courtesy of Luis Brandi, MD, Department of Pathology and Laboratory Medicine, University of Wisconsin School of Medicine and Public Health.)

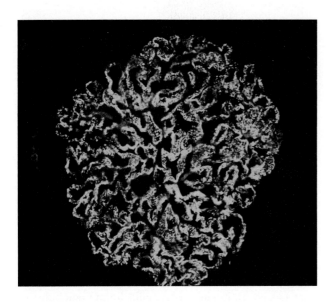

FIGURE 27–11 IgG antibodies in renal glomerulus demonstrated by immunofluorescence. (Courtesy of Dr. Weixiong Zhong, Department of Pathology, University of Wisconsin School of Medicine and Public Health)

when positive, a delayed (48 to 72 hours) inflammatory reaction ensues. Contact dermatitis is most often diagnosed by good detective work, but suspected allergens may be tested by placing them on the skin (patch test).

Autoimmune diseases are varied and complex, and their clinical features often overlap. Laboratory tests are confirmatory and best used when the pretest probability is high (clinical features suggest autoimmune disease prior to ordering the test). The **antinuclear antibody (ANA)** test detects antibodies against nuclei of tissue cells that are found in the serum of patients with autoimmune disease. The ANA test is elevated in most patients with connective tissue disease, including 98% of patients with systemic lupus erythematosus (SLE). However, the ANA may be abnormal in many other disease states (infection, cancer, drug induced), so it is not specific. There are other antibodies, such as anti-double-stranded DNA, Sm, and RNP, that are more specific for SLE. In rheumatoid arthritis, the detection of **rheumatoid factor (RF)** supports the diagnosis made on clinical features of the disease.

Lymphocytes can be tested for subtypes when this information is necessary. An example is in the diagnosis of AIDS, in which the T-helper subtype (CD4) concentration is disproportionately low.

Specific Diseases

Immune diseases are the result of excessive or deficient antibody or cellular immune response. They can take many forms, including developmental, inflammatory, and neoplastic conditions involving various organ systems. Specific diseases in this chapter are classified into the immune deficiencies and the four basic types

of allergy. Many of these diseases have already been encountered in other chapters.

Immune Deficiency Diseases

Immune deficiencies are manifested as an increased susceptibility to infections—that is, more frequent and severe infections. If the deficiency is in the immunoglobulins (B-cell system), infections such as pneumonia, produced by pyogenic bacteria, occur. If the deficiency is in the cell-mediated immune system, infections produced by a variety of weak pathogens, including bacteria, fungi, viruses, and protozoa, occur. Inherited deficiency of the immunoglobulin system can be substantiated by finding very low levels of serum gamma globulin (**agammaglobulinemia**). In acquired forms, the levels are not usually as low (**hypogammaglobulinemia**). Deficiencies of the T-cell immune system are demonstrated by absence of skin reactivity to substances that commonly cause a delayed hypersensitivity reaction. A delayed hypersensitivity skin test is performed by placing the antigen in or on the skin and checking in 1 to 2 days for the typical raised, firm, delayed hypersensitivity reaction. A person with a positive skin test for tuberculosis may later revert to a negative skin test following an acquired deficiency of T cell–mediated immunity. T-cell deficiencies can also adversely affect antibody production if the deficiency involves T-helper cells.

Acquired Immune Deficiency Syndrome

Acquired immune deficiency syndrome (AIDS) is now the most important and severe form of acquired immune deficiency.

Anaphylactic-Atopic Allergies (Type I)

Anaphylactic-atopic allergies are caused by the release of chemicals called vasoactive amines. These substances include histamine from tissue mast cells or blood basophils, which produce the most immediate reaction, and other substances that cause slightly more delayed reactions. As a group, these substances produce the following effects: (1) contraction of most nonvascular smooth muscle, producing effects such as bronchial constriction leading to asthmatic breathing; (2) vasodilation, which locally leads to increased blood flow and systemically may lead to shock; (3) increased vascular permeability, which leads to edema such as is seen in the raised wheals of urticaria of the skin or the swollen nasal mucosa of hay fever; and (4) stimulation of secretory activity of some glands, such as the increased mucus secretion in the bronchus in asthma and increased nasal secretions in hay fever. A typical laboratory finding in this group of diseases is an increase in eosinophils in the blood or tissue. Thus, **eosinophilia** suggests atopic allergy, but it also may be found in some immune complex diseases. Potential atopic allergens may be evaluated by skin testing. A raised edematous lesion with a red border (wheal and flare) reaches a maximum about 15 minutes after intradermal injection of the allergen being tested.

Asthma and Allergic Rhinitis (Hay Fever)

Because many allergens are airborne, the respiratory tract is a common site for hypersensitivity reactions to them. The portion of the tract affected presumably reflects individual differences of unknown nature. Both rhinitis and asthma can be triggered by nonallergic mechanisms in susceptible individuals. **Asthma** involves the lungs and produces three effects: (1) bronchoconstriction, resulting from the contraction of the smooth muscle layers of bronchial and bronchiolar segments of the tract; (2) edema, resulting from vasodilation and increased permeability of bronchial vessels; and (3) increased secretion of thick, tenacious mucoid material. If secretions are not removed by expectoration, their accumulation can impede air flow. The chief mechanical difficulty experienced in bronchial asthma is increased resistance to air flow manifested by wheezing. Generally, attacks are episodic, but the occasional asthma patient may experience a persistence of symptoms for 24 hours or more and fail to respond to medication. This condition of prolonged and unresponsive asthmatic distress is termed **status asthmaticus**. The patient exhibits very labored breathing with great respiratory effort, dyspnea, harassing cough, and sometimes cyanosis. Anxiety is great, and sleeplessness, extreme fatigue, exhaustion, dehydration, and disorientation develop.

BOX 27–1   Asthma

Cause

Type I allergy

Lesions

Spasm of bronchi

Thickened bronchi with increased mucus and eosinophils

Manifestations

Wheezing

Dyspnea

Cough

Positive skin test to allergen (some cases)

When allergic rhinitis is of short duration (days to a few weeks) and seasonal, the term **hay fever** is used. The allergens of hay fever are seasonal plant pollens including ragweed pollen (late summer and early autumn) and tree and grass pollens (spring and early summer). Ubiquitous allergens, such as those found in house dust, may produce a chronic condition lasting the year round that may be aggravated by factors such as high humidity, irritating vapors, and upper respiratory tract infections. Allergic rhinitis is marked by edema and hypersecretion by the mucosal lining of the nasopharyngeal cavities,

producing partial blockage of the airways with intense nasal and postnasal discharge. The involved nasopharyngeal mucosa appears pale and swollen. Edema may affect the mucosa of the paranasal sinuses, reducing their drainage, and it may close the eustachian tube. Secondary infection and inflammation of the sinuses (sinusitis) and the middle ear (otitis media) may result. After many years, allergic nasal polyps may develop. These are masses of redundant edematous mucosa, which may obstruct breathing and occur more frequently with nonallergic (intrinsic) rhinitis and asthma.

BOX 27–2   Allergic Rhinitis

Cause

Type I allergy

Lesions

Edematous nasal mucosa with eosinophils

Nasal polyps (late)

Manifestations

Nasal discharge

Partial obstruction

Complicated by:
  Sinusitis
  Otitis media
  Nasal polyps

Positive skin test to allergen

Urticaria (Hives) and Angioedema

Urticaria is a type I allergy that is recognized on the skin by slightly raised, flat, well-demarcated, edematous patches with a congested border (wheal and flare). Urticaria develops rapidly after exposure to an allergen and is associated with pruritus. Urticaria may be caused by an anaphylactic reaction in the skin to allergens that may have been introduced into the skin (injected drugs or insect stings) or, more often, by allergens that have been ingested and distributed throughout the body after alimentary absorption. A great variety of foods are known to cause urticaria—shellfish, strawberries, and tomatoes being common examples. Some contain histamine or histamine-releasing substances, thus causing urticaria by a nonspecific mechanism rather than an IgE-mediated mechanism. Mosquito bites cause a wheal as a result of nonspecific irritants in the saliva of the mosquito, whereas stinging insects (mainly *Trymenoptera*) inject allergens into the skin with rear stingers rather than mouth parts. Most chronic urticaria is idiopathic.

Angioedema is a more extreme skin manifestation of immediate hypersensitivity than is urticaria. It also is an edematous eruption, but it is more widespread and involves the deep dermis. Often it affects the lips, tongue, face, or even the pharynx, perhaps blocking the airway. Its causes are similar to those of urticaria.

Systemic Anaphylaxis

Anaphylaxis is one of the true medical emergencies. Within seconds to minutes after exposure to the allergen, the patient feels an itching of the scalp, tongue, and throat followed by generalized flushing and headache. Difficulty in breathing begins and is joined shortly thereafter by precipitous drop in blood pressure and body temperature. Shock and loss of consciousness occur within a short time. If early reversal is not instituted, the train of events may lead to death from shock within 15 minutes of allergic exposure. Treatment is immediate subcutaneous administration of epinephrine, which causes vasoconstriction, thereby reversing systemic shock. The more common allergens that cause anaphylaxis are pollens, foods, chemicals, venoms from stinging insects, foreign sera such as diphtheria or tetanus antitoxins, and drugs such as penicillin.

Gastrointestinal Food Allergies

Primary allergic reactions in the gastrointestinal tract are less common than skin reactions. A gastrointestinal reaction begins shortly after eating specific foods to which the person is allergic. Symptoms include diarrhea, vomiting, and cramps. Shellfish contain common allergens that can produce this reaction.

Cytotoxic Hypersensitivities (Type II)

Cytotoxic hypersensitivity reactions are usually manifested by low levels of specific types of blood cells because antibodies may form against red blood cells, platelets, or white blood cells and produce anemia, thrombocytopenia, or leukopenia, respectively. The direct Coombs test is used to detect antibodies on the surface of red blood cells.

Erythroblastosis Fetalis

The hemolytic disorder of the newborn known as **erythroblastosis fetalis** is caused by immunologic incompatibility between mother and child and usually involves the Rh antigen of red blood cells. This antigen is expressed as an autosomal dominant trait present on the erythrocytes of 85% of the population. When the fetus is Rh positive and the mother Rh negative, after delivery the mother will develop anti-Rh antibodies because some of the fetal erythrocytes will enter the mother's circulation at the time of birth. Consequently, the first pregnancy of a woman with an Rh-incompatible fetus is uncomplicated. If the sensitized mother has a subsequent pregnancy with an Rh-positive child, the transplacental passage of IgG brings anti-Rh to the child's blood. By the time of birth, the child has suffered from continuous hemolysis and may be jaundiced from excess bilirubin, as well as anemic and edematous. The hemolysis is often accentuated just after birth, at which time the infant no longer has the help of the placenta in removing bilirubin. Consequently, blood of the infant is often exchanged for Rh-negative blood in an exchange transfusion. Erythroblastosis fetalis can be prevented by injecting mothers with human gamma globulin containing anti-Rh antibodies within 72 hours after delivery of the first and subsequent Rh-positive children. This binds the antigens on the fetal red blood cells so that the mother's immune system does not recognize them as antigenic and, therefore, does not produce antibodies. Because of this now routine preventive measure, erythroblastosis fetalis is not nearly as common as it once was.

Blood Transfusion Reactions

There are many different antigen systems in red blood cells, of which the ABO and Rh systems are most important. An Rh-negative individual does not have anti-Rh antibodies unless previously sensitized. A person with the A antigen on red blood cells has anti-B antibody as a natural phenomenon. Conversely, persons with blood group B have anti-A antibodies; those with O blood have both anti-A and anti-B; and those with AB have neither antibody. Because the antibodies are normally present, transfused blood with an ABO incompatibility will produce immediate hemolysis of the transfused red blood cells, resulting in fever, chills, and possible renal failure. These **blood transfusion reactions** are prevented by typing and cross-matching of blood before transfusion. **Typing** refers to checking for major (ABO and Rh) blood groups to make sure that they are not incompatible, and **cross-matching** refers to mixing samples of donor and recipient blood to see if an *in vitro* (test tube) reaction occurs because of an unsuspected antibody (Coombs test; Figure 27–10).

Autoimmune Hemolytic Anemia and Thrombocytopenia

Many spontaneously occurring hemolytic anemias and thrombocytopenias are cytotoxic-type hypersensitivity reactions. The reactions may be mild, with agglutinated cells being prematurely removed by the spleen. In mild types, splenectomy may control the disease. Autoimmune hemolytic anemias can be detected by the direct Coombs test, in which red cells coated with

an antibody are observed to agglutinate *in vitro* with the addition of antihuman globulin serum. Sometimes drugs attach to the cell surface and become part of the antigen, in which case the drug is a hapten.

Immune Complex, or Arthus-Type, Hypersensitivities (Type III)

Immune complex hypersensitivity reactions produce vasculitis and, as a secondary phenomenon, edema because of the release of vasoactive substances. The frequent involvement of renal glomeruli in immune complex diseases is often associated with loss of protein and red blood cells in the urine and variable degrees of renal failure. Involvement of joint surfaces leads to joint swelling. More severe forms result in a generalized vasculitis with involvement of many organs.

Arthus Reaction

Arthus reaction is the prototype of immune complex hypersensitivity reactions and is an experimental reaction and not a naturally occurring disease. Local injection of soluble antigen in an animal previously sensitized by the same antigen produces an acute inflammation at the site of inoculation. Histologically, the reaction shows evidence of cell necrosis, infiltration with neutrophils, and vasculitis, all sequelae of the acute inflammatory reaction.

Serum Sickness

Serum sickness is the prototype of a systemic Arthus-type or immune complex reaction. Classically, it occurred after injection of horse serum. The horse serum was used as a source of antibodies to toxins such as tetanus toxin or diphtheria; however, the protective effect was often offset by the harmful effect produced when the patient developed antibodies to the horse serum. The horse serum (antigen) circulates in the patient's blood for a long time. As antibodies begin to develop after about 10 days, antigen–antibody complexes form, lodge in small vessels, and elicit the immune complex reaction at many sites. Although horse serum is rarely used anymore, the same reaction can be seen with drugs such as penicillin. The name serum sickness has been retained, although it is no longer appropriate. Symptoms are fever, painful joints, enlarged lymph nodes and spleen, and frequently an allergic urticaria. Usually, after suspending administration of the offending material, the patient recovers with no permanent damage.

Glomerulonephritis

Some forms of acute and chronic **glomerulonephritis** are mediated by immune complex reactions resulting from lodging of antigen–antibody complexes in the basement membrane of glomeruli (Figure 27–11). One form of glomerulonephritis, poststreptococcal glomerulonephritis, develops in association with the immune response to

BOX 27-7   Serum Sickness

Causes

Type III allergy (immune complex)

Mediated by horse serum or drugs

Lesions

Immune complex deposition in small vessels, with acute vasculitis

Manifestations

Fever

Painful joints

Enlarged lymph nodes and spleen

Urticaria

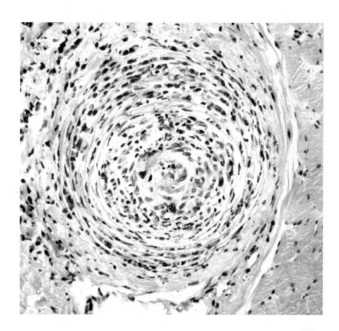

FIGURE 27-12 Polyarteritis nodosa. A cross section of a small artery; the vessel wall is intensely inflamed and necrotic. The lumen of the vessel is occluded by the necroinflammatory process.

infection by group A streptococci. The renal disturbance is first seen 1 to 4 weeks after apparent recovery from the acute streptococcal infection. Immune complexes are caught on the glomerular basement membrane, where they fix complement and promote an inflammatory process that compromises the filtering function of the glomerulus. The disease predominantly affects children, but some adults are also affected. Recovery is the rule, probably because the antigenic stimulation of the streptococcal infection subsides. Chronic glomerulonephritis results from a variety of antigens and is often low grade but persistent, eventually leading to renal failure.

Polyarteritis Nodosa

Polyarteritis nodosa is a severe but rare form of immune complex reaction producing widespread, multifocal, necrotizing vasculitis (**Figure 27–12**). It usually leads to organ failure and even fatal complications as a result of occlusion or rupture of vessels. The antigen is usually not identified, although hepatitis virus B or C is implicated in about 35% of cases. Medications, including penicillin, are occasionally implicated.

Delayed, or Cell-Mediated, Hypersensitivities (Type IV)

Delayed hypersensitivity reactions are manifested as subacute or chronic inflammation, with infiltration of the tissue by lymphocytes and macrophages and variable degrees of necrosis. The tuberculin skin test is an example of a typical subacute reaction, with development of a red, firm lump at the site of injection of tuberculin in a sensitized individual. The reaction reaches a peak at 2 days and gradually disappears. Contact dermatitis to a piece of jewelry is an example of a chronic reaction. Internal delayed hypersensitivity reactions are quite variable in appearance but are all characterized by a chronic inflammatory cell reaction, with predominance of lymphocytes and with variable degrees of tissue destruction. These

are often seen by the pathologist in tissues invaded by malignant neoplasms. The neoplastic cells carry antigens recognized as foreign that elicit delayed hypersensitivity.

Contact Dermatitis

Contact dermatitis is an acute or chronic delayed-type hypersensitive response to allergens placed on the skin surface. A notable example is poison ivy. However, the range of agents that cause contact dermatitis is very large and includes many topically applied drugs, cosmetics, paints, dyes, plastics, plants, and jewelry. The lesion varies from simple erythema discretely localized to the area of allergen contact to the more edematous, pruritic,

BOX 27-8   Contact Dermatitis

Causes

Type IV allergy (delayed hypersensitivity)

Caused by:

  Poison ivy (plants)

  Drugs

  Cosmetics

  Paints

  Dyes

  Jewelry

Lesions

Chronically inflamed skin

Manifestations

Skin erythema

Edema

Pruritus and vesicular eruptions

vesicular dermatitis seen with poison ivy. It is sometimes difficult to distinguish the reaction caused by direct irritants from that produced by allergens. Furthermore, it may be difficult to discover the allergen or to remove it from the environment once discovered. Treatment consists of removing the cause plus topical hydrocortisone ointments to reduce inflammation. If very severe, systemic steroids are sometimes used.

Infections Manifested Primarily as Delayed Hypersensitivity Reactions

Some microorganisms tend to stimulate cell-mediated immunity. Examples are the bacteria causing tuberculosis and leprosy, many fungi, and some viruses. A marshalling of sensitized T lymphocytes and macrophages into an infected tissue produces a picture of either chronic or granulomatous inflammation. In tuberculosis and fungal infection, the caseous necrosis is thought to be mediated by sensitized T lymphocytes. Manifestations of viral infections may be caused in part by delayed hypersensitivity reactions. Encephalitis occurring after a viral infection may also be a delayed hypersensitivity reaction.

Graft Rejection

The rejection of skin or a kidney grafted from one person to another is caused both by antibodies reacting against the tissue and by delayed hypersensitivity reaction. Different naturally occurring tissue antigens in the graft cause the development of sensitized lymphocytes in the person receiving the graft. The lymphocytes then can directly attack the graft and/or orchestrate the production of antibodies against the graft antigens. Such a reaction does not occur in identical twins because they have the same tissue antigens. Tissue typing, which is analogous to blood typing, is now used to match donor and recipient as closely as possible. The antigens that have to be matched between donor and recipient are histocompatibility antigens. Sometimes, lymphocytes in the graft proliferate after transplant and attack the recipient (host); this is referred to as graft-versus-host disease.

Autoimmune Diseases

Intolerance to self as a disease phenomenon requires an autoimmunization process in which sensitized lymphocytes or antibodies are developed against self-antigens. A number of relatively uncommon diseases appear to evolve as a result of such autoimmunization and its hypersensitive expression. Autoimmunity probably encompasses all four categories of hypersensitivity, but the most common types appear to be immune complex (type III) and hypersensitivity (type IV). Autoimmune hemolytic anemias are good examples of cytotoxic (type II) autoimmunity. A partial list of diseases thought to be autoimmune is given in **Table 27–1**. Of the numerous **autoimmune diseases**, only systemic lupus erythematosus is discussed here.

Systemic Lupus Erythematosus

Systemic lupus erythematosus (SLE), a moderately common systemic disease, may affect a number of different organ systems. A characteristic skin lesion, the butterfly rash, is an erythematous dermatitis that covers the bridge of the nose and extends bilaterally onto the cheeks (**Figure 27–13**). The skin is generally photosensitive; thus, rashes may appear after excessive exposure to sunlight. The joints may also be involved, producing complaints of arthritis. Muscles may become weak and atrophic. The kidneys develop a glomerulonephritis. The blood may show hypergammaglobulinemia, anemia, leukopenia, and thrombocytopenia. SLE predominantly affects young to middle-aged women and has a protracted but variable course that can end with renal insufficiency,

TABLE 27–1 Autoimmune Diseases

Disease	Organ or Tissue	Antigen
Hashimoto thyroiditis	Thyroid	Thyroglobulin
Pernicious anemia (vitamin B$_{12}$ deficiency)	Gastric mucosa	Intrinsic factor
Goodpasture syndrome	Kidney glomeruli and lung	Basement membrane
Autoimmune hemolytic anemia	Red cells	Red cell surface
Idiopathic thrombocytopenic purpura	Platelets	Platelet surface
Myasthenia gravis	Skeletal muscle	Acetylcholine receptors on muscle cells
Rheumatoid arthritis	Synovial membranes	Altered IgG
Systemic lupus erythematosus	Synovial membranes, kidney, skin, blood vessels	Many: DNA, DNA protein, RNA, cardiolipin
Multiple sclerosis	Brain white matter	Myelin proteins

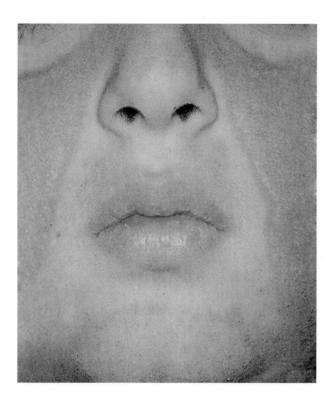

FIGURE 27–13 Butterfly rash of systemic lupus erythematosus.

bacterial endocarditis, cardiac failure, sepsis, or pneumonia. Neurologic problems including seizures or stroke may develop as a consequence of cerebral vasculitis or emboli from damaged heart valves. A number of different autoantibodies occur in lupus. The primary tissue damage is probably caused by cytotoxic antibodies and immune complexes, as well as by delayed hypersensitivity. Infiltrates of chronic inflammatory cells (lymphocytes and plasma cells) are found in many organs. Antinuclear antibody, an antibody directed against the body's own cell nuclei, provides the basis for the ANA test.

BOX 27–9   Systemic Lupus Erythematosus

Cause

Autoimmunity

Lesions

Varied: chronic inflammation in many organs

Manifestations

"Butterfly" rash

Photosensitivity

Arthritis

Muscle weakness

Glomerulonephritis

Anemia

Positive ANA, anti-double-stranded DNA, Sm, and RNP tests

Practice Questions

1. A 14-year-old boy complains of having episodes of sneezing and "runny" nose and generally feeling miserable every August and September. Skin tests are positive for ragweed pollen. This type of hypersensitivity is
   A. type I.
   B. type II.
   C. type III.
   D. type IV.

2. An infant does not suffer from any major infectious diseases during the first 6 months of her life. The most likely reason for this is because
   A. she is protected by her mother's IgM antibodies.
   B. she is protected by her mother's IgG antibodies.
   C. her immune system is at its strongest during her first 6 months.
   D. her parents have been careful to not expose her to infectious diseases.

3. A 28-year-old woman presents to her physician with a recent history of progressive weakness and a strange facial rash. She is found to have anemia, renal disease, and a positive ANA test. The type(s) of hypersensitivity this most likely represents is/are
   A. type IV.
   B. type III.
   C. types III and IV.
   D. types II, III, and IV.

4. Which of the following conditions is diagnosed by the cross-matching test?
   A. Asthma
   B. Transfusion reaction
   C. Contact dermatitis
   D. Urticaria

5. A 22-year-old man complains of a pruritic, red rash with small blisters underneath his watch band. This immune reaction is most likely mediated by
   A. IgG.
   B. lymphocytes.
   C. IgM.
   D. complement.
   E. cytotoxic T cells.

6. A type III hypersensitivity reaction always involves
   A. complement.
   B. IgM.
   C. mast cells.
   D. IgE.

7. Which of the following statements about erythroblastosis fetalis is true?
   A. The mother is Rh positive.
   B. The child is Rh negative.
   C. It occurs with the first pregnancy.
   D. The child suffers hemolysis of its red blood cells.

8. A 36-year-old woman who knows she is allergic to wasp venom is stung by a wasp. Within minutes she develops a severe headache, flushing of her face and neck, and difficult breathing followed by loss of consciousness and shock. This is an example of
   A. angioedema.
   B. serum sickness.
   C. anaphylaxis.
   D. autoimmune hemolytic anemia.

Physical Injury

OUTLINE

OBJECTIVES

1. Name and describe the three major categories of physical injury.
2. Identify the most common types of fatal accidents.
3. Understand the pathogenesis and appearance of contusions, abrasions, lacerations, and sharp force injuries.
4. Identify and describe the factors that determine the appearance and amount of damage caused by missile wounds.
5. Name the typical injuries of the abdomen, chest, spine, and head, and describe their complications.
6. Explain how the depth and extent of burns affect their course and treatment.
7. Describe the two major effects of electrical injury.
8. Describe the acute and chronic effects of sunlight, and exposure to extreme hot and cold temperatures.
9. Identify the tissues and neoplasms that are most and least sensitive to injury by radiation.
10. Describe the likely effects of a gradual rise in environmental radioactivity as compared to a massive nuclear accident.
11. Be able to define and use in context all words in headings and bold print throughout the chapter.

KEY TERMS

abrasion	paraplegia
abrasion collar	penetrating gunshot wound
contusion	perforating gunshot wound
decubitus ulcer	pneumothorax
electrical burn	quadriplegia
first-degree burn	radiosensitive
flail chest	second-degree burn
hemothorax	sharp force injury
herniation	stab wound
hypothermia	third-degree burn
incised wound	tracheostomy
laceration	trauma
malignant hyperpyrexia	ultraviolet radiation
manner of injury	

Most Frequent and Serious Problems

Major external agents causing physical injury fall into three general categories—mechanical, thermal, and radiation. The term **trauma** refers to injury caused by extrinsic forces, particularly when associated with an accident or violence. Overall, trauma is the fifth leading cause of death in the United States and is the most common cause of death in persons younger than 44 years of age. Trauma accounts for about 7% of patient visits to a physician, with half of these visits involving fractures and lacerations. The five most common types of fatal accidents are shown in **Figure 28–1**. Overall, automobile accidents are the most frequent cause of serious traumatic injury. Firearms are the second most frequent cause, and most of these are suicides. Other traumatic injuries not listed in the figure include thermal injuries, including burns, which are a serious threat to life if they cover a large surface area of the body, and radiation. Sunlight is the most common source of radiation injury. Radiation from sunlight affects all people, but fair-skinned people who spend a lot of time outdoors, in the sun, are more susceptible to sunburn and chronic skin changes. Ionizing radiation (x-ray and gamma-ray) injuries are immediately lethal only at the epicenter of a major nuclear disaster. At lower doses, ionizing radiation induces the development of cancer (leukemia, lung cancer, and thyroid cancer are most common). At the doses used for treatment of neoplasia, it causes connective tissue injury such as fibrosis and thrombosis of local blood vessels. The complications resulting from radiation therapy for treatment of cancer are the most common types of injury related to ionizing radiation.

The pattern of mortality from traumatic injury changes with age, sex, and race. The most common fatal injuries in the pediatric age group involve suffocation, drowning, and poisoning, while in young adults, especially young adult males, motor vehicle injuries and firearms account for the majority of deaths. In older adults, motor vehicle accidents and firearms are still leading causes of death, but deaths resulting from falls become much more common. Motor vehicle accidents are more frequent in American Indian populations than in white or black, while firearm-related deaths are more common in black than American Indian or white populations. Men are more likely to be involved in firearm fatalities, while women are slightly more prone to deaths resulting from poisonings and falls.

Traumatic deaths are classified not just as to the cause of the injury but the **manner of injury**: accident, suicide, homicide, or undetermined. By far, the majority of traumatic injuries are accidental. Differentiating accidents from suicides is often difficult, and usually relies on a suicide note left by the deceased or statements from people who knew the deceased as to his or her state of mental health prior to the fatal injury. These statistics are used by law enforcement, public health, and the justice system to identify and remedy harmful behaviors and social injustices so as to prevent similar deaths in the future.

Mechanical Injuries
Types of Simple Wounds

The cause of simple wounds can often be determined by their appearance. Common types include contusion, abrasion, laceration, incision, and puncture wounds.

A **contusion** is a bruise, caused by crushing, dislocation, or disruption of subsurface tissue by a blunt instrument that does not penetrate or break the skin surface (**Figure 28–2**). Blood released from broken vessels has no outlet and pools in the damaged tissue, causing gross discoloration. A "black eye" is a typical example. As the blood cells are phagocytosed and degraded, the bruise changes color, from red to purple, green, and yellow. The rate at which these color changes occur is quite variable, so they cannot be used to accurately date when an injury occurred.

An **abrasion** is a scraping or scuffing of the skin surface without full-thickness loss of skin (**Figure 28–3**). A **laceration** is a tear in the surface caused by shearing of tissue, leaving irregular, ragged wound margins (**Figure 28–4**). If caused by impact from a blunt object, there may be abrasion along the margins. Vessels and nerves tend to "bridge" the gap because they stretch rather than tear in response to the shearing force. This is called tissue bridging and helps differentiate lacerations from incisions.

Sharp force injuries are caused by trauma from a sharp-edged instrument or object, such as a knife or broken glass. The two general types of sharp force injury are **incised wounds** (or cuts) and **stab wounds**. Incised wounds are longer than they are deep, and stab wounds are deeper than they are long. An incision is a skin defect that differs from a laceration in that it has smooth, regular

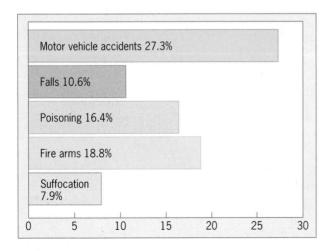

FIGURE 28–1 Percentage of traumatic deaths in the United States. (Data from the Centers for Disease Control and Prevention, 2002.)

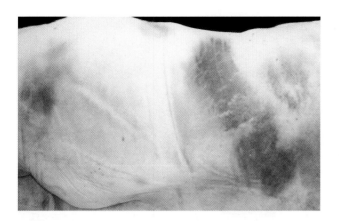

FIGURE 28–2 Contusion. Several contusions are present on the back, flank, and thigh. The yellow color around the periphery of especially the largest contusion indicates that this was incurred several days before the patient's death. (Courtesy of Dr. Robert F. Corliss, Department of Pathology and Laboratory Medicine, University of Wisconsin School of Medicine and Public Health.)

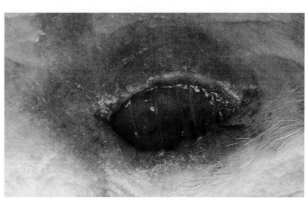

FIGURE 28–4 Laceration. This man fell forward onto the edge of a stair while suffering a cardiac arrest and incurred a laceration on his forehead, just above the eyebrow. This is not a lethal injury, but does indicate a forceful impact to the head. Note the stranding, or tissue bridging, across the base of the defect and the abrasion around it. (Courtesy of Dr. Robert F. Corliss, Department of Pathology and Laboratory Medicine, University of Wisconsin School of Medicine and Public Health.)

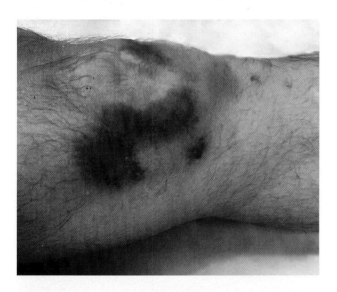

FIGURE 28–3 Abrasion. This knee was "skinned" or abraded several days before the man's death. The central area is covered with a crust, and the periphery is red. The injury here is superficial, the lower layers of the epidermis are still intact underneath the crust. (Courtesy of Dr. Robert F. Corliss, Department of Pathology and Laboratory Medicine, University of Wisconsin School of Medicine and Public Health.)

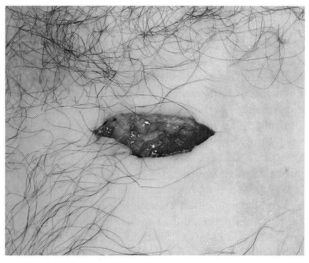

FIGURE 28–5 Incision. The wound has clean, sharp edges and is longer than it is deep. (Courtesy of Dr. Robert F. Corliss, Department of Pathology and Laboratory Medicine, University of Wisconsin School of Medicine and Public Health.)

edges (**Figure 28–5**). The underlying tissue, including blood vessels, is cleanly divided by the edge of the instrument. Thus, an incision has no bridging but more bleeding than a laceration.

Missile Wounds

A missile wound is a wound caused by a flying object such as a stone, arrow, or bullet. Gunshot wounds are the most common type. The nature of the injury produced by missiles depends on the mass of the object and the square of its velocity. Large, slowly moving missiles (such as the rotary blade of a lawnmower) produce much surface destruction and do not penetrate very deeply. High-velocity, small missiles such as rifle bullets may have a small entrance wound while producing much internal injury. The appearance of gunshot wounds, the location of entrance and exit wounds, and the location and extent of internal injury yield much information about the missile, type of gun, and its distance from the victim when it was shot.

A **penetrating gunshot wound** enters the body and does not exit, while a **perforating gunshot wound** passes through the body and leaves both entrance and exit defects. Distinguishing an entrance from an exit gunshot wound is not always easy. Entrance wounds often show an **abrasion collar** or ring, which is a marginal rim of abrasion around an entrance wound. This is caused by the projectile strafing the walls of a temporary tube of indented skin that forms following bullet impact and before skin penetration. Exit wounds are often slitlike or stellate in shape, but there is a wide variation in exit wound morphologies depending on projectile composition, integrity, positioning, and tissue properties.

Also important in examination of gunshot wounds is determination of range of fire (**Figure 28–6**). Gunshot wounds are broadly classified into contact, intermediate, and indeterminate ranges. Contact wounds may have a muzzle imprint or "stamp" from the end of the barrel (muzzle) being firmly applied to the skin at the time of discharge (Figure 28–6A). Other features of contact wounds include soot deposition or burning within or surrounding the entrance wound. Intermediate-range wounds by definition show stippling (Figure 28–6B), which consist of innumerable punctate abrasions of the skin around an entrance wound caused by unburned or burning gunpowder impacting the skin. The amount and pattern of stippling around a bullet wound depend on the distance the firearm was held from the skin, the length of the firearm barrel, the type of powder, the caliber of the weapon, and the load. In general terms, stippling occurs when the distance from the muzzle to the skin is no more than twice the length of the barrel, thus, a handgun must have been held closer to the victim than a rifle, if stippling is present. An intermediate-range gunshot wound results from a fairly close range shot—for most pistols generally less than 1 foot, and not beyond 3 to 6 feet. If the range of fire cannot be determined by wound examination because there is no evidence of contact or stippling, the wound is called indeterminate range (Figure 28–6C). This type of wound could have occurred from only a few inches away if there were an interposing object such as a leather jacket or windshield. The wound may also have been inflicted from several hundred feet away.

Types of Major Body Trauma

Major accidents, such as automobile accidents, often cause characteristic patterns of injury in various parts of the body. Injuries to the abdomen, chest, spine, and head are discussed here.

Abdominal Injury

Severe blows, sometimes even without any penetration, can produce significant injury to abdominal viscera. The most important effect of abdominal trauma is hemorrhage. Laceration or rupture of solid organs, such as the liver and spleen, is frequently seen in motor vehicle crashes and often leads to fatal internal hemorrhage. Internal injuries may go unrecognized until delayed complications arise. Fluid-filled and distended organs, such as

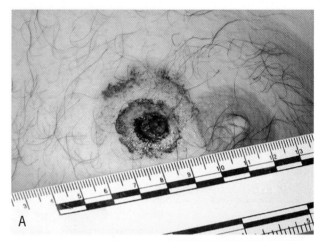

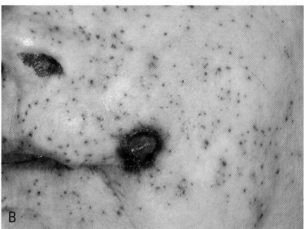

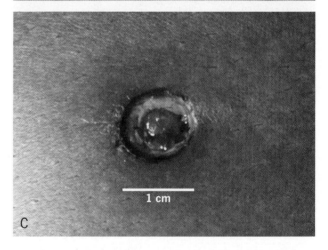

FIGURE 28–6 Range of fire of gunshot wounds. **A.** Contact gunshot wound. There is a "muzzle stamp" immediately around the wound. **B.** Intermediate-range gunshot wound. The skin around the entrance wound is "stippled," or covered with small abrasions resulting from gunpowder that spatters at the time of impact. **C.** Indeterminate-range gunshot wound. There is neither a muzzle stamp nor stippling around this entrance wound. (Courtesy of Dr. Robert F. Corliss, Department of Pathology and Laboratory Medicine, University of Wisconsin School of Medicine and Public Health.)

the bladder and the pregnant uterus, are prone to rupture with rapid pressure changes such as occur in automobile accidents. Because these serious abdominal injuries are likely to be fatal if not treated promptly, exploratory abdominal operations are often performed as a part of the diagnostic workup when serious abdominal injury is suspected.

Because of its muscularity, mobility, and serosal covering, the intestine may slide away from penetrating instruments such as needles, swords, and knives. If the intestines are ruptured, spillage of gastrointestinal contents into the peritoneal cavity causes an intense inflammatory reaction, or peritonitis, and the motility of the tract can become depressed, leading to functional obstruction, or ileus. Air may leak out of the ruptured viscus and accumulate under the diaphragm, where it can be detected by an abdominal x-ray.

Chest Injury

Major effects of chest trauma include fatal hemorrhage and interference with breathing. Fatal hemorrhage occurs from tears in the heart or great vessels produced by stab wounds, gunshot wounds, or rapid deceleration, as when the chest hits the steering wheel in an automobile accident. Laceration of the thoracic aorta following violent deceleration injuries in car crashes is not uncommon and is rapidly fatal because of the amount of blood lost in a short period of time.

Difficulty in breathing is produced by three mechanisms—obstruction of the tracheobronchial tree, material in the pleural space compressing the lungs, and multiple rib fractures resulting in an inability to move the chest cage, called **flail chest**. Obstruction of the tracheobronchial tree can be caused by accumulation of blood, an inhaled foreign body, or compression of the trachea. Creation of a surgical opening through the neck directly into the trachea (**tracheostomy**), and suction of the tracheal contents through it, can open the airway. The pleural space can traumatically become filled with air (**pneumothorax**) or blood (**hemothorax**). Either condition can be rapidly lethal. Hemothorax is caused by rupture of a blood vessel in the chest, such as the aorta or pulmonary artery. Open chest wounds must be closed to prevent sucking of air into the pleural space. A tube is placed in the pleural cavity under a water seal so that air is forced out of the pleural space with inhalation and cannot reenter the pleural space during expiration.

Flail chest caused by multiple rib fractures requires fixation of the sternum by wiring it to something external to prevent collapse of the chest with each inspiration. Artificial breathing may also be necessary. Severely displaced rib fractures result in sharp-edged rib fragments projecting into the chest cavity. These may cause pulmonary lacerations with hemorrhage, in which case a flail chest is complicated by a hemothorax and significant blood loss. Most deaths following automobile accidents are the result of chest trauma.

Spinal Injury

Fractures or extreme dislocations of vertebrae can shear the spinal cord, interrupting all neural connections below the damaged site. Injury to the lower cord causes **paraplegia**, or loss of control over the lower limbs and, usually, loss of bladder function. Injury of the spinal cord in the neck causes **quadriplegia**, or loss of control over all limbs. Major long-term complications of spinal cord injury include neurogenic bladder, with superimposed infection of the bladder and kidneys. With repeated bouts of kidney infection, kidney stones often form, and renal parenchyma is destroyed so that the kidney develops end-stage renal failure requiring dialysis or transplantation. **Decubitus ulcers**, or deep ulcers resulting from pressure on the skin, develop in patients who are so severely disabled that they cannot move their position frequently. Frequent changes of position through good nursing care prevent these ulcers from occurring over pressure points. Difficulty in breathing and pneumonia are also major complications of quadriplegia.

Head Injury

The brain is encased in a nonexpansive bony vault, the skull. If the contents of the cranial cavity expand, the skull cannot accommodate the increased mass. The two major mass-producing lesions of trauma are edema and hemorrhage. Edema may be localized or widespread, but, in either case, the increasing mass of the brain causes increased pressure throughout the cranial cavity. The increased pressure may affect neuronal function and compromise blood flow. **Herniation** of the brain through the foramen magnum into the spinal column causes secondary hemorrhages into the respiratory center of the brain stem, leading to death.

Thermal Injury
Burns

Minor small burns are very common and heal by regeneration of the surface epithelium without residual effects. The damage produced by larger burns depends on two major factors—the depth of the burn and the percentage of body surface involved.

The depth of the burn can be estimated by inspection. **First-degree burns** are limited to the epidermis and are red, painful, and dry. A sunburn is an example of a first-degree burn. Regeneration occurs rapidly from remaining epidermal cells. **Second-degree burns** destroy the epidermis and upper dermis and are red, moist, and often blister (**Figure 28–7**). Regeneration of the epidermis can occur because epithelial cells from sweat glands, sebaceous glands, and hair follicles in the dermis can proliferate and, with time, form new epidermis and remodel the skin appendages. Thus, second-degree burns heal without significant scarring.

Third-degree burns destroy epidermis and dermis down to the subcutaneous tissue and are charred and dry. Pain sensation is reduced because of destruction of sensory nerve endings in the skin. Because all epithelial cells are destroyed, regeneration of epidermis can occur

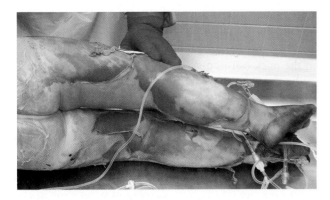

FIGURE 28–7 Extensive second-degree burns. The skin over the posterior legs and lateral thighs is red and there is extensive skin sloughage over the injured areas. Note the tangle of tubes around the patient's legs, indicating the patient was admitted to the hospital and receiving fluids in an attempt to replenish depleted fluid volumes. (Courtesy of Dr. Robert F. Corliss, Department of Pathology and Laboratory Medicine, University of Wisconsin School of Medicine and Public Health.)

only from the margins of the burn, and this type of regeneration can proceed only for a few centimeters into the injured area. Thus, third-degree burns cannot regenerate new epithelium, and skin grafting is required if the area is larger than a few centimeters. After granulation tissue has formed under the charred surface and the necrotic tissue is removed, postage stamp–sized pieces of skin are removed from a normal area of the body and placed on the granulation tissue. The graft grows, and the adjacent grafts fuse to form a new surface. The donor site also regenerates, because only a split thickness of skin is removed, leaving skin appendages behind to accomplish the regeneration of skin at the donor site. The grafted sites will not be normal because the burn will have provoked considerable scarring in the dermis and because the new epidermis will not be capable of regenerating skin appendages. Sometimes excessive scarring occurs.

The amount of body surface subjected to second- and third-degree burns correlates roughly with the chances of survival. The general health of the patient and quality of medical care are also very important determinants of survival with extensive burns. As a crude estimate, 30% body burns are serious and 60% body burns are fatal most of the time. The major complications of extensive burns are fluid loss from the exposed surface, leading to shock and infection developing in the burned skin and spreading to the bloodstream. *Pseudomonas* is a bacterium notorious for its occurrence in burns and its ability to produce fatal septicemia in patients with burns. Severely burned patients should be transferred to major treatment centers, where the skilled personnel and proper facilities are available to carry out the meticulous care needed to prevent dehydration and infection and to provide skin grafting and follow-up care.

Electrical Burns

Electricity produces two major effects—burns at entry and exit sites and electrical conduction changes, such as cardiac arrest. The amount of local injury depends on the amount of electrical energy and amount of electrical resistance in the tissue. Dry tissue, such as skin, is a poor conductor and therefore accumulates the energy and is burned (**Figure 28–8**). The effect of the electrical energy as it flows through the body in the shortest pathway from entry to exit site depends on the amount of energy absorbed at the entrance site and the location of entry and exit sites. As the electricity encounters resistance at the exit site, a burn also occurs there. The outcome is likely to be either sudden death or survival with burns at the entry and exit sites. Artificial respiration and cardiac resuscitation may be life saving. The burned tissue may be extensive and needs to be debrided to prevent secondary infection.

Excessive Heat Exposure

Prolonged exposure to hot weather can have two possible effects. Excessive sweating can cause dehydration and salt depletion leading to shock, with subsequent inadequate perfusion of vital organs. Salt and water replacement are necessary in this dire circumstance. The other effect is called **malignant hyperpyrexia** and is caused by a failure of sweating. The skin is hot and dry, and failure to lose heat by vaporization of sweat leads to a progressive rise in body temperature and death.

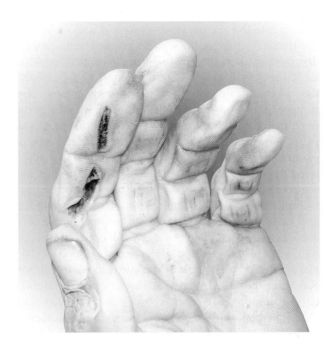

FIGURE 28–8 Electrical burn. Deep, linear burns are present on the index finger. There is soot from the combustion deposited on the ridges of the fingerprints. (Courtesy of Dr. Robert F. Corliss, Department of Pathology and Laboratory Medicine, University of Wisconsin School of Medicine and Public Health.)

Frostbite

Frostbite is simply necrosis of tissue caused by freezing. It occurs on exposed parts, such as feet, hands, and ears. The dead tissue demarcates from adjacent viable tissue in a few days and is either sloughed or removed surgically so that the remaining viable tissue can heal.

Excessive Cold Exposure (Hypothermia)

The body can tolerate moderate degrees of **hypothermia** for a considerable time, but when the body temperature falls to less than 33°C for a prolonged time, death occurs. Death is much more rapid in water and can occur with temperatures above freezing because water rapidly conducts heat from the body. In air, conduction of heat away from the body occurs more slowly.

Radiation Injury

Solar Radiation

The acute effect of solar radiation, or exposure to sunlight, is sunburn, a mild superficial injury of the epidermis. Much of the sunburn effect is caused by **ultraviolet radiation**, which can be blocked by sunscreen lotions. The chronic effects of sun exposure include a general deterioration in collagenous tissue of the skin termed solar elastosis. This accounts for the wrinkling and drooping of facial and hand skin. Sun exposure also relates to the frequency of premalignant skin lesions (senile or actinic keratoses) and skin cancers (basal cell carcinoma, squamous cell carcinoma, and malignant melanoma).

X-Radiation and Gamma Radiation

The basic effect of x-rays and gamma rays on cells is on the nucleus, with resultant death of the cells or interference with their ability to divide. Thus, continuously dividing cell lines are most susceptible to radiation injury. These include bone marrow, small intestinal epithelium, testes, and epidermis. Lymphocytes and ova are also very **radiosensitive**, or easily killed by radiation. Conversely, those cells least capable of cell division are least susceptible to radiation injury. Thus, very high doses are required to injure the brain or muscle. Other tissues are intermediate in their radiosensitivity.

In addition to the effects on specific tissues, radiation causes gradual changes in connective tissue and microvasculature that require months to years to develop. These effects include increased density of collagenous tissue, vascular changes leading to decreased blood supply, and ulceration of epithelial surfaces overlying the areas of connective tissue change.

The use of radiation therapy for the treatment of cancer is based on the fact that cancer cells are more radiosensitive than surrounding normal tissue is. The radiologist who performs radiation therapy is an expert at delivering the maximum dose of radiation to the cancer with as little damage to surrounding tissue as possible. Radiation therapy is provided in four forms. High-energy radioactive cobalt sources are available in major treatment centers and are used to deliver penetrating doses to deep-lying cancers. X-ray therapy machines are more widely available and are also used for treatment of solid cancer masses, although the lesser penetration of x-rays results in more tissue damage to the normal tissue lying in the treatment pathway. Radioactive substances that emit less-penetrating gamma rays can be selectively implanted near the cancer. For example, applicators containing radioactive cesium are implanted into the uterus for treatment of cervical and endometrial cancer, and radioactive gold is inserted into the prostate for treatment of prostatic cancer. Finally, radioactive compounds with particular chemical properties may be injected so that they will be localized in the target tissue. For example, radioactive iodine localizes in the thyroid gland and thus can be used to selectively treat hyperplasia of the thyroid or the occasional functional thyroid cancer.

Although most radiation injury develops as a complication of radiation therapy for serious disease, the effects of radiation used for diagnosis and of radiation encountered in the environment are of constant concern. The damaging effects of diagnostic x-rays appear to be very limited because of careful controls and knowledge gained from previous experiences. Radiologists no longer develop skin cancers on their hands because they wear protective gloves, and all radiology technicians are protected by lead aprons that absorb the x-rays before they can penetrate the tissue.

Injury from environmental radiation is of much greater long-range concern because of the massive number of people who might be involved and because radiation contamination of the environment lasts for years. A background level of atmospheric radiation is present from cosmic rays. The role of solar radiation in relation to the spontaneous occurrence of cancer and genetic defects is unknown. There is current concern that alteration of the stratosphere may lead to an increase in the background solar radiation. An increase in radioactive fallout from nuclear bombs or accidents is more likely to cause massive radioactive damage, however. The effects of nuclear disasters have been well documented from the atomic bombs dropped in Japan at the close of World War II, as well as from nuclear disasters such as at the Chernobyl nuclear power plant in the former Soviet Union. Immediate, or acute, effects include mechanical trauma and burns from the explosion and fire. Victims in the immediate vicinity of the disaster die immediately, and among those who survive, the severity of symptoms and diseases depends on how close they were to the epicenter of the explosion and how much radiation they were exposed to. Symptoms range from general malaise to anemia; hair loss; gastrointestinal upsets including nausea, vomiting, and diarrhea; headaches; and the development of leukemia. Children exposed to radiation are prone to developing papillary thyroid cancer, and women pregnant at the time of exposure may give birth to children with severe congenital anomalies.

Practice Questions

1. The most common cause of fatal accidents in young adult men is
   A. homicide.
   B. firearm injury.
   C. motor vehicle accident.
   D. traumatic fall.
   E. accidental poisoning.

2. A contusion is
   A. a defect in the superficial part of the skin, with sharp edges and tissue bridging.
   B. the same as a muzzle stamp.
   C. damage to subsurface tissue that does not break the surface of skin.
   D. a tear in a surface caused by shearing of tissue.
   E. the result of a sharp force injury.

3. A 24-year-old man drives his car into the pillar of a bridge. He was wearing his seat belt. When he is brought to the emergency room, he is neurologically intact and does not show much evidence of external trauma, but his hemoglobin is very low. His physician should
   A. send him home to get plenty of rest.
   B. give him blood transfusions and admit him for observation overnight.
   C. explore the possibility that he may have ruptured his spleen.
   D. explore the possibility that he may have an intracranial hemorrhage.
   E. give him blood transfusions and check his blood levels for drugs of abuse.

4. Police find a 43-year-old woman dead in the woods. Her hands are tied behind her back and there is an entrance gunshot wound on her right temple. The right cheek, forehead, neck, and shoulder are covered with punctate abrasions. The bullet that killed her was fired from
   A. a gun held in contact with her head.
   B. a gun held 6 feet away.
   C. an indeterminate range.
   D. a gun held a few inches away.
   E. an intermediate range.

5. Flail chest results from
   A. pneumothorax.
   B. hemothorax.
   C. multiple rib fractures.
   D. pleural effusion.
   E. abdominal injury.

6. A 25-year-old man sustains a spinal cord injury in a car crash that leaves him quadriplegic. Some of the complications he is likely to develop during his life include all of the following except
   A. decubitus ulcers.
   B. neurogenic bladder.
   C. pneumonia.
   D. gastroparesis.
   E. dialysis dependence.

Chemical Injury

OBJECTIVES

1. Identify the three general modes of chemical injury.
2. Describe the circumstances under which drugs can lead to injury.
3. Identify the chemical agents that account for the most serious and common medical and social problems.
4. Know what percentage of apparent poisonings lead to symptoms and to death.
5. Recognize the classes of agents most frequently involved in poisoning.
6. Recognize the ages at which poisoning are most likely to occur.
7. Identify the chemical agent that is the most important cause of cancer.
8. Describe the steps involved in the evaluation of a person suspected of having injury caused by a chemical agent.
9. Describe the role of laboratory tests in the diagnosis of poisoning.
10. Describe the type of injury associated with each of the chemical agents described in the text.
11. Be able to define and use in context all of the words in headings and bold print throughout the text.

KEY TERMS

acetaminophen
ammonia
anaphylaxis
aspirin
bone marrow suppression
carbon monoxide
chemical burn
cholinesterase inhibitor
cigarette smoke
cyanide
drug abuse
drug overdose

environmental
    accident
hypersensitivity
iron toxicity
lead poisoning
mercuric chloride
methyl alcohol
nitrogen dioxide
opioid analgesic
paraquat
pollution
renal tubular injury

Modes of Chemical Injury

The wide variety of chemical agents that are potentially harmful to humans produce diverse types of injury that are difficult to classify. Knowledge of the effects of each chemical agent is needed to provide the best treatment. Application of general principles along with knowledge of common agents allows the healthcare provider to make appropriate initial decisions in cases of chemical injury. Poison control centers provide ready access to information regarding more rarely encountered agents.

The mode of exposure to injurious chemicals provides the first clue to the likely agents involved. Three modes of chemical injury are considered: (1) overdose of a drug that a person is purposely taking for its effects; (2) exposure of an individual by accident or because of suicidal or homicidal intent; and (3) potential exposure of many people because of environmental pollution or accident.

Most drugs are potentially harmful if taken in sufficient dose. Often, the harmful dose is close to the therapeutic dose so that deleterious effects occur as a side effect of therapy. A second mode of **drug overdose** is miscalculation of the dose or misunderstanding by the patient of how much to take. **Drug abuse**, which involves self-administration of drugs for their psychological effects, is another mode of drug overdose.

Accidental exposure of an individual to harmful chemicals may occur by ingestion, by inhalation, or by contact with corrosive chemical agents. Agents selected for suicidal or homicidal purposes are likely to be strong agents that can be easily ingested, such as barbiturate drugs. **Environmental accidents** and **pollution** may be either acute or chronic. Carbon monoxide poisoning from car exhaust or fires is an example of acute environmental poisoning. Lead poisoning from eating paint or burning storage batteries is an example of chronic poisoning from environmental exposure.

Detection of chemical injury relates to the mode of exposure. Overdose of a therapeutic drug will be reported by the patient or observed by the physician. Drug abuse is a social problem that comes to attention in many ways—sometimes medical, sometimes criminal, and sometimes social in nature. Accidental poisoning brings patients to emergency rooms or poison control centers. Suicide and homicide are investigated by police, medical examiners, and forensic pathologists. Unsuccessful suicide and homicide attempts present as emergency medical problems. Acute environmental accidents are likely to be handled in emergency rooms and may involve enough victims to be considered a disaster. Chronic environmental injury is likely to go undetected until pilot cases are identified and the mechanism of exposure is brought to public attention through painstaking epidemiologic studies.

Most Frequent and Serious Problems

Toxicity as a side effect of therapeutic or prescription drugs is very common. Often, patients receive prescriptions from multiple physicians and multiple pharmacies for similar or additive drugs, and thus take a drug overdose. This is particularly likely to occur with patients who take tranquilizers, sedatives, and analgesics. Drug abuse with barbiturates, opiates, cocaine, and other drugs is a major medical and social problem involving millions of individuals, and in recent years has caused an increase in fatal overdose cases in young adults. Drug abuse is the most common cause of drug-related death, followed by suicide and accidental drug poisoning.

The frequency of poisoning is based on data reported to poison control centers. Those data give an approximation of emergency medical care problems relating to chemicals regardless of the mode of injury or potential

TABLE 29–1	Medical Outcome by Reason for Exposure in Human Poisoning Cases	
	Unintentional (%)	**Intentional (%)**
No effect	20	17
Minor effect	11.5	28
Moderate effect	2	21
Major effect	0.1	4
Death	0.01	0.3
No follow-up or unrelated effect	66	38

Data from Bronstein AC, Spyker DA, Cantilena LR, et al. *2008 annual report of the American Association of Poison Control Centers' National Poison Data System (NPDS): 26th annual report.* Alexandria, VA: American Association of Poison Control Centers; 2009. Available at: www.aapcc.org/dnn/Portals/0/2008annualreport.pdf.

injury. Most persons seeking medical care for poisoning are asymptomatic and few die (**Table 29–1**). Of the many agents that cause poisoning, drugs are collectively most common (**Table 29–2**), and of these, sedative/hypnotic agents cause the largest number of deaths (**Table 29–3**). More than 70% of reported poisonings occur in children younger than 6 years of age, and the agents responsible for these poisonings are similar to those causing poisoning in adults (**Table 29–4**). However, poisoning in children is usually accidental, whereas poisoning as a form of suicide is more common in adults. Overdoses of prescription drugs and "recreational" drugs, including opiates and street drugs, are more common in adults, especially young adults.

The importance of environmental injury by chemicals is difficult to assess because data are difficult to gather and effects may go undetected. Among acute cases of environmental chemicals causing death, carbon monoxide poisoning is common, whereas fatal poisoning from plants, such as mushrooms, is rare in the United States. Pesticides and herbicides are widely used and may produce acute injury when spilled on the skin or ingested. The long-term effects of many of these compounds in humans are unknown. Air pollutants, particularly hydrocarbons, which produce smog in large metropolitan areas, increase the frequency and severity of emphysema and other chronic lung diseases.

Examples of uncommon but serious exposure to gases include silo filler's disease and ammonia burns. In silo filler's disease, nitrogen dioxide produced in silos by fermentation is inhaled and results in acute and sometimes chronic damage to the lung. Ammonia burns the skin, eyes, and respiratory tract when leakage occurs from tanks of liquid ammonia.

Another large category of chronic environmental chemical injury relates to chemicals that induce cancer.

TABLE 29-2 Ten Substances Most Frequently Involved in Human Poison Exposures in the United States

	Substance	Number	Percentage
1	Analgesics	331,123	13.3
2	Cosmetics and personal care products	224,884	9.0
3	Household cleaning products	213,595	8.6
4	Sedatives/hypnotics/antipsychotics	165,539	6.6
5	Foreign bodies/toys	130,244	5.2
6	Topical preparations	114,024	4.6
7	Antidepressants	102,510	4.1
8	Cold and cough preparations	98,636	4.0
9	Pesticides (includes rodenticides)	93,998	3.8
10	Cardiovascular drugs	91,421	3.7

Data from Bronstein AC, Spyker DA, Cantilena LR, et al. *2008 annual report of the American Association of Poison Control Centers' National Poison Data System (NPDS): 26th annual report.* Alexandria, VA: American Association of Poison Control Centers; 2009. Available at: www.aapcc.org/dnn/Portals/0/2008annualreport.pdf.

TABLE 29-3 Drug or Poison Categories Associated with Largest Numbers of Deaths in the United States

1	Sedative/hypnotic/antipsychotic
2	Opioids
3	Antidepressants
4	Cardiovascular drugs
5	Acetaminophen combinations
6	Alcohols
7	Stimulants and street drugs
8	Acetaminophen alone
9	Antihistamines
10	Anticonvulsants

Data from Bronstein AC, Spyker DA, Cantilena LR, et al. *2008 annual report of the American Association of Poison Control Centers' National Poison Data System (NPDS): 26th annual report.* Alexandria, VA: American Association of Poison Control Centers; 2009. Available at: www.aapcc.org/dnn/Portals/0/2008annualreport.pdf.

TABLE 29-4 Ten Substances Most Frequently Involved in Pediatric Poison Exposures (Children 5 Years Old and Younger) in the United States

Substance	Number	Percentage
Cosmetics and personal care products	173,945	13.5
Analgesics	125,454	9.7
Cleaning substances	124,934	9.7
Foreign bodies	96,806	7.5
Topical preparations	89,730	6.9
Cough and cold preparations	52,723	4.1
Vitamins	50,836	3.9
Antihistamines	44,649	3.5
Pesticides (includes rodenticides)	43,526	3.4
Plants	43,398	3.4

Data from Bronstein AC, Spyker DA, Cantilena LR, et al. *2008 annual report of the American Association of Poison Control Centers' National Poison Data System (NPDS): 26th annual report.* Alexandria, VA: American Association of Poison Control Centers; 2009. Available at: www.aapcc.org/dnn/Portals/0/2008annualreport.pdf.

Cigarette smoke is the most well established and has the greatest impact because it is related to the development of lung cancer, squamous cell cancers of the oral region and esophagus, and urothelial carcinoma of the bladder. Our knowledge of cancer-causing chemicals is limited, although epidemiologic evidence suggests that they play a role in the development of a large number of cancers. Probably the most important injurious chemical is alcohol.

Symptoms, Signs, and Tests

The manifestations of chemical injury are dependent on numerous factors, including the route of exposure, the dose, the amount of absorption, the site of metabolism, the degree of excretion, and the specific chemical action of the agent involved. A discussion of these aspects of chemical injury is beyond the scope of this text. Only specific characteristics of individual agents are mentioned.

Some broad generalizations can be made about presentation of chemical injuries. From the data presented in the previous section, it is clear that the most common mode of presentation is the child younger than 6 years of age who has swallowed something and is brought to the emergency room. Examples of signs and symptoms of chemical injury include vomiting, burns, behavioral changes, and unconsciousness. The most important historical information is identification of the chemical agent to which the person was exposed. With knowledge of the agent, the physician can look for the specific signs and laboratory abnormalities caused by the agent and select the proper treatment.

Signs of chemical injury are usually not specific but may provide helpful clues. Nausea, vomiting, and diarrhea are observed with intestinal injury. Difficulty breathing occurs after inhalation of noxious fumes. Careful neurologic examination may detect changes caused by injury to the nervous system. Decreased urine output suggests severe renal injury.

Laboratory tests can help suggest whether injury has occurred, the likely site of injury, and sometimes the type and amount of the agent. General laboratory tests that may suggest whether injury has occurred include elevation of the white blood count, alteration in serum electrolytes, and elevation of serum enzymes, such as aspartate aminotransferase. Elevated blood urea nitrogen and creatinine levels suggest renal injury, high aspartate aminotransferase levels are found with liver damage, and altered levels of blood gases are associated with altered oxygen–carbon dioxide exchange in the lungs.

Many chemicals can be measured in samples of blood, urine, feces, or tissues. However, the laboratory needs a clue as to which chemical to look for among the myriad of possibilities. Extensive search for a poison is indicated only when the information will be of value in treatment or in criminal investigation.

Specific Diseases

The emphasis in this section is on representative specific agents and the type of injury they produce. Agents are grouped for discussion by mode of injury and/or similarities in patterns of injury. Effects of chemical agents on specific organs that have been previously discussed, such as pneumoconioses, are not repeated here. Other texts should be consulted for more comprehensive coverage of specific types of chemical injury.

Adverse Drug Reactions

Adverse drug reactions can occur during a usual course of therapy. In many instances, the adverse drug reaction is caused by **hypersensitivity**, usually an allergic reaction. In severe cases, this can result in **anaphylaxis**, or severe vasodilation resulting in shock and bronchoconstriction resulting in inability to breathe. Penicillin is probably the most well known for eliciting a hypersensitivity response,

but virtually any drug can do so, including aspirin and ibuprofen. It is essential that patients be asked about allergic reactions to drugs so that these can be avoided in treatment plans. However, most anaphylactic reactions occur in patients who have no known history of adverse drug reactions.

Other mechanisms of adverse drug reaction include use of drugs with a toxic dose range close to the therapeutic dose range, an enzyme deficiency that accentuates the effective dose of the drug, and renal or liver failure with decreased excretion or metabolism of the drug. The liver is also quite sensitive to numerous drugs that can adversely affect hepatocytes or bile production and clearance. Most of these reactions are idiosyncratic, or unpredictable. Discontinuation of the drug usually results in reversal of the abnormality.

Bone marrow suppression leading to leukopenia, thrombocytopenia, and/or anemia may occur as a hypersensitivity reaction to the antibiotic chloramphenicol or as a predictable action of anticancer drugs. **Renal tubular injury** is a complication of treatment with several antibiotic agents as well as other drugs. Other specific reactions worthy of special mention include hemorrhage resulting from anticoagulant drug therapy and malignant hyperthermia resulting from a rare enzyme defect that is manifested when patients are given succinylcholine, a muscle relaxant, in combination with halothane or certain other general anesthetic agents.

Drug Abuse

Agents involved in drug abuse include opiates, barbiturates, tranquilizers, hallucinogens, muscle relaxants, and stimulants such as amphetamines and cocaine. As mentioned earlier, these agents probably account for about 50% of drug-related deaths and for the high incidence of drug overdoses in adolescents and young adults. Death may occur because of overdose as a direct result of the pharmacologic effects of the drug, or it may be caused by other complications. The drugs themselves do not produce lesions, and most cause death by their effects on respiration and cardiac function.

Opiates such as heroin are frequently taken intravenously, leaving telltale lesions on the skin and occasionally leading to severe complications. Local lesions in drug addicts consist of inflammation at the injection sites caused by a granulomatous reaction to the talc or starch in the injection mixture or infection from failure to use sterile technique. Injected talc or starch is carried to the small vessels of the lung, where a granulomatous reaction occurs in small arterioles and may eventually lead to pulmonary hypertension and cor pulmonale because of the arteriolar obstruction. Allergic reactions can also occur to other ingredients in the injection mixture. Systemic infections, such as bacterial endocarditis and viral hepatitis, are more frequent in intravenous (IV) drug abusers, presumably because of direct injection of organisms into the bloodstream.

Symptoms of amphetamines and cocaine abuse include hypertension, acidosis, anxiety, agitation, psychosis, and, if severe, seizures, hyperthermia, and myocardial infarction from coronary artery spasm. Diagnosis is established by finding metabolites of these drugs in the blood or urine.

Accidental Poisonings

Because most accidental poisonings occur in children younger than 6 years of age, it is not surprising that the agents involved are those commonly found around the house (Table 29–4). Analgesics (aspirin, acetaminophen) and household cleaners are the most common accidentally ingested chemicals by children. The ingestion of both these types of substances can be decreased considerably by putting childproof locks on cabinet doors and by having childproof caps on medication bottles. Accidental poisonings usually occur when these safety measures are circumvented: a child is visiting in a home where there are no locks on cabinets, or the cap on a medicine bottle is not screwed on tightly. The major harmful effects of **aspirin** are metabolic, with an initial alkalosis caused by hyperventilation and later severe acidosis. **Acetaminophen** is toxic to hepatocytes if taken in too large a dose. Fulminant hepatitis can lead to death. The antidote to acetaminophen is acetylcysteine, which should be administered within 8 hours of an overdose for maximum protective effect. Accidental or suicidal ingestion of sedative drugs or **opioid analgesic** painkillers causes central nervous system and respiratory depression. Mothers of young children frequently take oral **iron** medications. Accidental ingestion of these iron compounds by a child leads to corrosive damage to the stomach and small intestine and toxic damage to various tissues such as the liver and heart.

There are hundreds of different chemicals in cleaning products, including such agents as acetone, chlorine, ammonia, formaldehyde, benzene, toluene, monoethanolamine, and naphthalene. They can be irritating to the skin and mucosa of the respiratory tract or eye; they can cause **chemical burns** when they come in contact with exposed tissue; they can cause damage to a variety of internal organs including the central nervous system, liver, kidney, and bone marrow; and they can interfere with hormone production. Many of them are also carcinogenic, causing malignant transformation of cells even years after the primary, acute exposure.

Carbon Monoxide Poisoning

Carbon monoxide is produced by incomplete combustion, and when inhaled, it preferentially combines with oxygen-carrying sites on hemoglobin molecules of red blood cells so that there is a resultant systemic anoxia. The anoxia may be fatal or may lead to permanent brain damage. Carbon monoxide levels are measured in blood and expressed as percentage of hemoglobin saturation. A carbon monoxide level of 50% saturation is considered lethal, although individuals with underlying cardiac or pulmonary disease may die at less than 50% saturation. Conversely, very healthy young individuals may survive carbon monoxide poisoning with levels significantly greater than 50% saturation, provided they are removed from the source of exposure before toxic systemic anoxia results.

Automobiles are a common source of carbon monoxide. This is why breathing automotive exhaust in an enclosed space can be lethal. Most deaths in cases of fire are the result of carbon monoxide poisoning because the air in and around a fire is rich in carbon monoxide. When investigating a fire-related fatality, elevated postmortem blood carbon monoxide levels allow the forensic pathologist to determine whether an individual was alive during a fire. Carbon monoxide is particularly dangerous because it is odorless and because initial symptoms of impaired mental function are not necessarily apparent to those affected. The effects of chronic low-level carbon monoxide poisoning resulting from smoking, smog, or automobile fumes have not been quantified. It is possible that mental impairment from mild carbon monoxide poisoning may cause some accidents.

Agricultural Chemical Injury

A number of chemicals encountered in farming cause rather specific types of damage. **Nitrogen dioxide**, produced by fermentation of silage, when inhaled causes severe, acute injury to the lining cells of the pulmonary alveoli. In mild cases of this condition, called silo filler's disease, the damage is gradually resolved, but in severe cases, damage to the alveolar walls leads to permanent fibrosis of the lungs and residual decreased breathing capacity.

Fertilizers, herbicides, and insecticides are human-made agricultural poisons. Liquid **ammonia**, when spilled, may lead to severe burns of the skin, eyes, and respiratory tract. Accidental exposure to agricultural anhydrous ammonia has increased in recent years as a result of illicit use of this compound in methamphetamine manufacture. **Paraquat** is a commonly used weed-killer that causes damage to the pulmonary alveoli regardless of whether it is ingested or inhaled. Acute damage may be fatal or may lead to pulmonary fibrosis. Many insecticides contain **cholinesterase inhibitors**, which may lead to depression of the central and autonomic nervous systems and motor nerve endings.

Injury by Other Agents

Cyanide poisoning may result from inhalation of hydrocyanic acid or ingestion of soluble inorganic cyanide salts or cyanide-releasing substances. Modes of cyanide poisoning include industrial accidents, ingestion of certain plants, suicide, homicide, and execution. Cyanide combines with cytochrome oxidase of cells throughout the body to prevent cellular oxygen utilization. Cyanide is extremely toxic and rapid in its effects.

Methyl alcohol (also called methanol or wood alcohol) is widely used as a solvent and denaturing agent for ethyl alcohol. The major adverse effect of nonfatal doses is blindness. Methyl alcohol is metabolized to formaldehyde, which in turn causes damage to the retina and optic nerve. Severe acidosis occurs in fatal methyl alcohol poisoning as a consequence of its metabolism to formic acid.

Lead poisoning is usually chronic and often occurs in children who eat paint that is peeling from walls or window frames. It may also follow exposure to burning lead batteries. Lead poisoning affects the brain, peripheral nerves, and bone marrow. Abdominal cramps or colic is a characteristic symptom of peripheral nerve involvement. Encephalopathy of varying degrees, with convulsions and behavioral changes, results from the brain damage. There may be permanent mental incapacity. A characteristic mild anemia in which red blood cells contain blue dots, or a "stippled" pattern, can occur with lead poisoning. A black line caused by deposition of lead sulfide along gingival margins is another characteristic physical finding.

Poisoning with **mercuric chloride** by ingestion leads to corrosive damage to the oral region and esophagus. The absorbed mercury is excreted by the renal tubules and colonic mucosa, where it produces renal tubular necrosis, leading to acute renal failure, and ulceration of the colon, leading to bloody diarrhea.

Practice Questions

1. Which of the following is not a usual mode of chemical injury?
   A. Taking antibiotics at the normal therapeutic dose when a patient does not have a bacterial infection
   B. Accidental overdose of an opioid analgesic
   C. Purposeful (suicidal or homicidal) exposure to carbon monoxide
   D. Ingestion of an industrial chemical that spilled into the drinking water
   E. Caustic burns from inappropriate use of household cleaners

2. Which of the following statements about chemical injury is true?
   A. Most chemicals exert their effect by causing caustic burns on exposed surfaces, such as the skin, oral or gastrointestinal mucosa, or eye.
   B. There are no known neurotoxic chemical agents.
   C. Most chemicals exert their effect by causing cancer many years after the acute exposure.
   D. Chemical injury is dependent on the dose, timing, and route of administration of the injurious agent.

3. Which of the following agents is the most common cause of death as a result of acute drug toxicity in adults?
   A. Sedative/hypnotic agent
   B. Alcohol
   C. Household cleaner
   D. Pesticide/herbicide
   E. Cosmetics and personal care products

4. Overdose of acetaminophen results in
   A. kidney failure.
   B. blindness.
   C. metabolic acidosis.
   D. hepatic failure.
   E. bone marrow failure.

5. Which of the following chemical agents is most strongly linked to cancers in many different organs in the body?
   A. Alcohol
   B. Opioid drugs
   C. Formaldehyde
   D. Cigarette smoke
   E. Nitrogen dioxide

6. The most important information to obtain in an acute poisoning case is
   A. how long ago the exposure occurred.
   B. the exact chemical the patient was exposed to.
   C. the patient's age.
   D. whether there was suicidal intent.
   E. whether the patient has an underlying disease.

7. Which one of the following people is most at risk for an adverse drug or poison exposure?
   A. An otherwise healthy 19-year-old college student who is given a prescription for opioid-containing analgesics after extraction of his wisdom teeth
   B. A 43-year-old woman who has a history of an allergic reaction to "an antibiotic" and is given penicillin for treatment of a skin abscess
   C. A 73-year-old woman who is taking warfarin for atrial fibrillation and routinely has a therapeutic-range INR
   D. A 3-year-old child living in a home where medications, cosmetics, and household cleaning products are kept in cabinets with childproof locks
   E. A 3-year-old child treated with pediatric doses of acetaminophen for a fever

8. Carbon monoxide is potentially lethal because it
   A. binds to hemoglobin, blocking sites on which oxygen is usually carried.
   B. interferes with oxidative phosphorylation in mitochondria.
   C. irreversibly binds oxygen to hemoglobin, so that it cannot dissociate in peripheral tissues.
   D. interferes with tissue utilization of oxygen.
   E. causes oxidative stress in renal tubular epithelial cells.

Nutritional Disorders

OBJECTIVES

1. Review basic and essential dietary elements, including why they are necessary to the proper functioning of the body and how nutrition affects health.
2. Recognize the serious burden of obesity and undernutrition around the world.
3. Identify the most common mineral deficiency states, recognize who is susceptible to developing them, and understand how to prevent their occurrence.
4. Recognize the threat of environmental pollutants on the food chain and their harmful effects on nutritional status.
5. Be able to match the fat- and water-soluble vitamins with their deficiency states.
6. Name the two most serious manifestations of undernutrition, and identify disease states that can lead to starvation, cachexia, or failure to thrive.
7. Describe some of the complications of alcoholism.
8. Describe how nutritive needs change during maturation, from the fetal period to aging, and identify some of the vitamin and mineral deficiency states people are prone to developing at different stages of their life.
9. Understand the pathophysiology of immune-mediated diseases that involve nutrition (e.g., food allergy, celiac disease, pernicious anemia).
10. Recognize the effect of deficient or absent digestive enzyme production on a patient's nutritive status, and name some of the diseases of enzymatic deficiency.
11. List the major causes and complications of obesity, and name some of the ways in which it can be treated.
12. Define and use in proper context all words and terms in headings and bold print in this chapter.

KEY TERMS

alcohol
amino acids
anorexia nervosa
bariatric surgery
beriberi
body mass index (BMI)
bulimia nervosa
cachexia
calorie
carbohydrate
celiac disease
environmental pollutant
essential dietary elements
failure to thrive
fat
fiber
food allergy
glucose
inborn errors of metabolism
iodine
iron-deficiency anemia
kwashiorkor
lactase deficiency
malnutrition
marasmus
minerals
neural tube defect
nutrition
obesity
osteomalacia
pancreatic insufficiency
pellagra
pernicious anemia
protein
rickets
scurvy
short bowel syndrome
starvation
total parenteral nutrition
undernutrition
vitamins
Wernicke-Korsakoff
    syndrome

Review of Function

Simply put, **nutrition** refers to food: to ingested substances that fuel metabolism, provide the substrate for growth, and maintain the function of tissues. Nutrition plays a significant role in health. It is required for reconstitution of cells that are lost due to physiologic processes or due to injury caused by disease, for nourishment of a growing fetus or nursing infant, and for obtaining molecules that the body does not produce itself but are necessary for physiologic processes.

Humans are omnivores and can digest and extract nutrients from a wide variety of food substances. In fact, the key to a healthy diet is variety: any restriction of food choices, whether optional (e.g., vegetarianism), imposed (e.g., food shortages), or due to a disease state (e.g., celiac disease) incurs the risk of creating deficiencies of essential nutrients, if conscious efforts to obtain these lacking substances through informed food choices or supplements are not made. Nutritional needs vary between sexes, and by age and degree of physical activity. Special nutritional needs arise during pregnancy and lactation, as the fetus and nursing infant acquire their nutrition from their mother. Infants and young children need relatively more calories, minerals, and vitamins than do adults, because their tissues are actively growing. The growth spurt and sexual characterizations at puberty also result in some special dietary needs. In the elderly, some specific nutritional requirements arise, primarily as older individuals' food choices often wane because of loss of taste for food and loss of appetite due to loneliness and inactivity.

Some general dietary guidelines, good for most every person, would be to (1) maintain ideal weight; (2) eat a variety of foods to meet vitamin and mineral needs; (3) avoid excessive fat, saturated fat, and cholesterol; (4) eat food with adequate fiber content; (5) avoid sugar; (6) avoid excessive sodium; and (7) avoid alcohol. For a thorough discussion of what makes a healthy diet, the interested reader is referred to any of several excellent texts, such as Wardlaw's *Perspectives in Nutrition*.[1]

The primary nutritional consideration in a diet is energy, expressed in terms of **calories**. One calorie (cal) is the amount of heat required to raise the temperature of 1,000 g of water from 15°C to 16°C. The caloric value of any food can be directly determined by oxidizing (burning) the food in a calorimeter chamber and measuring the amount of energy released. The energy released by this method is equivalent to the breakdown of the food in the human body, although the body utilizes food in a much more prolonged and complicated process than simple oxidation. The human body can obtain energy from **carbohydrates**, **proteins**, and **fats**. The caloric content of each of these three major food categories differs. Overall, carbohydrates yield 4.1 cal/g, protein 4.3 cal/g, and lipids 9.3 cal/g. Carbohydrates are the main source of readily available energy in the human diet. The metabolism of lipids, however, yields more than twice as many calories as either protein or carbohydrates, on a per-gram basis.

Carbohydrates include sugars, starch, and fiber. **Glucose**, a simple sugar, is the most important energy molecule in the body: almost all cells in the body have the enzymatic machinery to derive energy from glucose. Glucose is not ingested as such, but rather is derived from metabolism of more complex sugars, including starch. **Fiber** is not an energy source. Forming the bulk of plant foods, fiber also is responsible for the bulk of feces, thereby contributing to normal defecation and the health of the bowel. In addition, it helps regulate lipid absorption and blood glucose levels.

While proteins can be utilized for energy, their main functions are as building blocks of tissues and as enzymes in molecular pathways, including those involved in the production of energy and intercellular signaling. Proteins are made up of 20 different **amino acids**, each with a unique molecular structure that affects the manner in which the fully formed protein will fold into a complex three-dimensional structure capable of holding coenzymes, interacting with other proteins, and catalyzing enzymatic reactions. Many amino acids can be produced by the cell itself, but some must be taken in from dietary sources.

While lipids are an important source of energy, they also are important for other processes. They store energy, insulate the body, form the lipid bilayer of cell membranes, mediate the inflammatory response in the form of arachidonic acid metabolites, and—in the form of myelin—insulate nerve axons for effective transmission of nerve impulses.

Vitamins and **minerals** do not contribute calories to the human diet, but rather are utilized by the body in small amounts for many and varied functions (**Table 30–1**). Some of these nutrients are utilized as coenzymes, whereas others contribute to cell and tissue structure. Some vitamins are synthesized by intestinal bacteria, and a few are synthesized in the body by breakdown of other foods, but most need to be extracted from dietary sources. Minerals provide strength to bone (calcium and phosphorus), maintain the electric and osmotic gradients that differentiate intracellular from extracellular fluid (sodium and potassium), are the oxygen-carrying components of hemoglobin (iron) and are required for proper nerve and muscle function (magnesium) and thyroid hormone production (iodine), among other things.

The body can synthesize many of the carbohydrates, fats, and amino acids that serve as its building blocks and energy sources, but approximately 40 substances are considered essential, meaning they must be derived from dietary (exogenous) sources. These include nine amino acids (the building blocks of protein), two lipids, the vitamins, and minerals. Note that no carbohydrates are essential. **Table 30–2** lists **essential dietary elements**.

TABLE 30–1 Function and Source of Vitamins

Vitamin	Function	Source
Fat-soluble vitamins: stored in liver and adipose tissue		
A	• Development of major organ systems during embryonic period • Formation of epithelia • Cell differentiation, particularly in the eye (cornea, retina) • Vision, particularly night vision • Immune function	• Liver, fish oils, eggs • Sweet potato, carrots, kale, broccoli • Fortified foods (e.g., margarine, genetically engineered rice)
D	• Intestinal absorption of calcium and phosphorus • Bone mineralization • Maintenance of serum levels of calcium and phosphorus • Immune function	• Cod liver oil, fish • Synthesis from cholesterol derivative in skin if exposed to sunlight
E	• Antioxidant • Immune system	• Vegetable oils (e.g., sunflower oil, sunflower seeds) • Wheat germ, asparagus
K	• Synthesis of blood clotting factors	• Leafy green vegetables (kale, spinach, salad greens, brussels sprouts) • 10% produced by intestinal bacteria
Water-soluble vitamins: stored in limited amounts in tissues, mostly muscle and liver; readily excreted by the kidney		
B_1 (thiamin)	• Coenzyme for metabolism of glucose and certain amino acids	• Pork • Whole grains • Legumes • Enriched products (e.g., cereal)
B_2 (riboflavin)	• Coenzyme for numerous metabolic processes (glucose, fatty acids) • Formation of other active B vitamins (niacin, vitamin B_6, folate) • Antioxidant	• Milk and dairy products • Liver • Leafy green vegetables • Enriched wheat products
B_3 (niacin)	• Coenzyme in many pathways that produce ATP (oxidation–reduction pathways)	• Poultry, meat, fish • Enriched grain (particularly wheat) products • Synthesized in the body from the amino acid tryptophan • Pharmacologic preparations (for treatment of elevated HDL)
Pantothenic acid	• Part of coenzyme A, used to generate ATP or as a substrate for various fatty acid derivatives (cholesterol, bile acids, steroid hormones)	• Meat • Dairy or soy milk • Wide variety of vegetables • Enriched cereals
Biotin	• Coenzyme in metabolism of carbohydrates, proteins, and fats	• Whole grains • Poultry and fish • Peanuts • Legumes
B_6 (pyridoxine)	• Coenzyme in amino acid metabolism (synthesis of nonessential amino acids)	• Meat, fish, poultry • Whole grains • Carrots, potatoes, spinach, bananas, avocados
Folate	• Coenzyme in DNA synthesis • Amino acid metabolism • Synthesis of neurotransmitters	• Leafy green vegetables • Legumes • Liver • Avocados and oranges • Fortified foods
B_{12} (cobalamine)	• Coenzyme in production of amino acid methionine, which is required for regulation of DNA, RNA, and production of myelin • Production of folate	• Meat, poultry, fish • Dairy products

(continues)

TABLE 30-1 Function and Source of Vitamins (*continued*)

Vitamin	Function	Source
Choline	• Component of phospholipids (cell membranes, lipoproteins) • Precursor for the neurotransmitter acetylcholine	• Milk • Liver • Eggs • Peanuts • Foods enriched with lecithin
C	• Antioxidant • Collagen synthesis • Cofactor in synthesis of various amino acids, hormones, and neurotransmitters • Intestinal absorption of iron • Immune function	• Citrus fruits • Peppers • Other fruits (e.g., kiwi, strawberries, papaya) • Green vegetables

Because food is voluntarily ingested, food choices play a large role in the nutritional status of people living in areas where food is abundant. Food choices can be influenced by mental health or psychiatric conditions, such as with anorexia nervosa, and may be limited by economic resources. For the most part, however, food choices are learned in infancy and conditioned during social interactions. What counts as "tasty," desirable, valuable, "good," and appropriate as a food item is socioculturally defined. For example, in many areas of the world, insects are consumed in various preparations, ranging from snacks to main meals to desserts. Insects are excellent sources of protein. Yet despite all assurances of their nutritive benefits and great taste, it will probably take a while before McDonald's begins to serve locust burgers. Other food items carry a religious taboo, such as beef in parts of India and pork in Semitic cultures. The penchant for Americans to steer toward deep-fried or grilled red meat and starch-rich, sweet, and sugary foods is likewise a behavior learned in infancy and embedded in cultural values. Advising people on how to alter their eating habits so as to maintain a healthy body is therefore much more difficult than advising them on which car to buy or how to invest their money.

This chapter identifies some of the things that can go wrong when the body is deprived of or over-exposed to any of the nutrients mentioned earlier. Dietary "fads" abound, and the television and Internet are effective tools for promoting foods or dietary supplements that are supposed to give energy, improve the sex life, help lose weight, or supplement a critical dietary factor. The student of health sciences should be aware of the risks involved in taking foods or dietary supplements to the extreme, including excessive weight loss, vitamin over-supplementation, or consumption of a very restricted diet. In addition, many of the diseases that cause the majority of morbidity and mortality in the United States, including cardiovascular disease and diabetes, are treated and could to a large part be prevented with dietary modifications. Some individuals, such as those with "short gut," debilitation that interferes with the swallowing apparatus, or allergies such as celiac disease, require special diets or supplements that provide the nutrients essential to maintaining proper body functions.

TABLE 30-2 Essential Dietary Elements

Amino Acids	Fatty Acids	Minerals (Major)	Minerals (trace)	Vitamins
Histidine	Linoleic acid	Sodium	Iron	Water-soluble: B vitamins, vitamin C
Isoleucine	Alpha-linoleic acid	Potassium	Zinc	Fat-soluble: vitamins A, D, E, and K
Leucine		Chloride	Copper	
Lysine		Calcium	Manganese	
Methionine		Phosphorus	Iodine	
Phenylalanine		Magnesium	Selenium	
Threonine		Sulfur	Chromium	
Tryptophan			Fluoride	
Valine			Molybdenum	

Most Frequent and Serious Problems

Worldwide, the most serious problem related to nutrition is **obesity**, defined as body mass index (the measure of body fat based on height and weight; normal BMI is 18.5–24.9) greater than 30. More deaths are linked to the ill consequences of being overweight than underweight. Over the past decades, the rate of obesity in adults and children has skyrocketed, particularly in high- and middle-income countries. In the United States, more than 30% of adults and 15% of children are obese. Obesity is directly related to the most common causes of morbidity and mortality, including cardiovascular disease, diabetes, and stroke. It is also implicated in the development of certain cancers (e.g., endometrial cancer), and constitutes a major risk factor for the development of complications in surgical patients. The cost of treating obesity-related conditions is staggering—close to $150 billion in 2008 alone, and increasing as the rate of obesity continues to go up.

Undernutrition also is prevalent. It can be divided into primary undernutrition, in which there is a lack of a balanced diet and deficient total caloric intake, and secondary undernutrition, in which wasting results from a disease condition such as cancer, depression, or chronic disease. The latter instances need to be treated on a case-by-case basis with targeted nutritional supplements and supportive care, including treatment of the underlying disease. Primary undernutrition occurs in settings where access to the food supply is interrupted or the diet does not include all the essential nutrients. Examples include environmental catastrophes (e.g., drought), poverty, and war. The global burden of undernutrition is felt most heavily in middle- and low-income countries.

The effects of undernutrition are most severe in the developing fetus, infant, and child. Undernutrition refers to both deficient caloric intake and insufficient intake of essential vitamins and minerals, such as vitamin A, iron, calcium, or iodine. Poor nutrition stunts growth and development and increases susceptibility to infections, such as those causing diarrhea, pneumonia, and viral infections of childhood. Worldwide, undernutrition causes or contributes to approximately one-third (2 million) of all childhood deaths. A growing fetus already feels the effects of undernutrition: maternal undernutrition may result in restricted fetal growth and pregnancy complications. Delayed and restricted growth and development of the fetus and infant, if it does not result in death, typically causes lifelong disability, poor school performance, and reduced economic productivity.

Together, obesity and undernutrition are referred to as **malnutrition**. As you can deduce from the preceding discussion, malnutrition forms the major public health challenge, on a worldwide basis, in the early 21st century. In higher-income countries, people are eating themselves to death, while in lower-income countries, people are starving to death. Governments and international health agencies, such as the World Health Organization (WHO) and United Nations Children's Fund (UNICEF), are struggling to figure out how to set priorities for allocation of resources to tackle these problems. Finding the root cause of undernutrition is relatively easy, but getting adequate nutrition to the people in need often poses logistical and cultural challenges. In contrast, finding the root cause of obesity in an attempt to devise strategies for preventing it is not so easy, as individuals' food choices are linked in a complex manner to genetic, social, cultural, and environmental factors.

In comparison to overnutrition and undernutrition, excesses and deficiencies of vitamins and minerals, though prevalent, are much more manageable problems. Deficiencies of essential vitamins and minerals are part of the general problem of undernutrition. Where diet is adequate, only iron and iodine deficiencies pose a considerable health burden. Iron is required for the delivery of oxygen in the blood, and **iron-deficiency anemia** is one of the most prevalent causes of anemia worldwide. It primarily affects women of childbearing age, including pubertal and teenage girls. An estimated 2 billion people suffer from iron-deficiency anemia, and every second pregnant woman is iron deficient. Moreover, iron deficiency is not just a problem in resource-poor countries: in the United States, an estimated 9% of women of childbearing age are iron deficient. The primary source of iron in the diet is red meat. Where it is not readily available, the diet needs to be supplemented with alternative iron-rich foods, such as shellfish and certain legumes and vegetables. Iron fortification of foods (e.g., breakfast cereals, rice) and iron supplementation in the form of ferrous sulfate pills are relatively cheap and more reliable ways of preventing the development of iron deficiency, especially in vulnerable populations.

Iodine is required for the production of thyroid hormone. In the absence of iodine, the thyroid does not produce thyroid hormone, and the symptoms and consequences of hypothyroidism develop, including impaired brain development in children. The primary source of iodine is salt, but not all salt sources are naturally iodinated. Salt iodinization programs are cheap and effective at preventing iodine deficiency, and most countries have implemented such programs to ensure a supply of iodine to pregnant mothers and their growing children.

Alcohol is absorbed in the intestinal tract and has metabolic effects, so it could be considered a food item. However, its nutritive benefits, as a source of carbohydrates and in reducing LDL cholesterol, are far outweighed by its serious toxic consequences. The burden of excessive alcohol consumption, in the form of binge drinking, alcohol abuse, or alcohol dependence (alcoholism), is heavy worldwide. It is the third largest risk factor for disease and disability, a cause or risk factor for more than 200 diseases, and accounts for approximately 4% of deaths worldwide. In addition to its adverse biologic effects, alcohol dependence leads to serious social problems, including child abuse and neglect, violence, and absenteeism from work. Patients who depend on alcohol for their caloric intake become malnourished because they are not consuming essential nutrients, and those who have end-stage liver disease secondary to alcoholic injury not only have specific dietary requirements but also are at risk for developing side effects of liver disease (e.g., blood clotting disorders, ascites, impaired immunity, and hepatic encephalopathy) and experiencing premature death.

Ensuring a clean water supply for the world's population is one of the most significant public health challenges around the world. Microbial contaminants in water are one of the major causes of infant mortality and the outbreak of epidemic diseases, such as cholera. Just as harmful as infectious agents is contamination of water and soil by environmental pollutants. Industrial and agricultural waste and run-off tend to find their way into the water supply, from whence they are ingested directly or incorporated into the food chain. Even trace amounts of some of these chemicals in the water or diet can have serious adverse consequences on large numbers of people. Chemical water pollutants include heavy metals such as lead and mercury, as well as nonbiodegradable organic compounds such as benzene, trichloroethylene, and polychlorinated biphenyls.

Periodically, large-scale disasters—such as the mercury poisoning due to water contamination by methylmercury released by a chemical factory in Minamata, Japan (1960s), or the cyanide spill from a gold mining company in Romania in 2000 that killed 80% of aquatic life and contaminated the water supply of 2.5 million people—bring the risk of industrial pollutants to public attention. More insidious but just as harmful is the chronic, smaller-scale pollution that is covered up, denied, or blatantly ignored, as happens in many parts of the world where strict environmental protection guidelines are not enforced. While the health effects of chemicals in the food and water supply are difficult to determine through epidemiologic studies, many people blame the slowly but steadily increasing incidence of cancer on environmental pollutants.

Symptoms, Signs, and Tests

As with all conditions, a thorough history and physical exam are often the first lines of inquiry into the nature of nutritional disorders. These need to be followed by targeted laboratory tests. Overnutrition and undernutrition are readily evident at the time of physical examination. Laboratory tests are targeted to detecting substances that are often aberrant in these conditions, such as lipids in the case of obesity and electrolytes and iron in the case of undernutrition. If the patient has signs or symptoms related to specific deficiencies, such iodine or iron, the ensuing laboratory workup revolves around testing

for the levels of specific substances that are affected by those nutrients, such as thyroid hormone or hemoglobin and hematocrit. As shown in **Table 30–3**, vitamin deficiencies often cause specific signs and symptoms. These are usually sufficient to warrant replacement treatment without further diagnostic testing—for example, treatment of scurvy in the case of vitamin C deficiency. Most vitamins and heavy metals can be tested for in blood or tissues—for example, with suspected lead poisoning.

Routine laboratory work performed at the time of a physical examination includes testing for sodium, potassium, and calcium in the blood. The levels of these electrolytes are tightly regulated by the kidney, so they rarely reflect the individual's underlying nutritional status. Glucose also is measured during a routine laboratory workup. Elevated glucose levels should prompt more stringent testing of blood glucose control for the detection of diabetes mellitus. Nutritional disorders do not require imaging studies for diagnosis.

Specific Diseases

Many of the disease states resulting from poor nutrition have already been covered in this book—for example, iron-deficiency anemia, rickets, and heart disease (hypertension and atherosclerosis). This chapter gives an overview of diseases that relate to nutritional disorders, not so much in terms of specific deficiency states (these are outlined in Table 30–3), but with emphasis on diseases that affect the nutritional status of individuals.

Undernutrition

Undernutrition refers to caloric intake that is insufficient to meet the body's requirements, resulting in loss of weight beyond the accepted standard for height, age, and body build. The severest form of undernutrition is starvation. During undernutrition and starvation, fat and protein derived from the body's tissues are burned for energy. This process results in severe wasting, as adipose tissue and muscle are broken down to generate fuel. In addition, inadequate caloric intake is usually accompanied by inadequate intake of essential vitamins and minerals, resulting in specific deficiency states such as scurvy (vitamin C deficiency) and iron-deficiency anemia. Also, the perception of thirst is reduced, so even where adequate water is available, patients will develop dehydration. Starvation results in damage to all organs of the body, as tissues are deprived of the essential nutrients required for growth, adequate function, and regeneration.

The protein known as albumin is the main contributor to the oncotic pressure in blood: it prevents fluid from escaping the blood vessels. When albumin is not produced, fluid seeps from the liver and accumulates in the abdomen. This phenomenon is one of the reasons for the distended belly seen in starving children. Undernutrition also puts the individual at risk for developing infectious

TABLE 30–3 Signs, Symptoms, Causes and Risk Factors of Vitamin Deficiencies

Vitamin	Signs and Symptoms	Causes and Risk Factors of Deficiency
A	• Night blindness, complete blindness • Dry, rough skin as keratinocytes plug hair follicles • Impaired growth in children	• Dietary deficiency • Malabsorption (e.g., celiac disease, cystic fibrosis) • Liver disease • Preterm infants
D	• **Rickets**: deficient mineralization of bone in children—bowed long bones, stunted growth • **Osteomalacia**: softening of bones, impaired calcification of new bone (e.g., fractures)	• Dietary deficiency • Malabsorption • Lack of sun exposure
E	• Very rare: hemolytic anemia	• Malabsorption syndrome • Preterm infants • Smoking
K	• Hemorrhagic diathesis	• Prolonged antibiotic therapy • Newborn • Malabsorption
B_1 (thiamin)	• **Beriberi**: impairment of nervous, cardiovascular, and gastrointestinal systems—peripheral neuropathy, weakness, muscle pain, difficulty breathing, edema, anorexia, poor memory, confusion, congestive heart failure • Wernicke-Korsakoff syndrome: nervous system disorder—changes in vision, ataxia, decreased cognitive function	• Dietary deficiency (particularly when non-enriched white rice is the staple food) • Heavy alcohol consumption
B_2 (riboflavin)	• Inflammation of mouth or tongue (glossitis) • Painful cracks in corner of mouth (angular cheilitis) • Seborrheic dermatitis	• Dietary deficiency (most common in adolescent girls and elderly) • Malabsorption
B_3 (niacin)	• **Pellagra**: dermatitis (rough, scaly skin), diarrhea, dementia	• Dietary deficiency (especially when corn is the staple food)
Pantothenic acid	• Occurs only in experimental settings	
Biotin	• Very rare: rash, hair loss, stunted growth, convulsions	• Genetic deficiency of enzyme required for digestion of biotin precursor • Excessive consumption of raw eggs
B_6 (pyridoxine)	• Seborrheic dermatitis • Iron-deficiency anemia • Convulsions, depression, confusion	• Very restricted diet • Alcoholics • Certain drugs (L-dopa, isoniazid, theophylline)
B_{12} (cobalamine)	• Pernicious anemia • Subacute combined degeneration (neurological defects) • Elevated homocysteine levels	• Reduced production of intrinsic factor (required for absorption of vitamin B_{12}) • Malabsorption • Strictly vegan diet without vitamin B_{12} supplementation
Folate	• Neural tube defects in developing fetus • Megaloblastic anemia • Diarrhea and decreased absorptive capacity of GI tract • Susceptibility to infection • Often associated with vitamin B_{12} deficiency	• Pregnancy (increased needs of developing fetus) • Very restricted diet • Alcoholics • Chronic diarrhea • Chemotherapy
C	• **Scurvy**: pinpoint hemorrhages around hair follicles and in mouth, bleeding in gums and joints, impaired wound healing, weak bones, diarrhea, depression	• Dietary deficiency—infants are particularly susceptible

diseases, especially diarrhea, and compromises the body's ability to mount an effective antibody response, including to vaccinations. Infection is the usual cause of death in starving people. Besides the severe muscle atrophy, other signs of severe undernutrition include irritability, dry and cracked skin, skin sloughing and sores, and brittle hair.

In children, starvation manifests in two distinct ways. **Marasmus** refers to total caloric undernutrition, in which both calories and proteins are deficient in the diet. **Kwashiorkor** is caused by severe protein deficiency; in other words, caloric intake may be adequate, but there is no source of protein in the diet. It commonly occurs in areas with poor or marginal access to quality food sources after a child is weaned and put on a diet high in carbohydrates. Kwashiorkor is the type of starvation associated with abdominal swelling due to edema. Unfortunately, children who are severely undernourished and have signs of marasmus or kwashiorkor cannot digest and metabolize food once it is made available to them. They must be carefully treated, first with small sips of water to become rehydrated, then with the gradual addition of glucose (the most easily used source of energy); only gradually can carbohydrates and proteins be introduced. All of the tissues in the body of a severely undernourished patient have adapted to the starvation state, and the ability of the liver to handle complex metabolic processes is compromised. In very advanced cases, the tissues may have lost the ability to synthesize proteins; in this circumstance, the child will die even with protein and calorie replacement.

The effects of undernutrition in childhood are lifelong, even if the child does not die. This type of malnutrition results in stunted growth, delayed bone maturation, slowed mental processes, and retarded puberty. Mental retardation results from early-onset undernutrition with consequent failure of proper brain development.

Undernutrition is caused not only by poverty and famine but may also reflect underlying disease. In these situations, caloric intake may be adequate according to calculations based on the height and weight of the individual, but a hypermetabolic process occurring in the body starves the tissues of calories, so weight loss occurs. This type of undernutrition is called **cachexia**. It manifests with muscle wasting, weakness, skin rashes, diarrhea, loss of body hair, hepatomegaly, polyneuropathy, and signs and symptoms of vitamin and mineral deficiency, including anemia. Over time, the patient may develop outright aversion to food, or anorexia.

Many disease states can cause cachexia, with cancer and chronic infection (HIV, tuberculosis) being the most common. Patients with autoimmune diseases such as rheumatoid arthritis, or prolonged congestive heart failure, chronic obstructive pulmonary disease, or dialysis dependence, also often become cachectic. The pathophysiology in all these disease states involves the elaboration of cytokines by activated inflammatory cells. Cytokines are signaling molecules that effect a wide variety of changes during acute inflammatory events, from resetting the temperature set point (so patients develop fever) to decreasing appetite, inducing somnolence, increasing the release of cortisol, and up-regulating the production of white blood cells. They induce cachexia through a variety of mechanisms: by decreasing muscle protein synthesis and inducing targeted breakdown of muscle proteins; by increasing the resting metabolic rate; by reducing the activity of key hepatic enzymes involved in lipid metabolism; and by inducing anorexia and anhedonia, so voluntary food consumption is reduced.

In inflammatory conditions such as tuberculosis or rheumatoid arthritis, it is easy to see the connection between the condition, increased cytokine expression, and cachexia, but how and why cytokine production is increased in chronic heart, lung, or kidney disease is not well understood.

Anorexia nervosa and **bulimia nervosa** are eating disorders in which afflicted patients, usually adolescent girls, have an irrational fear of gaining weight, and voluntarily reduce their nutritional intake to effect severe weight loss. Anorexia nervosa refers to dietary restriction, sometimes accompanied by induced vomiting; patients with bulimia binge-eat and then purge by inducing vomiting, taking laxatives, or exercising excessively. Of all mental health conditions, anorexia nervosa is the most deadly: as many as 10% of patients die as a result of starvation. Patients also develop electrolyte disorders, resulting in cardiac arrhythmia or seizures, dehydration, hormonal disorders including amenorrhea and hypothyroidism, a decrease in immune function because of decreased production of white blood cells, liver damage (as reflected in elevated liver function tests), stunted growth and deficient mineralization of bone, and changes in the skin and hair. The most obvious sign is, of course, the extreme emaciation resulting from avoidance of food and often compulsive exercising.

What causes the irrational distortion of body image in anorexia nervosa and bulimia nervosa is not known. These disorders are more common in areas of the world where society places a high value on slender female bodies, and they appear to be more common in the wealthy, white demographic group. Nevertheless, development of these disorders cannot be blamed solely on exposure to unrealistic values. Genetic predisposition and hormonal imbalances also play a role. Some sources suggest that patients attempt to exercise "control" over one aspect of their life to compensate for other parts over which they feel they have no control. The disorders are often accompanied by other mental health conditions, including anxiety, obsessive–compulsive disorder, and depression.

Treatment of anorexia nervosa and bulimia nervosa is extremely difficult because patients must first be convinced that their behavior is irrational and harmful. Patients often are in denial that anything is wrong. Cognitive-behavioral therapy, therapy involving the whole family as a resource for change, and support groups are effective, but it may take a long time for patients to even accept the fact that they need to change their behavior, during which the serious complications mentioned above can develop. Patients may need the help of specialized treatment centers in which patients remain under medical observation while undergoing cognitive therapy. While in many instances the disease runs its course in two years or so, some patients may develop lifelong preoccupations with low body weight, or continue to experience anxiety and depression. Very few patients recover completely.

Failure to thrive is a term used to describe poor growth or weight loss. It is not a disease in itself, but rather reflects a wide variety of underlying conditions (**Table 30–4**). In the pediatric age group, failure to thrive refers to poor growth and weight gain as measured against standards of height and weight for age. In the geriatric population, it refers to a progressive decline in function, in which poor nutrition is accompanied by depression, impaired physical function, or cognitive impairment. In both age groups, determination of the cause of failure to thrive must include medical as well as psychosocial assessments, and treatment is geared toward correcting the underlying abnormality. If left to progress, patients will develop the symptoms and complications of starvation described earlier in this chapter.

Deficiencies and Excesses of Specific Vitamins and Minerals

Essential minerals and vitamins must be derived from exogenous sources. The bacteria in the gut produce a small amount of vitamin K, but this is insufficient to meet the needs of the body. Vitamin D can be synthesized in the skin when it is exposed to sunlight, but, especially in northern latitudes where people are indoors

TABLE 30–4 Causes of Failure to Thrive

Pediatric

Endogenous

Genetic
- Inborn errors of metabolism
- Cystic fibrosis
- Down syndrome

Congenital
- Cleft palate
- Hiatal hernia/gastroesophageal reflux
- Heart disease (valve defects)
- Cerebral palsy

Allergies
- Celiac disease
- Milk allergies

Infection

Exogenous

- Poverty
- Improper administration of formula
- Diet insufficient in calories
- Inability to meet special needs of child (e.g., tube feedings)
- Emotional deprivation
- Child abuse or neglect

Geriatric

- Social isolation
- Poor self-care
- Depression
- Cognitive impairment
- Medical conditions (e.g., lung, liver, or kidney disease; stroke; rheumatologic diseases)
- Medications

and habitually wear clothes that cover most of the skin most of the year, endogenous vitamin D production is also insufficient. While nutritionists recommend that all essential vitamins and minerals be obtained from a well-balanced diet, this is actually difficult for most people to achieve. Doing so requires consumption of a large variety of foodstuffs, particularly fresh fruit and vegetables, that people may not be able (because of their cost, for example) or willing to consume. Vegetarians, pregnant women, children, and people older than age 50 are most vulnerable to developing vitamin and mineral deficiencies if they rely on dietary sources alone. Multivitamin supplements are a cheap and convenient source of vitamins, and they often contain essential minerals, such as iodine and iron, as well. Vitamins and minerals are also available as individual preparations for people with specific deficiencies, such as ferrous sulfate for patients with iron-deficiency anemia or vitamin B_{12} for patients with megaloblastic anemia.

The wide variety of foodstuffs available in the North American market, combined with the fortification of many types of foods with essential nutrients (e.g., milk with vitamin D, breakfast cereals with iron and B vitamins, salt with iodine), makes overt manifestation of vitamin and mineral deficiency states rare in this geographic region. In the past, it was much more common for people to develop scurvy, rickets, pellagra, or pernicious anemia (see Table 30–3 for descriptions of these conditions) due to deficiencies in consumption of essential nutrients. Nowadays, these conditions develop only rarely; moreover, when they do occur, they can easily be treated with supplements.

Relatively cheap and convenient access to vitamin and mineral supplements also makes it easier for people to be exposed to toxic quantities, however. People are easily swayed by the idea that "more is better," which may encourage them to consume greater than the recommended dose in the hope of deriving some added benefit. Water-soluble vitamins (vitamin C and the B-complex group) are cleared by the body when ingested in excess amounts. Nevertheless, excess vitamin C ingestion can lead to the development of kidney stones. Minerals are stored in the liver and released in very small amounts to meet the needs of the tissues, or are chelated (bound to a substance that makes them inert) and excreted through the kidney. Pharmaceutical chelating agents can also be used to remove some of these minerals, if laboratory tests demonstrate that they are present in excess. Excess iron deposition may be treated with phlebotomy, as loss of red blood cells and the iron they contain stimulates the mobilization of stored iron for the synthesis of new hemoglobin. Mineral toxicities are usually seen in the setting of environmental contamination, and most of their toxic effects involve the brain.

Vitamins A, D, E, and K are fat soluble, so their absorption and metabolism are linked to that of fatty acids; consequently, only very small amounts of these vitamins are excreted through the kidney. They are stored primarily in the liver, and to a smaller extent in fatty tissues. Usually the body stores sufficient amounts of these vitamins to maintain tissue function for several months after complete dietary deficiency occurs. Toxicity is not a concern when their only source is a well-balanced diet. Excess supplementation can cause problems, especially with vitamins A and D. Chronic vitamin A toxicity can cause bone and joint pain, liver damage, skin disorders, and hair loss, among other effects, and in very severe instances can cause death. Vitamin A, in the form of retinoic acid, is effective in treating skin disorders such as acne and psoriasis, but retinoic acid is a potent teratogen: women should be counseled against using this therapy during pregnancy, because it can lead to neural crest defects and spontaneous abortion of the fetus. Vitamin D supplementation may lead to excessive absorption of calcium, with subsequent deposition of calcium in tissues and bone demineralization.

Table 30–3 describes specific vitamin deficiency states. It is beyond the scope of this text to go into these imbalances in greater detail. Instead, diseases and conditions that predispose individuals to specific deficiency states are discussed here.

Patients who have undergone surgical resection of their small intestine (for conditions such as Crohn disease, necrotizing enterocolitis, or volvulus of the small intestine) suffer from **short bowel syndrome**. The small intestine absorbs most, if not all, ingested nutrients; thus, with decreased surface area available for absorption, the gastrointestinal tract cannot digest a normal diet. Depending on how much of the small intestine is left, patients may require supplementation not only of vitamins and minerals but also of calories, fiber, and proteins. This is often achieved only with **total parenteral nutrition**, or intravenous administration of nutritive solutions. Selective resection of parts of the small intestine also can cause deficiency states: resection of the duodenum causes iron deficiency, as iron is primarily absorbed in the duodenum, while resection of the terminal ileum can cause vitamin B_{12} deficiency. Selective supplementation is required in these conditions.

Alcoholics ingest the majority of their calories in the form of alcohol, which provides carbohydrates but not much else by way of nutritive benefit. In other words, alcoholics consume a very restricted diet and are predisposed to developing protein-energy undernutrition (kwashiorkor) as well as symptoms of vitamin and mineral deficiencies. Thiamin (one of the B-complex vitamins) deficiency leads to progressive, irreversible atrophic changes in areas of the brain related to memory, balance, and the ability to concentrate and perform higher, or "executive," functions. This disorder, called **Wernicke-Korsakoff syndrome**, has been described in other conditions in which there is defective consumption of thiamin. Various forms of anemia develop in alcoholics secondary to deficiencies in other B-complex

vitamins. Alcohol also does serious damage to the gastrointestinal tract and liver, further compromising the ability to absorb and metabolize essential nutrients. Chronic liver disease results in impaired absorption of the fat-soluble vitamins, with subsequent impaired night vision, bone mineralization, and blood clotting. It also causes damage to the small intestine, leading to impaired iron absorption and the development of iron-deficiency anemia. Finally, alcohol is a potent teratogen. Consumption of alcohol during pregnancy can cause serious developmental disturbances in the fetus, which may be manifested in the form of the *fetal alcohol syndrome*. Children with this syndrome exhibit characteristic facial features, such as depressed nasal bridge, inner canthal folds, and small eyes; absence of a philtrum and thin upper lip; and mental retardation resulting from impaired brain development.

Women are prone to developing iron-deficiency anemia. In particular, menstruation, pregnancy, and lactation pose considerable nutritional challenges. Menstruating women need to replace iron lost through the menstrual purge. Pregnant and lactating women need to ingest sufficient nutrients not only for themselves, but also for the growing fetus and nursing infant. Iron-deficiency anemia is the most common nutritional deficiency state occurring during pregnancy.

The developing fetus and growing infant and child have special nutritional needs. Pregnant women are urged to consume folate to prevent the development of **neural tube defects** in infancy. Folate is found in high concentrations in legumes and leafy green vegetables, such as spinach and kale. It also is an ingredient in the multivitamin pills that are designed specifically for pregnant women. Other foodstuffs may be teratogens when ingested during pregnancy—the harmful effects of retinoic acid and alcohol on the fetus have already been mentioned. The fastest rates of growth occur during infancy and adolescence. While human milk or formula provides all the nutrients an infant needs during the first six months or so of life, weaning and the introduction of solid foods are fraught with nutritional challenges. The diet must contain not only carbohydrates for fuel but also sufficient proteins and essential vitamins and minerals to promote brain development, bone maturation, and muscle growth. The same is true during puberty, when rapid growth requires consumption of much larger quantities of foods than the individual was used to consuming during childhood. The growing boy or girl requires good nutritional counseling during this period so as to make wise food choices and not just satisfy his or her hunger with foods that have poor nutritional quality.

Nutritional needs change during a person's lifetime. While aging adults often restrict their diet in response to their gradually slowing metabolism, the need for a healthy diet and sufficient, clean water never goes away. In fact, older adults may require more supplementation or a shift in their dietary consumption to make up for increased needs. Certainly the need for iron, calcium, and the B-complex vitamins never disappears, and it may actually increase due to diseases of the small intestine that compromise the absorption of these essential nutrients. A deficiency state that tends to be seen more often in older individuals than in their younger counterparts is vitamin B_{12} deficiency, which causes anemia, sensorimotor deficiencies (delayed or absent reflexes, diminished sensation of vibration and soft touch), and, if not detected and corrected in a timely manner, irreversible injury to the spinal cord and dementia.

Chronic diseases, pharmaceutical drugs, and medical interventions can also induce special dietary needs. For example, thiazide diuretics are effective in controlling hypertension because they rid the body of excess water, but in the process potassium is also lost. Patients taking these medications must supplement their diet with foods high in potassium, such as bananas, to prevent a deficiency state. Patients with chronic kidney disease are at greater risk of developing bone disorders because of impaired regulation of calcium and phosphorus by the kidney. Chronic liver disease is associated with impaired absorption of fats, so patients risk developing deficiencies of the fat-soluble vitamins. Treating patients with these conditions therefore requires not only gaining control of the underlying mechanism of disease, but also counseling them on special dietary needs.

Immune-Mediated Disorders

The intestines are an important immunological organ. They contain large numbers of lymphocytes and macrophages (approximately as many as the spleen), which are actively engaged in presenting antigens derived from substances in the lumen of the gut to macrophages to induce the production of cytotoxic T cells and B cells. It is a wonder that the immune system so rarely overreacts to ingested substances, given the vast quantity and variety of molecules to which it is exposed on a daily basis.

The simplest form of hyperreactivity of the immune system in the gut is **food allergy**. This Type 1 hypersensitivity reaction is mediated by an antigen derived from a particular food item, which cross-links immunoglobulin E (IgE) antibodies present on mast cells to cause their rapid degranulation. Release of histamine results in an immediate acute inflammatory response—in other words, vasodilation and increased vascular permeability, often accompanied by itching, wheezing, or abdominal pain. The symptoms of food allergies can range from mild (rash, hives, or "flare and wheal" reactions in the skin) to lethal (due to generalized tissue swelling with constriction of the larynx, bronchoconstriction, and coronary artery muscle spasm). The list of foods that can stimulate a Type 1 allergic reaction is long, but the most common culprits are peanuts, eggs, shellfish, tree nuts, soy, and wheat. Food allergies are more common in children, who may even outgrow them, but they can develop at any time, even in adults who have eaten the offending food

item all their lives with no problems. The only means of preventing these allergic symptoms is to avoid eating the food that triggers them.

Celiac disease is a relatively common, immunologically mediated disease linked to ingestion of *gluten*, a protein found in wheat, barley, and rye. It is estimated that approximately 1% of the U.S. population has celiac disease, and this condition is more common in people of Northern European descent. While celiac disease was first diagnosed in children, it has become abundantly clear that adults also can develop it. The pathophysiology involves both autoimmune and delayed-type hypersensitivity reactions. Through direct and indirect processes, one of the molecules produced during the digestion of gluten, called *gliadin*, activates T cells. Cytotoxic T cells cause injury to the epithelial cells on intestinal villi. At the same time, helper T cells stimulate B cells to produce antibodies against gliadin and certain other molecules involved in the processing of gliadin. These cells also incite an inflammatory reaction against the epithelial lining of the villi. Over time, the epithelial cells become damaged to such an extent that the intestinal villi become severely blunted and the small intestine loses its absorptive ability.

Patients with celiac disease develop symptoms related to impaired digestion and absorption and, if their condition is not treated, can suffer starvation. Symptoms include bloating, diarrhea, and abdominal pain as well as irritability, anorexia, muscle wasting, and failure to thrive. In addition, patients with celiac disease may develop extra-intestinal manifestations, such as an itchy, blistering rash called *dermatitis herpetiformis*. The incidence of other autoimmune diseases, including diabetes and thyroid disease, is more common in patients with celiac disease than in the general population.

There is no pharmacologic treatment for celiac disease; the only effective treatment is complete withdrawal of gluten from the diet. This is easier said than done. It is bad enough that wheat is a staple in the North American diet: finding tasty substitutes for bread, noodles, and beer (malt is derived from barley) is already a challenge. But gluten also is commonly used as a food additive: it imparts a chewy, elastic quality to foods, thickens sauces, and stabilizes foods. Gluten is added to a wide variety of products, from baked beans to ice cream and ketchup, to shampoo and toothpaste, and it is even used as "filler" in multivitamin pills and other medications. Gluten does not need to be disclosed on food labels, so people with celiac disease need to become experts at detecting gluten lurking in the ingredients listed on food labels. For patients with very severe celiac disease, "gluten-free" products that were processed in the same plant or with the same machinery as wheat products can contain enough trace gluten to cause disease symptoms. Even toasting gluten-free and wheat bread in the same toaster can cause problems.

Another autoimmune disease linked to digestion and absorption is **pernicious anemia**. Epithelial cells in the stomach produce a protein called *intrinsic factor*, which binds to vitamin B_{12} in the duodenum and facilitates its absorption in the ileum. Without intrinsic factor, vitamin B_{12} is absorbed very poorly. In pernicious anemia, an autoimmune reaction destroys the epithelial cells in the stomach, so the production of intrinsic factor declines. Once the body uses up its stores of vitamin B_{12}, the patient begins to develop symptoms of vitamin B_{12} deficiency. Pernicious anemia is most common in the elderly population (the median age of diagnosis is 60 years), and it can develop in conjunction with other conditions in which the epithelial cells of the stomach are damaged (e.g., achlorhydria, chronic inflammation) or surgically removed (e.g., for bariatric surgery).

Pernicious anemia develops insidiously and, if untreated, progresses relentlessly to cause irreversible neurologic damage and death. Before overt symptoms develop, routine laboratory testing may detect megaloblastic anemia. The diagnosis is confirmed with additional laboratory findings: leukopenia, low serum vitamin B_{12}, and increased levels of metabolites usually processed by the enzyme of which vitamin B_{12} is the cofactor. If the diagnosis is made early enough and treatment begun quickly, the symptoms may never develop. The classic triad of symptoms associated with pernicious anemia is glossitis (large, sore, and red tongue with a smooth surface), paresthesias (numbness and tingling of the hands and feet), and weakness. This type of anemia can also cause fatigue, rapid heart rate, heart murmurs, shortness of breath, and, if severe and prolonged, frank congestive heart failure. The neurologic damage is due to degeneration of axons in the spinal tract. It initially causes paresthesias in the hands and feet, which then progresses to absent reflexes, difficulty walking, and eventually paraplegia.

There is no cure for pernicious anemia: the epithelial cells of the stomach, once irreparably damaged, cannot be stimulated to produce intrinsic factor again. Also, because oral vitamin B_{12} is absorbed very poorly in the absence of intrinsic factor, oral administration of this nutrient alone is insufficient to bring the body stores of vitamin B_{12} back up to safe levels. Patients with vitamin B_{12} deficiency are initially treated with daily, intramuscular injection of high doses of vitamin B_{12}. Once the serum levels of vitamin B_{12} are sufficiently high, the patient can be maintained on monthly injections. If caught early enough, pernicious anemia is reversible, and signs of anemia and neurological damage do not develop.

Enzyme Deficiencies

Digestion and absorption of nutrients require the action of numerous enzymes, as well as lubrication by secretions produced by various glands in the upper digestive tract and participation of the indigenous intestinal flora. Amylase, an enzyme that digests starch, is produced by the salivary glands and begins to digest food while it is being masticated in the mouth. Destruction of the salivary glands—for example, by an autoimmune disorder—can lead to problems with nutrition, both because of the reduced activity of salivary amylase and because of reduced production of saliva. Without saliva, food loses its taste and is difficult to chew, and the mouth has a dry and uncomfortable sensation that precludes the desire to eat.

Pancreatic insufficiency also causes poor digestion and absorption. The pancreas makes digestive enzymes capable of breaking up fats, proteins, and starches. In addition, it produces insulin, the hormone responsible for regulating the metabolism of glucose. Patients with diseases affecting the pancreas, such as cystic fibrosis or pancreatitis, or who have had part or the entire pancreas surgically removed for cancer treatment, require supplementation of the pancreatic enzymes via the diet, and need to control their blood glucose with frequent blood sugar checks and insulin administration. If untreated, pancreatic enzyme insufficiency results in a variety of symptoms: diarrhea, weight loss, fatigue, and failure to thrive, secondary to the body's inability to derive nutrition from the food that is ingested; flatulence and abdominal distention, as bacteria ferment the unabsorbed food particles in the intestine; steatorrhea, as undigested fat causes the stool to be bulky and foul smelling; and specific nutrient deficiencies such as anemia (deficiency of iron and/or vitamin B_{12}), bleeding disorders (deficiency of vitamin K), night blindness (deficiency of vitamin A), impaired bone mineralization (deficiency of calcium and vitamin D), and paresthesias (deficiency of vitamin B_{12} and folate), among others.

Nutrients are absorbed from the intestinal lumen primarily by epithelial cells of the small intestine. These cells also contribute to digestion by producing certain enzymes, such as lactase. **Lactase deficiency**, also called *lactose intolerance*, develops after infancy as the production of lactase in intestinal epithelial cells is downregulated. Lactose is the main type of sugar present in dairy products. Patients with lactose intolerance develop abdominal bloating and flatulence after ingestion of dairy products, as lactose remains undigested in the gut lumen and bacteria use it as a substrate for fermentation. The enzyme lactase can be added to dairy products to make them digestible for patients with lactase deficiency, and various pharmaceutical lactase preparations (pills and tablets) can be taken with dairy products to help digest them. Dairy products are excellent sources of calcium, so patients who avoid them should make an effort to acquire calcium and vitamin D from other sources. Lactase deficiency is not as common among Caucasians as it is in Native American and Asian populations.

Fructose intolerance causes symptoms similar to those associated with lactose intolerance (i.e., abdominal pain, bloating, flatulence), but after ingestion of foods that either are high in fructose content, such as prepared foods containing high-fructose corn syrup as an additive, or contain more fructose than glucose (certain fruits, such as apples, pears, mango, and honey). In this case, the symptoms are not caused by a deficient enzyme but rather by deficient absorption of fructose by small intestinal epithelial cells. Fructose does not require enzymatic digestion, but diffuses into the epithelial cells along a concentration gradient with the help of a cotransport molecule, or by attaching to glucose, which freely diffuses across the lipid bilayer. If the amount of ingested fructose is more than the diffusion process can handle—in other words, when the cotransport molecule is saturated and there is insufficient glucose to bind to—fructose stays within the gut lumen and is fermented by bacteria.

Inborn errors of metabolism are genetic diseases in which the proteins necessary for the complete metabolism of specific molecules are not produced, or are produced in insufficient quantities, such that the molecules accumulate and lead to progressive decline in function of tissues. Although these disorders involve metabolism rather than digestion and absorption, the treatment of patients with inborn errors of metabolism often requires specific dietary restrictions. For example, patients with *phenylketonuria* (PKU) are incapable of fully metabolizing the essential amino acid phenylalanine to tyrosine. As phenylalanine builds up in the blood, it saturates proteins at the blood–brain barrier that transport amino acids into the brain. The brain in essence suffers amino acid starvation, resulting in impaired neurologic development. Because of the serious consequences of undetected PKU, infants are tested for this disorder at birth. Treatment of this condition requires strict avoidance of phenylalanine in the diet, which means essentially following a vegan diet (no dairy products, eggs, meat, poultry, or fish), with additional restrictions on consumption of vegetables with a high protein content, such as potatoes, peas, and legumes. A phenylalanine-free diet is especially important for infants and children, because the brain experiences its greatest rate of development during this phase of life.

Some of the other inborn errors of metabolism can be similarly treated; for example, *galactosemia*, resulting from a deficiency of enzymes responsible for digestion of galactose, is treated with complete avoidance of milk and dairy products, which are high in galactose. For many of the other disorders, dietary modifications have not been shown to be of benefit.

Obesity

As mentioned in the section on most frequent and serious problems related to nutrition, obesity is by far the most important nutritional disorder in the world today. Obesity is measured in terms of **body mass index (BMI)**, which relates a person's weight to his or her height. BMI is a crude estimate of body fat because weight may be increased secondary to increased muscle mass (e.g., in athletes) rather than fat. Other measurements that give a crude estimate of obesity are skin fold calipers and measurement of waist circumference. More reliable methods are cumbersome and involve estimating the ratio of fat to lean tissue. Despite many people's objections to the use of BMI, it is the accepted standard for measuring and recording obesity. A BMI greater than or equal to 30 is considered obese; a BMI in the range 25–30 is overweight; and a BMI less than 18.5 is underweight. New categories are being defined for patients with a BMI greater than 30, as more and more patients are becoming "severely" obese, "morbidly" obese, and "super" obese.

The pathophysiology of obesity is extremely complex. At a basic level, it results from an imbalance in calories ingested versus calories expended. A ubiquitous, relatively cheap food supply rich in carbohydrates and simple sugars, coupled with an increasingly sedentary lifestyle, is undoubtedly a major factor contributing to obesity in upper- and middle-income nations. However, the development of obesity is also linked to genetic variability in metabolism. Aging is accompanied by slowing of the metabolism, so some patients gain weight beginning in their midlife, even when their diet and energy expenditure stay the same. Certain populations are predisposed to obesity, such as Native Americans. It is thought that these populations are genetically predisposed to metabolize food very effectively, perhaps due to evolutionary selection for efficient metabolism during food shortages in American prehistory. Tall people with increased body surface area have a faster rate of metabolism than do short people, so they are less inclined to gain weight. Also, there are likely genetic differences in people's sensations of hunger and satiety, which are hormonally and neurally regulated, such that some people have a greater tolerance for hunger or feel satiety with fewer calories consumed compared to others.

In addition, environmental factors play a significant role in development of obesity. Children tend to acquire a body habitus similar to that of their parents, so children of obese parents are already predisposed to becoming obese themselves. This pattern could in part be due to genetics, but it also has to do with learning about food choices and values. If socializing revolves around high-calorie snacks or "all you can eat dinners" at a favorite restaurant, all members of the social circle will be more likely to be obese than if socializing includes going for a bike ride or a run. The taste for fatty foods is acquired through conditioning—that is, through repeated exposure accompanied by positive reinforcement, such as hearing "This is so good" or "This is comfort food," or simply eating the foods with people one depends on (parents) or admires (social group). Certain pharmaceutical compounds that people take for treatment of illness are known to cause an increase in weight, including steroids (e.g., for autoimmune diseases) and selective serotonin uptake inhibitors (e.g., for depression).

Some epidemiologists believe that environmental toxins are responsible for the worldwide increase in obesity.

They argue that the rate of weight gain documented all over the world in the past few decades has been too rapid to be explained by genetic and dietary factors alone. They claim instead that exposure to synthetic organic and inorganic chemicals that are known to have weight-promoting effects in experimental settings is responsible for this trend. It is postulated that these so-called *obesogens* exert their effects by controlling the rate of transcription of proteins involved in lipid metabolism, altering the ratio of sex steroids so accumulation of lipid is favored over its mobilization from adipose tissue, or altering the neurohormonal control of appetite. Much more research on these molecules and their effects on weight control needs to be done before solid evidence-based public health interventions can be implemented.

In the meantime, treatment of obesity is put squarely on the shoulders of the affected individual—and anyone who has tried to lose weight will recognize the enormity of the problem these individuals face. Some are obstinately in denial that they have a problem because everyone in their social network is obese and the wider cultural value placed on "normal" weight appears unrealistic; for others, the changes in lifestyle that weight reduction would require are literally unpalatable; and some simply do not lose significant weight however valiantly they try. Nutritional counseling and programs such as Weight Watchers that provide support and advice from others going through the same transition can be very effective. Patients who have repeatedly been unsuccessful in their attempt to lose weight may opt for **bariatric surgery**, or surgical reduction of the volume of the stomach. With a reduced stomach volume, smaller amounts of food are required for the stomach to become full and give the sensation of satiety. Bariatric surgery performed in experienced centers is reportedly successful in achieving long-term weight reduction in as many as 70% of patients. In addition, it reduces the risk of developing obesity-related diseases in patients who experience significant weight loss. However, bariatric surgery is expensive and associated with a 10% risk of developing surgical complications, so it is not a solution for the global obesity epidemic.

Obesity is a problem because it is associated with numerous serious health hazards that collectively reduce life expectancy. **Table 30–5** lists some of the known complications of obesity. Life expectancy is reduced by as much as 10 years in patients who are obese, in comparison to normal-weight nonsmokers. In addition, quality of life is reduced secondary to the development of diseases including type 2 diabetes mellitus and its complications, osteoarthritis, and sleep apnea. Not only is obesity harmful to individuals' health, but it also costs a staggering amount of money: according to the Centers for Disease Control and Prevention, the direct and indirect costs of medical care for obesity in the United States in 2008 totaled $147 billion. It is estimated that obesity and its complications will soon account for at least 20% of U.S. healthcare expenditures.

TABLE 30–5 Complications of Obesity
Cardiovascular disease and its risk factors
Coronary atherosclerosis
Hypertension
Dyslipidemia
Aortic aneurysm
Stroke
Pulmonary embolism
Disorders of insulin regulation
• Insulin resistance
• Diabetes mellitus (type 2)
Neoplasia
• Endometrial carcinoma
• Breast cancer
• Others (less strong association: pancreas, colon, gallbladder)
Respiratory problems
• Sleep apnea
• Restrictive lung function
• Asthma
• Complications during general anesthesia
Gastrointestinal problems
• Gastroesophageal reflux
Fatty liver disease
• Hepatic fibrosis and cirrhosis
• Gallstones
Joint disease
Osteoarthritis
Gout
Low back pain
Skin problems
• Lymphedema
• Cellulitis
• Hirsutism
• Rash between skin folds (intertrigo)
Gynecologic problems
• Irregular menses
• Infertility
• Pregnancy complications
Urologic problems
• Urinary incontinence
• Chronic renal failure
• Buried penis
• Hypogonadism
• Erectile dysfunction
Psychiatric conditions
• Depression
• Social stigmatization
Reduced life expectancy

Clearly, obesity is one of the major public health challenges not only in the United States but throughout the world. It will take the concerted effort of policy makers, doctors, researchers, nutritionists, teachers, and a well-educated public to make any kind of dent in the rising trend of obesity. Our major challenge is to remember to make healthy food choices in an unhealthy environment.

REFERENCE

1. Byrd-Brenner, Carol, et al. *Wardlaw's Perspectives in Nutrition*, 8th ed. New York, NY: McGraw-Hill; 2007.

Practice Questions

1. Which of the following is the largest threat to health in the world today?
   A. HIV/AIDS
   B. Malnutrition
   C. Iron-deficiency anemia
   D. Contaminated drinking water

2. Which of the following nutritional deficiency states is usually not seen in alcoholics?
   A. Calorie malnutrition (starvation)
   B. Protein malnutrition (kwashiorkor)
   C. Thiamin deficiency (Wernicke-Korsakoff syndrome)
   D. Deficiencies of vitamins A, D, E, and K

3. Teratogens include all of the following except
   A. Alcohol.
   B. Folate deficiency.
   C. Retinoic acid (vitamin A).
   D. B vitamins.

4. Iron-deficiency anemia is most likely to develop in
   A. The developing fetus.
   B. Children.
   C. Women of childbearing age.
   D. The elderly.

5. Celiac disease is
   A. A Type 1 food allergy.
   B. An immune reaction against a protein found in wheat, barley, and rye.
   C. A disease of childhood.
   D. Easily prevented because gluten is not a common ingredient in foods.

6. Pancreatic enzyme deficiency results in all of the following except
   A. Steatorrhea, flatulence, and abdominal pain.
   B. Stunted growth and development.
   C. Impaired digestion of fats, carbohydrates, and proteins.
   D. Gallstones.

7. Which of the following is not a cause of decreased quality of life in obesity?
   A. Joint pain
   B. Sleep apnea
   C. Erectile dysfunction
   D. Decreased night vision

Glossary

A

Abrasion A scraping or scuffing of the skin surface without full-thickness loss.

Abrasion collar A marginal rim of abrasion around an entrance wound.

Abscess A localized collection of pus.

Accessory breast tissue Mammary tissue found in locations other than the breast.

Accommodation Ability of the eye to adjust its focusing power.

Acetabulum The hip socket.

Acetaminophen A drug commonly used to control pain and fever that can have a toxic effect on the liver if overused.

Acidosis Increased acidity of the blood, which is incompatible with the physiologic function of cells.

Acinus Grape-shaped secretory apparatus of certain glands such as the breast and pancreas.

Acquired immune system A defense mechanism that requires previous exposure to the offending agent and entails antibody or cellular specificity.

Acquired immunodeficiency syndrome (AIDS) The final and most severe stage of HIV (human immunodeficiency virus) disease.

Acral lentiginous melanoma A melanoma that occurs on the palms and soles, and in or around the nail unit.

Acromegaly A clinical condition of excess growth hormone causing thickening of soft tissue and bones.

Acrophobia Fear of high places.

Actin One of the two primary proteins that make up muscle.

Actinic Early skin lesions occurring on surfaces exposed to the sun.

Actinic keratoses Skin changes caused by solar damage.

Activated partial thromboplastin time (aPTT) A test for deficiencies in the intrinsic pathway of the coagulation mechanism.

Acute abdomen Sudden severe abdominal pain of unknown origin.

Acute appendicitis Inflammation of the appendix.

Acute bacterial prostatitis Inflammation of the prostate caused by the same organisms that cause urinary tract infections, which manifests with urgency, frequency, and perineal pain.

Acute mastitis Acute inflammation of the breast caused by bacteria entering through cracks in the nipple or areola of a lactating woman.

Acute necrotizing ulcerative gingivitis A particularly severe type of gingivitis, manifested by ulcerated and bleeding gingivae.

Acute pancreatitis Inflammation of the pancreas.

Acute rejection   Organ rejection that begins about one to six weeks after transplantation. It is caused by a mismatch between donor and recipient antigens.

Acute respiratory stress syndrome (ARDS)   A disease where the epithelial cells lining the pulmonary alveoli become damaged and the lungs fill with edema fluid and blood, thereby severely hampering respiration.

Acute salpingitis   Infection and inflammation of the fallopian tubes.

Adaptive immune system   An internal chemical system whose purpose is to enhance specific reactivity to materials that are foreign to the body.

Adenoids   The lymphoid tissue of the nasopharynx.

Adenomas   Usually benign tumors of glandular origin.

ADHD   (*see* Attention deficit hyperactivity disorder)

Adhesion   Usually refers to the process of platelets or leukocytes sticking to endothelium.

Adiposity   An increased storage of fat in fat cells.

Adolescence   The final developmental period before the process of aging begins.

Adrenal cortex   Outer part of the adrenal gland that mediates the stress response through the production of mineralcorticoids and glucocorticoids.

Adrenal medulla   The center of the adrenal gland responsible for secreting epinephrine, norepinephrine, and dopamine.

Adrenocorticotropic hormone (ACTH)   A hormone secreted by the anterior pituitary gland in response to stress.

Adynamic ileus   The delayed movement and emptying of the gut due to paralyzed gastrointestinal musculature rather than to a physical obstruction.

Agammaglobulinemia   Very low levels of serum gamma globulin due to an inherited deficiency.

Age-dependent   Diseases that occur to some extent in all individuals with time.

Age-related   Diseases that occur in the elderly but are not part of the aging process, as they do not occur in all individuals.

Agoraphobia   Fear of being alone.

AIDS   (*see* Acquired immunodeficiency syndrome)

Albinism   An uncommon autosomal recessive hereditary condition in which melanocytes are unable to produce normal amounts of melanin pigment. Patients lack normal pigmentation in skin, hair, and irides.

Albumin   A serum protein that maintains osmotic pressure and can carry nonsoluble molecules such as unconjugated bilirubin in the blood.

Alcohol   A colorless, volatile liquid.

Aldosterone   A steroid secreted by the cortex of the adrenal gland that increases the resorption of sodium and water by the renal tubules and thus expands blood volume.

Alkaline phosphatase   An enzyme produced by osteoblasts that is elevated in many bone diseases that involve proliferation of osteoblasts.

Alleles   Alternative forms of a gene (one member of a pair) located at specific positions on specific chromosomes.

Allergies   Disorders of the immune system; a form of hypersensitivity.

Allopathic medicine   Conventional practice of medicine with biological bases for treatment.

Alopecia   Hair loss.

Alpha-1 antitrypsin deficiency disease   A type of emphysema caused by the destruction of alveolar walls by uninhibited inflammatory enzymes.

Alveoli   Thin-walled sacs in the lungs through the walls of which gas is exchanged.

Alzheimer disease   A specific type of dementia.

Amebiasis   Disease caused by an intestinal organism that invades and produces colonic ulcers and, occasionally, liver abscesses.

Amenorrhea   The absence of menstruation.

Amniocentesis   Transabdominal aspiration of amniotic fluid for testing.

Amylase   Enzyme that digests carbohydrates, fats, and proteins.

Amyloid   A hyaline deposit that stains with the dye Congo red.

Anaerobic   Bacteria that grow in environments in which there is little or no oxygen.

Anaphylaxis   Severe acute hypersensitivity with vasodilation resulting in shock and bronchoconstriction resulting in inability to breathe.

Anaplasia   Loss of cellular differentiation; seen in malignant neoplasms.

Anasarca   Edema generalized throughout the body.

Anatomic pathology   Medical specialty involved with performing autopsies and examining tissues and fluids removed from live patients for the purpose of diagnosis.

Androgens   A group of chemically related male sex hormones.

Anemia   A decrease in the circulating red blood cell mass.

Anemia of chronic disease   A common type of anemia caused by a chronic medical condition that affects the production and life span of red blood cells and is unresponsive to therapy.

Anencephaly   A severe malformation in which the entire forebrain is missing.

Aneurysm   An abnormal widening or ballooning of a portion of an artery due to weakness in the wall.

Angina pectoris   Cardiac chest pain brought on by exercise or emotional stress and relieved by rest or vasodilator drugs.

Angiogram   A type of x-ray test to reveal the anatomy of the blood vessels and thereby detect abnormalities in the route of blood flow. Radiopaque dyes are injected directly into the coronary arteries to outline atherosclerotic plaques.

Angiography   X-rays taken after radiopaque dye is injected into arteries to show the caliber of the vessels and distribution of blood flow.

Angioplasty   Reconstruction or recanalization of a blood vessel.

Angiotensin   A peptide that stimulates vasoconstriction of vessels throughout the body and thereby elevates the blood pressure.

Angiotensin-converting enzyme (ACE)   An enzyme that coverts angiotensin I to angiotension II.

Ankylosing spondylitis   An inflammatory arthritis predominantly involving the spine and sacroiliac joints, and resulting in ankylosis.

Ankylosis   Joint rigidity.

Anorexia   Loss of appetite.

Anoxia   Absence of oxygen.

Anthracosis   Pneumoconiosis from carbon accumulation in the lungs and draining of lymph nodes.

Antibodies   Gamma globulin proteins that are found in blood or other fluids, used by the immune system to neutralize foreign materials.

Antidiuretic hormone   A hormone released to act on the epithelial cells of the collecting duct to increase their permeability so more water is resorbed back into the bloodstream.

Antigen   Material recognized as foreign by the immune system.

Antigen-presenting cells (APC)   Specialized cells that present antigens to T lymphocytes.

Antinuclear antibody (ANA)   A test that detects antibodies against nuclei of tissue cells that are found in the serum of patients with certain autoimmune diseases.

Antithrombin   A small protein molecule that inactivates several enzymes of the coagulation system.

Antrum   A portion of the lower part of the stomach.

Anuria   Complete absence of urine production.

Anus   The termination of the digestive tract; controls the expulsion of feces.

Aorta   The largest artery in the body arising from the left ventricle; pumps blood to the entire body.

Aortic dissection   A life-threatening condition where there is bleeding into and along the wall of the aorta.

Aortic stenosis   Marked narrowing of the aortic valve.

Aphasia   Disorder resulting from damage in the areas of the brain controlling language.

Aplastic anemia   A blood disorder in which the body's bone marrow does not make enough new red blood cells.

Apocrine glands   One of three types of sweat glands (*see* Sebaceous glands, Eccrine glands); are located in restricted areas of the body: underarms, genitals, eyelids, perianal, areole, periumbilical, and ear canals.

Apoptosis   Programmed cell death that occurs in multicellular organisms.

Appendix   A nonfunctional vestigial structure attached to the cecum.

Aqueous humor   Watery fluid within the anterior chamber of the eye.

Arachidonic acid   A phospholipid-rich fatty acid present in the membranes of the body's cells.

Areolae   Pigmented skin surrounding the nipple.

Aromatase   An enzyme that converts circulating androgens to estrogenic hormones.

Arrhythmias   Abnormal heart rhythms.

Arteries   Blood vessels that carry blood away from the heart.

Arteriography   A procedure in which radiopaque dye is injected into arteries and successive x-ray films are taken to show the caliber of the vessels and distribution of blood flow.

Arterioles   Very small arteries.

Arteriolosclerosis   Hardening of arterioles.

Arthritis   Inflammation of the joints.

Arthroscopy   Insertion of a fiber-optic scope into a joint cavity to visualize the joint structures, perform repairs of ligaments, remove loose cartilaginous fragments, or take biopsies.

Arthus-type hypersensitivity   A complement-mediated reaction to precipitates of antigen and antibody in vessel walls.

Asbestosis   A disease caused by the inhalation of fibrous silicates resulting in interstitial pulmonary fibrosis.

Ascites   Edema in the abdominal cavity.

Aspartate aminotransferase (AST)   A test performed to assess the status of the liver.

Asperger syndrome   A condition related to autism characterized by intact intelligence, but problems with communication and behavior, impaired school functioning and interpersonal relationships.

Aspergillus   Fungus found in soil that can cause infections, especially opportunistic.

Aspiration pneumonia   A bronchopneumonia caused by inhalation of particulate material carrying bacteria, usually from the mouth or stomach, that settles in the lower, more dependent lung lobes.

Asthma   A nondestructive lung disease caused by hypersensitivity or environmental factors, most common in children and young adults. Excess, tenacious secretions and bronchial smooth muscle constrictions impede the airway.

Astrocytes   Spider-like processes that provide structural and metabolic support to the central nervous system.

Astrocytoma   A brain tumor composed of astrocytes that can be slow growing or malignant.

Atelectasis   Collapse of the lung.

Atheroma   A fibrofatty deposit in the intima of blood vessels, particularly in the major muscular arteries; more commonly called plaque.

Atherosclerosis   Disease of the major blood vessels manifested as fibrofatty plaques in the vessel wall.

Atopic asthma   Asthma caused by allergies.

Atopic dermatitis   A chronic, relapsing form of dermatitis with a genetic basis.

Atrium   A blood-receiving chamber in the heart.

Atriventricular node   Part of the electrical system of the heart that carries the electrical impulse from the sinoatrial node to the ventricles.

Atrophy   A partial or complete wasting away of a cell or organ.

Attention deficit hyperactivity disorder (ADHD)   A commonly diagnosed disorder in children that includes either inattention symptoms or hyperactivity-impulsivity symptoms, or both.

Audiometers   Devices that generate auditory stimuli and then assess how well the patient responds to the tones produced.

Auscultation   Using a stethoscope to listen to heart and lung sounds.

Autism   A pervasive developmental disorder that starts before 36 months of age and is marked by sustained impairment of verbal and nonverbal communication skills with repetitive patterns of behavior.

Autoimmune gastritis   Immune-mediated chronic inflammation of the fundus, which is where the acid- and enzyme-producing cells are located.

Autoimmune hepatitis   An autoimmune disorder that targets hepatocytes in the portal areas, causing their death and eventual replacement by fibrosis.

Autoimmune reaction   The body's immune system reacts to its own tissues, producing destructive diseases.

Autopsy   The postmortem examination of a body.

Autosomal   Relating to genes that are located on any of the chromosomes other than the X or Y chromosome.

Autosomal dominant polycystic kidney disease   A relatively common form of polycystic kidneys that presents in adults.

Autosomal recessive polycystic kidney disease   Genetic disorder appearing in neonates and infants; characterized by the growth of numerous cysts in the kidneys that fill with fluid, thus reducing the capability of the organ to function, and that can lead to renal failure and death. The liver also may be involved.

B

B lymphocytes   Lymphocytes that are capable of developing into plasma cells to produce immunoglobulins.

Bacillary   Pertaining to elongated bacteria.

Bacterial culture   A method of multiplying bacteria by letting them reproduce in a controlled environment.

Band   An immature form of neutrophil.

Bariatric surgery   Surgery to reduce the size of the stomach in an effort to curb the appetite in obese patients.

Barium enema   Insertion of barium into the colon followed by radiologic examination of the rectum and colon.

Barrett's esophagus   A condition in which the gastric mucosa undergoes a second metaplastic alteration to intestinal-type epithelium, complete with intestinal absorptive and mucus cells.

Bartholin's glands   Glands located at the outlet of the vagina that produce a mucoid secretion lubricating the vagina during sexual intercourse.

Basal layer   The deepest layer of the skin; a single layer of predominantly cuboidal germinative cells that gives rise to all other epidermal cells by mitotic division.

Basophil   A type of of white blood cell; usually makes up 1% or less of the total white cell count.

Benign   Refers to a condition that will not likely kill the organism that harbors it.

Benign prostatic hypertrophy   Enlarged prostate that causes obstruction of the outflow of urine from the bladder, resulting in increased urgency to urinate, incontinence, and nocturia.

Bicuspid (mitral)   The valve between the left atrium and the left ventricle.

Bile   Excretory product of the liver.

Bile salts   The main constituents of bile produced by the liver; they emulsify lipids into small water-soluble packets so they can be transported and digested.

Biliary atresia   Progressive obstruction of the extrahepatic biliary tree in the first three months of life.

Biliary colic   Severe right upper quadrant and flank pain caused by acute cholecystitis or obstruction of the biliary ductal system by stones.

Bilirubin   The major product of red blood cell breakdown.

Biopsy   Surgical procedure for obtaining small specimens of a lesion.

Biopsychosocial model   A model that postulates illness arises from a complex interplay among biological, psychological, and social factors.

Bipolar   (also, biopolar affective disorder, manic depression illness, mood swings) A brain disorder characterized by unusually intense shifts in energy, activity, and ability to carry out daily tasks; most cases begin in teens to age 25; this mental condition is treatable.

Blastocyst   The fertilized egg that has gone through meiosis and started undergoing mitotic divisions.

Blastomycosis   A fungal infection common in the southeastern and midwestern United States caused by *Blastomyces dermatiditis.*

Blood bank (transfusion medicine)   The branch of medicine concerned with the administration of blood and blood products.

Blood–brain barrier   The capillary endothelium that separates blood constituents from the brain parenchyma.

Blood coagulation   (also, blood clotting) The process of converting plasma from a liquid to a solid.

Blood pressure   Measurement of force applied to arterial walls as the heart pumps blood through the circulatory system and the arteries' resistance to the blood flow.

Blood smear   A blood test that gives information about the number and shape of blood cells.

Boil   A skin abcess involving an entire hair follicle and nearby skin tissue.

Borderline malignant potential   A tumor that is not clearly "benign" and not really "malignant" when examined under the microscope.

Botulism   A disease caused by *Clostridium botulinum*, a serious infection that can lead to paralysis by secretion of a neurotoxin.

Bradykinin   A peptide that causes vasodilation and increased vascular permeability.

BRCA   Breast cancer tumor suppressor gene.

Bronchopneumonia   An infection of the lungs usually centered on the bronchi, involving multiple areas of one or both lungs, and usually caused by bacteria.

Bronchoscopy   Endoscopic examination of the trachea and bronchi.

Brown atrophy   The brown color of the heart and the liver that develops with aging due to the accumulation of lipofuscin pigment in myocardial fibers and hepatocytes.

Buccal smear   A process in which epithelial cells are scraped from inside the mouth and examined under a microscope to determine sex chromosome numbers.

Buffy coat   A thin white layer of leukocytes between the serum and red blood cells in a tube of blood.

Bullous emphysema   The formation of blebs or grossly visible bubbles in the lung due to grossly expanded alveoli.

C

Calcitonin   A hormone that antagonizes the effect of parathormone by stimulating calcium uptake by bone.

Calcium   A mineral essential for life, incorporated into bones and teeth.

Canaliculi   Tiny canals that carry bile to the portal area.

Cancer   Disease characterized by the development of abnormal cells that divide uncontrollably and have the ability to destroy normal body tissue.

Candidiasis   An infection commonly referred to as a yeast infection, caused by a fungus, *Candida albicans*, normally present in the vagina.

Capillaries   The smallest of the body's blood vessels and part of the microcirculation. They connect arterioles and venules.

Carbohydrates   The main source of readily available energy in the form of sugars and complex chains of sugars.

Carbuncle   A group of abcesses with associated connecting sinus tracts and multiple openings on the skin.

Carcinogens   Agents known to initiate cells to develop cancer.

Carcinoid tumors   Neoplasms that can arise in several places throughout the body and secrete various hormones.

Carcinoma   A malignant neoplasm of epithelial tissues.

Carcinoma *in situ*   Early stage of cancer limited to the place where it began and has not yet begun to spread.

Cardiac catheterization   An invasive procedure in which catheters are threaded through the vessels and into the heart to measure pressures in various chambers and to allow injection of radiopaque dyes for the purpose of diagnosis.

Cardinal signs of inflammation   Redness, swelling, heat, pain, and loss of function.

Cardiogenic shock   Shock caused by failure of the heart.

Cardiomyopathy   Intrinsic disease of the heart muscle.

Carrier   A host that can carry and transfer a disease to another host without overt signs of infection.

Caseous necrosis   A form of tissue death in a granuloma, meaning it has a cheese-like appearance; fairly specific for tuberculosis.

Casts   Tightly packed collections of proteins, lipids, or cellular debris that precipitated in renal tubules or collecting ducts and may be washed out by the flow of urine. Usually associated with kidney disease.

Celiac disease   A malabsorption syndrome in which gluten, a protein present in grains, induces injury to the mucosa of the small intestine.

Cell membrane   A covering that protects the cell from physical injury and selectively regulates the entrance and exit of various ions and nutrients.

Cellular atypia   The degree to which cells morphologically differ from normal.

Cellular basis of disease   The tracing of disease to deranged structures or functions of cells.

Cellular immune system   A system of lymphocytes with immune functions.

Cellulitis   A spreading infection of soft tissue.

Cerebral palsy   A condition characterized by nonprogressive abnormal muscular coordination with or without mental retardation or seizure disorders, sometimes caused by brain damage in the late fetal or perinatal period.

Cerebral vascular accident (CVA)   Clinically referred to as a "stroke," and resulting from interruption of the blood supply to the brain, either by a vascular obstruction or bleeding.

Cervical canal   The channel between the uterine cavity and the cevical os.

Cervical os   Opening of the cervical canal into the vagina.

Cervix   The distal, narrow portion of the uterus that projects into the vagina.

Chagas disease   A chronic destructive disease, caused by *Trypanosoma cruzi*, that causes severe damage to the heart and esophagus.

Chancre   The primary lesion of syphilis, a painless ulcer.

Chemical burns   Burns caused by exposure of the skin or tissues to various chemicals.

Chemical carcinogens   Chemicals known to initiate cells to develop cancer.

Chemistry   Biochemical tests on blood to determine organ function.

Chemokines   Small proteins produced by the body during the inflammatory response.

Chemotaxis   The movement of white blood cells in response to a chemical gradient.

Chemotherapy   Treatment of cancer through chemicals.

Chlamydia   A group of parasites that cause a variety of human diseases, including trachoma and several sexually transmitted diseases of the urinary tract.

Cholangiocarcinoma   Gallbladder cancer and cancer of the intrahepatic biliary tree.

Cholecystectomy   Removal of the gallbladder.

Cholesteatoma   A mass of keratinized tissue within the middle ear, which can become infected or erode the structures of the middle ear, resulting in hearing loss; caused by chronic low-grade otitis media.

Cholesterol   A waxy metabolite found in cell membranes, it is important and necessary for vitamin manufacturing.

Chondrocytes   Mature cells found in cartilage that can proliferate to form new cartilage or bone after an injury or fracture.

Chorioamnionitis   Infection of the placental membranes.

Choriocarcinoma   A malignant neoplasm growing from the placenta.

Choroid plexus   A group of cells in the venticles of the brain that secrete cerebrospinal fluid.

Chronic gastritis   Chronic inflammation of the stomach mucosa.

Chronic kidney failure   A long-standing disease resulting in scarring in the kidney, permanently altering function.

Chronic obstructive pulmonary disease (COPD)   The combination of chronic bronchitis and emphysema that occurs almost exclusively in smokers, causing significant morbidity and disability.

Chronic pelvic pain syndrome   Having symptoms of frequency, urgency, and perineal pain, but no infectious organisms that can be cultured.

Chronic rejection   Organ rejection occuring years after a transplant. The mechanism by which it occurs is not known: it appears to be a mixture of smoldering acute rejection and additional immune injury.

Circle of Willis   An arterial circle at the base of the brain that distributes blood to the various cerebral arteries.

Cirrhosis   Scarring of the liver, leading to poor liver function.

Claustrophobia   Fear of tight places.

Clinical pathologist   A physician who analyzes various specimens removed from patients such as blood, urine, and sputum to determine the type and cause of disease.

Closed-angle glaucoma   Obstruction of the angle where the iris meets the corneal–scleral junction by the iris.

Closed fractures   Broken bones that do not disrupt the skin.

Clostridium difficile   A bacterium that produces an enterotoxin that causes irreversible damage to the colonic epithelial cells.

Clotting factors   Blood proteins that aid in coagulation.

Coagulation necrosis   A type of cell death typically caused by ischemia or infarction.

Coagulation (clotting) system   The system in the body responsible for clot formation and hemostasis.

Coagulopathy   An abnormality in the coagulation mechanism leading to either excessive bleeding or excessive clotting.

Coarctation   A narrow fibrous constriction in the thoracic aorta.

Cocci   Round-shaped type of bacteria.

Coccidioidomycosis   A fungal infection common in the southwestern United States caused by *Coccidioides immitis.*

Cochlea   The auditory portion of the inner ear.

Cognitive   Pertaining to memory and intellect.

Collagen   A group of naturally occurring proteins found in connective tissue.

Colon   The large intestine.

Colonoscopy   A procedure used to visualize and biopsy lesions of the entire colon and distal ileum.

Colostomy   A surgical procedure in which an opening is formed between the large intestine and the abdominal wall.

Colposcope   A diagnostic procedure to examine an illuminated, magnified view of the cervix and vagina.

Columnar epithelium   The cellular lining of body surfaces composed of elongated cells.

Coma   Loss of consciousness.

Comedones   (*also*, pimples) The basic lesion of acne; blackheads and whiteheads.

Commensals   Viruses or other organisms that live a long time in host cells without doing harm; analagous to indigenous bacterial flora.

Comminuted fractures   Fractures in which more than two fragments are produced.

Common bile duct   The connection between the cystic duct and the papilla of Vater.

Complement   A group of special serum proteins that often take part in antigen–antibody reactions.

Complete blood count (CBC)   A measurement of hemoglobin, counting of white and red blood cells, and microscopic evaluation for morphologic changes in the blood cells.

Complete fractures   Fractures in which the bone is separated into two or more parts.

Compound nevus   Nevus composed of clusters of melanocytes present at the junction of the epidermis and the dermis as well as in the dermis.

Compression fractures   Fractures in which the bones are pushed together rather than pulled apart.

Computerized tomography (CT scan)   A radiologic procedure that combines a series of x-ray views taken from many different angles to produce cross-sectional images of the body.

Computerized tomography (CT) colonoscopy   Use of CT imaging to build high-resolution images of the inside of the intestine.

Conductive   Hearing loss in which the external or middle ear is damaged.

Condyloma acuminatum   Genital wart caused by human papillomavirus.

Cone biopsy   The removal of a cone of tissue, including the cervical os and endocervical lining, for systematic histologic evaluation.

Congenital   Present at birth, but not necessarily genetic in origin.

Congestion   Distention of veins and capillaries due to increased venous pressure.

Congestive heart failure   A disease in which the heart can no longer pump enough blood to the rest of the body.

Conjunctiva   A mucous membrane forming the inner layer of the eyelid.

Connective tissue   An aggregation of fibrocytes and similarly specialized cells that constitute the structural framework of organs and tissues.

Consumption coagulopathy   A coagulopathy resulting in bleeding, caused by the aberrant consumption of coagulation factors.

Contrecoup lesions   Contusions occurring on the opposite side of the brain from the initial trauma.

Contusion   A bruise, caused by crushing, dislocation, or disruption of subsurface tissue by a blunt instrument that does not penetrate or break the surface.

Conversion disorder   A form of a somatization disorder in which there is involuntary loss of a specific function suggestive of physical illness such as paralysis, loss of voice, blindness, anesthesia, or incoordination.

Cor pulmonale   Failure of the right side of the heart secondary to pulmonary hypertension.

Cornea   The transparent structure through which light first passes into the eye.

Cornified layer   Outermost layer of skin.

Coronary artery bypass graft (CABG)   A surgical procedure that utilizes a segment of either an artery or a vein to divert blood flow around the diseased portion of the coronary artery.

Corpus luteum   The empty follicle in the ovary following ovulation; it continues to grow into a large mass of lipid-rich cells.

Cortex   The outer portion of organs.

Coryza   Profuse nasal discharge; usually associated with a "cold."

Coup lesions   Contusions occurring on the same side of the brain as the trauma.

Coxsackievirus   An enterovirus family virus that can cause myocarditis.

Cradle cap   Seborrheic dermatitis that usually begins in childhood as fine scaling of the scalp.

Creatine kinase   An enzyme normally involved in the metabolism of muscle that is elevated in the serum following disorders that damage muscle.

Creatinine   A substance in the blood that is excreted by filtration through the glomerulus, giving an indication of renal function.

Creatinine phosphokinase (CK)   Enzyme released from the heart when it is damaged.

Crohn disease   A chronic inflammatory bowel disease.

Cross-match   The *in vitro* mixing of samples of donor and recipient blood to determine compatibility.

Croup   A laryngeal spasm characterized by a loud, high-pitched, inspiratory sound.

Cryptococcosis   A fungal infection, affecting the lungs and meninges, caused by *Cryptococcus neoformans*.

Cryptosporidiosis   A diarrheal illness caused by *Cryptosporidium parvum*.

CT colonoscopy   (*see* Computerized tomography colonoscopy)

Culture   A method of multiplying microorganisms by letting them reproduce in a controlled environment.

Curative therapy   A medicine or therapy that attempts to permanently cure disease or relieve pain; the attempt to remove all of a cancer.

Cushing syndrome   A constellation of physical and physiological findings caused by excess corticosteroids, most commonly induced by the administration of corticosteroids for treatment of various illnesses.

Cyanosis   Decreased oxygenation of the blood that results in the skin having a blue hue.

Cyclopia   A brain malformation in which a single, malformed eye is centrally situated.

Cystic duct   The connection between the gallbladder and the papilla of Vater.

Cystic fibrosis   An autosomal recessive disorder caused by mutations in a gene that encodes the cystic fibrosis transmembrane regulator conductor (CFTR). The CFTR regulates chloride ions, which affect the viscosity of mucus.

Cystic hygroma   Dilated masses of lymphatics that occur in the neck of an infant.

Cysticercosis   An infection by a tapeworm of the *Taenia* species. Infection with *Taenia solium*, the pork tapeworm, can result in muscle, brain, and eye cysts.

Cystogram   A radiologic technique used to assess the size and shape of the bladder and the pattern of flow of urine.

Cystoscopy   Insertion of tubes fitted with lenses and lights through the urethra to visualize the urethra and bladder.

Cytochrome p450   An enzyme that catalyzes the first step in the clearance of many drugs.

Cytogenetics   The science of examining the chromosomal and genetic makeup of cells to diagnose and detect disorders such as trisomies, translocations, and deletions known to cause disease.

Cytokines   Small proteins secreted by specific cells of the immune system that initiate or modify inflammatory responses.

Cytology   The study of cells in terms of their structure, function, and chemistry.

Cytopathology   The study of cellular changes for the diagnosis of disease.

Cytoplasmic organelles   The membrane-bound structures in a cell.

Cytotoxic T cells   Lymphocytes that directly kill other cells possesing foreign or altered antigens, such as neoplastic cells or cells infected with viruses.

Cytotoxic-type hypersensitivity   The destruction of host cells either by agglutination and phagocytosis or by lysis of the cell membrane as a consequence of complement fixation.

D

Debridement   Removal of foreign material and necrotic tissue.

Decubitus ulcers   Ulcers resulting from pressure on the skin.

Degeneration   Mild forms of injury that produce sublethal cell or tissue injury without necrosis.

Degenerative joint disease   An erosion of the articular joint cartilage, with subsequent deformity of the cartilage and bone, resulting in stiffness and decreased motion.

Deglutition   The act or process of swallowing.

Delayed hypersensitivity   A cell-mediated hypersensitivity (undesirable reaction), resulting in the harmful destruction of tissue by T lymphocytes and macrophages.

Delirium tremens (DTs)   A state of delirium in which the patient experiences frightening visual hallucinations; caused by the acute withdrawal of excessive alcoholic intake.

Dementia   A decrease in cognitive function, usually accompanied by loss of memory for recent events.

Denervation atrophy   Muscle cell degeneration resulting from loss of nervous stimulation.

Dental caries   Cavities in the teeth created by bacteria.

Dental plaque   A mass of adherent bacteria and debris on the tooth surface.

Dental pulp   The central connective tissue core of a tooth.

Depression   A sad or melancholy state with either decreased activity or agitation.

Dermatitis   Inflammation of the skin.

Dermis   The underlying layer of the skin composed of fibrous connective tissue, and containing the hair follicles, sebaceous and sweat glands, blood vessels, and sensory nerves.

Desensitization   Repeated exposure to minute amounts of allerogenic antigen resulting in a relative tolerance to the antigen.

Developmental abnormality   Abnormalities of development that may be due to altered genetic structure or environmental effects, or a combination of the two.

Diabetes mellitus   A metabolic disease manifested as high blood sugar levels due to either insulin deficiency or insulin resistance.

Diabetic ketoacidosis   A medical emergency characterized by dehydration and acidosis in the setting of severe hyperglycemia.

Diagnosis   Observation, history, and laboratory results used to determine the specific disease being experienced by a patient.

Dialysis   A filtration procedure to separate waste products from blood or body fluids; an artificial kidney function.

Diaphysis   The long, tubular shaft of bone.

Diarrhea   Passage of abnormally frequent and liquid stools.

Diastole   Relaxation phase of the heart ventricles.

Diastolic pressure   Measurement of the lowest force of blood circulating through arteries when the heart is resting between contractions (*see* Blood pressure, Arterial pressure).

Differential diagnosis   A list of possible diagnoses that fit the physical and historical presentation of a patient's illness.

Differential white blood cell count   Determination of the percentages of each type of white blood cell present.

Differentiation   The maturation from a nonspecific cell type to a specialized cell.

Diffuse idiopathic pulmonary fibrosis   A clinical term that refers to a distinct pattern of lung injury whose cause is not known. The fibrosing process begins at the periphery of the lung and moves inward to the hilar region.

Diffuse Lewy body disease   A common neurodegenerative disease, related to Parkinson and Alzheimer diseases, that produces dementia, psychosis, and abnormalities of movement.

Diffusion   Process of gas passing from air to blood or from blood to air.

Diffusion capacity   Facility with which gases cross the alveolar walls.

Digital rectal examination (DRE)   Palpation of the posterior of the prostate by a gloved, lubricated finger inserted into the rectum to check for abnormalities.

Dilation and curettage (D&C)   A surgical procedure that involves dilating the cervical os and scraping out tissue from the uterus with a curette.

Diplopia   Double vision.

Dipstick   A piece of paper with reagents on it that change color in the presence of certain chemicals in the urine; it can be used to detect specific gravity, pH, and the presence of protein, sugar, nitrites, ketones, or leukocyte esterase.

Direct Coombs test   Addition of antihuman gamma globulin to a test tube of washed erythrocytes. If the erythrocytes have been coated with cytotoxic or other antibodies, they will agglutinate upon addition of the antihuman gamma globulin.

Disseminated intravascular coagulation (DIC)   A condition in which damage to endothelial cells causes widespread activation of the clotting cascade with subsequent formation of microthrombi in small vessels.

Disuse atrophy   Loss of muscle mass and strength due to a prolonged period of immobility.

Diverticulitis   Inflammation of diverticulae in the intestine.

Dominant   Expression of an allele to the exclusion of a contrasting (recessive) allele.

Down syndrome   A chromosomal abnormality in which persons have three copies (trisomy) of chromosome 21, and manifested as mental retardation and other dysmorphic features.

Dry gangrene   An infarct of the foot caused by atherosclerosis in the arteries of the lower extremity.

Duchenne muscular dystrophy   A sex-linked disorder with an abnormality in or absence of a muscle protein (dystrophin) that leads to muscular weakness.

Ductal carcinoma   Carcinoma of the breast that arises from the ductal epithelium.

Ductal hyperplasia   A proliferation in the number of layers of epithelial cells lining the duct.

Duodenum   The first section of the small intestine.

Duplication   Abnormal copying of fragments of chromosomes, resulting in extra genetic material in the daughter cells.

Dysentery   Severe diarrhea with mucus and/or blood in the feces.

Dysesthesias   Distortion of the sense of touch.

Dysfunctional uterine bleeding   Excessive bleeding, often due to an imbalance of hormones.

Dysmenorrhea   Cramping pain during menstruation.

Dysphagia   Swallowing with pain or discomfort.

Dysplasia   Atypical cell growth that has acquired some of the genetic alterations for the development of malignancy, but is localized to the tissue of origin.

Dysplastic nevi   Clinically atypical moles with irregular pigmentation or ill-defined borders, thought to be markers for moderately increased risk for developing melanoma.

Dyspnea   Shortness of breath of which the patient is aware.

Dystrophic calcification   Calcium deposits in an abnormal location.

Dystrophy   Any condition of abnormal development, usually referring to muscle.

Dysuria   Painful urination.

E

Ecchymoses   Large areas of hemorrhage into the skin.

Eccrine glands   Glands present in the deep dermis over nearly the entire surface of the body that are responsible for the production of sweat in response to heat stress.

Echocardiography   A noninvasive procedure that provides an image of the heart based on ultrasound waves that are reflected at tissue interphases.

Eclampsia   Maternal hypertension, proteinuria, edema, and seizures.

Eczema   A chronic, relapsing form of dermatitis with a genetic basis.

Edema   Leakage of fluid into tissue.

Elastin   A tightly coiled protein that can stretch under pressure; found in the wall of the aorta and other organs.

Elective abortion   The terminating of pregnancy through artificial measures.

Electrocardiography   A noninvasive procedure that records electrical activity of the heart at electrodes placed at standard locations on the body surface.

Electroencephalogram   A device for evaluating electrical activity in various areas of the brain.

Electromyography A procedure in which the electrical activity of the muscle is recorded.

Electrophoresis A method of separating substances, especially proteins, and analyzing molecular structure based on the rate of movement of each component in a colloidal suspension while under the influence of an electrical field.

Elephantiasis A marked enlargement of affected tissues, resulting from lymphatic channel blockage.

Embolus Any particulate object (usually clotted blood) that travels in the bloodstream from one site to another.

Embryonic development The first 8 weeks after fertilization.

Emigration A process by which leukocytes exit from the vascular space.

Emphysema Permanent enlargement of air spaces in the lung due to destruction of their walls.

Empyema A collection of pus between the chest wall and lung.

End-stage renal disease (ESRD) Irreversible loss of renal function.

Endarterectomy Removal of material from the inside of an artery; especially a surgical procedure used to prevent stroke by correcting stenosis in the carotid artery.

Endocarditis Inflammation of the inner lining of the heart.

Endocrine system Includes those organs, or tissues within organs, that secrete their cellular products into the bloodstream rather than into viscera, cavities, or outside the body.

Endogenous Agents acting from inside the body.

Endometrium Glandular mucosa lining the uterine cavity.

Endoplasmic reticulum Divided into rough and smooth; the rough's function is to process newly synthesized peptides from ribosomes, and the smooth's is to synthesize and metabolize lipids.

Endoscopy The use of a tube or flexible scope to look inside a body passageway.

Endothelium The continuous lining of blood vessels.

Endotoxic shock A profound hemodynamic and metabolic disturbance elicited by the release of endotoxins from gram-negative enteric organisms.

Endotoxin Toxins found in the bacterial cell wall of gram-negative enteric organisms.

Enterotoxin A toxin specific for the cells of the intestinal mucosa.

Enucleation Removal of the eye.

Enzymatic fat necrosis Necrosis resulting from the action of pancreatic lipase on fat.

Eosinophilia Increased levels of eosinophils in the blood or tissue.

Eosinophils White blood cells that respond to multicellular parasites and some immunologic conditions.

Ephelides (*also*, freckles) Focal areas of hyperpigmentation that occur in response to sunlight.

Epidermis The outer covering of stratified squamous epithelium on the skin.

Epididymis An organ of the male reproductive system that partially surrounds the testes; it transports and stores sperm.

Epigenetic phenomena Modification of the DNA by methylation or addition of protein groups to certain portions of genes prior to coding for RNA.

Epiglottis A thick flap of tissue that folds over the larynx during swallowing to prevent aspiration into the trachea.

Epiphyseal plate A cartilaginous piece between the epiphysis and metaphysis.

Epiphysis The end of a bone that articulates with another bone.

Epistaxis Nose bleed.

Epithelial cells Cells that work together to carry out specialized functions, such as protection of body surfaces, secretion of specific products, and special metabolic functions.

Epithelioid cells Activated macrophages that resemble epithelial cells.

Epithelium A tissue composed of cells that line the cavities and structures throughout the body.

Epitope The site on the antigen to which an antibody binds.

Epstein-Barr virus (EBV) A member of the herpes virus family; one of the most common viruses worldwide; a common cause of infectious mononucleosis.

ER positive (*see* Estrogen receptor positive)

Eruptive xanthoma An eruption of small yellow papules on the extensor surfaces of the extremities and buttocks, usually indicative of a significant elevation in plasma triglyceride levels as can be seen in hereditary disorders of lipid metabolism or uncontrolled diabetes.

Erythroblastosis fetalis A fatal disease caused by the mother producing antibodies to the fetus's red blood cells.

Erythrocyte sedimentation rate   A test that serves as an indicator of inflammation and is useful in following patients with rheumatoid arthritis.

Erythropoiesis   The production of erythrocytes; normally in the bone marrow.

Erythropoietin   A hormone, released from the kidney, that stimulates erythropoiesis.

Esophageal atresia   The absence of part of the esophagus so that the upper esophagus ends as a blind pouch.

Esophageal varices   Permanently dilated venous channels of the lower esophagus.

Essential hypertension   Primary or idiopathic hypertensive disease.

Estrogen   A hormone primarily produced by the ovaries and adrenals that stimulates female secondary sexual characteristics.

Estrogen receptor (ER) positive   Cells that express estrogen receptor.

Etiology   Cause of diseases.

Eustachian tubes   Tubes that connect the middle ear with the nasal cavity and serve as pressure equalizers for the middle ears.

Evidence-based medicine   Guidelines for treatment based on the empirical evidence and advice issued by experts.

Ewing sarcoma   The most common type of non–metastatic (primary) cancer in children and adolescents; occurs primarily in bone.

Exfoliative   Sloughing of the skin.

Exogenous   Agents acting from outside the body.

Exophthalmos   Protrusion of the eye.

Exotoxins   Proteinaceous poisons secreted by virulent organisms.

Experimental pathology   (*also*, investigative pathology) Science that seeks to link the presentation of a disease in a whole organism with its fundamental molecular and cellular mechanisms, with the research findings being applied to its diagnosis and treatment.

External agents   Physical, chemical, or microbial causes of injury.

Extrinsic pathway   The tissue factor pathway of the coagulation cascade.

Exudates   Extravascular fluid that is protein rich and cloudy and produced in pathologic conditions.

F

Factor XII   (Hageman factor) A plasma protein in the coagulation cascade.

Factor XIII   Fibrin stabilizing factor.

Fallopian tubes   (*also*, uterine tubes) Two channels leading from the ovaries to the uterus.

Familial adenomatous polyposis   An inherited condition resulting in the growth of numerous polyps in the lower intestine.

Familial diseases   Genetic or environmental diseases that occur more often in family members than by chance alone.

Fascicles   A bundle of skeletal muscle fibers enclosed in connective tissue.

Fats   (lipids) Components of all cell membranes, an important source of energy because their metabolism in the body yields more than twice as many calories as either protein or carbohydrates. One or two naturally occurring lipids need to be ingested, but all the others can be synthesized from proteins.

Fatty change   Accumulation of lipids within cells.

Fatty streaks   The earliest visible lesions of an atheroma that are composed of lipid.

Ferritin   A protein that binds free iron.

Fertilization   The uniting of a sperm and an ovum, creating a zygote.

Fetal alcohol syndrome   A condition caused by alcohol use during pregnancy; characterized by abnormal facial features, impaired growth during infancy and childhood, and neurological problems, including mental retardation and impaired socialization.

Fetal period   The eighth week after fertilization to birth.

FEV$_1$ The volume of air that can be moved out of the lungs under maximal effort in one second.

Fever   An elevated body temperature.

Fibrin   A filamentous protein involved in the clotting of blood.

Fibrin degradation products/D-dimer   A small protein fragment present in the blood after a blood clot has been degraded by fibrinolysis.

Fibrinogen   A soluble blood protein that may leak into an inflamed site and be converted to fibrin.

Fibrinolytic system   Responsible for the removal of a clot by breaking down fibrin so tissue can be repaired; opposite of coagulation.

Fibrinous exudate   Material noted after severe injury when large molecules such as fibrinogen and fibrin pass through the vascular barrier and deposit in the extracellular space.

Fibroadenoma   A benign neoplasm derived from glandular epithelium; commonly occurs in the breast.

Fibrocystic change   A term encompassing a variety of alterations that occur in the epithelial and stromal compartments of the breast.

Fibromas   A benign stromal tumor that arises from the fibrous tissue in several organs.

Fibrous connective tissue repair   A biochemical and cellular process in which damaged tissue is replaced by scar.

Filariasis   A disease caused by a helminthic worm found in the tropics that causes chronic lymphedema.

Fine-needle aspiration (FNA)   A technique that uses a small-caliber needle to obtain aspirated tissue for cytological examination.

First-degree burns   Burns that are limited to the epidermis and are red, painful, and dry.

Fistula   An abnormal connection between two organs.

Flail chest   The result of three or more ribs broken in two or more places that leads to a segment of the chest being separated from the rest of the chest wall.

Flat bones   Bones such as ribs, sternum, pelvis, and cranium that serve to protect the thorax, abdomen, and brain.

Flow cytometry   A technique by which blood cells can be tested for antigenic composition as well as size and cytoplasmic granularity.

Fluoroscope   An instrument that uses a fluorescent plate to detect x-rays.

Focal segmental glomerular sclerosis   A special type of scarring process in the glomeruli.

Folic acid deficiency   A type of anemia characterized by red blood cells that are larger than normal, have a deformed shape, and a shortened life span. The rate of production of red blood cells is also diminished.

Follicle-stimulating hormone (FSH)   A hormone secreted by the anterior pituitary gland that regulates the growth, development, pubertal maturation, and reproductive processes of the body.

Follicles   Specialized structures where the ova rest in the ovarian cortex.

Follicular carcinoma   A rare form of thyroid carcinoma.

Foramen ovale   A hole in the fetal heart in the septum between the right and left atria.

Forced vital capacity (FVC)   The maximum amount of air that can be taken in and exhaled under strenuous effort.

Foreign body granulomas   A reaction to foreign or endogenous material too large to be ingested by macrophages.

Forensic pathology   A subfield of pathology in which accidental and criminal deaths are investigated.

Fovea   The central portion of the macula of the eye.

Fragile X syndrome   A genetic condition that involves changes in part of the X chromosome; it produces mild-to-moderate mental retardation and is the most common genetic cause of mental retardation in males. It is caused by trinucleotide repeats, which increase in length in successive generations.

Free oxygen radicals   Unstable oxygen molecules that have only a single unpaired electron in their outer orbit and that are generated by the reduction of molecular oxygen to water. They react with proteins, lipids, and carbohydrates, releasing energy that damages membranes and DNA.

Frequency   The number of occurrences of a repeating event.

Frozen section   A pathological laboratory procedure to perform rapid microscopic analysis of a specimen.

Fulguration   Destruction of tissue by means of an electrical current.

Fundoscopic examination   Visualization of the retina with the ophthalmoscope.

Fundus   The body of the stomach.

Funduscopic examination   An examination of the back of the eye with an ophthalmoscope.

Furuncle   A small abscess centered about a hair follicle.

G

Galactorrhea   Production of milk unassociated with pregnancy.

Gallbladder   A reservoir where bile from the liver is stored.

Gallstones   Pebble-like stones found in the gallbladder.

Gamete   A reproductive cell, essentially a sperm or an ovum.

Ganglion cells   Nerve cell bodies in various organs.

Gangrenous necrosis (gangrene)   Coagulation necrosis with superimposed decomposition by saprophytic bacteria.

Gas gangrene   As the organism *C. perfringens* breaks down proteins in dead tissue, it produces a foul-smelling gas. The resultant tissue distention compresses blood vessels, which in turn induces more tissue anoxia and tissue necrosis.

Gastric analysis   Measurement of acid in the stomach.

Gastroesophageal reflux disease (GERD)   A condition of highly acidic gastric contents slipping back into the esophagus. The symptom this causes is commonly referred to as "heartburn."

Generalized anxiety disorder (GAD)   Chronic worry that is difficult to control.

Genes DNA arranged into specific sequences that defines the subunits of a chromosome.

Genetic analysis The analysis of a sample of DNA to look for mutations or translocations.

Genetic disease Disease caused by an abnormal gene.

Genetic mutation Changes in a genomic sequence that can keep a gene from functioning properly.

Genotype The genetic makeup of an individual.

Germ cells Cells that give rise to the gametes of organisms that reproduce sexually.

Gestational age The length of a pregnancy; the fertilization period plus two weeks.

Ghon complex The combination of a peripheral lung nodule and enlarged lymph node secondary to tuberculous infection.

Giant cells A mass formed by the union of several distinct cells, usually in response to an infection or foreign body.

Giardiasis A diarrheal illness due to intestinal infection by the protozoan *Giardia lamblia*.

Gigantism A condition caused by excess secretion of growth hormone, resulting in thickening of soft tissue and lengthening of bones in children with open growth plates.

Gingiva The supporting tissues of teeth.

Gleason score A grading system to determine the severity of a cancer (i.e., how aggressive it appears under the microscope). There are five grades of cancer, scored from 1 to 5.

Glioblastoma A malignant, high-grade astrocytoma; the most common brain tumor in adults, which usually results in death within a year or two following diagnosis.

Glomeruli The major functional units of the kidney.

Glomerulonephritis Inflammatory damage to the glomeruli.

Glomerulosclerosis Scarring of the glomeruli.

Glucagon A hormone secreted by alpha cells in the islets of Langerhans.

Glucose-6-phosphate dehydrogenase (G6PD) deficiency A genetic enzyme defect that only becomes apparent when persons with the defect are exposed to fava beans or certain oxidant drugs such as antimalarial drugs, sulfas, nitrofurantoin, aspirin, and other analgesics. These patients have a mutant enzyme that becomes deficient in older red blood cells, allowing oxidants to damage the cell membrane and produce hemolysis.

Glucose tolerance test A test to measure the ability of cells to utilize glucose. After fasting, the patient is given a standardized glucose solution to drink, and the blood glucose is measured two hours later.

Glycogen storage disease An accumulation of carbohydrates; there are several variants of the disease.

Goiter An enlarged thyroid.

Golgi apparatus Major site in a cell for sorting and modifications of proteins and lipids.

Gonorrhea A sexually transmitted disease, caused by *Neisseria gonorrhoeae*, that can cause abscesses in organs and can disseminate to other tissues, primarily the joints.

Grade An assessment of how aggressive a tumor appears under the microscope.

Graft-versus-host disease (GVHD) A disease occurring when donor lymphocytes from transplanted organs mount an attack against the recipient's tissues.

Gram-negative shock Shock elicited by the release of endotoxins from gram-negative enteric organisms.

Gram stains A microbiology procedure used to divide bacteria into gram negative or positive, and coccal or bacillary.

Granular layer The middle layer of the epidermis.

Granulation tissue The tissue composed of blood cells, capillaries, and fibrous connective tissue that replaces a fibrin clot in healing wounds.

Granulocyte A type of white blood cell that includes neutrophils, eosinophils, and basophils.

Granulocytosis Increased production of granulocytes, usually a sign of acute inflammation.

Granuloma An aggregate of macrophages lymphocytes, the purpose of which is to seal bacteria off from the surrounding tissue, preventing them from spreading.

Graves disease An autoimmune disorder that causes hyperthyroidism.

Growth hormone (GH) A hormone secreted by the pituitary gland that stimulates growth, cell reproduction, and regeneration.

Gut microflora Bacteria that colonize the gut shortly after birth to aid in digestion, produce nutrients, and influence the development of the gastrointestinal immune system.

Gynecomastia Enlargement of the male breast.

H

Hageman factor (*also*, Factor XII) A plasma protein in the coagulation cascade.

Halothane   An anesthetic drug that can cause liver damage.

Haptens   Incomplete antigens.

Hashimoto thyroiditis   An autoimmune process that causes hypothyroidism.

Hay fever   Allergic rhinitis that is of short duration and seasonal.

HDL   (*see* High-density lipoprotein)

Heart disease   A broad term used to describe a range of diseases affecting the heart.

Helicobacter pylori   A bacterium that causes gastritis and ulcers of the stomach and duodenum.

Hemangiomas   Local proliferations of capillaries that may be present at birth.

Hematemesis   Vomiting of blood.

Hematochezia   Bright red blood in feces.

Hematocrit   The percentage of the red blood cells, compared with all other blood elements.

Hematology   The study of blood, blood-forming organs, and blood diseases.

Hematoma   A localized collection of blood.

Hematopoiesis   Blood cell formation.

Hematopoietic system   The system of organs and tissues, primarily the bone marrow, spleen, tonsils, and lymph nodes, involved in the production of blood.

Hematuria   Blood in the urine.

Hemiparesis   Weakness of one side of the body.

Hemochromatosis   Excessive iron accumulation in tissues associated with tissue damage.

Hemodialysis   A mechanism to remove waste products by which blood is filtered through an external device and returned to the patient's bloodstream.

Hemoglobin   The protein molecule in red blood cells to which oxygen binds.

Hemoglobin A1C   A test that gives an impression of the average glucose level in the blood over the past four months.

Hemoglobinopathies   Genetic conditions that produce abnormal hemoglobins and can cause anemia.

Hemolytic anemia   The destruction of red blood cells within the vascular or mononuclear phagocytic systems.

Hemolytic uremic syndrome (HUS)   A disease characterized by the acute onset of microangiopathic hemolytic anemia, renal injury, and low platelet count; similar to thrombotic thrombocytopenic purpura.

Hemophilia A   A sex-linked clotting disorder referred to as "classical hemophilia" that is caused by a deficiency of factor VIII.

Hemophilia B   (*also*, Christmas disease) A sex-linked clotting disorder caused by a deficiency of factor IX.

Hemoptysis   Coughing up blood.

Hemorrhagic diathesis   A tendency to bleed, whether known by a history of bleeding or by abnormal laboratory tests.

Hemorrhagic disease of the newborn   A bleeding disorder that develops in infants due to a deficiency of vitamin K.

Hemorrhagic pancreatitis   A surgical emergency caused by bleeding into a pseudocyst or into damaged pancreatic tissue.

Hemorrhoids   Permanently dilated venous channels surrounding the anus.

Hemosiderosis   A genetic disorder affecting iron storage.

Hemostasis   The stoppage of bleeding.

Hemothorax   Blood-filled pleural space.

Henoch-Schönlein purpura   A systemic vaculitis characterized by deposition of immune complexes containing the antibody IgA in the skin and kidney. It causes a palpable purpura.

Heparin   A pharmacologic anticoagulant that enhances the function of antithrombin.

Hepatic encephalopathy   Depression of the central nervous system caused by hyperammonemia.

Hepatitis   Inflammation of the liver.

Hepatitis A virus (HAV)   The most prevalent of the hepatitis viruses, which mostly causes a benign illness.

Hepatitis B virus (HBV)   The cause of an acute illness that manifests with fever, malaise, and jaundice; the main cause of chronic liver disease and hepatocellular carcinoma worldwide. It is spread by feces, urine body secretions, and parenterally.

Hepatitis C virus (HCV)   The major cause of chronic viral hepatitis in the United States; spreads parenterally.

Hepatitis D virus (HDV)   A defective strand of RNA that requires the cellular synthetic machinery of HBV to replicate.

Hepatitis E virus (HEV)   An enterally transmitted cause of acute hepatitis; a zoonotic disease (the primary reservoir for the virus is in animals).

Hepatocellular carcinoma   The most common primary neoplasm of the liver, which tends to arise in cirrhotic livers.

Hepatocytes   The parenchymal cells of the liver.

Hepatomegaly   Increase in liver size.

Hepatosplenomegaly   Enlargement of the liver and spleen.

Her2/neu   A growth factor receptor that can be blocked with the agent trastuzumab.

Hereditary spherocytosis   A genetic defect of the red blood cell membrane with an autosomal dominant inheritance pattern. The abnormal red blood cells are spherical rather than the normal flat, biconcave disks.

Hernia   Protrusion of a structure through the tissues normally containing it.

Herpes simplex type I   A virus that lies dormant in facial nerves and produces painful blisters in and around the oral cavity.

Herpes simplex type II   A virus that causes blistering lesions in the genital areas.

Herpes zoster   A blistering, painful skin rash (shingles) caused by the varicella-zoster virus.

Hiatal hernia   A disorder of the diaphragm allowing the stomach to slide up through the diaphragm into the thorax.

High-density lipoproteins (HDL)   (*also*, "good" cholesterol) A lipid that scavenges cholesterol in blood, carrying it to various points in the body and then transporting it to the liver, where it is broken down and eliminated.

Hirsutism   The growth of male-pattern facial hair.

Histamine   A vasoactive and bronchoconstricting amine.

Histiocytes   Tissue macrophages.

Histologic examination   The study of a tissue sample under a microscope.

Histoplasmosis   A fungal infection common in the central United States caused by *Histoplasma capsulatum*.

History   Listening to the patient or patient's relatives to ascertain the symptoms, and reviewing any other past or present medical problems that might relate to them.

HLA   (*see* Human leukocyte antigens)

Hodgkin lymphoma   A lymphoma characterized by a large, malignant (Reed-Sternberg) cell with a multilobed nucleus containing prominent nucleoli.

Homeostasis   The body's ability to physiologically regulate itself, to adapt to minor fluctuations.

Homologous   Belonging to the same pair of chromosomes.

Honeycomb lung   An appearance on a chest x-ray showing large air spaces that are separated from one another by fibrous bands.

Hormonal therapy   The use of hormones in medical treatment either by administering the hormones or by removing glands that produce hormones.

Hormone   A chemical released by a cell or gland in one part of the body that sends out messages that affect cells in other parts of the body.

Human chorionic gonadotropin (HCG)   A hormone produced by the embryo/placenta to maintain the corpus luteum.

Human immunodeficiency virus (HIV)   The virus that causes AIDS; it infects lymphocytes and destroys them at a rate that exceeds the ability of the body to replace them.

Human leukocyte antigens (HLA)   The major histocompatibility complex (MHC) in humans; these are determined when matching patients for transplant.

Human papillomavirus (HPV)   A sexually transmitted virus; infection with HPV can lead to the development of cervical cancer.

Humoral immunity   Immunity mediated by secreted antibodies.

Hyaline   A dense, homogeneous, eosinophilic deposit in tissue.

Hydatid cysts   Large cysts that develop in involved organs in *Echinococcus* infection, usually in the liver.

Hydatidiform mole   Benign trophoblastic neoplasm forming in the uterus from aberrant products of conception.

Hydronephrosis   Massive dilation of the urinary system proximal to a blockage.

Hydrothorax   Fluid in the chest cavity.

Hyperacute rejection   Organ rejection occurring following a major mismatch between the donor and the recipient; the recipient already has circulating antibodies against donor antigens that cause immediate immune attack of the donor organ.

Hypercalcemia   Increased levels of serum calcium.

Hypercapnia   High blood carbon dioxide levels.

Hyperemia   Increased blood flow in dilated vessels.

Hyperhomocysteinemia   An amino acid involved in conversion of methionine to cysteine. When found in elevated levels in blood, it is associated with accelerated atherosclerosis and venous thrombosis.

Hyperlipidemia   High cholesterol, triglyceride, and low-density lipoprotein (LDL) levels.

Hyperparathyroidism   Excessive production of parathyroid hormone by the parathyroid gland.

Hyperplasia   The abnormal proliferation of cells within an organ or tissue resulting in an increase in cells.

Hypersensitivity   Overactive immune response.

Hypersplenism   A disorder that causes the spleen to rapidly and prematurely destroy blood cells.

Hypertension   High blood pressure.

Hypertensive heart disease   Heart disease caused by high blood pressure.

Hypertrophy   Increase in size of cells or organs.

Hypogammaglobulinemia   An acquired form of very low levels of serum gamma globulin.

Hypoglycemia   Low blood glucose levels.

Hypotension   Low blood pressure.

Hypothalamus   A portion of the brain that contains a number of small nuclei secreting hormones that primarily regulate the endocrine system.

Hypoxemia   Decreased level of oxygen in the blood.

Hypoxia   Reduced oxygen.

Hysterectomy   Surgical removal of the uterus.

I

Iatrogenic   Adverse reactions resulting from treatment applied by a healthcare provider.

Idiopathic   Disease of unknown causes.

Idiopathic thrombocytopenia purpura (ITP)   A blood clotting disorder resulting in excessive bleeding or bruising; uncertain cause but believed to be due to antibodies in platelets in most instances.

Idiosyncratic   An unpredictable result.

IgA, IgD, IgE, IgG, and IgM   (*see* Immunoglobulin)

Ileostomy   A surgical opening made in the end of the small intestine to allow for defecation.

Ileum   The final section of the small intestine.

Ileus   A functional obstruction of the bowel caused by decreased motility.

Immune complex   The binding of an antibody to a soluble antigen.

Immune surveillance   Surveillance provided by natural killer and other cells that continually destroy foreign antigens and neoplastic cells before they can accumulate.

Immunity   The resistance to or protection from an individual's environment.

Immunization   Injection of a (usually) denatured antigen that primes the body to recognize particular foreign antigens and immediately produce antibodies to them on re-exposure.

Immunodiffusion   Tests in which prepared antibodies are reacted against IgG, IgA, IgM, IgE, and IgD. The reaction product precipitates in a gel medium and can then be stained and quantified.

Immunofluorescence   An imaging test in which a section of tissue (biopsy) from a diseased organ is overlain with fluorescent-tagged antibodies to specific immunoglobulin or complement. The fluorescent-tagged antibody will form a complex with the deposited immunoglobulin or complement and fluoresce a bright yellow-green color under a special blue light.

Immunoglobulin A (IgA)   An immunoglobulin secreted into body fluids such as tears, milk, saliva, bronchi, and the intestinal tract, where it may interact with antigens before they can enter the body's tissues.

Immunoglobulin D (IgD)   An antigen receptor on the surface of mature B cells; found in small amounts in the chest and belly.

Immunoglobulin E (IgE)   A class of antibody attached to basophils in the bloodstream and mast cells in tissues. When antigen reacts with IgE on the surface of basophils or mast cells, the cells release histamine.

Immunoglobulin G (IgG)   The smallest and most abundant of the immunoglobulins; IgG antibodies appear in all body fluids with the purpose of fighting viral and bacterial infections. This is the only antibody small enough to cross the mother's placental barrier to protect the fetus.

Immunoglobulin M (IgM)   The largest of the antibodies (5 times the size of IgG antibodies), and the first type to develop following antigenic stimulation to combat bacterial infection and stimulate other immune system cells to destroy foreign substances such as incompatible red blood cells.

Immunoglobulins   Antibodies produced by plasma cells that are released into the blood, where they circulate freely as part of the gamma-globulin fraction of serum proteins.

Immunohistochemistry   Testing for antigens in tissue by tagging with chromogen-labeled antibodies.

Immunologic diseases   Diseases caused by aberrations of the immune system.

Immunopathology   The branch of medicine that studies immune responses associated with disease.

Imperforate anus   Failure of the anus to connect with the rectum.

Impetigo   A superficial skin infection caused by *Staphylococcus* or *Streptococcus* species.

Imprinting   Learning characterized by occurrence early in life.

Inborn errors of metabolism   Enzymatic defects of carbohydrate, protein, lipid, or mineral metabolism.

Incidence   A measure of the number of newly diagnosed patients with a given disease in a given time period.

Incomplete fractures   Fractures without manifest separation of the bone.

Indigenous flora   Microorganisms that live on the skin and in the alimentary tract without producing ill effects and that are sometimes helpful.

Indirect Coombs test   A test to detect serum antibodies having the potential to react with erythrocytes.

Infancy   One month to 1 year of age.

Infarcts   Areas of tissue death due to occlusive conditions of the arteries.

Infections   Microbiologic injury caused by organisms of bacterial, viral, fungal, or protozoan origin.

Infectious disease   Any disease directly caused by pathogens.

Infectious mononucleosis   An infection commonly caused by the Epstein-Barr virus resulting in dysfunction of the hematopoietic system.

Infertility   The inability to achieve pregnancy after one year of unprotected sex.

Inflammation   The vascular and cellular response to necrosis or sublethal cell injury that is the body's mechanism of limiting the spread of injury.

Inflammatory breast cancer   Breast cancer in which malignant cells have diffusely infiltrated the lymphatics of the skin, giving the impression of inflammatory change.

Inguinal hernia   An outpouching of the abdominal cavity into the groin into which loops of bowel can slip and become entrapped.

Initiation   The beginning of alteration of cells to acquire autonomous growth potential.

Innate immunity   The way the body responds to foreign agents short of the immune response; composed of the skin, the inflammatory response, and natural killer cells, among other things.

Insulin   A hormone secreted by beta cells in the islets of Langerhans that regulates blood sugar levels.

Insulinoma   A neoplasm of the beta cells that produce insulin.

Interferon   A protein that prevents viral replication.

Intermittent claudication   Pain and atrophy of the leg muscles associated with gradual ischemic changes in the arteries to the lower extremities, relieved by rest.

International Normalized Ratio (INR)   A test that compares the patient's prothrombin time to that of the "normal" population recorded by the same test in the same laboratory.

Interstitial pneumonia   An inflammatory process affecting the alveolar walls.

Interventricular septum   The wall between the left and right ventricles.

Intradermal nevus   Nevus composed of cells that have migrated into the dermis.

Intraductal papilloma   A localized growth of epithelial cells around slender fibrovascular cores within a large duct.

Intravenous pyelogram   A test in which dye is injected in the body to look for gross structural changes in the kidneys and ureters.

Intrinsic factor   A protein that is required for absorption of vitamin B_{12} in the ileum.

Intrinsic pathway   The contact activation pathway that begins with factor X, and is another part of the clotting cascade.

Invasive   Cancer that infiltrates the surrounding tissue.

Iodine   A mineral that is a necessary constituent of thyroid hormone.

Iron   A mineral that is a component of hemoglobin and myoglobin. Blood loss and pregnancy increase dietary iron needs.

Iron-deficiency anemia   Anemia caused by loss of iron or inadequate intake of iron (*see* Anemia).

Irritable bowel syndrome   A disorder that affects the large intestine, causing cramping, abdominal pain, bloating, gas, diarrhea, and constipation.

Ischemia   Localized hypoxia due to poor blood flow.

Ischemic atrophy   Gradual loss of tissue due to insufficient blood supply.

Islets of Langerhans   The regions of the pancreas that contain its insulin- and glucagon-secreting cells.

J

Jaundice   A yellow color seen in the eyes, skin, and internal organs when bilirubin is present in excess.

Jejunum   The middle section of the small intestine.

Junctional nevus   A nevus in which the melanocytes or nevus cells proliferate at the junction of the epidermis and dermis.

Juvenile arthritis   Arthritis that occurs very early in life and can be very severe.

Juxtaglomerular apparatus   A collection of kidney cells that are stimulated to secrete renin either by the sympathetic nervous system or by a perceived decrease in the rate of filtration by the glomeruli.

K

Karyolysis   The breakdown or fading of the nucleus of a cell.

Karyorrhexis   The fragmentation of the nucleus of a cell.

Karyotyping   The process of inducing cells to grow in cell culture, arresting the dividing cells during mitosis, and squashing and staining the cells so that the chromosomes can be seen under a microscope.

Keratinocytes   The stratified squamous epithelium cells that compose the epidermis.

Keratitis   Corneal inflammation.

Keratoses   Patches of thickened skin.

Kidney stones   Solid masses of tiny crystals that form when urine contains too much of certain substances. They may block the flow of urine and are extraordinarily painful.

Kinin system   A poorly delineated system of blood proteins that plays a role in inflammation, blood pressure control, homeostasis, coagulation, and pain.

Klinefelter syndrome   A disorder that occurs in males who are born with one Y and two X chromosomes; technically a sex chromosome trisomy.

Koilocytosis   The appearance of a cell in which the nucleus becomes large and swollen or contracted and wrinkled, and is often surrounded by a "halo" of cytoplasmic clearing.

Korsakoff dementia   A condition accompanied by severe memory loss and organic psychosis due to degenerative changes in the thalamus of alcoholics.

Kupffer cells   Cells within the sinusoids of the liver that phagocytose particulate matter present in the blood.

Kwashiorkor   A severe protein deficiency, with or without caloric deficiency, characterized by generalized edema and fatty liver.

L

Labile cells   Cells that multiply constantly throughout life.

Laboratory findings   Observations made by the application of tests or special procedures.

Laboratory medicine   Branch of pathology that examines and tests specimens of tissue, fluid, or other body substances outside of the body, usually in a laboratory.

Laceration   A tear in the surface caused by shearing of tissue, leaving irregular, ragged wound margins.

Lactase deficiency   The lack of a functioning lactase enzyme that affects the digestion of dairy products.

Lactation   The secretion of milk from mammary glands.

Lactiferous duct   A tube that leads from the lobules of the mammary gland to the tip of the nipple.

Lamina propria   Loose connective tissue underlying mucosa.

Laparoscopy   The insertion of an endoscope into the peritoneal cavity through an incision at the umbilicus.

Laryngitis   Inflammation of the larynx.

Laryngoscopes   Instruments that employ fiber-optic technology to access the curved nasopharyngeal passages to visualize the mucous membranes of the upper respiratory tract.

Larynx   The air passage to the lungs; contains the vocal cords.

LDL   (*see* Low-density lipoproteins)

Lead poisoning   Usually a chronic condition that can affect the brain, peripheral nerves, and bone marrow.

LEEP   (*see* Loop electrocautery excision procedure)

Left heart failure   Increased venous pressure in the lungs resulting from backup of blood due to failure of the left ventricle.

Left ventricular assist devices   Mechanical pumps that siphon blood from the left ventricle and pump it into the aorta through a tube. They are used as temporizing measures until a donor heart becomes available.

Legal blindness   Visual acuity of 20/200 or less in the better eye with best correction.

Legionnaire disease   A bronchopneumonia caused by inhalation of the bacterium *Legionella pneumophila*, which lives in water storage tanks and cooling systems.

Leiomyoma   (*also*, fibroid) A nodular overgrowth of smooth muscle cells in the uterus.

Leishmaniasis   A disease of the mononuclear phagocytic systems and skin caused by several types of the protozoa *Leishmania*.

Lens   The transparent body situated anteriorly in the eye that allows light to enter.

Lentigo   Areas of increased skin pigmentation.

Lentigo maligna melanoma   A clinical variant of melanoma *in situ* that classically develops as a slowly expanding tan-brown patch with pigmentary variations on the face of an elderly individual.

Lesions   Structural changes within the body caused by disease.

Leukemia   Cancer of the white cell or red cell elements of the blood or bone marrow.

Leukocytes   White blood cells, including lymphocytes and granulocytes.

Leukocytosis   Elevated white blood cell count.

Leukopenia   Decreased white blood cell count.

Leukoplakia   A thickened white patch on the oral mucosa, often the first sign of squamous cell carcinoma.

Leukotriene   A metabolite of arachidonic acid produced locally by cells that act as a short-range hormone, especially in inflammation.

Lewy body   Abnormal aggregates of proteins that develop inside nerve cells in Parkinson's disease.

Lichen sclerosus   A condition in which the epidermis becomes very thin, almost parchment paper-like, while the underlying dermis becomes thickened with fibrosis; occurs most commonly on the vulva.

Lichen simplex chronicus   Extreme vulvar pruritus that often occurs with decreased levels of estrogen after menopause. In this condition, the epidermis becomes hyperplastic, or thickened, because of rubbing or scratching of the vulvar skin.

Life expectancy   The amount of time an individual can expect to live.

Lipases   Lipid-splitting enzymes released by the pancreas to aid in digestion.

Lipofuscin pigment   A pigment composed of lipid, carbohydrate, and protein, which is the residue of lysosomal digestion of cellular debris. It has no clinical significance other than being a marker for aging or increased cellular damage.

Lipoproteins   The major carriers of cholesterol in the serum.

Liquefaction necrosis   A type of necrosis characteristic of focal bacterial or fungal infections.

Liquid ammonia   A compound of nitrogen and hydrogen that burns the skin, eyes, and respiratory tract, commonly found in fertilizers, herbicides, and insecticides.

Lithotripsy   A method of treating kidney stones; stones are shattered by externally applied, high-intensity shock waves.

Liver   Glandular organ with an excretory duct emptying into the duodenum. It filters and detoxifies the blood coming from the digestive tract before distribution to other parts of the body, secretes bile, and produces numerous proteins.

Lobar pneumonia   An infection of a discrete area of lung, often a single lobe.

Lobular carcinoma   Carcinoma of the breast that arises from the lobular epithelium.

Lobules   Glandular units of the breast and other organs.

Loop electrocautery excision procedure (LEEP)   Surgical procedure for treatment of cervical lesions.

Low birth weight   Babies born weighing less than 5 pounds 8 ounces.

Low-density lipoproteins (LDL)   (*also,* "bad" cholesterol) A molecule that combines lipid with proteins; LDL transports cholesterol to the body's tissues. High levels generally are associated with more severe atherosclerosis.

Lumbar   Lower part of the spine.

Lumen   The space in the center of a tube.

Lumpectomy   Removal of the cancer and a rim of benign mammary tissue around it.

Luteinizing hormone (LH)   A hormone secreted by the anterior pituitary gland that triggers ovulation.

Lyme disease   An infectious disease caused by a spirochete carried by a tick, resulting in acute and chronic involvement of numerous organ systems.

Lymphangioma   Dilated mass of lymphatic vessels.

Lymphatic vessels   Blind-ended, thin-walled channels carrying lymphatic fluid that drain local tissues and extend to lymph nodes.

Lymphedema   Chronic edema resulting from obstruction and failure of the lymphatic system.

Lymphocyte   A type of white blood cell that is part of the immune system and collectively has multiple functions.

Lymphocytosis   An increased production of lymphocytes, usually a sign of chronic inflammation.

Lymphogranuloma venereum   An acute and chronic sexually transmitted disease caused by a strain of *Chlamydia* and characterized by a primary genital lesion followed by lymph node enlargement and possible draining sinuses and rectal strictures.

Lymphoma   White blood cell cancer characterized by involvement of sites other than the bone marrow or blood.

Lysis   Cell breakage.

Lysosomes   Organelles responsible for the degradation of various macromolecules in the cell.

M

Macrocytic, normochromic anemia   Anemia due to vitamin B_{12} or folic acid deficiency.

Macrophages   Types of white blood cells that destroy foreign material and secrete cytokines.

Macula   The spot on the retina of greatest visual acuity.

Macular   Lesions that are flat.

Magnesium   A mineral important for nerve and muscle physiology; normal diets provide adequate amounts.

Magnetic resonance imaging (MRI)   A type of image produced by displacing protons in atomic nuclei with radio-frequency signals while the body is surrounded by a strong magnet.

Major histocompatibility complex (MHC)   The genes that control the expression of both self antigens on cell surfaces of most cells in the body; MHC antigens must be compatible between donor and recipient for organ transplant, analogous to cross-matching for blood transfusions.

Malabsorption   Failure to absorb the nutrients in food.

Malaise   A feeling of tiredness and lethargy.

Malaria   A parasitic disease endemic in some parts of the world that infects red blood cells and causes their periodic destruction.

Malignant   The ability to cause death of the organism.

Malignant hyperpyrexia   The failure of sweating that does not allow the body to lose heat and leads to a progressive rise in body temperature and death.

Malingering   Feigning illness to avoid an obvious external circumstance.

MALT   (*see* Mucosa-associated lymphoid tissue)

Mammography   A radiographic procedure that detects lesions in the breast.

Managed   Controlling a chronic disease by limiting complications and delaying progression of the disease.

Mania   A hyperactive state.

Mantoux test   A procedure to test for the presence of tuberculosis exposure. It involves the instillation of a small amount of inactive *Mycobacterium* antigen under the skin and produces a large wheal in patients who have previously been infected with the bacterium.

Marasmus   A total caloric malnutrition associated with severe wasting but without specific effects of serum protein deficiency.

Margination   Movement of leukocytes from the bloodstream to the endothelium in preparation for emigration from the vessel as part of the inflammatory process.

Marsupialization   Exteriorization of an enclosed cavity and suturing the exposed flap to adjacent tissue, so the cyst is open and can drain to the surface.

Mast cells   Bone-marrow–derived cells found in several different types of tissues and that contain vasoactive amines and other inflammatory mediators.

Mastectomy   Surgical removal of a breast.

Mastication   Chewing.

Mean corpuscular hemoglobin concentration (MCHC)   Calculated by dividing the hemoglobin by the hematocrit, this is the concentration of hemoglobin in packed red blood cells.

Mean corpuscular volume (MCV)   A measure of red blood cell size that is calculated by dividing the hematocrit by the red blood cell count.

Meckel diverticulum   An outpouching of the distal small intestine. It is a remnant of an embryonic connection between the intestine and the yolk sac.

Medial sclerosis   The calcification of the media of large arteries.

Medulla   The central part of an organ.

Medullary carcinoma   A type of thyroid carcinoma that arises from the calcitonin-secreting cells that reside in the connective tissue of the thyroid gland.

Medulloblastoma   A common brain tumor in children that arises in the cerebellum from primitive cells.

Megacolon   Massive distention of the colon.

Megakaryocyte   A bone marrow cell that produces platelets.

Meiosis   A special type of cell division of germ cells that develop into sperm and ova.

Melanin   A brown pigment that helps protect the skin from sunlight damage and contributes to skin color.

Melanocyte-stimulating hormone (MSH)   A hormone secreted by the pituitary gland that regulates skin color.

Melanocytes   Large, pale cells located in the basal layer of skin that contain melanin.

Melanocytic nevus   The common nevus that results from a benign proliferation of melanocytes of the epidermis.

Melanoma   A malignant neoplasm of melanocytes.

Melanoma *in situ*   Melanoma that is confined to the epidermis, and therefore has a better prognosis as compared to invasive lesions.

Melasma   A patchy pigmentation of the exposed areas of the skin; seen most commonly during pregnancy.

Melena   Black, tarry-appearing stools, due to alteration of the blood as it passes down the gastrointestinal tract.

Membrane attack complex   An aggregate of activated complement proteins that kill cells by damaging the cell membrane.

Membranous glomerlulonephritis   A kidney disease in which antigen–antibody complexes are deposited on the glomerular basement membrane, disturbing its permeability.

Memory cells   Special lymphocytes that are long-lived and programmed to proliferate rapidly after a second encounter with an antigen.

Menarche   The first menstrual period of a pubertal girl.

Ménière disease (*also*, endolymphatic hydrops) A degenerative disease of the vestibular apparatus in the ear.

Meninges   The system of membranes that envelopes the central nervous system.

Meningioma   A benign neoplasm that arises from the dura; it is usually slow growing and well circumscribed.

Meningomyelocele   An outpouching of the spinal cord and its covering, the meninges, through a defect in the bony structure of vertebrae.

Menisci   Fibrocartilaginous pads in knee joints.

Menopause   The permanent cessation of menstruation.

Menorrhagia   Excessive menstrual bleeding.

Menses   Normal menstrual hemorrhage.

Menstrual cycles   A series of changes a woman's body goes through approximately every month in which the endometrium is stimulated to proliferate; if no egg is fertilized, it sloughs.

Menstrual history   Information on the length of the menstrual cycle, the duration of menses, the amount of menstrual blood flow, and the regularity of the cycles.

Mental retardation   Below normal intelligence (IQ less than 70) occurring before age 18.

Mercuric chloride   A poison that causes corrosive damage to the oral region and esophagus. The absorbed mercury is excreted by the renal tubules and colonic mucosa, where it produces renal tubular necrosis, leading to acute renal failure, and ulceration of the colon, leading to bloody diarrhea.

Merozoites   An asexual form of sporozoites released by protozoas.

Mesangium   Specialized cells that hold together the renal capillary tufts.

Mesentery   The connective tissue attachment of the bowel that contains blood vessels, lymphatics, and nerves.

Metabolic diseases   Biochemical disorders involving lipids, carbohydrates, proteins, minerals, or vitamins.

Metabolic syndrome   The constellation of central (abdominal) obesity, type 2 diabetes mellitus, hypertension, and dyslipidemia.

Metaphysis   A section of bone between the diaphysis and epiphysis.

Metaplasia   The replacement of one tissue type by another.

Metaplastic bone formation   Bone formation at sites far away from bone, such as in severely stenotic aortic valves or at sites of soft-tissue injury.

Metastasis   The spread of disease from one part of the body to another.

Metastatic calcification   Calcium accumulation in normal tissues, especially those that excrete acid from the body such as renal tubules, lung, and gastric mucosa.

Metastatic cancer   Cancer that has spread from the site of origin.

Methyl alcohol   A toxic alcohol that, when metabolized to formaldehyde, causes damage to the retina and optic nerve. Severe acidosis occurs in fatal methyl alcohol poisoning as a consequence of its metabolism to formic acid.

Metrorrhagia   Irregular bleeding from the uterus between menses.

Micelles   Spherical masses with lipids inside and a water-soluble outside.

Microangiopathic hemolytic anemia   The fragmentation of red blood cells because of narrowing or obstruction of small blood vessels.

Microangiopathy   Disease of small vessels, often due to narrowing.

Microbiology   The study of microorganisms.

Microcytic, hypochromic anemia   Anemia that occurs with iron deficiency.

Microhemorrhages   Vascular lesions in the retina associated with diabetes that can lead to vision loss.

Micturition   The act of urination.

Miliary tuberculosis   The collection of tiny granulomas in multiple organs from disseminated tuberculosis infection.

Minimal change disease (MCD)   A renal disease that may lead to the nephrotic syndrome.

Mitochondria   Complex, membranous cell organelles that generate energy for use by the cell.

Mitochondrial diseases   Diseases that primarily affect the energy-producing mitochondria.

Mitosis   The process of cell division.

Mole   The common nevus that results from a benign proliferation of melanocytes of the epidermis.

Monocyte   A type of leukocyte in the blood that is called a macrophage or histiocyte in tissue.

Monocytosis   An increase in the number of monocytes; usually a sign of chronic inflammation.

Monogenetic   Single gene.

Monosomy   A zygote that has formed from only one homologous chromosome.

Morbid obesity   A body mass index (BMI) of greater than 40, or greater than 35 with an obesity-related illness.

Morbidity   The frequency of disability within a population.

Mortality rate   A measure of the number of people dying from a disease in a given time period.

Mosaicism   Abnormalities occurring in the first or second cell division after fertilization, resulting in an individual with cells of differing chromosomal makeup.

MRSA   Methicillin-resistant *Staphylococcus aureus*.

Mucociliary escalator   A specialized epithelial lining of the bronchial tree composed of columnar cells, some containing cilia on the lumenal surface and others producing mucus. The mucus traps inhaled particles, and the cilia convey the mucus upward toward the mouth, from whence it is swallowed or expectorated.

Mucoepidermoid carcinoma   A malignant neoplasm of the salivary glands.

Mucosa   The mucosal layer.

Multiple endocrine neoplasia 1 (MEN1)   An autosomal dominant disease in which affected patients develop hyperplasia of the parathyroid glands and tumors of the islet cells of the pancreas and/or anterior pituitary.

Multiple myeloma   A cancer of plasma cells, usually arising in the bone marrow.

Multiple organ system failure   When multiple organs cease to function properly.

Mumps   A viral infectious disease that causes painful swelling of the salivary glands and testes.

Mumps virus   An RNA virus that causes mumps by infecting preferentially the salivary glands and the testes.

Mural thrombosis   The formation of a blood clot on the endocardium, usually overlying an infarct.

Murmurs   Abnormal sounds of the heart heard with the aid of a stethoscope.

Muscle cells   Cells that contain contractile fragments.

Muscle fibers   Cells that are highly specialized for the active generation of force for contraction.

Muscularis mucosae   A unique thin muscular layer in the gastrointestinal tract.

Muscularis propria   The deep muscle layer of the gastrointestinal tract that contracts rhythmically to move materials through the alimentary tract.

Mutation   Alteration in gene expression, caused by alteration in a sequence of DNA.

Muzzle imprint   A contact wound from the barrel of the gun being firmly applied to the skin at the time of discharge.

Mycosis   (*also*, mycotic) An infection by a fungus.

Myelophthisic anemia   Anemia caused by replacement of the bone marrow by diseased tissue such as cancer or fibrous tissue.

Myocardial infarction   (*also*, heart attack) Occurs when blood vessels that supply the heart become blocked, preventing oxygen from getting to the heart. The muscle either dies or becomes permanently damaged.

Myopathic   Disease of muscle.

Myosin   One of the two primary proteins of muscle, the other being actin.

Myotonia   Inability to release contraction, a feature of myotonic dystrophy.

Myxedema   An edema of "doughy" consistency, often resulting from hypothyroidism.

N

Narcosis   Confused or stuporous state caused by elevated levels of carbon dioxide.

Natural killer cells (NK cells)   Lymphocytes that destroy other cells in the absence of any known antigenic stimulation.

Necrosis   The death of cells or tissue due to an endogenous or exogenous injury.

Necrotizing fasciitis   A rare soft-tissue infection that leads to the destruction of muscle, skin, and underlying tissue.

Negri bodies   Round or oval inclusion bodies seen in the cytoplasm of neurons of rabies victims.

Neonatal period   The time from birth to 4 weeks after birth.

Neoplasia   The abnormal proliferation of cells.

Neoplasm   Abnormal mass of tissue; tumor.

Nephroblastoma   (*also*, Wilm's tumor) A solid malignant tumor commonly found in children and derived from primitive cells in the renal cortex.

Nephron   The basic functional unit of the kidney.

Nephrotic syndrome   A group of symptoms that include protein in the urine, high cholesterol levels, high triglyceride levels, low blood protein levels, and edema.

Nervous tissue cells   Cells derived from neuroectoderm.

Neuroblastoma   A malignancy of children arising from the adrenal medulla or sympathetic ganglia.

Neurofibromas   Neoplasms that arise anywhere along the course of peripheral nerves; usually benign.

Neurogenic bladder   A condition in which the bladder does not empty completely, promoting infections of the bladder and kidneys.

Neurogenic shock   The sudden loss of the autonomic nervous system signals to the smooth muscle in vessel walls that leads to vasodilation.

Neuron   A cell in the central and peripheral nervous systems that conducts nervous impulses.

Neutrophils   The most common type of white blood cells, capable of phagocytosis.

Nevocellular nevus   A common nevus that results from a benign proliferation of melanocytes of the epidermis.

Nipple   A projection on the breast from which milk is discharged.

Nitrogen   A gaseous element that binds to proteins.

Nocturia   Increased nighttime urination.

Nodes of Ranvier   Small gaps formed in the myelin sheath along axons of peripheral nerves.

Nodular melanoma   A melanotic neoplasm that grows primarily downward, into the dermis rather than along the epidermis, and expands outward to form a nodule.

Nonatopic asthma   (*also*, intrinsic asthma) Airway hyperactivity not caused by allergies.

Nondisjunction   An abnormality in the chromosome number in which two chromosomes of the same type go to one gamete.

Nonmelanoma skin cancers   Basal cell carcinoma and squamous cell carcinoma.

Non-Mendelian inheritance   A term that refers to any pattern of inheritance in which traits do not separate in accordance with Mendel's laws.

Nonpenetrance   An abnormal dominant gene or pairs of abnormal recessive genes that fail to result in an abnormal trait.

Normocytic, normochromic anemia   Anemia in which the red blood cell size remains normal but the overall amount of hemoglobin is reduced.

Nosocomial   Disease acquired from a hospital environment.

Nuclear medicine   A subspecialty that involves the injection of various radioactive materials into the bloodstream and subsequently determining their degree of localization within tissue.

Nucleic acid sequencing   A method of identifying genes and their abnormalities.

Nucleus pulposis   The jelly-like substance in the middle of the spinal disk.

Nystagmus   Flickering eye movements.

O

Obsessive–compulsive disorder (OCD)   A mental disorder typified by recurrent intrusive thoughts accompanied by compensatory behaviors.

Obstructive lung diseases   Diseases that prevent the outflow of air through the bronchial tree, so air becomes trapped within the distal branches.

Obstructive sleep apnea   A debilitating condition in which patients repeatedly stop breathing for as long as one minute during their sleep. The resultant hypoxia interrupts their sleep as they awaken or semi-awaken to resume breathing.

Occult blood   Blood present in feces that is not visibly apparent.

Occult fecal blood test   A blood test on feces to detect blood not visible.

Oligodendroglia   CNS cells that manufacture and maintain the myelin sheath that surrounds and protects axons and dendrites.

Oliguria   Decreased urine output.

Oncogenes   Genes encoding proteins that are involved in cell growth and regulation; may foster neoplastic growth under certain conditions.

Oncogenic viruses   Viruses capable of inducing the formation of tumors.

Oophorectomy   Surgical removal of ovaries.

Open-angle glaucoma   Gross or microscopic abnormalities of the angle tissues of the eye. Open-angle glaucoma is more common than closed-angle glaucoma and is chronic and insidious in onset.

Open fractures   Fractures that cause disruption of the skin.

Ophthalmoscope   A hand-held, light-projecting instrument used to examine the retina by utilizing lenses of various refractive powers.

Opioid analgesics   (*also*, narcotic analgesics, painkillers) The most powerful group of drugs used for pain relief medication; they are potentially addictive and if overused can cause central nervous system and respiratory depression.

Opportunistic infections   Infections that do not normally produce illness in healthy people, but can colonize and infect immunocompromised people.

Opsonins   Phagocytosis-promoting antibodies.

Opsonization   A process that promotes phagocytosis by leukocytes.

Oral cavity   Includes the teeth, tongue, and walls of the mouth; it is part of the digestive system and respiratory system, and is a phonetic box for speech.

Organ   One or more tissues arranged into a structure that carries out a major body function.

Organic diseases   Diseases characterized by structural changes within the body.

Organization   The process of fibrous repair.

Organized thrombus   A thrombus converted to scar tissue.

Orthopnea   Difficulty breathing while in a recumbent position.

Ossicles   The tiny bones of the auditory apparatus that are found in the middle ear.

Ossification   Bone formation.

Osteitis deformans   A localized or multifocal enlargement of bone of unknown cause that affects about 2 percent of the population, typically in persons over 40 years of age.

Osteitis fibrosa cystica   Bone lesions characterized by the presence of giant multinucleated osteoclasts, fibrosis, and cyst formation.

Osteoarthritis   Degenerative joint disease.

Osteoblasts   Cells that form bone.

Osteoclasts   Multinucleated cells that dissolve the mineral matrix of bone in response to hormonal signals.

Osteoid   The unmineralized, organic portion of the bone matrix that forms prior to the maturation of bone tissue.

Osteopenia   Generalized loss of bone.

Osteophytes   Protrusions of bone in a degenerative joint.

Osteoporosis   The thinning of bone tissue and loss of bone density over time.

Osteosarcoma   The most common type of bone cancer in children and adolescents.

Otitis media   Inflammation of the middle ear.

Otosclerosis   The growth of new bone in the middle ear that can impede the vibration of the ossicles, resulting in a mechanical loss of hearing.

Otoscope   A device that allows inspection of the external ear and external surface of the tympanic membrane.

Ova (parasites)   Intestinal parasites that can be found in feces.

Ovaries   Reproductive organs responsible for producing ova.

Ovulation   Release of a mature ovum from its follicle; the ovum is then expelled from the surface of the ovary.

Ovum   A fertilized egg.

Oxytocin   A hormone, produced in the pituitary gland, that stimulates contraction of the myoepithelial cells so that milk is expressed into the ducts and transported to the nipple.

P

Pain   An unpleasant sensory and emotional experience associated with actual or potential tissue damage.

Palliative   Type of treatment or therapy to reduce pain, symptoms, and stress that is provided when a cure is not expected.

Palpation   Applying gentle digital pressure to feel for abnormal growths.

Pancreas   Glandular organ with excretory ducts emptying into the second portion of the duodenum.

Panhypopituitarism   Decreased secretion of most pituitary hormones.

Panic disorder   Mental illness characterized by repeated bouts of severe anxiety.

Pannus   An inflammatory membrane overlying the synovial cells on the inside of a joint.

Pap smear   (*also*, Papanicolau test, cervical smear, smear test) A type of screening test using a sample of cells that is scraped from the cervix and examined microscopically for abnormalities.

Papillary carcinoma   A well-differentiated cancer of the thyroid.

Papilledema   Swelling of the head of the optic nerve as seen through the ophthalmoscope.

Papular   Lesions that are raised.

Paralysis   Loss of muscle function for one or more muscles.

Paraneoplastic syndrome   Ectopic hormone production by a neoplasm with associated symptoms.

Paraplegia   The loss of voluntary control over the lower limbs.

Paraquat   A commonly used weed killer that causes damage to the pulmonary alveoli when ingested or inhaled.

Parathormone   A hormone secreted by the parathyroid epithelial cells that regulates the balance of calcium and phosphorus in the body.

Parathyroid   Small endocrine glands in the neck that produce parathormone.

Parenchymal   The cells and tissues that carry out the main function of an organ and are usually the most abundant and unique to an organ.

Paresis   Weakness.

Paresthesia   Altered sensation; a usually benign sensation of tingling, pricking, or numbness of a person's skin.

Parietal cell   Cell that produces gastric acid.

Paronychia   A skin infection that occurs around the fingernails.

Parotitis   Painful swelling of the parotid gland.

Pathogenesis   Structural and functional mechanisms leading to disease.

Pathogens   Microorganisms that produce disease when they elaborate a toxin or gain entrance to a host tissue.

Pathology   The study of disease.

Pathophysiology   Derangement of function in disease.

Pelvic examination   Direct inspection of the vulva, examination of the vagina and cervix, and bimanual palpation of the uterus, fallopian tubes, and ovaries.

Pelvic inflammary disease   Infection of the cervix and urethra with extension to the fallopian tubes; most commonly caused by gonorrhea or chlamydial infection.

Pelvic pain   Pain in the pelvic region that may originate in the reproductive organs.

Penis   External sexual organ of the male.

Percussion   The tapping on a finger placed against the chest; may reveal dull or low-pitched sounds suggestive of underlying pulmonary consolidation or pleural effusion.

Perforating   A wound that enters and exits the body.

Perfusion   Blood flow per unit volume of tissue.

Perinatal period   The period from 2 weeks before birth to 4 weeks after birth.

Periodontal disease   Inflammation of the gums; can lead to tooth loss.

Periosteum   A tough, fibrous membrane that covers and supplies blood to bone.

Peripheral edema   Edema of the extremities.

Peristalsis   Waves of muscle contractions that carry materials through the gastrointestinal tract.

Peritonitis   An inflammatory reaction in the peritoneal cavity.

Permanent cells   Cells that do not divide once they reach maturity.

Pernicious anemia   Anemia caused by the failure to absorb vitamin B_{12} from the gastrointestinal tract; vitamin B_{12} is necessary to properly develop red blood cells.

Petechiae   Pinpoint hemorrhages in the skin or on mucosal surfaces.

Phagocytes   Neutrophils and macrophages.

Phagocytosis   The act of engulfing particulate matter.

Pharmacogenomics   Predicting a particular patient's response to particular drugs on the basis of their genetic makeup.

Pharyngitis   Inflammation of the pharynx.

Pharynx   A passageway for air that provides the musculature for swallowing; also contains abundant lymphoid tissue, including the tonsils, which aids in the recognition of antigens such as foreign materials and microorganisms that enter the body via the air or food.

Phenotype   The physical and functional manifestation of genetic traits.

Phenylketonuria   An autosomal recessive disease caused by an absence of the enzyme phenylalanine hydroxylase, which metabolizes phenylalanine to tyrosine, resulting in phenylalanine accumulation.

Pheochromocytoma   A neoplasm of the chromaffin cells of the adrenal medulla; it may produce catecholamines in an unregulated fashion.

Phlebothrombosis   A thrombus in a vein.

Phosphorus   A mineral essential for life, which is incorporated into bone.

Photophobia   Uncomfortable sensitivity to light.

Physical examination   The process by which a healthcare specialist examines the body for signs of disease.

Physiologic hypertrophy   An exaggerated response to a normal physiologic demand, resulting in enlargement in size.

Pia-arachnoid   An inner lace-like membrane that lies directly over the cortex of the brain.

Pilonidal cyst   An abscess occurring around ingrown hair in the skin just above the gluteal fold.

Pituitary   A gland located at the base of the brain that produces many types of regulating hormones as part of the endocrine system.

Placenta   An organ that connects a developing fetus to the uterine wall to allow nutrient uptake, waste elimination, and gas exchange.

Placenta previa   A condition in which the placenta is implanted low in the uterine cavity and can partially or completely cover the cervical os, resulting in difficult childbirth.

Placental abruption   Separation of the placenta from its attachment to the uterus.

Plaque   A raised patch on a surface.

Plasma   The liquid component of blood.

Plasma cells   Antibody-producing cells derived from lymphocytes.

Plasmin   An enzyme formed from plasminogen in the presence of a variety of activators. Plasmin breaks down the insoluble fibrin clot into soluble fragments called fibrin-split products.

Platelet count   The number of platelets present in blood.

Platelet function analyzer   An instrument that measures platelet-dependent coagulation under flow conditions.

Platelets   Irregularly shaped, colorless bodies present in blood and derived from megakayocytes. They have a sticky surface that helps form clots to stop bleeding.

Pleural effusion   Fluid in the pleural space.

Pleural space   The space between the lungs and the chest wall.

Pluripotent   Able to differentiate into many different types of adult cells.

Pneumoconiosis   Environmentally induced pulmonary fibrosis resulting from inhalation of particulate matter.

Pneumonia   Infection of the lungs.

Pneumonitis   Inflammation of the lung, usually limited to the interstitium.

Pneumothorax   Air in the pleural space.

Pollution   Environmental contaminants that may cause harm to individuals.

Polyarteritis nodosa   A type of vasculitis that results in nodular inflammatory thickenings of medium-sized arteries, particularly those of the kidneys, intestines, and skeletal muscles.

Polycythemia vera   An abnormal increase in the number of red blood cells, of unknown origin.

Polydypsia   Excessive drinking, usually of water.

Polygenetic   Multiple genes.

Polymerase chain reaction (PCR)   A technique of molecular biology to amplify a single or few copies of a segment of DNA.

Polymyositis   An autoimmune inflammatory disease that affects skeletal muscle in preference to other organs and is characterized by a lymphocytic infiltrate.

Polyps   Any abnormal protusion from a mucosal surface.

Polyuria   Excessive urination.

Port wine stain   A vascular birth mark on the skin made up of capillary malformations.

Portal hypertension   Increased blood pressure in the portal vein due to increased resistance to blood flow through damaged veins in the liver.

Portal triad   A triad composed of branches of the hepatic artery, portal vein, and bile ducts.

Portal vein   A vein that collects blood from most of the intestinal tract and spleen and carries it to the liver, where nutrients and metabolic products are removed.

Positive-pressure ventilator   A machine that pushes air into a patient's airway to keep it from collapsing.

Positron emission tomography (PET)   The injection of positron-emitting radio nucleotides, such as carbon, nitrogen, or oxygen, into the body. The body is then scanned to view where the nucleotides are deposited.

Post-traumatic stress disorder (PTSD)   A mental disorder typified by hyperarousal and reexperiencing and avoidance of psychologically painful stimuli following a traumatic event.

Potter syndrome   A collection of symptoms including impaired lung development, impaired growth of the fetus, limb deformities, and characteristic facial features. Not compatible with life.

Premalignant lesion   An area of increased likelihood of cancer developing compared to adjacent tissues.

Prematurity   Refers to births that occur 3 weeks or more prior to term (37 weeks, gestational age or less).

Presbycusis   Hearing loss occurring with increasing age.

Pressure atrophy   Atrophy resulting from steady pressure on a tissue.

Prevalence   The number of persons with a disease at any one time, regardless of when they were diagnosed.

Preventive medicine   A specialty dedicated to the prevention of disease.

Primary atypical pneumonia   (*also*, walking pneumonia) A smoldering infection for many months with low-grade symptoms such as coughing, shortness of breath, and fatigue; commonly found in children and adolescents, and often caused by *Mycoplasma pneumoniae.*

Primary biliary cirrhosis   A disease that primarily affects women. It is attributed to an autoimmune reaction to the bile ductular epithelium. The intrahepatic bile ducts are destroyed and become obliterated by fibrous tissue.

Primary hyperparathyroidism   A disease occurring when the production of parathormone by the parathyroid glands is not controlled by normal feedback mechanisms.

Primary sclerosing cholangitis   A disease that is very strongly associated with ulcerative colitis. The bile ducts are the targets of the inflammation, but the pattern of injury is different from that seen in primary biliary cirrhosis. Both intrahepatic and extrahepatic bile ducts are affected in a discontinuous fashion.

Prion   Abnormal protein found in the brain in association with Creutzfeldt-Jacob dementia.

Progesterone   A hormone that encourages the endometrium to undergo secretory changes that make it hospitable to the blastocyst.

Prognosis   A prediction about the course a disease will take.

Progression   The acquisition of additional DNA mutations that results in multiple clones creating a neoplasm.

Prolactin   A hormone produced by the pituitary gland during pregnancy that stimulates the secretion of milk.

Proliferative glomerulonephritis   Inflammation in which the glomeruli are infiltrated by leukocytes, making them appear hypercellular.

Promotion   Selective growth of initiated cells that does not involve new mutations.

Prostacyclin   An inhibitor of platelet aggregation and vasodilator; derived from arachadonic acid.

Prostaglandins   Metabolite of arachidonic acid produced locally by cells and influencing inflammation.

Prostate gland   Exocrine gland of the male reproductive system.

Prostate-specific antigen (PSA)   A screening test for prostate cancer that checks a blood level.

Protein C   A protein that, in its activated form, plays an important role in the clotting of blood.

Proteins   Aggregates of individual amino acids that can be synthesized in the body.

Proteolytic enzymes   Enzymes that break down proteins.

Proteomics   The mapping of the patterns of proteins in health and disease.

Prothrombin time (PT)   A test that assesses disorders of the extrinsic pathway of coagulation.

Pruritus   Itching of the skin.

Pseudocysts   Cavitary lesions filled with necrotic debris that are caused by the autodigestion of the pancreas and the surrounding tissues.

Pseudomembrane   A false membrane that forms over infected tissue; composed of fibrin and inflammatory cells.

Psychosis   A mental disorder in which the personality is seriously disorganized and contact with reality is impaired.

Psychosomatic   Physical symptoms caused by mental or emotional disturbances.

Pulmonary arteries   Arteries that carry deoxygenated blood to the lungs.

Pulmonary edema   Seepage of fluid into the pulmonary air spaces.

Pulmonary embolism (PE)   A condition in which emboli break away from thrombi in deep peripheral veins and are carried through the veins to the right side of the heart, where they are pumped into the branches of the pulmonary arteries, causing obstruction of blood flow to portions of the lungs.

Pulmonary hypertension   Elevated vascular pressures in the pulmonary blood system.

Pulmonary valve   The valve between the right ventricle and the pulmonary trunk.

Pulmonary veins   Veins that carry oxygenated blood to the left side of the heart.

Pulpitis   Infection and necrosis of dental pulp.

Pupil   Aperture of the eye.

Purpura   Larger collections of blood in the skin that are red-purple in color.

Purulent exudate   (*also*, pus) A thick, creamy mixture of fluids, dead tissue, and neutrophils.

Pyelonephritis   Infection of the renal parenchyma, calyces, and pelvis.

Pyknosis   Condensation of the nucleus of a cell.

Pylorus   A muscular sphincter that controls the rate of emptying of the stomach into the small intestine.

Pyogenic   Eliciting of a neutrophilic inflammatory response with purulent exudate (pus generating).

Pyuria   Pus-filled urine.

Q

Quad test   A test performed on the serum of pregnant women to check for fetal abnormalities; it measures alpha fetoprotein, human chorionic gonadotropin, inhibin-A, and estriol.

Quadriplegia   The loss of voluntary control over all limbs.

R

Radiation Divergence in all directions from a center, especially referring to x-rays.

Radiation therapy The medical use of ionizing radiation as part of a cancer treatment.

Radiculopathy Pain in the tissues serviced by a nerve.

Radiography The use of x-rays to view tissue.

Radiology The discipline of medicine that uses techniques such as x-rays, computed tomography (CT) scans, ultrasound (US), and nuclear medicine to diagnose disease.

Radiosensitive Easily damaged by radiation.

Rales An abnormal breath sound caused by fluid-filled alveoli opening during inhalation.

Range of fire Distance from which a gunshot was fired.

Rapid strep test A test rapidly performed in a doctor's office to detect a carbohydrate produced by *Streptococcus* and not by other organisms.

Rash Any eruption on the skin.

Raynaud's phenomenon Constriction of the small vessels of the extremities, usually the hands, in an exaggerated response to cold, leaving the fingers or toes cold and blue.

Recessive Pattern of inheritance pertaining to a defect on an allele that will result in disease only if both alleles are defective.

Red blood cells (RBCs) (*also*, erythrocytes) Specialized cells that have no nucleus and whose hemoglobin-filled cytoplasm is shaped like a biconcave disk; their principal function is oxygen transport.

Reed-Sternberg cell A type of giant cell seen in patients with Hodgkin disease.

Refractive error Degree by which the cornea and lens fail to focus light rays on the retina.

Regeneration The replacement of the destroyed tissue by cells similar to those previously present.

Regression Return to an earlier state; the spontaneous disappearance of neoplasms.

Regurgitation Backward flow; backflow of blood in the heart due to an incompetent or stenosed valve.

Renal cell carcinoma A type of kidney cancer arising from abnormal tubular cells.

Renin An enzyme secreted by the kidney when decreased blood flow is sensed.

Repair The body's attempt to replace dead cells, whether by regeneration of the original tissue or by replacement with connective scar tissue.

Resection The removal of large specimens by surgery.

Resolution The removal of dead tissue and particulate material by macrophages following inflammation.

Resorption Passage of substances from the tubules to capillaries in the kidney.

Restrictive lung diseases Diseases that destroy the lungs' elastic property.

Reticulocytes Immature red blood cells that retain basophilic material in their cytoplasm.

Reticulocytosis An increase in the production and release of reticulocytes.

Retinal layer Inner layer of the globe of the eye on which images are focused.

Rhabdomyosarcoma A rare primary malignant neoplasm of skeletal muscle.

Rheumatic fever An inflammatory disease that may develop after an infection with certain strains of *Streptococcus*, characterized by myocarditis and arthritis.

Rheumatic heart disease An inflammatory disease following rheumatic fever that can affect connective tissues, such as the heart valves.

Rheumatoid factor (RF) An antibody directed at the body's own tissues; present in high levels in rheumatoid arthritis.

Rhinitis Inflammation of the nose, with discharge.

Ribosomes Cell organelles that make proteins from amino acids.

Rickets A bone disease caused by vitamin D deficiency.

Right and left coronary arteries Two medium-sized arteries that supply blood to the cardiac muscle.

Right heart failure Failure of the right ventricle to adequately pump.

Ringworm Superficial fungal infection of the skin also known as tinea.

Risk factors Conditions that, when present, will render an individual more susceptible to development of the disease.

Rocky Mountain spotted fever A rickettsial infection in which the organism is transmitted by a tick.

S

Salivary glands Glands in the oral cavity that provide moisture to soften and add carbohydrate-digesting enzymes to food; includes the parotid.

Saprophytes Microorganisms that specialize in biodegrading dead animals or other organic material.

Sarcoidosis   A generalized, noncaseating granulomatous disease of unknown cause and with varying clinical manifestations. The organs most commonly involved are lung and lymph nodes.

Sarcoma   Term used to decribe neoplasms arising from mesenchymal tissue.

Scar   A tough mass of collagen.

Scarlet fever   An uncommon systemic streptococcal infection so named because the effect of one of the bacteria's toxins is to produce a scarlet rash.

Schwannomas   Common tumors, usually benign, that arise anywhere along the course of peripheral nerves.

Sciatica   Shooting pain in the leg, which may extend all the way down to the foot, when the sciatic nerve is pinched.

Sclera   The outer layer of the eye, a tough fibrous coating.

Scoliosis   Curvature of the spine.

Screening procedures   Tests to identify different types of disease at treatable stages.

Scurvy   A disease caused by vitamin C deficiency.

Sebaceous gland   Gland attached to each hair follicle that secretes lipid-rich sebum. Sebum waterproofs skin and hair, and protects them from dehydration.

Seborrheic keratoses   Usually multiple brown-black–colored, stuck-on–appearing, warty lesions commonly occurring on the face, trunk, and extremities of persons past middle age.

Second-degree burns   Burns that destroy the epidermis and upper dermis; they are red and moist, and often blister.

Secondary hyperparathyroidism   A condition associated with low serum calcium, most often caused by chronic renal failure or vitamin D deficiency.

Secondary hypertension   Hypertensive disease in which a cause, such as a tumor that is producing adrenalin, is evident.

Secondary infection   An infection that is reactivated after a period of time; often refers to tuberculosis.

Secondary response   A subsequent encounter with the same antigen that is associated with a more rapid production of antibodies.

Seminal vesicles   Small tubes behind the prostate that provide fluid to mix with sperm.

Seminoma   A germ cell tumor of the testes.

Senile atrophy   Wasting or diminution of tissues characterized by advanced age.

Senile elastosis   The degeneration of dermal collagen and elastic fibers, which results in excessive wrinkling of the skin, usually due to chronic sun exposure.

Senile macular degeneration (SMD)   (*also*, age-related macular degeneration) Characterized by damage to retinal pigment epithelium with underlying vascular proliferation.

Sensorineural   Refers to hearing loss in which the cochlea and/or auditory nerve is damaged.

Sentinel lymph node   The first lymph node that receives lymph drainage from the area of the cancer; biopsied preferentially in cases of breast cancer.

Septic shock   Systemic shock caused by overwhelming infection and toxins produced by bacteria.

Septicemia   Systemic blood contamination with toxic products of microorganisms.

Serosa   A thin, smooth membrane present on the outer surface of those parts of the alimentary tract that lie within the abdominal cavity.

Serum   Fluid remaining after fibrin is removed from blood.

Serum iron-binding capacity   A test to measure the amount of the protein that carries iron in the blood.

Sex-linked   Genes located on the X or Y chromosome.

Sexually transmitted disease (STD)   Disease transmitted through sexual encounters; includes chlamydia, genital herpes, gonorrhea, syphilis, bacterial vaginosis, human papillomavirus, and others.

Sheehan syndrome   Postpartum infarction of the pituitary gland.

Shingles   (*see* Herpes zoster) A painful rash that follows a peripheral nerve distribution; caused by the varicella-zoster virus, which also causes chickenpox.

Shock   Failure of the cardiovascular system to maintain adequate blood pressure.

Short bowel syndrome   A condition in which more than one-half to two-thirds of the small intestine is surgically removed or severely diseased, allowing malabsorption to occur.

Sialoliths   Stones that form in salivary glands and cause obstruction of ducts, also resulting in pain and swelling.

Sickle cell anemia   A genetic abnormality of the hemoglobin structure that leads to red blood cells becoming crescent shaped in times of low oxygen tension.

Sigmoidoscopy   The most common endoscopic procedure; used to visualize the rectum and lower sigmoid colon.

Signs   Physical observations made by the examiner of the patient.

Sinoatrial node   A pacemaker focus in the atria of the heart that generates an electrical pulse.

Sinuses   Air-filled spaces in bones in the skull that help with the heating and humidification of inspired air.

Sinusitis   Infection of the sinuses.

Sinusoids   Dilated capillaries that are more continuously open to blood flow than ordinary capillaries; found in selected organs such as the liver.

Sjögren's syndrome   An autoimmune disease that causes destruction of the cells that produce tears in the lacrimal gland and saliva in the salivary glands.

Slit-lamp   A binocular magnifying instrument that projects a focused beam of light into the eye and is used for detailed examination of the cornea, anterior chamber, iris, and lens.

Small cell (neuroendocrine) carcinoma   A cancer composed of sheets of poorly cohesive cells with scanty cytoplasm and numerous mitotic figures and areas of necrosis. In the lung it is a more aggressive form of cancer strongly associated with smoking.

Small intestine   The part of the digestive tract between the stomach and colon; comprises the duodenum, jejunem, and ileum.

Social phobia   Anxiety in social settings.

Sociopathic   Having antisocial personality disorder.

Solar elastosis   Degeneration of dermal collagen and elastic fibers that results in excessive wrinkling of the skin.

Solar keratosis   (*also*, actinic keratosis) Scaly lesion on skin exposed to sun; develops into squamous cell carcinoma in approximately 25 percent of cases.

Solar lentigines   Dark brown skin lesions in adults after chronic sun exposure.

Somatic   Relating to the body of an organism.

Speculum   Device that spreads the walls of the vagina apart so that the inner vagina and cervix can be seen.

Spherocytes   Spherical red blood cells.

Sphygmomanometer   Device used to measure blood pressure manually.

Spina bifida   Birth defect in which there is an absence of the posterior arches and spines of some vertebrae.

Spirometry   Pulmonary function testing.

Spontaneous abortion   Commonly referred to as a miscarriage, usually within the first 12 gestational weeks.

Spontaneous bacterial peritonitis   Inflammation resulting from the bacteria in the gut infecting abdominal fluid.

Sporozoites   The motile infective stage of certain protozoa.

Sprain   Traumatic injury to a ligament as the result of overstretching.

Sputum   The mucoid material coughed up from the lungs.

Squamous cell carcinoma   A form of cancer that may develop in many different organs; strongly associated with cigarette smoking in the lung.

Squamous metaplasia   Transformation of glandular epithelium to squamous.

Stable cells   Cells that divide only in response to injury.

Stage   A definition of the extent of a cancer in the body. It is based on whether the cancer is invasive/noninvasive, if lymph nodes are involved, and if abnormal cells have spread to other parts of the body.

Staging   Studies performed to determine the extent of cancer spreading to other tissues in the body.

Starches   Complex chains of carbohydrates.

Stasis   Pooling or slower than normal flow of liquid; usually refers to blood.

Status asthmaticus   A prolonged asthma attack not responsive to traditional therapy.

STD   (*see* Sexually transmitted disease)

Steatorrhea   The passage of greasy, smelly stools that often float in toilet water; indicative of malabsorption of fats.

Steatosis   The accumulation of fat in hepatocytes.

Stem cells   Undifferentiated cells capable of renewing themselves through mitotic cell division and differentiating into specialized cell types.

Stenosis   Narrowing of a vessel or valve.

Stent   A cast that is placed inside a hollow tube to brace the lumen open.

Stippling   Punctate abrasions of the skin around an entrance wound caused by unburned or burning gunpowder impacting the skin. It is seen in an intermediate-range wound.

Stratified squamous epithelium   The cellular covering of the body surface.

Stress test   A test that determines the effectiveness of oxygen delivery to myocardial tissue, either at rest or with exercise, real or simulated.

Stroke   Common name for cerebral vascular accident.

Stroma   The fibrous connective tissue component of an organ.

Structural barriers   A defense mechanism that exists between the host and the environment, such as the skin and mucous membranes of the gastrointestinal tract and lungs.

Subacute bacterial endocarditis   A smoldering infection on a heart valve that gradually destroys the valve.

Subcutaneous   (*also*, subcutis) Refers to tissue underlying the epidermis.

Sublethal (reversible) cell injury   Where the cells are damaged but capable of repair.

Subluxation   A partial dislocation of bones from joint sockets.

Submucosa   A layer of deep tissue beneath the mucosa of the gastrointestinal tract that provides structural support to the mucosa.

Sudden cardiac death   (*also*, cardiac arrest) The abrupt loss of heart function occurring within an hour of the onset of symptoms, resulting in rapid cessation of blood circulation and death.

Sunburn   A first-degree burn.

Superficial spreading melanoma   The most common type of skin cancer; characterized by spreading growth of malignant cells within the epidermis and superficial dermis, producing a flat to slightly raised lesion, often with a variegated color pattern.

Suppurative inflammation   An inflammatory reaction with purulent exudate.

Surfactant   A phospholipid that lowers the surface tension of the alveolar lining fluid, preventing the alveolus from collapsing during exhalation.

Surgical pathology   A branch of pathology that makes diagnoses based on gross, microscopic, and other tests on tissue removed from live patients during surgery; used to develop treatment strategies.

Survival rate   Percentage of people with a particular condition who live for a given period of time after diagnosis.

Susceptibility   How vulnerable a microorganism is to specific drugs.

Symptoms   Evidence of disease perceived by the patient.

Syncope   Fainting caused by the pooling of blood in the lower body.

Syndrome   A cluster of findings commonly encountered with more than one disease.

Synostosis   The abnormal fusion of neighboring bones.

Synovial fluid   Lubricating fluid in synovial joints secreted by the synovial membrane.

Synovial joints   Joints between two articulating bones that have synovial membranes.

Syphilis   A sexually transmitted disease that can affect several organs in several stages and produces varying symptoms in males and females; caused by *Trepomema pallidum*, a spirochete.

Systemic lupus erythematosus (SLE)   An autoimmune disease that can affect a large number of organ systems, from the skin to the nervous system, hematologic system, joints, kidneys, and serosal surfaces.

Systole   Contraction of the ventricle of the heart.

Systolic pressure   The maximum pressure as the heart muscle contracts; first number typically recorded in a blood pressure measurement.

T

T-helper cells   Type of cells that physically deliver information about antigens to B cells so as to aid B cells in the production of antibodies.

T lymphocyte   A type of lymphocytes so named because its production is initially programmed by the thymus.

T-score   The result of a dual energy x–ray absorptiometry, which relates the measured bone density to normal values.

T suppressor cells   Type of cells that suppress other T cells to down-regulate the immune response and suppress B cells so as to prevent the production of excess antibody; they also prevent the production of antibodies to the body's own tissues.

T1 images   Images produced by a magnetic resonance image that gives a strong signal for lipid.

T2 images   Images produced by a magnetic resonance image that gives a strong signal for water.

Tachypnea   A respiratory rate faster than normal.

Targeted therapy   Treatment with particular drugs if the substrate on which they act is known to be present.

Telangiectasia   Collections of small blood vessels.

Temporal ateritis (giant cell arteritis)   A specific type of inflammation and damage to blood vessels that supply the head area.

Teratogens   Environmental factors that can interfere with the development of the embryo or fetus.

Teratoma   An encapsulated tumor with tissue or organ components resembling normal derivatives of all three germ layers.

Test   A critical analysis.

Testes   Bilateral organs, sitting in the scrotum slightly outside the body cavity, where sperm are produced.

Tetanus   (*also*, lockjaw) A disease caused by *Clostridium tetani*, a soil bacterium, manifested as painful, generalized muscle spasms.

Tetany   Prolonged contraction of a muscle after a single stimulus.

Tetralogy of Fallot   A congenital heart defect with four abnormalities: ventricular septal defect, overriding aorta, right ventricular hypertrophy, and pulmonary stenosis.

Thalassemia   A genetic defect affecting the rate of synthesis of hemoglobin A due to a deficient production of alpha or beta globin.

Thalidomide   A hypnotic drug prescribed worldwide to women from 1957 to 1961 to treat the nausea of pregnancy; banned due to the resulting severe, sometimes life-threatening birth defects.

Third-degree burns   Burns that destroy epidermis and dermis down to the subcutaneous tissue; the skin is charred and dry.

Thrombin   An enzyme in the clotting cascade that converts fibrinogen to fibrin.

Thrombocytopenia   A disorder marked by a decreased number of platelets.

Thrombocytosis   Excessive numbers of platelets defined by platelet counts exceeding 500,000 per microliter of blood.

Thrombophlebitis   (*also*, phlebothrombosis) Thrombosis in an inflamed vein.

Thrombosis   Process of coagulation occurring in a blood vessel, resulting in a blood clot.

Thrombotic thrombocytopenia purpura (TTP)   A rare disorder of the blood-coagulation system causing extensive microscopic thromboses to form in small blood vessels throughout the body.

Thrombus   A blood clot that forms during life in a blood vessel due to activation of the coagulation mechanism.

Thyroid   The largest endocrine gland in the body; located in the neck and secretes thyroxin.

Thyroid-stimulating hormone (TSH)   A hormone secreted by the anterior pituitary gland to regulate the endocrine function of the thyroid gland.

Tinea   (*also*, ringworm) Various superficial fungal infections.

Tinea barbae   Superficial fungal infection of the beard.

Tinea capitis   Superficial fungal infection of the scalp.

Tinea cruris   (*also*, jock itch) Superficial fungal infection involving the perineum, buttocks, and/or inner thighs.

Tinea pedis   (*also*, athlete's foot) Superficial fungal infection that affects the soles and interdigital spaces of the feet.

Tinnitus   The sensation of ringing in the ears.

Tissue   A functional grouping of cells and intercellular substances.

Tissue diagnosis   Diagnosis based on microscopic examination of a biopsy sample.

Tissue factor   A protein present in tissues, and necessary to start the extrinsic pathway of the coagulation cascade.

Tissue plasminogen activator   A drug that breaks down thrombi and emboli; a natural and synthetic chemical.

TNM system   A staging system for cancer, where T describes the tumor, N describes lymph node involvement, and M describes whether there is distant metastasis.

Tonometer   A small instrument placed directly on the eyeball to measure the intraocular pressure.

Tonsillitis   Inflammation of the pharyngeal tonsils.

Tonsils   Structures in the pharynx that aid in the recognition of antigens such as foreign materials and microorganisms that enter the body via the air or food.

Tophi   Lumps of crystallized uric acid that appear on joints affected by gout.

TORCH   Acronym; diagnostic test for toxoplasma, other (syphilis), rubella, cytomegalovirus, and herpes simplex virus.

Torsion   Twisting of a structure, including an organ, around its vascular stalk with resultant ischemic injury.

Total parenteral nutrition (TPN)   The administration of carbohydrates, lipids, salts, proteins, and essential minerals and vitamins through the bloodstream.

Toxemia   A condition caused by release of toxins into the blood.

Toxic epidermal necrolysis   Sloughing of portions of the epidermis that can be a life-threatening condition.

Toxic megacolon   An acute form of colonic distention.

Toxic shock syndrome (TSS)   A severe illness caused by an exotoxin secreted by *Staphylococcus aureus* that involves fever, shock, and problems with the function of several body organs.

Tracheostomy   A surgical opening into the trachea directly through the anterior portion of the neck.

Trachoma   A chlamydial disease of the eye resulting in blindness.

Transformation   Process by which normal cells lose important checks on their growth, eventually leading to cancer.

Transitional epithelium   The lining of hollow organs such as the urinary bladder that are subject to contraction and distention.

Translocations   Fragments of chromosomes that exchange places with sequences on nonhomologous chromosomes.

Transplantation   Surgical moving of an organ from one body to another or from one location to another.

Transudate   The edema fluid produced by increased hydrostatic pressure or decreased osmotic pressure in the blood that has a low protein content.

Trauma   Injury caused by extrinsic forces.

Traveler's diarrhea   Any acute diarrheal illness in travelers to foreign countries.

Trichomoniasis   A sexually transmitted disease caused by the protozoan parasite *Trichomonas vaginalis*.

Tricuspid   Valve between the right atrium and the right ventricle of the mammalian heart.

Triglycerides   The chemical form in which most fat exists in food as well as in the body.

Triple negative   Breast cancers that do not express ER/PR or Her2/neu.

Triple screen test   A measure of three substances (alpha fetoprotein, human chorionic gonadotropin, and estriol) in the serum of pregnant women to test for fetal abnormalities.

Trisomy   Three homologous chromosomes.

Trophic hormones   Hormones that stimulate growth and development in other tissues.

Trophoblast   The layer of cells that immediately surrounds an embryo and develops into the villi of the placenta.

Trophozoites   The proliferative forms of protozoa.

Troponins   Enzymes released from the heart when it is damaged.

Trypsin   Enzyme that digests carbohydrates, fats, and proteins.

TSS   (*see* Toxic shock syndrome)

Tubal ligation   Surgical interruption of the uterine tubes performed for birth control.

Tube feedings   A medical device that conveys nutrients to the stomach if caloric supplementation is required.

Tuberculin   Inactive *Mycobacterium tuberculosis* antigen that is injected under the skin and produces a large wheal in patients who have previously been infected with the TB bacillus (tuberculin skin test).

Tubular adenoma   A type of benign tumor; small, usually less than 2 centimeters, pedunculated, composed predominantly of glands; uncommonly contains cancer at the time it is removed.

Tubules   Minute tubes; contain a filtrate that eventually becomes urine in the kidney (renal); microscopic channels in dentin (dental canaliculi), testis (seminiferous), and other structures.

Tumor suppressor cells   Cells that normally keep oncogenes in check.

Tunica adventitia   Outer layer of a blood vessel.

Tunica intima   Innermost lining of an artery or vein.

Tunica media   Middle layer of an artery or vein.

Turner syndrome   A sex chromosome monosomy. Affected individuals are females with a single X chromosome.

Tympanic membrane   (*also*, eardrum) A membrane separating the middle ear and the external ear.

Type I allergy   A reaction mediated by IgE antibody that involves release of vasoactive chemicals from tissue mast cells or blood basophilic leukocytes.

Type II allergy   The destruction of host cells either by agglutination and phagocytosis or by lysis of the cell membrane as a consequence of complement fixation. Red blood cells are commonly targets of this type of hypersensitivity, and the antigens are either the red blood cell membrane itself or a foreign chemical, such as a drug, that adheres to the red cell membrane as a hapten.

Type III allergy   A complement-mediated reaction to precipitates of antigen and antibody. The antigen–antibody complexes lodge in vessel walls, and the activation of certain inflammation-inducing components of complement results in release of vasoactive substances from mast cells and attraction of polymorphonuclear leukocytes to the site. The acute inflammatory reaction takes several hours to develop and may be prolonged if the amount of antibody is small.

Type IV allergy   Cell-mediated hypersensitivity; it is the harmful destruction of tissue by T lymphocytes and macrophages.

Typhus   A disease caused by rickettsia that are transmitted to a human by the body louse.

Typing   The process of checking for major (ABO and Rh) blood groups prior to transfusion to ensure that they are compatible.

U

Ulcer   A local excavation of an epithelium, such as skin or mucous membranes.

Ulcerative colitis   An inflammatory bowel disease that causes chronic inflammation of the digestive tract.

Ultrasound   A diagnostic test that measures the reflection of high-frequency sound waves as they pass through body tissues.

Ultraviolet radiation   The portion of the electromagnetic spectrum between x-rays and visible light, which causes the most solar skin damage.

Undescended testis   A testicle that has not descend into the scrotum before birth.

Undulant fever   (brucellosis; *also* Crimean fever, Malta fever, Mediterranean fever) Infectious disease caused by contact with an animal carrying the *Brucella* bacterium; so named because of the waxing and waning of febrile episodes.

Unstable angina   Cardiac chest pain not relieved by rest.

Upper GI series   Radiologic examination of the esophagus, stomach, and upper small intestine.

Upper respiratory infections   Illnesses of the upper respiratory tract, involving the nose, sinuses, pharynx, or larynx.

Urea   Chemical compound found in urine; the breakdown product of proteins.

Uremia   Accumulation of waste products in the blood due to severe renal failure.

Ureters   Tubes that carry urine from the kidney to the bladder.

Urethra   Tube that drains urine from the bladder.

Urethritis   Inflammation of the urethra.

Urgency   Medical condition of pressing importance: almost continuous urge to urinate (urinary); severe untreated high blood pressure (hypertensive).

Uric acid   A chemical present in elevated amounts in gout.

Urinalysis   Analysis of urine to detect the presence of many common urinary tract disorders.

Urothelium   The lining of the bladder; transitional epithelium.

Uterus   (*also*, womb) The organ in which the fetus develops prior to birth.

Uvea   (*also*, choroid) The middle layer of the eye, which includes the iris and ciliary body.

V

Vagina   A fibromuscular tubular tract leading from the uterus to the exterior of the body.

Vaginal speculum   A device that allows for the visual inspection of the upper vagina and outer cervix.

Valves   Fibrous pieces of tissue that separate the atria and ventricles of the heart; also present in large veins.

Valvulitis   Inflammation of the heart valves.

Variable expressivity   An abnormal trait that may be expressed differently in individuals with an identical genotype for the alleles responsible for the trait.

Varices   (*also*, varicosities) Permanently dilated venous channels.

Varicose veins   Permanently dilated venous channels in the legs.

Vas deferens   Part of the male reproductive system that transports sperm from the epididymis.

Vasculitis   A disease characterized by inflammation of the blood vessels.

Vasoactive amine   A chemical containing amino groups that acts on blood vessels to alter their permeability or cause vasodilation.

Vasoconstriction   (*see* vasospasm) Decreased caliber of a vessel.

Vasodilation   Increase in caliber of a vessel.

Vasopressin   A hormone that regulates blood pressure.

Vasospasm   Severe narrowing of a blood vessel due to a contraction of the vessel's muscle.

Vector   An organism (such as an insect) that transports a pathogen to a host.

Veins   Blood vessels that carry deoxygenated blood to the heart.

Vena cava   The large vein that returns deoxygenated blood to the heart.

Venereal disease   Disease acquired through sexual contact; also called sexually transmitted disease (STD).

Ventilation   Process of moving air from the atmosphere to the terminal units of the lung.

Ventricle   Pumping chamber of the heart.

Ventricular fibrillation   An uncoordinated, ineffective, weak contraction of ventricular muscle due to spontaneous generation of impulses within the muscle cells themselves rather than coordinated electrical stimulation through the conduction system.

Venules   Smaller veins that carry deoxygenated blood from the capillaries to the veins.

Verruca plana   Flat wart.

Verruca vulgaris   Common wart.

Vertebral body   The weight-supporting solid central part of the vertebra.

Vertigo   Dizziness or spinning sensation.

Very-low-density lipoproteins (VLDL)   One of the five lipoproteins; made by the liver and containing a very large ratio of lipids to proteins and carrying the most cholesterol; generally associated with more severe atherosclerosis.

Vesicoureteral reflux A condition in which the usual anatomic and functional relationship of the ureters to the bladder is disturbed, allowing urine to flow back up from the bladder to the kidneys.

Vestibular apparatus A sensory organ for body equilibrium found in the inner ear.

Video capture endoscopy A diagnostic procedure that entails swallowing a small camera, about the size of a pill, that takes photographs as it is pushed through the gastrointestinal tract via normal peristalsis.

Villous adenomas Usually larger than 2 centimeters; grow as a raised, broad-based mass; and are composed predominantly of villous-type epithelium or long, papillary fronds. About 20 percent contain cancer at the time of their removal, and the likelihood that they harbor cancer increases with their size.

Viral enteritis (*also*, intestinal flu) A sudden infection affecting the stomach and colon, caused by a virus.

Virchow's triad Three factors thought to contribute to the formation of a thrombus: circulatory stasis, hypercoagulability, and endothelial injury.

Viremia Virus in the blood, resulting from the virus's exit from cells.

Virilization Biologic development of sex differences; in boys includes development of androgenic features such as facial hair, atrophy of the breasts, and changes in voice. Abnormal in girls.

Virulence The degree to which a pathogen elicits a response from the organism it is invading.

Visual acuity Clarity of vision; the ability to distinctly focus an image on the retina.

Visual field tests A test in which the person being examined is asked to focus on a small stationary spot while a test spot is moved to different points of a circular map. In those areas where the person cannot see the test spot, he or she has a visual field defect.

Vitamin B$_{12}$ deficiency anemia (*also*, pernicious anemia) Caused by failure to absorb vitamin B$_{12}$ from the intestinal tract; vitamin B$_{12}$ is necessary to properly develop red blood cells.

Vitamin D A vitamin that promotes bone mineralization.

Vitamin K A fat-soluble vitamin produced by bacteria in the intestines.

Vitreous humor A clear gelatinous substance in the vitreous cavity behind the lens of the eye.

VLDL (*see* Very-low-density lipoproteins)

Von Hippel–Lindau disease A syndrome in which patients develop cysts and neoplasms in various tissues in the body, including the eyes, brain, adrenal gland, spinal cord, pancreas, and kidney.

Von Willebrand disease An autosomal dominant disease due to lack of von Willebrand factor, a plasma factor mediating platelet adhesion that needs to bind to factor VIII for it to become functional. Patients with this disease have abnormal tests of both platelet function and coagulation function.

Vulva The external genital organs of the female.

W

Warfarin A pharmacologic anticoagulant that inhibits plasma proteins involved in thrombosis by reducing the amount of vitamin K available for use by the liver enzymes that produce coagulation factors. The name is derived from the Wisconsin Alumni Research Foundation (WARF), where it was developed.

Werdnig-Hoffman disease Disease of dying motor neurons that occurs in infants and small children.

Wernicke encephalopathy The degeneration of several regions in the center of the brain, producing incoordination and mental confusion, usually caused by thiamine deficiency.

Wheal An acute patchy eruption with raised edematous areas surrounded by erythema.

Wheezes An abnormal breath sound indicative of airway obstruction.

Whiplash injury A type of trauma caused by sudden extension of the neck; a sprain in which ligaments and other tissues supporting the cervical spine are torn.

White blood cells (*also*, leukocytes) Mobile connective tissue-type cells that are specialized to attack foreign substances.

Wilm's tumor (*also*, nephroblastoma) A solid tumor commonly found in children; a malignancy derived from primitive cells in the renal cortex.

Workup Investigation of a patient's symptoms to determine the cause of the ailment.

X

X-ray The net amount of x-radiation that passes through the body and exposes film to produce a roentgenogram.

Xeroderma pigmentosum A rare autosomal recessive condition characterized by intolerance of skin and eyes to sunlight, with development of skin cancers in childhood or early adult life. Affected patients lack the enzymes necessary to repair damage to DNA caused by sunlight.

Z

Zygote The group of cells formed by the unification of a sperm and an ovum.

Index